Fundamentals of

Children and Young People's Applied Pathophysiology

Fundamentals of

Children and Young People's Applied Pathophysiology

For Nursing and Healthcare Students

SECOND EDITION

EDITED BY

Elizabeth Gormley-Fleming, RGN, RSCN, RNT, PGCert (Herts), PGDip HE (Herts), BSc (Hons), MA (Keele), SFHEA

Associate Director of Academic Quality Assurance, Centre for Academic Quality Assurance, University of Hertfordshire, UK

Ian Peate, OBE, FRCN, EN(G), RGN, DipN (Lond), RNT, BEd (Hons), MA (Lond), LLM, Hon DUniv (BNU)

Visiting Professor, Northumbria University; Visiting Professor, Buckinghamshire New University; Visiting Senior Clinical Fellow, University of Hertfordshire; Editor-in-Chief, *British Journal of Nursing*; Consultant Editor, *Journal of Paramedic Practice*; Consultant Editor, *International Journal for Advancing Practice*

WILEY

This edition first published 2026

Edition History
John Wiley & Sons Ltd (1e, 2019)

Registered Offices
John Wiley & Sons, Inc., 111 River Street, Hoboken, NJ 07030, USA
John Wiley & Sons Ltd, New Era House, 8 Oldlands Way, Bognor Regis, West Sussex, PO22 9NQ, UK

For details of our global editorial offices, customer services, and more information about Wiley products visit us at www.wiley.com.

The manufacturer's authorized representative according to the EU General Product Safety Regulation is Wiley-VCH GmbH, Boschstr. 12, 69469 Weinheim, Germany, e-mail: Product_Safety@wiley.com.

Wiley also publishes its books in a variety of electronic formats and by print-on-demand. Some content that appears in standard print versions of this book may not be available in other formats.

Library of Congress Cataloging-in-Publication Data

Names: Gormley-Fleming, Elizabeth editor | Peate, Ian editor
Title: Fundamentals of children and young people's applied pathophysiology : for nursing and healthcare students / edited by Elizabeth Gormley-Fleming and Ian Peate
Description: Second edition. | Hoboken, NJ, USA : John Wiley & Sons, Inc, 2026. | Includes bibliographical references and index.
Identifiers: LCCN 2025047247 (print) | LCCN 2025047248 (ebook) | ISBN 9781394240951 Paperback | ISBN 9781394240975 adobe pdf | ISBN 9781394240968 epub
Subjects: LCSH: Pediatric pathology–Study and teaching | Pediatric nursing–Study and teaching
Classification: LCC RJ49 .F86 2026 (print) | LCC RJ49 (ebook)
LC record available at https://lccn.loc.gov/2025047247
LC ebook record available at https://lccn.loc.gov/2025047248

Cover Design: Wiley
Cover Image: © PIXOLOGICSTUDIO/SCIENCE PHOTO LIBRARY/Getty Images

Set in 9.5/12.5pt Source Sans Pro by Straive, Pondicherry, India

Printed and bound by CPI Group (UK) Ltd, Croydon, CR0 4YY

C9781394240951_020726

To the student nurses who are learning to turn science into comfort, watchfulness into healing, and complexity into compassionate care. May this book help you connect knowledge with kindness and guide you towards a future where every child is met with the care, dignity, and understanding they deserve.

Contents

About the editors

Elizabeth Gormley-Fleming RGN, RSCN, RNT, PGCert (Herts), PGDip HE (Herts), BSc (Hons), MA (Keele), SFHEA
Associate Director of Academic Quality Assurance, Centre for Academic Quality Assurance, University of Hertfordshire, UK
Liz commenced her nursing career in Ireland where she qualified as an RGN and RSCN. Initially working in paediatric oncology and bone marrow transplant, Liz moved to London and has held a variety of senior clinical nursing and leadership roles across a range of NHS Trusts both in the acute care setting and in the community. Liz has worked in education since 2001, initially as a clinical facilitator before moving into full-time higher education in 2003.

Liz has held a number of senior leadership positions in higher education: Head of Nursing (Children's, Learning Disability, Mental Health), Social Work Associate Dean of School and Principal Lecturer in Learning and Teaching. Her areas of interest are care of the acutely ill child, healthcare law and ethics, the use of technology in higher education, curriculum development and work-based learning

Ian Peate OBE, FRCN, EN(G), RGN, DipN (Lond), RNT, BEd (Hons), MA (Lond), LLM, Hon DUniv (BNU)
Visiting Professor, Northumbria University; Visiting Professor, Buckinghamshire New University; Visiting Senior Clinical Fellow. University of Hertfordshire; Editor-in-Chief, British Journal of Nursing; Consultant Editor, Journal of Paramedic Practice; Consultant Editor, International Journal for Advancing Practice
Ian began his nursing career at Central Middlesex Hospital, becoming an Enrolled Nurse practising in an intensive care unit. He later undertook three years' student nurse training at Central Middlesex and Northwick Park Hospitals, becoming a Staff Nurse and then a Charge Nurse. He has worked in nurse education since 1989. His key areas of interest are nursing practice and theory. Ian has published widely. He has been granted an Honorary Doctorate by Buckinghamshire New University. He was awarded an OBE for his services to Nursing and Nurse Education and was bestowed a Fellowship from the Royal College of Nursing in 2017.

Contributors

Nikki Beill

Nikki Beill is a Senior Lecturer at Buckinghamshire New University with a specialist background in children's community nursing, including oncology, haematology and end-of-life care. Transitioning into academia, she completed an MA in Education, where her research explored the challenges faced by Nursing Associate students in clinical practice, informing her teaching and programme leadership.

Mary Brady RN, RSCN, CHSM, BSc (Hons), PGCHE, MSc Senior Fellow HEA

Retired Senior Lecturer, Kingston University Teaching and Learning Fellowship

Mary has extensive knowledge of the clinical care of neonates, children and young people. Moving into Higher Education, she held a variety of posts and taught pre- and post-registration students. Her scholarly activity included working with the RCN Children and Young People's Professional Interests Forum, creating publications and two external examiner posts.

Her research interests have been regarding children's perceptions of the 'good nurse', increasing mental health education within children's nursing curricula and the challenges of research productivity amongst nurse academics.

Most recently, she has become the membership Officer of the Association of Paediatric Nurses' Membership Working Group.

Sarah Brazel-Terris

Sarah is a Lecturer in Children's Nursing at the University of Hertfordshire, alongside her role as a Specialist Nurse in Bone Marrow Transplant at Great Ormond Street Hospital in London.

Sarah completed her Children's Nursing degree at King's College London and began her career on the children's ward at the Royal Brompton Hospital. In 2014, Sarah began working at Great Ormond Street Hospital, caring for and treating children undergoing allogeneic and autologous Haematopoietic Stem Cell Transplants. Due to Sarah's interest in the speciality, she progressed to become a Specialist Nurse in Bone Marrow Transplant, a role she continues to hold alongside her academic work. Sarah continues to be passionate about her work within clinical practice.

Sarah has always endeavoured to support student nurses whilst in practice. She realised that she particularly enjoyed sharing information, knowledge and good practice with others and decided to make the transition into teaching and academia.

Emily Burke

Emily qualified as a mental health nurse in 2022. She began working as a Specialist ADHD Nurse in a children and young people's neurodiversity service, managing a caseload of children on ADHD medication, supporting families and conducting medication reviews. Emily is now a Senior Nurse specializing in assessing and diagnosing ADHD. Alongside her work, she is also a Trustee for the charity Autistic Girls Network and uses her own lived experience as a passionate speaker and author. Her debut book was a Sunday Times bestseller.

Gemma Bush RMN, FHEA

Having completed a degree in Psychology and English at Keele University, Gemma completed her nursing training at the University of Hertfordshire. Upon qualification, she began her nursing career within private Inpatient Eating Disorder Services. Following this, Gemma practiced at Great Ormond Street Hospital in both the therapeutic milieu of the Mildred Creak Unit and the Outpatient Eating Disorder Team. Gemma worked in the Children's and Young Peoples Community Eating Disorder Services in Hertfordshire before her current position as Senior Lecturer of Mental Health Nursing at the University of Hertfordshire.

Simon Dean RCN (BSc Hons), MMedSci, FHEA
Paediatric advanced clinical practitioner (ACP) in Paediatric Haematology and Oncology
Simon studied paediatric nursing at the University of the West of England from 2001 until 2004. Since qualifying, he has worked on a Bone Marrow Transplant unit, paediatric surgery ward and paediatric oncology wards across the United Kingdom. He is currently practising as an ACP in paediatric oncology and haematology in Leeds Children's Hospital, having completed his master's qualification in paediatric advanced practice in 2018 at Sheffield University. He has also been the paediatric pathway lead on the MMedSci Advanced Clinical Practice (Paediatrics) Programme at Sheffield University since 2022.

Kate Heaton-Stockton Registered Nurse Adult, Learning Disabilities and Children, BSc (Hons), MSc, FHEA
Senior Lecturer in Clinical Skills and Simulation Sheffield Hallam University, Sheffield, UK
Immunisation Nurse, School Age Immunisation Team, Derbyshire, UK
Kate's career began in 1982, undertaking RNMH training (now RNLD) at Whittington Hall Hospital, Chesterfield. Subsequently training as an RGN and RSCN, Kate's practice since 1991 has been predominantly in children's nursing. She has worked and trained in the Sheffield Hospitals as a Staff Nurse and then as a Sister in acute and ED settings. In 1998, Kate took up a post as Senior Sister at Chesterfield Royal Hospital and, successively, positions of Practice Development Advisor, Matron and Senior Matron. In 2007, to pursue her interest in nurse education, Kate joined Sheffield Hallam University as a Senior Lecturer in Children's nursing, concurrently maintaining clinical skills by working as a staff nurse on the acute children's ward at Chesterfield Royal Hospital. In 2020, Kate retired from Sheffield Hallam University and returned to practice during the pandemic, undertaking Covid vaccination and community work for adults and children, at the same time returning to Sheffield Hallam University to provide clinical skills training for nursing students in practice. Since 2023, Kate has rejoined Sheffield Hallam University as part of the clinical skills and simulation team and continues to practise with the school-age immunisation team in Derbyshire.

Laura Lowe BSc, MSc, RMN, SFHEA
Laura Lowe has a degree in psychology and later trained as a mental health nurse at the University of Hertfordshire. She has extensive experience working with young people and families in Hertfordshire and in Great Ormond Street Hospital. Alongside working as a mental health nurse, Laura has worked in nurse education since 2010 and has a particular interest in therapeutic approaches (including therapeutic milieu), children and young people's mental health and authentic approaches to learning and teaching. Laura is currently Head of Undergraduate Curriculum for the School of Health, Medicine and Life Sciences at the University of Hertfordshire.

Sarah McDonald RSCN, BA (Hons), PGCert, MSc, FHEA
Associate Head of School Health and Social Care, Sheffield Hallam University
Sarah began her nursing career after earning an RSCN Honours Degree from Sheffield Hallam University in 1995. She initially worked in paediatric medicine at Rotherham District General Hospital before progressing to Staff Nurse and Senior Staff Nurse roles at Sheffield Children's Hospital. Her clinical experience includes leadership as Sister in Outpatient Theatres and Post-Anaesthetic Care, followed by a role as Clinical Nurse Educator in orthopaedics, plastics and burns. In 2014, Sarah transitioned into nurse education, completing an MSc in Health and Social Care Education and gaining Fellowship of the Higher Education Academy. She is currently Associate Head of the School of Health and Social Care at Sheffield Hallam University. Her professional interests focus on nursing education and practice-based learning. Sarah has contributed to nursing textbooks and published work on clinical skills.

Louise McLaughlin RN (Child), BSc (Hons), MSc, PG Cert, FHEA
Louise McLaughlin is a Senior Lecturer in the Children's Nursing team at the University of Hertfordshire. She has a keen interest in children's palliative care, having worked in Children's Hospices across the East of England for 15 years, working in inpatient units, community and symptom management teams. Louise left her role as a Children's Palliative Care Clinical Nurse Specialist in 2022 to pursue her passion for education. She is currently involved in the teaching and assessment of undergraduate and postgraduate students, including Nursing Associates, Children's Nurses and postgraduate nurses studying for their Specialist Practice Qualification (SPQ) and non-medical prescribing qualification.

Elizabeth Mills
Liz began her nursing career at Halifax Royal Infirmary as a registered nurse practising in the emergency department in 1995, moving into general paediatric nursing with a strong focus on paediatric respiratory nursing in 1996. After studying the RSCN conversation course in 1997 and developing a passion for neonatal nursing, Liz moved to neonatal nursing.

Liz continued to work in neonatal care in both district general and sub-regional hospitals. Liz's career progressed to becoming a senior lecturer in children's nursing in 2008 at the Sheffield Hallam University before moving to the University of Sheffield in 2021 as a Senior University Teacher and programme lead for Advanced Clinical Practice.

Helen Monks RGN, RSCN, BSc (Hons), RNT, MSc, FHEA
Associate Lecturer in Children's Nursing, Sheffield Hallam University, Sheffield, UK
Helen commenced her nursing career in 1986, gaining her RGN qualification at Bradford School of Nursing, followed a few years later by her RSCN qualification in Manchester. Her clinical experience includes caring for children and families in general surgery, plastic surgery and general medicine.

Her career progressed to Ward Manager, with her final leadership role in the NHS being that of Practice Development Nurse. She began lecturing at the University of Bradford in 1997 and in 2008, moved to teach at Sheffield Hallam University.

Helen has held several senior leadership positions within higher education and retired from her Principal Lecturer post in 2023. Since retiring, she has taken on a casual Researcher role and a part-time Associate Lecturer position, and she continues to work as a bank nurse for a local seasonal immunisation service.

She has published works arising from research projects with Roald Dahl's Marvellous Children's Charity, the Admiral Nursing Service and a Digibete Chatbot feasibility study. Helen is passionate about helping students develop an appreciation for the value, methodologies and interpretation of research.

Alison Mosenthal RGN, RSCN, RNT, MSc
Visiting Lecturer, Children's Nursing, School of Health and Social Work, University of Hertfordshire, Hatfield, UK
Alison commenced her nursing career in London, where she qualified as a registered nurse at St Thomas' Hospital, London, and a registered children's nurse at Great Ormond Street Hospital. She subsequently worked in paediatric respiratory intensive care before moving into nurse education in the School of Nursing at Great Ormond Street Hospital. Following a career break, she returned to clinical nursing, working as a clinical nurse specialist in paediatric immunology nursing at St George's Healthcare NHS Trust. In 2010, she returned to teaching in higher education at the University of Hertfordshire and currently works there as a visiting lecturer for the Children's Nursing programme.

Michele O'Grady RGN, RSCN, MSc, PGCert
Michele O'Grady is a Senior Lecturer at the University of Hertfordshire. She trained in Dublin and worked as a qualified nurse until she went to Sudan with the voluntary agency GOAL, running a primary care programme. She moved to the United Kingdom in 1987 where she worked in several hospitals before moving to Oxford where she became the HIV Liaison Officer for five years. Michele returned to the NHS where she was a Senior Sister and an Emergency Nurse Practitioner in the Children's Emergency Department in Watford General Hospital. Michele joined the child nursing lecturing team in 2015.

Michele has had an interest in sexual health and health promotion since her time in Sudan. Michele is responsible for introducing Schwartz rounds to the University of Hertfordshire students and is a trained Schwartz Round Facilitator.

Dr. Julia Petty
Associate Professor (learning and teaching), Senior Lecturer in Children's Nursing, School of Health, Medicine and Life Sciences, University of Hertfordshire, England, UK
After achieving a degree in Psychology in 1987, Julia began her children's nursing career at Great Ormond Street Hospital, London, United Kingdom. After a period in paediatric and neonatal clinical practice and education, she moved into higher education and worked as a Senior Lecturer at City University, London for 12 years, where she taught the neonatal nursing post-qualification programme. She commenced her current role at the University of Hertfordshire in 2013 and has been an Associate Professor since 2020. She undertakes narrative-based research as part of her education role, having gained her doctorate in 2020, and is widely published in the field of neonatal and children's nursing.

Cathy Poole RGN, RSCN, MSc, PGDip
Cathy Poole has worked for many years with children and adults with renal disease. This has allowed her to develop her passion for renal care and management in public and private healthcare settings. She loves to share this passion and has been fortunate to work as a paediatric lecturer practitioner developing and delivering a paediatric renal course, as a training and education manager for Fresenius Medical Care (world's largest dialysis company) as well as working as a senior lecturer at Birmingham City University ensuring renal care was included in the curriculum.

Sheila Roberts RGN, RSCN, RNT, BA (Hons), MA

Sheila is currently a Senior Lecturer in Children's Nursing, School of Health, Medicine and Life Science, University of Hertfordshire, Hatfield, UK. Prior to moving into nurse education, Sheila trained as an RSCN/RN at the Queen Elizabeth School of Nursing, Birmingham, and worked primarily at Birmingham Children's Hospital before holding a variety of posts within acute paediatric care. Sheila has an interest in service-user involvement and has been involved in ensuring the voice of the child and young person is embedded in the pre-registration curriculum.

Karen Roberts-Edema Dip HE(Child), BSc Professional Practice (Children's Nursing), MSc Contemporary Nursing, PG Cert (Registered NMC Teacher) and FHEA

Senior Lecturer in Children's Nursing

Karen is a qualified Children's Nurse with 26 years of experience across a range of clinical settings, including inpatient wards, outpatient departments, A&E, and community services. Her most recent clinical role was as a Community Children's Nurse, supporting children with complex healthcare needs—a role she was deeply passionate about. For the past seven and a half years, Karen has served as a Senior Lecturer in Children's Nursing at the University of Hertfordshire. Her responsibilities include leading Level 5 and Level 6 clinical practice modules and collaborating with the practice placements team to ensure effective student placement allocation. In addition, she acts as a personal tutor and Academic Assessor for Level 6 students. Karen is also actively involved in the university's Race and Ethnicity Equality Staff Network. She has a strong interest in authoring academic chapters and is currently pursuing research into the support needs of international student nurses in higher education.

Amsale Wamburu BSc, MSc, PGcert, FHEA

Amsale Wamburu is a Senior Lecturer and Programme Lead in Adult Nursing at Buckinghamshire New University, with master's degrees in Human Biology & Genetics and Advanced Practice Nursing (MSc). Her background spans specialist practice in haematology, cardiology, respiratory, and infectious diseases, as well as roles in clinical education. She is currently undertaking a PhD exploring first-year nursing students' clinical placement experiences to inform educational practice and enhance student learning, support, and retention.

Megan White RSCN, SCPHN (HV), Bsc (HONS), PG DIP, AFHEA

Megan White is a lecturer in Child Nursing at Buckinghamshire New University, with a background in Emergency Care, Health Visiting and Infant Feeding. She is currently undertaking her MSc in Healthcare and Medical Education.

Michelle White BSc Children's Nursing and PG Cert (Registered NMC Teacher) and FHEA

Senior Lecturer in Children's Nursing, University of Hertfordshire

Michelle earned her degree in Children's Nursing from the University of Hertfordshire and began her career at the Royal National Orthopaedic Hospital, where she gained experience in high dependency and intensive care settings. She later progressed to the role of Clinical Nurse Specialist for Children and Young People with Spinal Cord Injuries. Throughout her clinical career, Michelle also worked in a children's hospice, providing care for children and young people with life-limiting conditions and those receiving end-of-life care.

In 2020, Michelle transitioned into higher education and has since served as a Senior Lecturer in Children's Nursing at the University of Hertfordshire. Her current responsibilities include leading Level 4 and Level 5 modules, delivering simulated practice learning, and acting as a personal tutor for Level 6 students and Academic Assessor for Level 4 students.

Michelle has a particular interest in the mental health of children and young people, which has led her to undertake additional training to deepen her expertise in this area.

Preface

We are very pleased to have been invited to edit a second edition of the popular *Fundamentals of Children's Applied Pathophysiology*. The new edition, *Fundamentals of Children and Young People's Applied Pathophysiology*, has been thoroughly updated and revised to ensure it aligns with the evolving needs of its readers. This edition now includes 20 chapters, with the addition of five new chapters that reflect recent developments in practice and advances in the field. Learning the Language, a chapter that focuses on the terminology associated with pathophysiology, is available online. These changes to the book aim to enhance the relevance and applicability of the content, ensuring that readers are equipped with the most up-to-date knowledge and insights to inform their practice and improve care for children and young people.

To ensure the delivery of safe and effective care to children, young people and their families, it is vital that caregivers understand the underlying pathophysiology of the child or young person's condition. The primary aim of this book is to make the complex subject of pathophysiology more accessible and engaging, enabling readers to apply their knowledge across various care contexts. The body has an extraordinary ability to respond to disease through various physiological and psychological processes, compensating for changes caused by disease; these are the pathophysiological mechanisms. The *Fundamentals of Children and Young People's Applied Pathophysiology* will help you develop critical thinking skills, fostering innovation and creativity in relation to the health and well-being of those you offer care and support to.

Designed with the reader in mind, *Fundamentals of Children and Young People's Applied Pathophysiology* encourages deeper exploration, discovery and the cultivation of curiosity. Numerous illustrations are included to explain and clarify the complex disease patterns being discussed. A fundamental approach will equip you with a solid understanding of applied pathophysiology while always keeping the child, young person and their family at the centre of care.

The *Fundamentals of Children and Young People's Applied Pathophysiology* offers a series of activities designed to engage you actively and assist you in applying your knowledge in various care settings. It provides a current overview of pathophysiology and the key issues involved in care provision. The importance of considering the broader context of care delivery is emphasised, recognising the expansion of the professional base beyond nursing. An integrated, multidisciplinary approach is crucial for contemporary, safe and effective care, and healthcare students play an important role in any multidisciplinary team. It is also important to acknowledge that care is delivered in ever-changing environments to diverse children, young people, families, communities and circumstances.

Most of the chapters include case studies that are relevant to the content, designed to stimulate reflection and further understanding. All names used in these case studies are pseudonyms to maintain confidentiality, as nurses have a duty to protect patient privacy (Nursing and Midwifery Council, 2018); all healthcare providers must maintain confidentiality. Many case studies are extended, including vital signs and blood analysis, which can help relate key concepts to care and provide deeper insight into the patient's condition and needs. Some case studies also include the Paediatric Early Warning Score (PEWS).

In the United Kingdom, different care providers use different PEWS charts, and they may calculate PEWS in varied ways. The PEWS charts included in this book are examples, and it is essential to become familiar with the PEWS chart that is used in your workplace. Where relevant, key information is highlighted in boxed sections, such as red, yellow and green flags or medicines management, to aid in delivering care to vulnerable and anxious children, young people and families.

Most chapters feature an 'investigations box', which discusses a specific test or investigation linked to the chapter's content, prompting you to consider pre-, peri- and post-procedural care for the child, young person and their family. New resources include a consideration of growth and development, a discussion that centres on 'special' considerations, along with the provision of 10 multiple choice questions that can help in self-testing learning and understanding. Each chapter begins with questions designed to test your knowledge before you commence your reading. You will find a glossary of terms assisting you in further expanding your learning online.

Pathophysiology explores the cellular and organ changes that occur when disease is present and how these changes affect a person's ability to function. When normal physiological functioning is disrupted by disease, it becomes a pathophysiological issue. It is important to recognise that 'normal' health can vary from one child or young person to another, so this term should be used with caution. Understanding the concepts of 'normal' and 'abnormal' in pathophysiology will help healthcare students provide care that is compassionate, sensitive and holistic.

This book serves as a foundational resource to support your personal and professional growth in care provision. It is primarily aimed at those who care for children and young people with various health conditions in both hospital and community settings. Illness and disease are explicitly discussed, emphasising that children and young people do get sick and experience disease.

The *Fundamentals of Children and Young People's Applied Pathophysiology* has been designed for flexible reading, encouraging you to explore it as needed rather than from cover to cover. The goal is to inspire curiosity and motivate further reading, nurturing a deeper understanding of the subject.

Liz Gormley-Fleming, Hertfordshire
Ian Peate, London

Reference

Nursing & Midwifery Council (NMC) (2018). The Code. Professional standards of practice and behaviour for nurses, midwives and nursing associates. Available at: https://www.nmc.org.uk/globalassets/sitedocuments/nmc-publications/nmc-code.pdf (accessed March 2025).

Acknowledgements

Liz would like to thank her family, her husband, Kieran, and her daughters, Kate and Eilis. Thank you all for being you and providing me with real-life case studies.

Ian would like to thank his partner, Jussi Lahtinen, for his support and encouragement.

We extend our sincere thanks to all the contributors to this edition and to those who contributed to earlier editions. Their valuable insights and efforts have significantly enriched the content and helped make this work possible.

How to use your textbook

Features contained within your textbook

Learning outcome boxes give a summary of the topics covered in a chapter.

LEARNING OUTCOMES

On completion of this chapter, the reader will be able to:

- Outline the structure and function of a human cell.
- Name and describe the functions of the organelles.
- Explain the cellular transport system.
- Describe the structures and functions of the various tissues of the body, namely epithelial, connective, muscle and nervous tissues.

Keyword boxes give a summary of the keywords covered in a chapter.

KEYWORDS

- heart
- circulation
- congenital
- acquired
- disorders
- heart failure

Every chapter contains **'Test your prior knowledge' questions**.

Test your prior knowledge

1. Name three different treatment approaches for childhood cancer.
2. Name the most common form of childhood cancer.
3. What percentage of children with cancer are now cured? (a) > 60%, (b) > 70% or (c) > 80%.
4. What is the difference between a malignant tumour and a benign tumour?
5. What are the differences between chemotherapy and radiotherapy?

Case studies give an up-close, in-depth and detailed examination of a subject.

Case study 1

Sophie is 11 and is admitted to the hospital for the first time in her life with abdominal pain. Her Mum is with her and is understandably anxious to find out what is causing Sophie's pain. She cannot stay long as she has to get back to nursery to collect Sophie's younger brother, Danny. She will come back later after taking Danny to her estranged husband's flat.

1. What pain tools are appropriate to help assess Sophie's pain?
2. What other factors would need to be considered?
3. What non-pharmacological methods could be used to help Sophie?

Red flags provide quick summaries of alert signs and symptoms.

Nursing considerations

Because this is a potentially fatal condition, nurses need to be alert to older children presenting with a more chronic picture of diarrhoea, anorexia, weight loss, periodic pain and vomiting.

Green flags relate to growing up healthy, safe and strong.

Children on high-dose steroids should receive a Steroid Emergency Card to show any healthcare professional if they become ill. Steroids can cause adrenal insufficiency, reducing the ability to fight infection and increasing risk of allergic reactions. During sudden illness or severe injury, additional support or medications may be needed to help the child's nervous system respond.

Yellow flags identify any potential psychological or social factors that may cause the person to recover slower or differently as would be expected.

Traumatic brain injury is a leading cause of death and disability in children and young people. Those from lower socioeconomic backgrounds are at higher risk of falls (Lawrence *et al.*, 2016), highlighting the importance of targeted prevention, such as home safety and cycle safety measures.

Amber flags indicate potential clinical concern that is not immediately life-threatening, but could deteriorate if not addressed.

If children present with evidence of faltering growth, developmental delay or concerns about their well-being, which may indicate systemic disease, then they should be referred for specialist assessments for testing GI disorders such as coeliac disease.

Your textbook is full of **illustrations and tables**.

TABLE 8.2 Size and speed of first-order sensory fibres

Sensory fibre	Diameter (µm)	Myelinated	Speed of conduction (m/s)
A-beta (Aβ) fibres	6–12	Yes	35–75
A-delta (Aδ) fibres	1–5	Yes	5–35
C fibres	0.2–1.5	No	0.5–2

Source: Peate (2021).

Gate control theory

A number of theories exist to explain how pain is experienced, but the one continuing to hold widespread support is the gate control theory (Fig. 8.4) (Melzack & Wall, 1965).

In essence, the theory is that the pain impulse has to pass through a theoretical gate to enable the brain to receive, perceive and interpret the impulse as painful. Broadly, the theory works on the basis that stimulation of A-delta fibres and C fibres pushes the gate open, and the stimulation of A-beta fibres pushes the gate closed, but also the presence (or absence) of other factors like fear or distraction may open or close the gate (McCaffery & Beebe,1989).

Effects of pain on vital signs

Pain involves more than anatomical and physiological processes, and its effects extend beyond physical reactions. However, it can still significantly impact children's vital signs. Common deviations in vital signs can be:

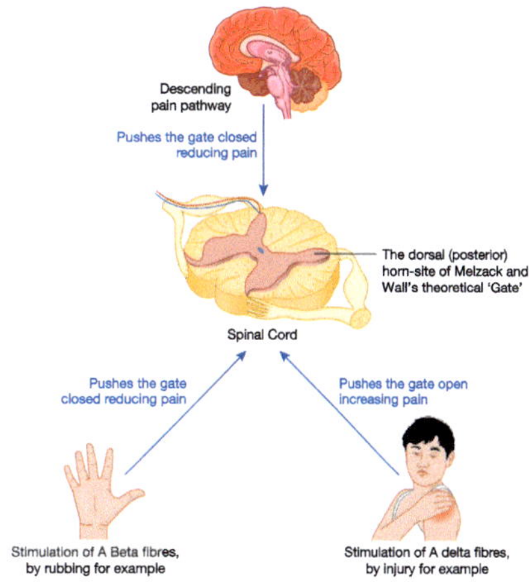

FIGURE 8.4 The gate control theory of pain.

About the companion website

This book is accompanied by a companion website.

www.wiley.com/go/fundamentalsofchildpatho2e

To access the website materials, click on the link under Related Resources on the book's page on wiley.com. You can also find this by searching www.wiley.com for the ISBN 9781394240951.

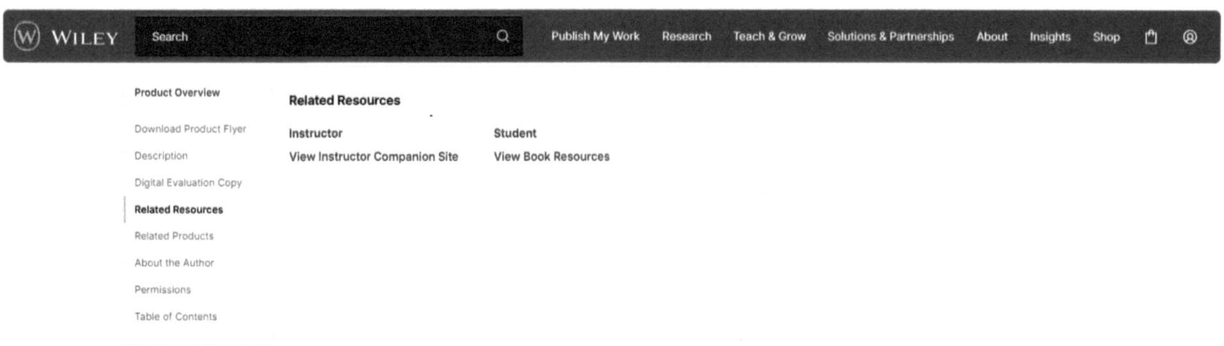

This website includes:

Learning the Language – a dedicated, online-only chapter that focuses on the terminology associated with pathophysiology
Further Reading
Glossary
Multiple-choice questions
Answers to Multiple-choice questions

CHAPTER 1

The cell and body tissue

Megan White, Nikki Beill, and Amsale Wamburu

AIM

The aim of this chapter is to introduce the reader to the cells and tissues of the developing human body, with a focus on childhood growth and development.

LEARNING OUTCOMES

On completion of this chapter, the reader will be able to:

- Outline the structure and function of a human cell, with reference to the developing child.
- Name and describe the functions of the main organelles within cells.
- Explain the cellular transport system and how it supports tissue growth in children.
- Describe the structure and function of the major tissue types in the body – epithelial, connective, muscle and nervous – with examples relevant to childhood.

KEYWORDS

- cytoplasm
- plasma membrane
- organelles
- nucleus
- passive transport
- active transport
- epithelial tissue
- muscle tissue
- connective tissue
- mitochondria
- mitosis
- growth plate
- myelination

Test your prior knowledge

1. What are the characteristics of human cells?
2. Describe the ways in which substances can pass through the cell membrane.
3. What is the role of the cell nucleus?
4. What are the four main roles of connective tissue?
5. How many different types of muscle tissue are there, and what are their various roles?
6. Where is epithelial tissue to be found within the body?

Cells

Introduction

Cells are the basic structural and functional units of life, forming and developing the human body. In children, they are especially active, supporting rapid growth, tissue formation and physiological change from infancy through adolescence. Many cell types exist, each with distinct roles: some create protective tissues like skin, others provide structural support such as bone, and specialised cells form organs including the heart, brain and muscles, enabling key functions such as circulation, immunity and movement.

All body cells originate from two parent cells: the ovum and the sperm. At conception, they fuse to form a single cell containing the full genetic code for human development. This cell then divides and specialises to create the diverse tissues and systems of the growing child. This genetically regulated process of growth and differentiation is particularly active in early life.

This chapter outlines cell structure and function in the context of child development, explaining how cells form tissues and what can happen when normal cellular function is disrupted. The chapter begins by outlining the common features shared by all human cells (Fig. 1.1).

Characteristics of cells

- Cells are active – carrying out specific functions.
- Cells need nutrients to survive and function. Through endocytosis, they surround and absorb substances such as bacteria to obtain the nutrients required for energy, growth and repair. In children, stem cells are especially active; these undifferentiated cells divide and develop into specialised types, supporting tissue formation, immune development and organ growth throughout infancy and adolescence.
- Cells reproduce asexually by doubling their organelles and then dividing so each new cell has the

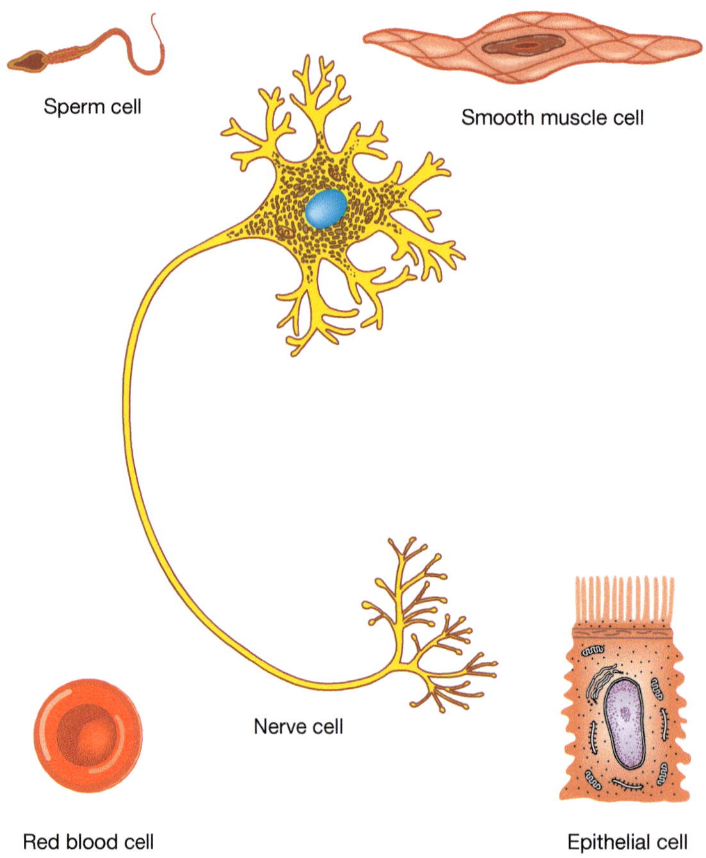

FIGURE 1.1 Examples of different types of cells in the body.
Source: Reproduced with permission of Peate & Gormley-Fleming (2015)/John Wiley & Sons.

same structures, a process known as simple fission. In children, this occurs more frequently to support growth, tissue repair and the development of new structures such as bone and muscle.
- Cells excrete waste products.
- Cells react to things that irritate or stimulate them – for example, in response to threats from chemicals and viruses.

The structure of the cell

There are four main compartments of the cell:

- cell membrane
- cytoplasm
- nucleus
- nucleoplasm.

Within these compartments are many organelles (or small organs). These organelles perform numerous roles to keep cells alive and functioning.

The cell membrane

As can be seen in Fig. 1.2, the various structures of the cell are contained within a cell membrane (also known as the plasma membrane). This cell membrane is a semi-permeable biological membrane separating the interior of the cell from the outside environment and protecting the cell from its surrounding environment. It is semi-permeable because it allows only certain substances to pass through it for the benefit of the cell itself. For example, it is selectively permeable to certain ions and molecules (Alberts *et al.*, 2022). Inside the cells are the cytoplasm and the organelles, which include, for example, the lysosomes, mitochondria and the nucleus of the cell.

The cell membrane varies in thickness from approximately 7.5 to 10 nm (Peate, 2021) and is composed of a self-sealing phospholipid bilayer with interspersed protein molecules (Fig. 1.3). Each phospholipid consists of a hydrophilic (water-attracting) polar head and hydrophobic (water-repelling) non-polar fatty acid tails. In the bilayer, the hydrophilic heads face both the extracellular and intracellular environments, while the hydrophobic tails orient towards the centre of the membrane. This arrangement creates a barrier that prevents the passive movement of water-soluble substances (Marieb, 2021).

The cell membrane contains phospholipids, proteins and lipids that support transport, signalling and structural integrity. Plasma membrane proteins (PMPs) are either integral or peripheral. Integral PMPs are embedded in the lipid bilayer, some forming channels for selective transport,

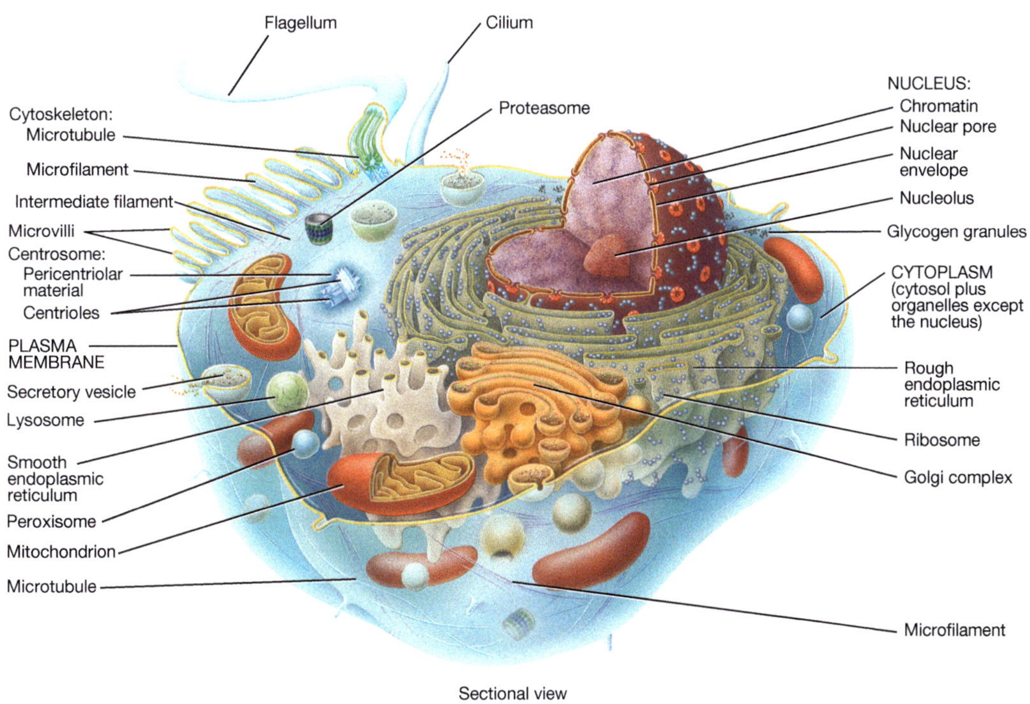

FIGURE 1.2 Structure of the cell.
Source: Reproduced with permission of Peate & Gormley-Fleming (2015)/John Wiley & Sons.

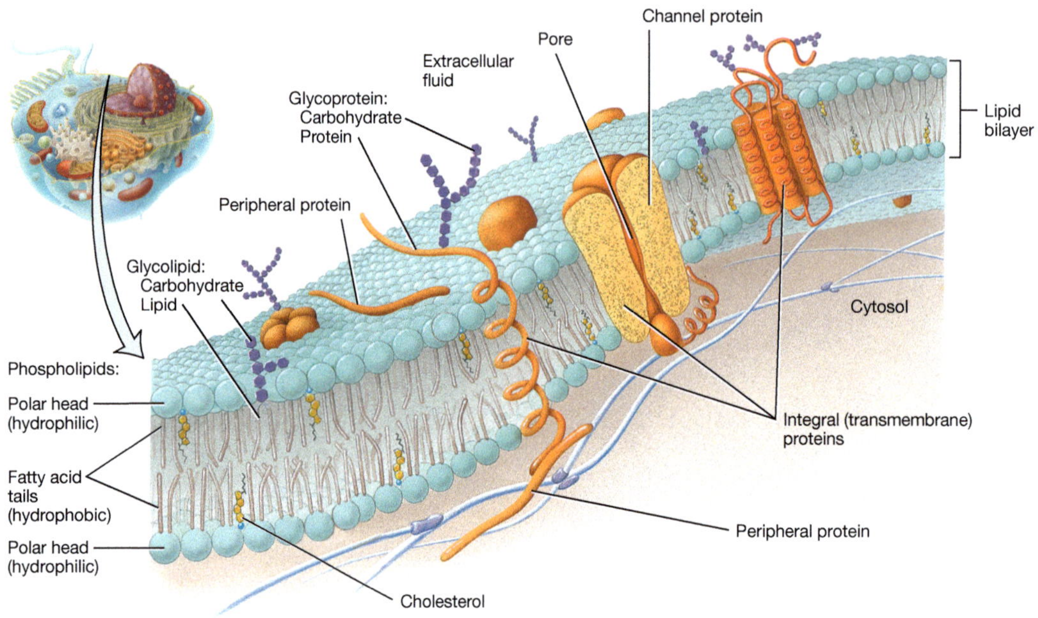

FIGURE 1.3 Cell membrane.
Source: Reproduced with permission of Peate & Gormley-Fleming (2015)/John Wiley & Sons.

others acting as receptors for molecules like insulin, neurotransmitters or bacterial components. Peripheral PMPs are loosely attached to the membrane surface and aid in cell signalling and enzymatic reactions.

Functions of the cell membrane

The cell membrane has several important physiological functions, particularly in regulating transport into and out of the cell. Two of the most significant are endocytosis and exocytosis.

Endocytosis refers to the process by which fluids and particles are taken into the cell. There are three main types:

- Phagocytosis – the ingestion of large particles, such as microbes
- Pinocytosis – the ingestion of smaller particles and extracellular fluid
- Receptor-mediated endocytosis – the highly selective uptake of specific substances, such as proteins, via membrane receptors.

During endocytosis, the cell membrane folds inward to enclose material, forming a vesicle that pinches off inside the cell. The vesicle may fuse with a lysosome to break down its contents. This process is vital for human cells and is also used by simple organisms like amoebae to obtain nutrients.

Exocytosis is the reverse process. It involves the removal of waste products or the export of substances, such as hormones or enzymes, by fusing intracellular vesicles with the cell membrane and releasing their contents outside the cell.

The cell membrane and transport

The cell membrane's selective permeability controls what enters and exits the cell. Its hydrophobic phospholipid bilayer blocks water-soluble substances, which instead pass through specialised channels or carrier proteins.

The membrane performs several transport-related roles:

- Regulates metabolism by controlling the flow of glucose and other molecules
- Maintains ion gradients, which store energy and support cell function
- Controls the rate of ion movement, ensuring precise regulation of intracellular conditions.

The controlled movement of ions and molecules supports key physiological functions:

- Nutrient uptake from the surrounding extracellular fluid
- Electrical signalling in nerve and muscle cells (nerve excitability)
- Regulation of cell volume by managing osmotic balance.

Together, these mechanisms ensure the cell can respond appropriately to its environment, maintain internal stability and carry out its specialised roles.

Cell membrane permeability
There are four factors involved in the degree of permeability of a cell membrane, namely:

1. The size of molecules – large molecules cannot pass through the integral membrane proteins, whilst small molecules (e.g., water and amino acids) can.
2. Solubility in lipids (fats) – substances that easily dissolve in lipids (e.g., oxygen, carbon dioxide and steroid hormones) can pass through the membrane more easily than non-lipid-soluble substances can.
3. If an ion has an electrical charge that is the opposite of that found in the membrane, then it is attracted to the membrane and so can more easily pass through it.
4. Carrier integral proteins can bind to substances and carry them across the membrane, regardless of the aforementioned three processes, i.e., size, ability to dissolve in lipids or membrane electrical charge.

Movement of substances across the membrane
There are two ways for this to occur, namely, passive and active.

Passive processes

A passive process is one in which the substances move under their own volition down a concentration gradient from an area of high concentration to an area of lower concentration. In this process, the cell expends little energy on the process (like rolling down a hill).

There are four types of passive transport processes, namely:

- diffusion
- facilitated diffusion
- osmosis
- filtration.

Diffusion is the most common form of passive transport. A substance in an area of higher concentration moves to an area of lower concentration (Colbert *et al.*, 2019). The difference seen between areas of different concentrations is known as the concentration gradient. This passive transport process is essential for respiration. It is through diffusion that oxygen is transported from the lungs to the blood and carbon dioxide from the blood into the lungs.

Although similar to diffusion, facilitated diffusion differs from it by the use of a substance (a facilitator) to help in the process (see Fig. 1.4). As an example, glucose is moved using this process. To be able to pass through a membrane, glucose needs to attach itself to a carrier/transport protein (McCance & Huether, 2022).

Osmosis is the process by which water travels through a selectively permeable membrane so that concentrations of a solute (a substance that is soluble in water) are equal on both sides of the membrane. This gives rise to osmotic pressure. The higher the concentration of the solute on one side of the membrane, the higher the osmotic pressure available for the movement of water (Colbert *et al.*, 2019).

If osmotic pressure rises too much, then it can cause damage to the cell membrane. So, the body attempts to ensure that there is always a reasonably constant pressure between the cell's internal and external environments.

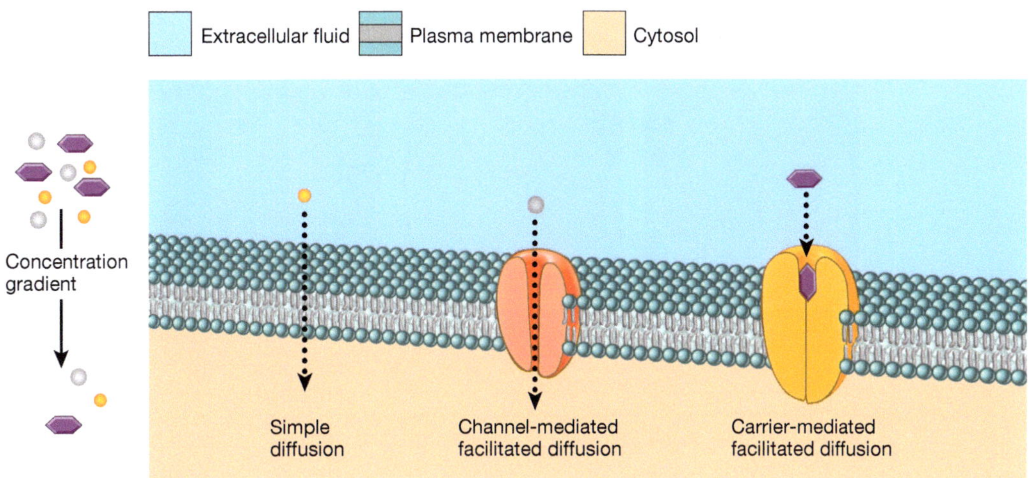

FIGURE 1.4 Facilitated diffusion.
Source: Reproduced with permission of Peate & Gormley-Fleming (2015)/John Wiley & Sons.

We can see the possible damage if, for example, a red blood cell is placed in a low-concentration solute; then it will undergo haemolysis. On the other hand, if it is placed in a highly concentrated solute, the result will be a crenulated cell. If the red blood cell is placed in a solution with a relatively constant osmotic pressure, it will not be affected because the net movement of water in and out of the red blood cell is minimal.

Filtration is similar to osmosis, with the exception that physical pressure is used in order to push water and solutes across a cell membrane. This is seen in renal filtration, where the heart beating exerts pressure as it pushes blood into the kidneys, where filtration of the blood can then take place to remove any impurities (Colbert *et al.*, 2019).

Active processes

Active processes are:

- active transport pumps
- endocytosis
- exocytosis.

An active process is one in which substances move against a concentration gradient from an area of lower to higher concentration. In order for this to happen, the cell must expend energy, which is released by the splitting of adenosine triphosphate (ATP) into adenosine diphosphate (ADP) and phosphate.

ATP is a compound of a base, a sugar and three phosphate groups (triphosphate) and is held together by phosphate bonds, which release a high level of energy when they are broken. Once one of the phosphate bonds is broken and phosphate has been released, that compound then becomes ADP. The 'spare' phosphate will then join another ADP group, so forming ATP (with energy stored in the phosphate bond). This process is continually recurring within the body.

Active transport pumps need energy to be able to function. This energy occurs as a result of the reaction mentioned earlier. It is necessary when the body is attempting to move an area that already has a high concentration of that substance. The higher the concentration already present, the more energy is required to move further molecules of that substance into that area. Fig. 1.5 demonstrates the effect of solute concentration on a red blood cell.

The organelles

These are rather like small 'organs' within the cells. The following sections give a brief overview of the many cell organelles and their functions.

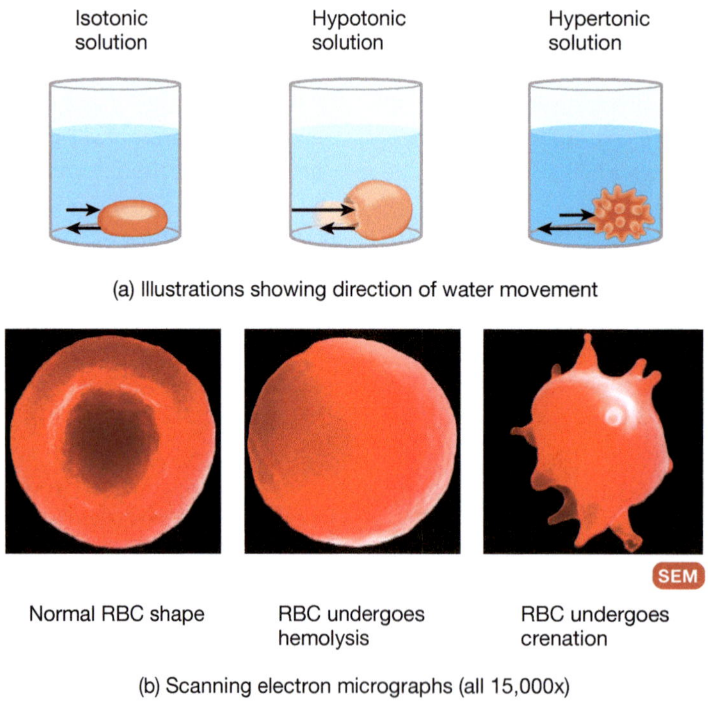

FIGURE 1.5 Effect of solute concentration on a red blood cell.
Source: Reproduced with permission of Peate & Gormley-Fleming (2015)/John Wiley & Sons.

Cytoplasm

Although not strictly an organelle, the cytoplasm is a vital part of the cell, forming the matrix in which cellular components are suspended. Part of the protoplasm, it is a thick, semi-transparent, elastic fluid containing the cytoskeleton, which provides structure and aids movement within the cell. Chemically, it consists of 75–90% water plus carbohydrates, lipids and inorganic compounds.

The role of the cytoplasm

- Cytoplasm is the substance within the cell in which chemical reactions occur.
- It receives raw materials from the external environment (e.g., from digested food) and converts them/breaks them down into usable energy by means of decomposition reactions.
- It is the site where new substances are synthesised (produced), which can then be used by the cell for its various functions.
- It is the place where various essential chemicals are packaged either for use by itself or to be transported out for other cells of the body to use.
- The cytoplasm is also the place where various chemicals help with the excretion of waste materials.

The nucleus (see Fig. 1.2)

The nucleus is the control centre of eukaryotic cells, found in animals and plants. Prokaryotic cells, such as bacteria, are simpler and often smaller. Not all human cells have a nucleus; for example, mature red blood cells lack a nucleus and are concave in shape.

There are also some human cells (some muscle fibre cells) that have more than one nucleus (see Fig. 1.1).

Some facts about the nucleus

- The nucleus is the largest structure in a human cell.
- It is surrounded by a nuclear membrane (just as the cell is surrounded by a cell membrane).
- It has its own protoplasm, although rather than 'cytoplasm', it is called 'nucleoplasm'.
- The nucleus is responsible for the reproduction of the cell and for making us what we are (see later) – it is where the processes of meiosis and mitosis take place.
- Within the nucleus is found all our genetic material, including DNA, leading to chromosomes.
- In humans, there are normally 23 pairs of chromosomes in each cell that contains a chromosome, apart from sperms and ova, which only have 23 single chromosomes.

Cell reproduction

For the body to grow and replace damaged or dying cells, cells must reproduce accurately to preserve their genetic information. Human cells with a nucleus contain 23 pairs of chromosomes. Cells reproduce via mitosis, which occurs in most cells or meiosis, which is limited to reproductive cells (sperm and ova).

Cells reproduced by mitosis are exact copies of the parent cell, with the full 23 pairs of chromosomes, whereas cells from meiosis contain only one of each chromosome. In childhood, mitosis is vital for rapidly expanding cell populations, supporting organ and tissue development and helping the body meet increasing functional demands.

In mitosis, chromosomes replicate before the cell divides, ensuring each new cell receives a full set of chromosomes. In meiosis, although the process starts similarly, additional steps result in cells with only one copy of each chromosome, which is essential for human reproduction.

In human reproduction, a sperm penetrates an egg, combining its DNA with the egg's genetic material. Sperm and egg cells carry only one copy of each chromosome due to meiosis, which halves the chromosome number. Without meiosis, fertilisation would produce cells with four copies of each chromosome, causing a genetic imbalance. Meiosis ensures the embryo has the correct two copies, maintaining genetic stability.

In children, hormones such as growth hormone, thyroid hormones and sex hormones regulate the rate and timing of cell reproduction, especially during key developmental stages and puberty.

Other organelles

All cells contain many organelles, and these are discussed in the following sections.

Endoplasmic reticulum

The endoplasmic reticulum (ER) consists of membranes that form a series of channels known as cisternae (see Fig. 1.6).

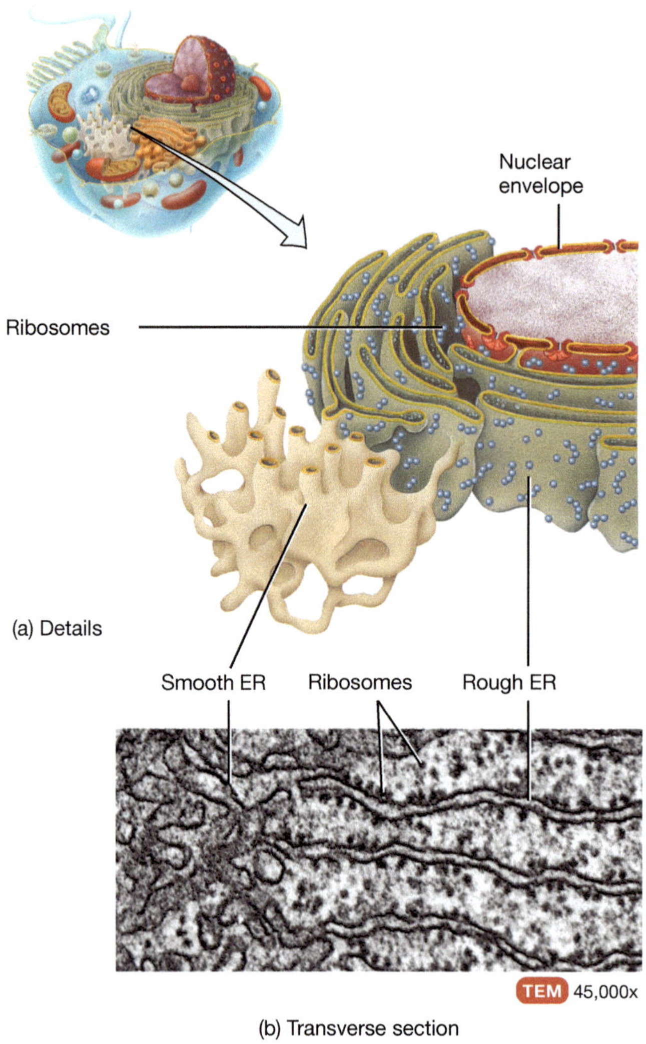

FIGURE 1.6 Endoplasmic reticulum.
Source: Reproduced with permission of Peate & Gormley-Fleming (2015)/John Wiley & Sons.

These divide the cytoplasm into compartments. There are two types of cisternae:

1. granular ER (rough), which is associated with ribosomes
2. agranular ER (smooth), which is free of ribosomes.

Ribosomes include tiny particles of RNA – these are formed in the cell nuclei and are associated with the synthesis of proteins needed by the cell.

- The membranes of the ER contain many enzymes that speed up chemical reactions within the cells.
- ER consists of a series of channels (cisternae), which are concerned with the transport of materials – particularly proteins.
- ER contains a number of enzymes that are important for cell metabolism – such as digestive enzymes, enzymes that are involved in the synthesis (production) of steroids and enzymes that lead to the removal of toxic substances from the cell (McCance & Huether, 2022).
- The alteration/addition of proteins exported from the cell also occurs in the cisternae.
- ER is also present in liver cells, where it has a role to play in drug detoxification.
- Granular ER is particularly found in cells that actively synthesise and export proteins.
- Agranular ER is found in steroid hormone-secreting cells, such as the cells of the adrenal cortex or, in males, the testes.

Golgi complex (Fig. 1.2)

The Golgi complex (also known as the Golgi apparatus) is a collection of membranous tubes and elongated sacs. These are actually flattened cisternae that are stacked together. The Golgi complex has two major roles:

1. Helping to concentrate and package some of the substances that are made in the cell itself, for example, lysosomal enzymes.
2. Helping with the assembly of substances for secretion outside of the cell. Secretory cells (such as those found in the mucous membrane) have many Golgi stacks, whilst non-secretory cells have few Golgi stacks per cell.

Proteins destined for export are first synthesised on ribosomes, then pass through the ER to Golgi vesicles. These vesicles fuse with the cell membrane via exocytosis, releasing their contents outside the cell. The Golgi complex also helps form glycoproteins.

Lysosomes (Fig. 1.2)

Lysosomes are organelles that are bound to the cell membrane, and they contain a variety of enzymes. They have a number of functions:

- They are responsible for the digestion of material (e.g., pathogenic organisms) taken up by the process of endocytosis.
- They are capable of breaking down components within a cell when they are not needed. For example, during human embryonic development, the fingers and toes of the embryo are connected by tissue and appear webbed, and the lysosomal enzymes facilitate the removal of these cells making up the webbing from between the digits separated.
- After the baby's birth, the uterus (which can weigh around 2 kg at full term) is invaded by phagocytic cells that are rich in lysosomes. These then reduce the uterus to its non-pregnant weight of approximately 50 g within about 9 days.
- In normal cells, some of the synthesised proteins may be faulty, and so, consequently, it is the lysosomes that are responsible for their removal and destruction.

It is vital that lysosomes do not rupture within living cells, as their enzymes could digest and destroy the cell, contributing to degenerative diseases such as rheumatoid arthritis. Lysosomal rupture in macrophages may drive the destruction of essential cells and tissues. Lysosomes also aid hormone production, including thyroxine, which regulates physiological activities such as metabolism.

Peroxisomes (Fig. 1.2)

Peroxisomes are small, lysosome-like organelles, abundant in liver cells, containing enzymes that can be toxic to the body. Their main role is detoxifying harmful substances, such as alcohol and formaldehyde, and neutralising dangerous free radicals – highly reactive chemicals that can damage molecules. Peroxisomes are organelles that are similar in structure to lysosomes. However, they are much smaller. These organelles are particularly abundant in the cells of the liver, and they contain several enzymes that are toxic to cells of the body.

The role of peroxisomes in cells appears to be one of detoxification of harmful substances – such as alcohol and formaldehyde – within the cell. Importantly, they also neutralise dangerous free radicals. Free radicals are highly reactive chemicals that contain electrons that have not been 'paired off' and so are 'free' to disrupt the structure of molecules (Marieb, 2021).

Mitochondria (Fig. 1.2)

Mitochondria, the cell's 'powerhouses', produce most of the cell's ATP energy and are concentrated in areas of high metabolic activity. Anatomically, mitochondria consist of two membranes (an inner and an outer) and an intermembrane space.

The inner membrane has many folds (cristae) that increase the surface area available for chemical reactions to occur, such as the production of ATP (a coenzyme used as an energy carrier in the cells of all known organisms, which is responsible for the process by which energy is moved throughout the cell). This process is collectively known as internal respiration. The inner membrane is of the same thickness as the outer membrane and is responsible for oxidative phosphorylation.

The mitochondrial matrix is the name given to the space that is surrounded by the inner membrane. It contains enzymes of the tricarboxylic acid (TCA) cycle, as well as those enzymes involved in fatty acid oxidation. In children, mitochondria are especially important due to their role in meeting the high energy demands of growth, repair, learning and physical activity. Their increased metabolic rate relies on efficient mitochondrial energy production. About two-thirds of the total protein is found in mitochondria, and, with the inner membrane, they play an important role in the production of ATP and contain a very concentrated mixture of hundreds of enzymes.

The intermembrane space: Because the outer membrane is freely permeable to small molecules, there is a high concentration of small molecules, such as ions and sugars. However, larger molecules cannot enter this space unless they possess a specific signalling code that allows them to be able to pass through the outer membrane.

The outer mitochondrial membrane encloses the entire organelle. It contains large numbers of integral membrane proteins, known as porins, which form channels in the membrane to allow small molecules to diffuse easily from outside the mitochondria to the intermembrane space, and vice versa. Any disruption of the outer membrane allows proteins in the intermembrane space to leak into the intercellular fluid in the cell (cytosol), leading to certain cell death.

Mitochondria generate the cell's energy by converting the chemical energy in food into ATP. This process occurs in multiple enzyme-driven stages, with enzymes arranged in the mitochondrial membranes to ensure reactions happen in the correct sequence, preventing potentially harmful errors.

Mitochondria are self-replicating, in that, although most of a cell's DNA is contained in the cell nucleus, the mitochondrion has its own independent genetic organisation that is really quite similar to that of bacteria. DNA that is incorporated into the mitochondrial structure controls its own replication system.

The cytoskeleton

The cytoskeleton is a lattice-like collection of fibres and fine tubes, and these are found in the cytoplasm of the cell. It is involved with the cell's ability to maintain and alter its shape as required (see Fig. 1.7).

There are three components that make up the cytoskeleton:

- microfilaments
- microtubules
- intermediate filaments.

Microfilaments

Microfilaments are rod-like structures that are approximately 6 nanometres (6 nm) in diameter and are made of a protein called actin. In muscles, both actin (which is thick) and another protein – myosin (which is thin) – combine together to allow the contraction of muscle fibres. In non-muscle cells, microfilaments help to provide support and shape to the cell. Microfilaments also assist in the movement of the cells themselves, as well as movement within the cells.

Microtubules

Microtubules are relatively straight, slender, cylindrical tubules that range in diameter from 18 to 30 nm. They consist of another protein – tubulin.

- Microtubules and microfilaments help provide shape and support for cells.
- They provide conducting channels – like tunnels – through which various substances can move through the cytoplasm.

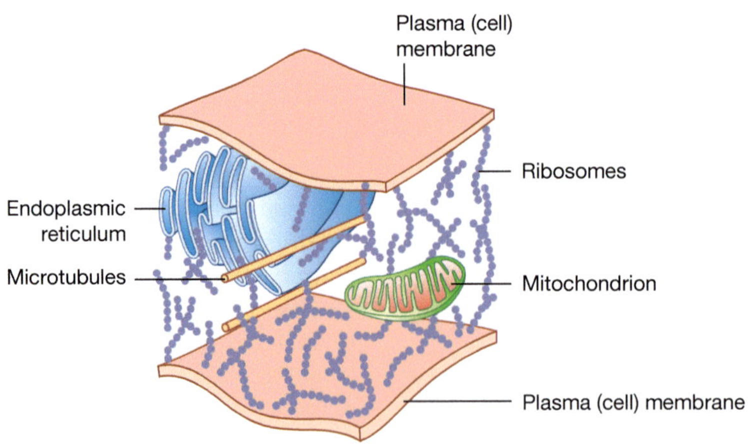

FIGURE 1.7 The cytoskeleton.
Source: Reproduced with permission of Peate & Gormley-Fleming (2015)/John Wiley & Sons.

- They also assist in the movement of pseudopodia (false arms/legs) – temporary projections of eukaryotic cell membranes. The functions of pseudopodia include locomotion (movement) and the capturing of prey. Pseudopodia sense prey that can then be engulfed. The engulfing pseudopodia are used by phagocytic white cells.

Intermediate filaments

These help determine the shape of a cell and range in size from 8 to 12 nm. Examples of intermediate filaments are neurofilaments, which are found in nerves.

Centrioles

These cylindrical structures are found in most animal cells and are composed of nine sets of microtubule cylinders arranged in a circular pattern. They are particularly involved in cell reproduction. Centrioles are involved in the organisation of the mitotic spindle.

Cilia and flagella

These 'hair-like' structures extend from the surface of some cells. They possess the facility to bend, which causes the cells to move.

In humans, cilia generally have the function of moving fluid or particulates over the surface of the cells. However, ciliated cells of the respiratory tract have a very important role to play in our immune and respiratory system in that they are able to move mucus that has trapped foreign particles, including bacteria and viruses, over the surface of respiratory tissues and towards the mouth or nose, thus preventing them from causing illness.

A flagellum (singular of flagella) is usually a much larger structure than a cilium (singular of cilia), and it is often used like a fish's tail to propel the cell forward. The only example of a human cell with a flagellum is a spermatozoon, where the flagellum acts as a tail and propels the spermatozoon towards an ovum.

Conclusion

This concludes the section on cells. Understanding their structure and function is essential for grasping how the human body works. The next section will examine the body's organs and structures, all composed of billions of cells.

Tissues

Introduction

Each human begins as a single fertilised egg, which divides to form an embryo, then a foetus and finally a baby. Cells divide in a controlled way, becoming specialised, such as muscle, skin or blood cells, and group into tissues, which combine to form the body. Tissues are groups of similar cells performing the same functions (McCance & Huether, 2022).

There are four primary types of tissues:

- epithelial
- connective
- muscle
- nervous.

These four primary tissue types then interweave to form the fabric of the body (Marieb, 2021). Each of the four types of tissue has a specific role to perform within the body. In simple terms:

- Epithelial tissue is concerned with covering and/or lining the body, both internally and externally.
- Connective tissue is concerned with supporting the body and the tissues and organs that make up the body.
- Muscle tissue is concerned with movement – both of the body and within the body.
- Nervous tissue is concerned with the control of the body – both internally and externally (Marieb, 2021).

These specialist cells form themselves into tissues in one of two ways:

1. The first way is by means of a process known as 'mitosis'. Cells formed as a result of the process of mitosis are clones of the original cell. Therefore, if one cell with a specialised function undergoes mitosis, and subsequent generations of daughter cells continue to undergo mitosis, then the resulting hundreds and thousands of cells will all be identical and of the same type, meaning that they will all have the same function. If these identical cells join together, they will become a specialised tissue. So, for example, epithelial cell sheets (such as skin) are formed as a result of mitosis (McCance & Huether, 2022).
2. The second way is by migrating to the site of tissue formation and assembling with other cells to form a tissue. This is particularly seen during the development of the embryo when, for example, cells migrate

to sites in the embryo where they differentiate and assemble into a variety of tissues (McCance & Huether, 2022). This movement of cells is known as 'chemotaxis'. Chemotaxis is the movement of cells along a chemical gradient caused by chemical attraction (McCance & Huether, 2022).

Types of tissues

Epithelial tissue

Epithelial tissue lines and covers areas of the body – both outside and inside – as well as forming the glandular tissue of the body. Thus, the exterior of the body (i.e., skin) is covered by one type of epithelial tissue, whilst other types of epithelial tissue line digestive organs, such as the stomach and the small intestines, along with the kidneys, and so on. So it can be seen that epithelial tissue covers or lines most of the internal and external surfaces of the body.

Classification

Epithelial tissue is classified in two ways:

1. The number of cell layers:
   - simple – where the epithelium is formed by a single layer of cells (Fig. 1.8)
   - stratified – where the epithelium has two or more layers of cells (Fig. 1.9).
2. Shape:
   - squamous
   - cuboidal
   - columnar.

Simple epithelial tissue is most concerned with absorption, secretion and filtration of fluids and particulates. However, because this tissue is usually very thin, it is not involved in protection.

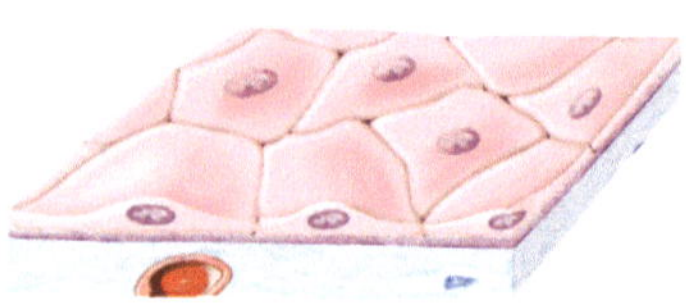

FIGURE 1.8 Simple epithelium.
Source: Peate & Gormley-Fleming (2015)/with permission of John Wiley & Sons.

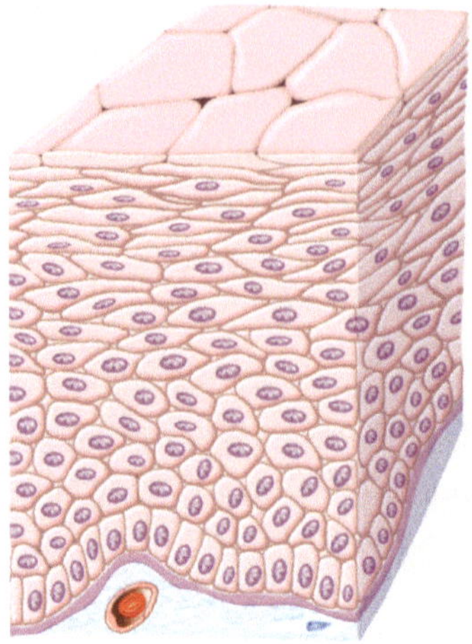

FIGURE 1.9 Stratified epithelium.
Source: Peate & Gormley-Fleming (2015)/with permission of John Wiley & Sons.

Simple squamous epithelium rests on a basal layer known as the 'basement membrane'. This is composed of a structural material that is secreted by the cells themselves (Marieb, 2021). The basement membranes provide a layer of cells that supports and separates epithelial tissue from the underlying connective tissue (Fig. 1.10). The squamous epithelial cells fit very closely together to give a thin sheet forming the tissue. This type of epithelial tissue is found in the alveoli of the lungs as well as in the walls of capillaries. It is this very thin tissue that easily allows for rapid diffusion into and out of the cell, thus facilitating oxygen and carbon dioxide exchange through the epithelial tissue that is lining the alveoli of the lungs and allowing nutrients and gases to pass easily through the epithelial tissue from the cells into the capillaries – and vice versa.

Simple squamous epithelial cells also form the serous membranes that line certain body cavities and organs.

Simple cuboidal epithelial tissue consists of one layer of cells resting on a basement membrane (Fig. 1.11). However, because cuboidal epithelial cells are thicker than squamous epithelial cells, they are found in different places within the body and also perform different functions. This type of epithelial tissue is found in glands, such as the salivary glands and the pancreas. In addition, they form the walls of the kidney tubules as well as covering the surface of the ovaries (Marieb, 2021).

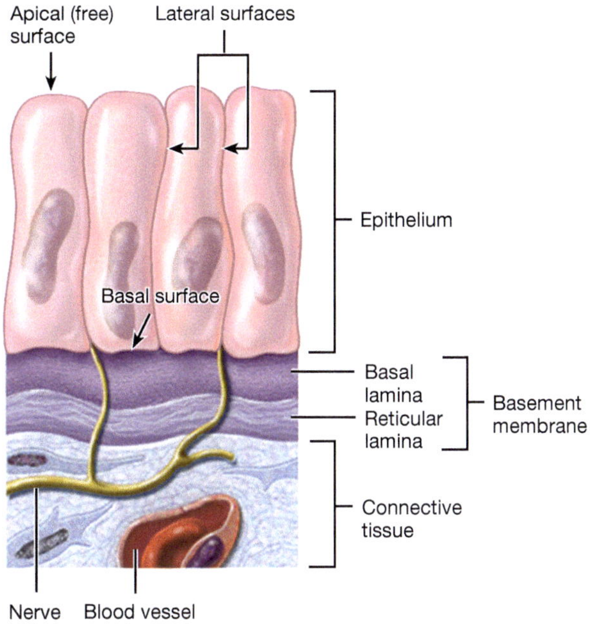

FIGURE 1.10 Connective tissue reinforces epithelial tissue.
Source: Reproduced with permission of Peate & Gormley-Fleming (2015)/John Wiley & Sons.

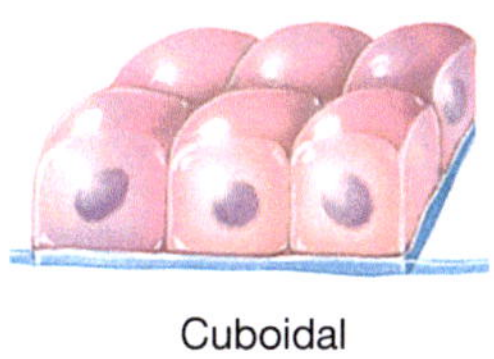

FIGURE 1.11 Simple cuboidal.
Source: Reproduced with permission of Peate & Gormley-Fleming (2015)/John Wiley & Sons.

Simple columnar epithelium (Fig. 1.12) is the third type of simple epithelial tissue. Like the other types of simple epithelium, it is composed of a single layer of cells, although these cells are relatively tall. However, similar to the other types, they still fit closely together. It is this type of epithelial tissue, which also contains goblet cells, that lines the entire length of the digestive tract from the stomach to the anus. Goblet cells produce mucus and, so, consequently, the simple columnar epithelial tissues that line all the body cavities that are open to the exterior of the body are known as mucous membranes (Marieb, 2021).

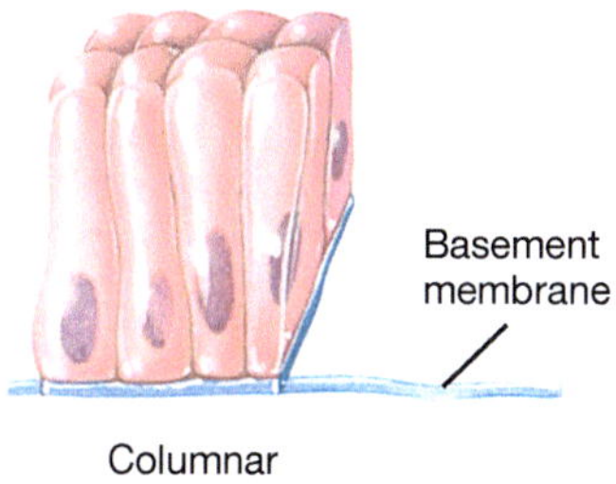

FIGURE 1.12 Simple columnar.
Source: Reproduced with permission of Peate & Gormley-Fleming (2015)/John Wiley & Sons.

Stratified epithelial tissue, unlike simple epithelial tissue, consists of two or more cell layers – so they lie in strata (hence the name). Because these stratified epithelial tissues have more than one layer of cells, they are stronger and harder than simple epithelia. As a consequence, a primary function of stratified epithelia is protection.

Stratified squamous epithelial tissue consists of several layers of cells and is the most common stratified epithelium found within the human body (Marieb, 2021). Despite being called 'squamous epithelium', it is not composed entirely of squamous cells. Only the cells at the free edges of the epithelial tissue are squamous, while those cells that are close to the basement membrane are made up of either cuboidal or columnar cells. This tissue is to be found in parts of the body that are most at risk of everyday damage, such as the oesophagus, the mouth and the outer layer of the skin.

Stratified cuboidal epithelial tissue has just two layers of cells and is only found in the ducts of large glands, such as the sweat glands, mammary glands and salivary glands, where its role is to protect the ducts of these glands.

Stratified columnar epithelial tissue is also found only in a few particular places in the body, such as in the conjunctiva of the eye, parts of the pharynx and anus, the uterus and the male urethra and vas deferens. It is also found in ducts located within the salivary glands.

Transitional epithelium, a specialised stratified squamous epithelium, lines the urinary bladder, ureters and part of the urethra. It allows these organs to stretch: when empty, the tissue has many layers with rounded surface cells; when distended with urine, the cells flatten and slide past each other, enabling expansion and greater urine storage until micturition.

Case study: epidermolysis bullosa (EB)

Patient profile

Emily, a 6-month-old infant, was admitted to the hospital with persistent blistering of the skin following minimal friction. Initially, concerns were raised about potential non-accidental injury, leading to a referral to Social Services.

Diagnosis

An experienced paediatric dermatologist recognised the clinical presentation as indicative of *junctional epidermolysis bullosa* (JEB), a rare genetic skin disorder. JEB is characterised by mutations affecting proteins that anchor the epidermis to the dermis, resulting in skin fragility and blister formation upon minor trauma.

Epidemiology

In the United Kingdom, the prevalence of all EB types is approximately 34.8 per million people. JEB accounts for about 1 per million, making it one of the rarer subtypes.

Pathophysiology

Human skin comprises two primary layers: the epidermis (outer layer) and the dermis (inner layer), connected by anchoring proteins. In JEB, mutations in genes such as *LAMA3*, *LAMB3* or *LAMC2* disrupt these connections, leading to skin separation and blistering.

Clinical implications

Beyond skin involvement, JEB can affect mucous membranes, leading to complications in the mouth, oesophagus and gastrointestinal tract. There is also an increased risk of developing squamous cell carcinoma in severe cases.

Advancements in treatment

Recent developments have introduced promising therapies:

- **Zevaskyn™ (prademagene zamikeracel or pz-cel):** Approved by the Food and Drug Administration (FDA) in April 2025, this autologous, cell-based gene therapy targets the underlying genetic defects in recessive dystrophic EB (RDEB) by correcting the *COL7A1* gene.
- **Vyjuvek™ (beremagene geperpavec):** A topical gene therapy approved in 2023, delivering functional *COL7A1* genes to promote wound healing in dystrophic EB patients.
- **Filsuvez® (birch triterpenes):** A topical gel approved in the EU in 2022 for treating partial-thickness wounds in both dystrophic and junctional EB.

Multidisciplinary care approach

Management of EB requires a comprehensive, multidisciplinary team, including:

- **Dermatologists:** For diagnosis and ongoing skin management.
- **Nurses:** Specialised in wound care and patient education.
- **Genetic counsellors:** To advise families on inheritance patterns and future family planning.
- **Psychologists and social workers:** Providing emotional support and resources.
- **Educational staff:** Assisting with school integration and accommodations.

Investigations

Diagnosis is confirmed through:

1. **Skin Biopsy:** Histological examination reveals sub-epidermal blistering with neutrophil infiltration.
2. **Direct Immunofluorescence (DIF):** Perilesional skin samples may show deposits of immunoglobulins (IgG, IgM and IgA), aiding in subtype classification.

Red Flag

Due to the rarity of EB, its symptoms can be mistaken for signs of abuse. Healthcare professionals must approach such cases with sensitivity, ensuring accurate diagnosis to prevent unwarranted social interventions.

Conclusion

Although there is no cure for EB, advances in gene therapy and supportive care have improved outcomes. Early diagnosis and a holistic care approach are key to managing the condition and enhancing the quality of life for patients and their families.

Glandular epithelium

Glandular epithelial tissue is found within the glands. According to Marieb (2021), a gland consists of several cells that make and secrete a particular product.

There are two major types of glands developed from sheets of epithelial cells:

- exocrine glands
- endocrine glands.

Exocrine glands have ducts that carry secretions to epithelial surfaces, such as sweat glands, the liver and the pancreas. Endocrine glands lack ducts; their secretions, hormones, diffuse directly into blood vessels and include the thyroid, adrenal and pituitary glands.

Connective tissue

Connective tissue is found throughout the body and, as the name suggests, it connects and supports other tissues and organs (see Fig. 1.10). It is the most abundant of the four primary tissue types.

Despite its varied structure, connective tissue shares four main functions:

- Protection
- Support
- Binding together of other tissues (Marieb, 2021)
- Storage of nutrients (McCance & Huether, 2022).

Its most common role is to act as a framework on which other tissues, like epithelium, are built to form organs (McCance & Huether, 2022).

Connective tissue contains fewer cells than other tissues, with a large extracellular matrix that provides strength and flexibility. The matrix is made of:

- Ground substance (mainly water, proteins and large sugar molecules)
- Fibres, produced by cells called fibroblasts.

There are three types of fibres in connective tissue:

- Collagen fibres – strong and supportive
- Elastic fibres – stretchy and able to recoil
- Reticular fibres – form delicate networks in soft organs like the spleen.

The ground substance varies from fluid to a jelly-like consistency. It acts as a water reservoir and supports cell attachment.

Connective tissue also acts as a protective layer around organs and helps the body absorb mechanical stress. It can withstand weight, stretching and pressure. Different types of connective tissue vary in strength and flexibility. For example:

- Fat tissue contains mostly cells and a soft matrix.
- Bone and cartilage contain fewer cells but a hard matrix, making them strong.

Blood supply also varies as:

- Most connective tissues (like bone) have a good blood supply and heal quickly.
- Tendons and ligaments have limited blood supply and heal more slowly.
- Cartilage has no direct blood supply, which makes healing very slow (Marieb, 2021).

Types of connective tissue

Bone

Bone, the most rigid connective tissue, consists of bone cells in a hard matrix of calcium and collagen, providing protection, support and muscle attachment. In children and adolescents, bones lengthen at epiphyseal (growth) plates, where cartilage is gradually replaced by bone through endochondral ossification until the plates close in late adolescence.

Cartilage

Cartilage is not as hard as bone, but it is more flexible. It is found in only a few places in the body (see Fig. 1.13). For example, hyaline cartilage supports the structures of the larynx. It also attaches the ribs to the sternum and covers the ends of bones where they form joints. Another type of cartilage is fibrocartilage, which can be compressed and forms the discs between the spinal and neck vertebrae. Elastic cartilage is found in the external ear, where a degree of elasticity is necessary.

Dense connective tissue

This forms strong, stringy structures such as tendons (which attach skeletal muscles to bones) and the more elastic ligaments (which connect bones to other bones at joints). Dense connective tissue also makes up the lower layers of skin (the dermis). These tissues have collagen fibres as the main matrix element, with many fibroblasts found between the collagen fibres. Fibroblasts are involved in the manufacturing of fibres.

Loose connective tissue

These tissues are softer and contain fewer fibres but more cells than other types of connective tissue (with the exception of blood). There are four types of connective tissue:

- areolar tissue
- adipose tissue
- reticular tissue
- blood.

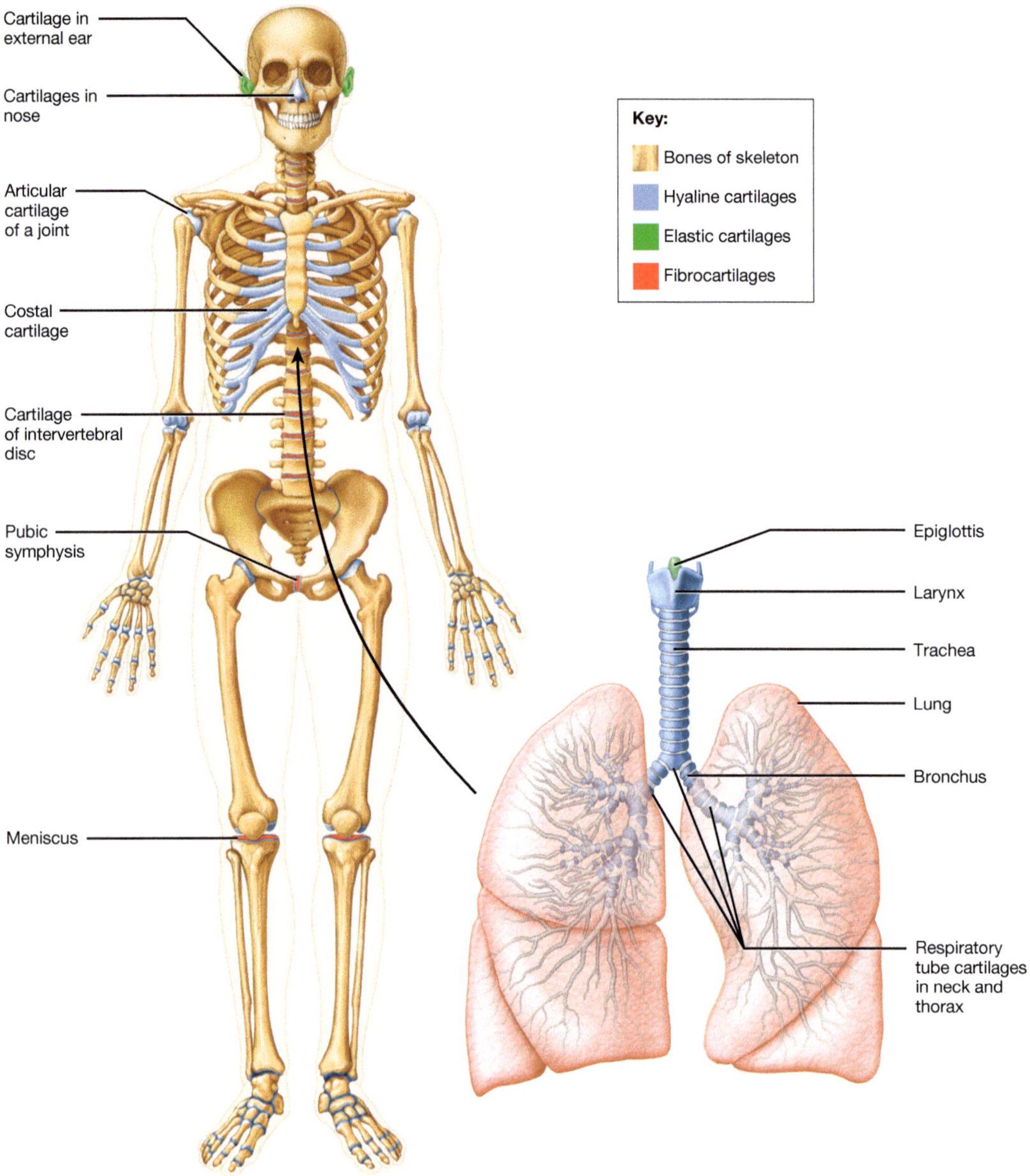

FIGURE 1.13 Where cartilage is found in the body.
Source: Reproduced with permission of Peate & Gormley-Fleming (2015)/John Wiley & Sons.

Areolar tissue

Areolar tissue, the most widely distributed connective tissue, cushions and protects organs, holds them together and has a loose, fibre-filled matrix that provides softness, pliability and a reservoir of water and salts for surrounding tissues.

All body cells obtain their nutrients from this tissue fluid, and they also release their waste into it. It is in this area that, following injury, swelling (oedema) can occur because the areolar tissue soaks up the excess fluid, causing it to become puffy (Marieb, 2021).

Adipose tissue

Adipose tissue, commonly known as 'fat', consists mainly of fat cells. It forms the subcutaneous layer beneath the skin, insulating the body, protecting against temperature extremes and cushioning organs like the kidneys and eyes.

Reticular connective tissue
This tissue consists of a delicate network of reticular fibres that are associated with reticular cells. It forms an internal framework to support many free blood cells – mainly the lymphocytes – in the lymphoid organs, such as the lymph nodes, spleen and bone marrow.

Blood
Blood, a connective tissue, consists of cells suspended in a non-living fluid matrix called plasma. It transports nutrients, waste, gases and other substances. In children, blood-forming tissues such as bone marrow are highly active, and the immune system matures with increasing white blood cell production to combat infections.

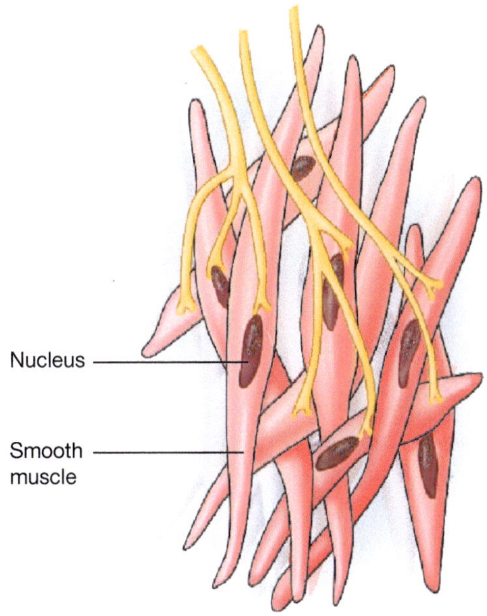

FIGURE 1.15 Smooth muscle.
Source: Peate & Gormley-Fleming (2015)/with permission of John Wiley & Sons.

Muscle tissue

There are three types of muscle tissue. These are responsible for helping the body to move and for moving substances around the body. The three types of muscle tissue are:

- skeletal muscle
- cardiac muscle
- smooth muscle.

See Figs. 1.14 and 1.15 for examples of skeletal muscle cells and smooth muscle.

Skeletal muscle
Skeletal muscle is attached to bones and is involved in the movements of the skeleton. These muscles can be controlled voluntarily and form the 'bulk' of the body – the flesh. The cells of skeletal muscles are long and cylindrical and have several nuclei (Fig. 1.12). In addition, they appear striated (striped). They work by contracting and relaxing, with pairs working antagonistically against each other – i.e., one muscle contracts and the opposite muscle relaxes. So, if the muscles in the front of the arm contract, then the ones at the back relax, which causes the arm to bend.

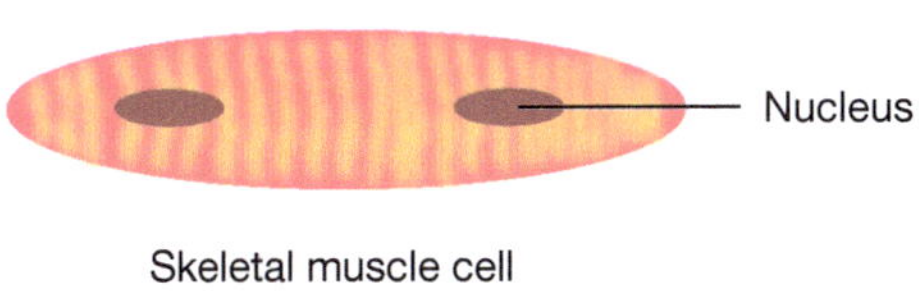

FIGURE 1.14 Skeletal muscle cells.
Source: Peate & Gormley-Fleming (2015)/with permission of John Wiley & Sons.

Cardiac muscle
Cardiac muscle is only found in the heart, and its role is to pump blood around the body. It also achieves this by contracting and relaxing. However, unlike skeletal muscles, cardiac muscle works in an involuntary way – the activity cannot be consciously controlled. The cells of the muscle do not have a nucleus.

Smooth muscle
Also known as visceral muscle, smooth muscle is found in the walls of hollow organs – for example, the stomach, bladder, uterus and blood vessels. Like cardiac muscle, smooth muscle works in an involuntary way. It causes movement in the hollow organs; for example, as smooth muscle contracts, the cavity of the organ constricts – becomes small in volume – and when it relaxes, the organ

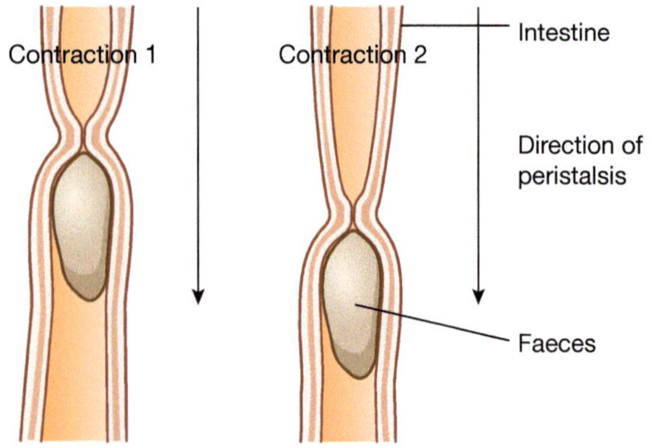

FIGURE 1.16 Peristalsis.
Source: Reproduced with permission of Peate & Gormley-Fleming (2015)/John Wiley & Sons.

becomes larger in volume (dilates). This allows substances to be propelled through the organ in the right direction, for example, faeces in the intestine. As smooth muscle contracts and relaxes, it forms a wave-like motion (peristalsis) to push the faeces through the intestines to the rectum (see Fig. 1.16).

Nervous tissue

Nervous tissue is concerned with control and communication within the body by means of electrical signals. The neurone (Fig. 1.17) is the main type of cell found in nervous tissue.

All neurones receive and conduct electrochemical impulses around the body. The structure of neurones is very different from that of other cells. The cytoplasm is found within long processes or extensions; some in the leg are more than a metre long. These neurones receive and transmit electrical impulses very rapidly from one to the other across junctions (known as synapses). Synapses also allow electric impulses to pass from neurones to muscle cells. The total number of neurones is fixed at birth and cannot be replaced if lost or damaged (McCance & Huether, 2022). Although the number of neurones is fixed, the development of the nervous system continues throughout childhood. In particular, the process of myelination – where nerve fibres are coated in an insulating layer to increase transmission speed – is ongoing during infancy and early childhood, supporting improvements in coordination, motor skills and cognitive development.

In addition to neurones, nervous tissue includes some cells known as neuroglia (supporting cells). These

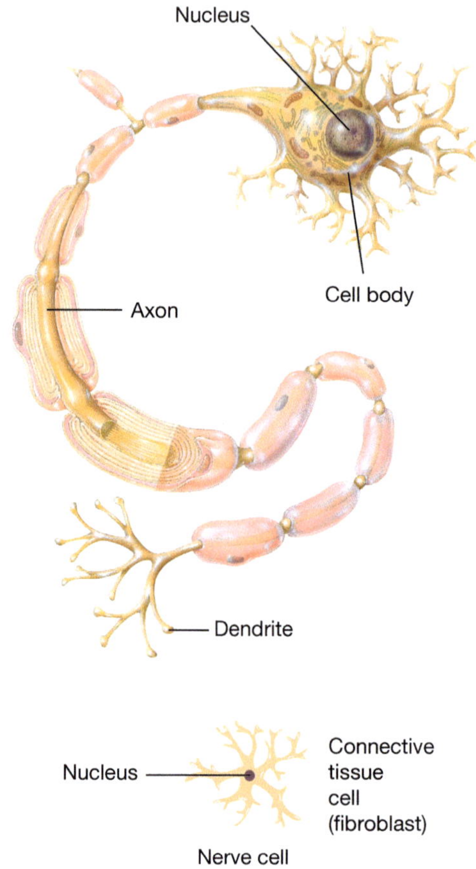

FIGURE 1.17 Nerve cell.
Source: Peate & Gormley-Fleming (2015)/with permission of John Wiley & Sons.

cells insulate, support and protect the delicate neurones. The neurones and supporting cells comprise the structures of the nervous system, namely:

- brain
- spinal cord
- nerves.

Tissue repair

The many tissues of the body are always at risk of injury or disease. Inflammation is the body's immediate reaction to tissue injury or damage because when this occurs, it stimulates the body's inflammatory and immune responses to spring into action so that the healing process can begin almost immediately. In children, tissues generally have greater plasticity and healing capacity than in adults. This means that many injuries, particularly to skin, bone and muscle, heal more quickly and with less scarring. This regenerative advantage gradually decreases with age.

Conclusion

This chapter has examined the building blocks of the human body: cells and tissues. Understanding cells and their functions is key to understanding how the body works. Cells form tissues, which build the body's structures, systems and organs. The rest of the book will explore these systems and organs, their functions and potential disorders.

Test your knowledge

1. How many primary tissue groups are there?
2. What is the difference between an exocrine and an endocrine gland?
3. What is the function of muscle tissue?
4. Discuss the two main classifications of cells: the prokaryotes and eukaryotes.
5. Each cell is surrounded by a membrane, what is the function of this membrane?

References

Alberts, B., Johnson, A., Lewis, J., *et al.* (2022). *Molecular Biology of the Cell*, 7th edn. Garland Science, New York.

Colbert, B.J., Ankney, J., Lee, K.T., *et al.* (2019). *Anatomy and Physiology for Nursing and Healthcare Professionals*, 4th edn. Pearson Education, Harlow.

Gormley-Fleming, E., & Peate, I. (2015). In: Tortora, G.J. & Derrickson, B.H. (eds). *Principles of Anatomy and Physiology*, 14th edn. Wiley, Hoboken: New Jersey.

Marieb, E.N. (2021). *Essentials of Human Anatomy and Physiology*, 13th edn. Pearson Education, New Jersey.

McCance, K.L., & Huether, S.E. (2022). *Pathophysiology: The Biologic Basis for Disease in Adults and Children*, 9th edn. (ebook). Mosby, St. Louis.

Peate, I. (2021). *Fundamentals of Applied Pathophysiology*, 4th edn. Wiley, Oxford.

Peate, I., & Gormley-Fleming, E. (eds) (2015). *Fundamentals of Children's Anatomy and Physiology: A Textbook for Nursing and Healthcare Students*, 1st edn. Wiley-Blackwell, Chichester.

CHAPTER 2

Genetics

Ian Peate and Elizabeth Gormley-Fleming

AIM

To introduce students to the important subject of genetics, providing the knowledge needed to understand many illnesses with a genetic basis.

LEARNING OUTCOMES

On completion of this chapter, the reader will be able to:

- Describe the anatomy and functions of chromosomes, and explain the role of genes and their importance.
- Describe the structure of the DNA double helix and its bases.
- Identify the differences between DNA and RNA, and explain protein synthesis and cell division.
- Explain the modes of inheritance.
- Describe genetic mutations and their potential effects on health and child development.

KEYWORDS

- genes
- chromosomes
- DNA
- RNA
- mutation
- inheritance
- traits
- genetic variation
- genetic disorders

Test your prior knowledge

1. Which process is responsible for the transfer of genetic information from parents to offspring?
2. What is the role of chromosomes?
3. What is the function of genes, and how does a genotype differ from a phenotype?
4. What is a genetic mutation, and in what ways can it impact a child's health and development?
5. What are the key stages of mitosis and meiosis, and how do they contribute to growth and reproduction?

The cell nucleus and DNA

Fig. 2.1 provides an overview of the cell nucleus and DNA.

Introduction

Genetics is an increasingly important area in healthcare, requiring nurses to have a solid understanding of its principles and applications. Often called 'the century of genetics', this field has expanded rapidly, enabling the manipulation of human, animal and plant genes to tackle major health challenges, including disease prevention and hunger alleviation. Clinical genetic services began in the United Kingdom in the 1950s, initially limited in scope (Patch & Skirton, 2009; NHS England, 2023). Understanding genetics is crucial, especially in children's and young people's health, as many conditions have a genetic component. This knowledge helps healthcare professionals recognise inherited conditions, support early intervention, provide genetic counselling and promote informed decision-making in patient care.

Genes

Genes are subdivisions of deoxyribonucleic acid (DNA) that are carried within chromosomes. These genes contain sets of instructions related to our bodies and how they function. Almost all the genes that we possess have been inherited from our parents (apart from any spontaneous mutations), who in turn inherited theirs from their parents, and so on.

Here are some technical definitions that will help you understand this chapter on genetics:

- Deoxyribonucleic acid (DNA): It is the essential ingredient of heredity. It comprises the basic units of hereditary material – our genes. The ability of DNA to replicate itself is the basis of hereditary transmission, and it organises and produces our genetic code by acting as a template for the synthesis of messenger ribonucleic acid (mRNA).
- Ribonucleic acid (RNA) and mRNA: These determine the amino acid composition of proteins, which in turn determines the function of that protein, and therefore the function of that particular cell.
- Chromosome: It is a long strand of DNA and protein. Each chromosome is made up of two chromatids

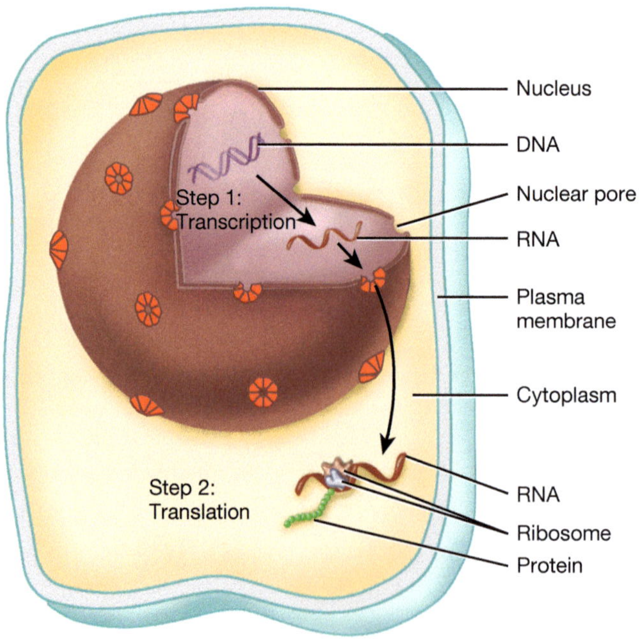

FIGURE 2.1 The cell nucleus.
Source: Reproduced with permission of Peate & Gormley-Fleming (2015)/John Wiley & Sons.

joined by a centromere. Each nucleated cell in our body contains, within its genes, all the genetic material to make an entire human being.

The double helix

The double helix was identified in the 1950s by James Watson and Francis Crick (Patch & Skirton, 2009).

The double helix is made up of two strands of DNA and phosphate. It is a spiral-shaped molecule, resembling a corkscrew ladder, whose rungs are pairs of bases. Within the double helix, the genetic information is encoded in a linear sequence of chemical subunits called nucleotides (see Fig. 2.2).

Deoxyribonucleotides

Deoxyribonucleotides consist of three molecules:

- deoxyribose
- phosphate
- nitrogenous base.

The bases are those elements of the double helix that carry the genetic code. They are arranged in different sequences along the deoxyribose–phosphate strands of the double helix. Each deoxyribonucleotide comprises three parts: a nitrogenous base, a deoxyribose sugar and one phosphate group.

Bases

There are four different bases found in DNA, namely:

- adenine (A)
- thymine (T)

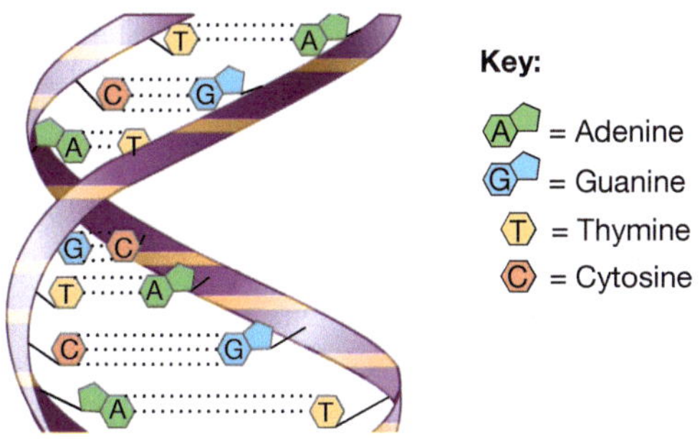

FIGURE 2.2 A pictorial representation of a portion of the double helix.
Source: Reproduced with permission of Peate & Gormley-Fleming (2015)/John Wiley & Sons.

- guanine (G)
- cytosine (C)

The order in which the bases are organised along the length of the DNA molecule provides the variation that allows for the storage of genetic information.

Look again at Fig. 2.2, the double helix; each strand carries different bases. These bases join together and make the molecule stable. However, these bases do not just pair off haphazardly; they can only pair up with bases that match them so that they will fit together (like jigsaw pieces). This limitation means that each base pairs with only one specific partner, according to the golden rule of DNA pairing:

- **adenine (A)** always pairs with **thymine (T)**
- **guanine (G)** always pairs with **cytosine (C)**

So, if one half of the DNA has a base sequence

AGGCAGTGC

then the opposite side of the DNA will always have the complementary base sequence

TCCGTCACG

The bases join together by means of hydrogen/polar bonding, and the individual bases are connected to the deoxyribose of the strands by means of covalent bonds. This is important because hydrogen bonds are not as strong as covalent bonds, and thus can separate more easily. The importance of this will become apparent when DNA replication and protein synthesis are discussed (Jorde *et al.*, 2019).

Chromosomes

A chromosome is made of DNA combined with proteins called histones. Together, they form nucleosomes within the nucleus, and this DNA–histone complex is called chromatin.

This vast amount of DNA and histones fits into each cell because it is neatly folded; without this precise organisation, it would not fit and errors would likely occur (Bywater, 2025). Consequently, the chromosomes twist on one another before being arranged into loops and super loops, until they assume the shape that is recognisable as a chromosome – i.e., the X-shape that can be seen in a human cell (Fig. 2.3) (Jorde *et al.*, 2019).

Each chromosome is made up of two chromatids joined by a centromere to make an 'X' shape. Each half of the chromosome is a chromatid, and where they join near the top of the X, that is the centromere (Fig. 2.3).

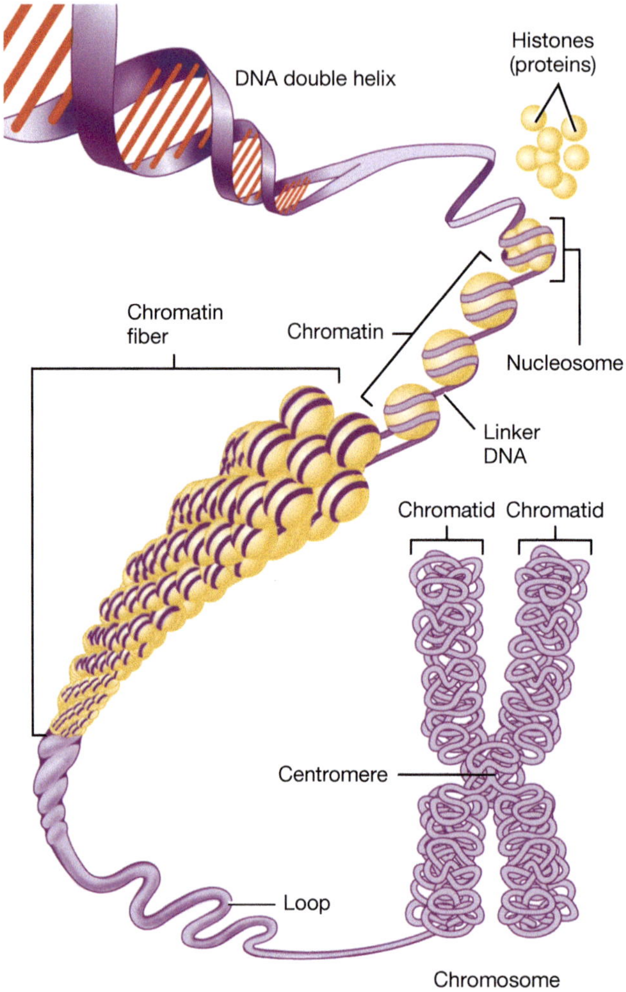

FIGURE 2.3 DNA from double helix to chromosome.
Source: Reproduced with permission of Peate & Gormley-Fleming (2015)/John Wiley & Sons.

In most humans, each nucleated body cell (i.e., each body cell with a nucleus) has 46 chromosomes, arranged in 23 pairs. Of those 23 pairs, one pair determines the gender of the person. These sex chromosomes are designated as X and Y chromosomes (all the others have numbers from 1 to 22), as can be seen in Fig. 2.4.

- Females have a matched homologous (similar) pair of X chromosomes, i.e., XX.
- Males have an unmatched heterologous (different) pair – one X and one Y chromosome.
- The remaining 22 pairs of chromosomes are known as autosomes. In biology, the word 'some' means body, so an autosome means 'self-body'.
- Autosomes determine physical/body characteristics – in other words, all characteristics of a person that are not connected with gender.

Each chromosome pair includes one chromosome from the mother and one from the father. A gene's position on a chromosome is called a locus, which acts like an address on 'Chromosome Street', indicating where that gene is located.

Genes at corresponding loci that code for the same trait are called alleles. Each allele occupies the same position on the two corresponding chromatids and determines an alternative form of a characteristic, such as hair colour, eye colour or susceptibility to certain diseases.

Example

A person's hair colour gene is located at the same position on each of the two chromatids, with one copy inherited

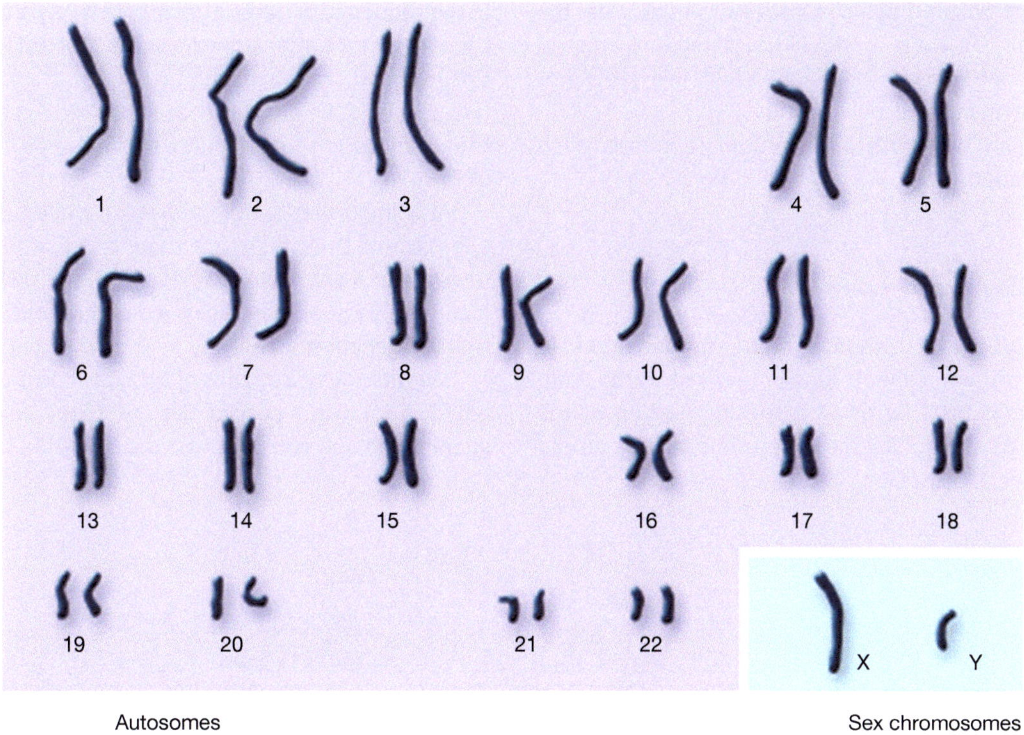

FIGURE 2.4 Male human chromosomes.
Source: Lister Hill National Center for Biomedical Communications (2010)/with permission of Lister Hill National Center for Biomedical Communications (2010).

from each parent. If the parents have different hair colours, such as red and brown, the child may inherit either trait. Factors determining which trait is expressed are discussed later in this chapter.

This principle applies to each of a person's characteristics, for example, eye colour or height. A person with a pair of identical alleles for a particular gene locus is said to be homozygous for that gene, whilst someone with a dissimilar pair is said to be heterozygous for that gene.

There are two other very important facts to mention about genes: some genes are 'recessive' and some genes are 'dominant'.

- A dominant gene is one that exerts its effect when it is present on only one of the chromosomes. (The name 'genotype' is given to the type of genes found in the body, whilst the name 'phenotype' is given to any gene that is manifested in the person.)
- A recessive gene (genotype), however, must be present on both inherited chromosomes in order to manifest itself (phenotype).

This is a very important concept to grasp because of the significance that it brings to bear on hereditary disorders.

From DNA to proteins

Returning to the biology of genetics, nucleic acids are components of DNA, and they have two major functions:

1. The direction of all protein synthesis (i.e., the production of protein).
2. The accurate transmission of this information from one generation to the next (from parents to their children) and, within the body, from one cell to its daughter cells.

Protein synthesis

Synthesis means 'production', for example, the production of protein from raw materials. All the genetic instructions for making proteins are found in DNA, but in order to synthesise these proteins, the genetic information encoded in the DNA must first be translated into RNA and then into a protein.

Initially, all of the genetic information in a region of DNA has to be copied in order to produce a specific molecule of RNA.

Then, through a complex series of procedures, the information contained in RNA is translated into a corresponding specific sequence of amino acids in a newly produced protein molecule.

There are two parts to this procedure: transcription and translation.

Transcription

In transcription, the DNA must be transcribed into RNA because protein cannot be synthesised (produced) directly from DNA. By using a specific portion of the cell's DNA as a template, the genetic information stored in the sequence of bases of that DNA is rewritten so that the same information appears in the bases of RNA. To do this, the two strands of the DNA first have to separate (Fig. 2.5), and the bases that are attached to each strand then pair up with bases that are attached to strands of RNA.

It is important to note here that, while there is only one form of DNA, there are three types of RNA: mRNA (messenger RNA), tRNA (transfer RNA) and rRNA (ribosomal RNA). Each of these plays a different role in the synthesis of genetic material.

As with the two strands of DNA, the bases of DNA can only join up with a specific base of mRNA. As with DNA, guanine can only join up with cytosine in RNA, but in RNA,

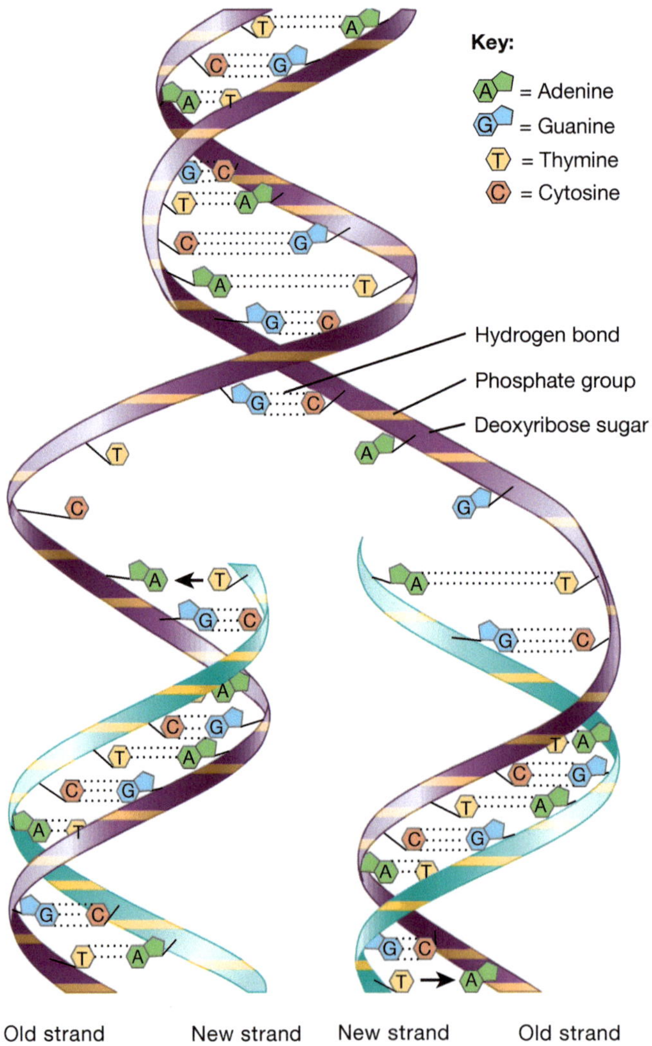

FIGURE 2.5 The separation of DNA and production of further DNA.
Source: Reproduced with permission of Peate & Gormley-Fleming (2015)/John Wiley & Sons.

the adenine in DNA can only join to uracil (U) in the RNA, because there is no thymine in RNA:

DNA		mRNA
guanine (G)	–	cytosine (C)
cytosine (C)	–	guanine (G)
thymine (T)	–	adenine (A)
adenine (A)	–	uracil (U)

For example,

- if DNA has a base sequence **AGGCAGTGC**
- then mRNA will have a complementary base sequence **UCCGUCACG**

Figure 2.5 shows how the DNA separates and makes more DNA. This same process occurs during transcription, except that the new strand with its bases is RNA rather than DNA.

Question 1

In the DNA sequence given herewith, what should the RNA bases be?

C A G C T G C A

(Answer at the end of this section)

Thus, DNA acts as a template for mRNA (Bywater, 2025). However, in addition to serving as the template for the synthesis of mRNA, DNA also synthesises two other kinds of RNA: rRNA and tRNA.

- rRNA = ribosomal RNA – rRNA, together with ribosomal proteins, makes up the ribosomes.
- tRNA = transfer RNA – this is responsible for matching the code of the mRNA with amino acids.

Once ready, mRNA, rRNA and tRNA leave the nucleus of the cell and in the cytoplasm of the cell commence the next step in protein synthesis, namely translation (Fig. 2.6).

Answer to Question 1

G U C G A C G U

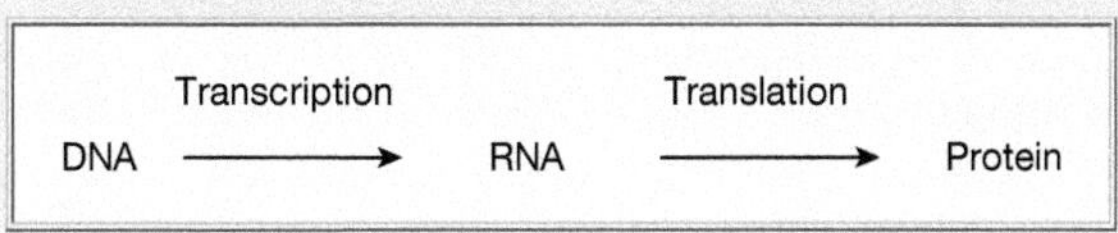

FIGURE 2.6 Brief summary of protein synthesis.
Source: Reproduced with permission of Peate & Gormley-Fleming (2015)/John Wiley & Sons.

Genetic mutations

During transcription, translation and protein synthesis, errors (mutations) can occur due to the speed and complexity of these processes. Such mutations may cause cell death or malfunctioning genes, affecting health and development depending on their location and impact on essential proteins (National Library of Medicine, 2025).

The DNA sequence of a gene can be changed in several different ways, of which a few are discussed in the following sections.

Missense mutation

This occurs when there is a change in one DNA base pair, which leads to the replacement of one amino acid with another in the protein for which that gene is an important component.

DNA bases	TAG	TTC	AGC	TAG
Amino acids	1	2	3	1

If, in the aforementioned gene sequence, one of the nucleotides is altered so that the sequence becomes:

DNA bases	TAG	TGC	AGC	TAG
Amino acids	1	4	3	1

Then that change in the sequence causes that triplet to code for a different amino acid, and hence, a different protein is formed. So, the gene does not make sense – hence 'missense'.

An example of a genetic disorder caused by a missense mutation is sickle cell anaemia.

Nonsense mutation

When a nonsense mutation occurs, there is also a change in one DNA pair. However, rather than substituting one DNA base pair for another, this type of mutation sends a signal for the sequence to be prematurely concluded. This leads to a shortened protein which may, or may not, function properly, or even may not function at all.

DNA bases	TAG	TTC	AGC	TAG
Amino acids	1	2	3	1

If, in the aforementioned gene sequence, one of the nucleotides is altered so that the sequence becomes:

DNA bases	TAG	TGC	AGC	TAT
Amino acids	1	2	3	end

Then the sequence for this gene is altered in such a way that the production of the protein is terminated prematurely. The subsequent resulting shortened protein may not function as it should or may not even function at all.

Cystic fibrosis is an example of a disease caused by a nonsense mutation.

Deletion

A deletion mutation happens when DNA bases are lost, ranging from a few base pairs to an entire gene or multiple genes. This can alter the function of the resulting protein(s).

22q11.2 deletion syndrome is one such disease caused by this mutation. It is caused by the deletion of just a small section of chromosome 22. There are many health problems with this deletion mutation, including cleft palate, heart defects and autoimmune disorders, to name just a few. The symptoms differ widely between children and may also be associated with learning difficulties and mental health conditions.

Other problems caused by genes are as follows:

- **Insertion:** This occurs where the number of DNA bases are increased by adding a piece of DNA to the sequence. Examples of diseases caused by this mutation include Fragile X syndrome and Huntington's disease.
- **Frameshift mutation:** This is a mutation that is caused by an insertion or deletion of a nucleotide, which causes a shift in the translational reading frame (the groups of three nucleotide bases that each code for one amino acid). This results in the moving of one nucleotide forward or back within one triplet so that the resultant triplets are out of synchronisation. This usually results in a non-functioning protein – hence the body is missing that protein. Tay–Sachs disease is caused by frameshift mutations, which can also contribute to some cancers.
- **Duplication:** Sometimes a mutation can occur when a piece of DNA is copied wrongly so that there is more than one copy of it. This can lead to altered functioning in the resulting protein. One such disease caused as a result of duplication is Charcot–Marie–Tooth disease type 1, which leads to disorders of the peripheral nervous system, causing progressive loss of muscle tissue and loss of touch sensation.

In healthcare, the clinical application of genetics involves a multidisciplinary team, including doctors, genetic scientists and nurses. A central aspect of this care, support and counselling falls primarily to nurses, especially those working with children and young people, as most genetic conditions present in infancy or childhood.

While genetic counsellors provide families with initial guidance, their contact is limited. Nurses, in contrast, have ongoing interactions with the child and family, often extending into the community if home care is required. Nurses, therefore, need not only knowledge of the child's condition but also an understanding of the underlying genetics to confidently support the family and child as they process the diagnosis and its long-term implications. Empathy and strong listening skills are essential, particularly when the condition is inherited, and parents may feel guilty. Nurses also reinforce discussions from genetic counsellors regarding future children.

Nurse responsibilities

- Acquire thorough knowledge of the child's condition, genetics, treatment options, prognosis and potential impact on the child, parents, siblings and extended family.
- Show consistent empathy while providing honest information. Children often cope well with full honesty, while parents may struggle but rely on accurate guidance.
- Explain clearly and repeatedly what has happened, what is happening and what may happen, using language appropriate for the child, family and siblings.
- Collaborate with genetic counsellors to support informed and independent family decisions about the current and future implications of the condition.
- Provide presence and support while managing other patients, offering families private time and space to process information.

- Be honest about potential consequences while emphasising positive aspects where possible – for example, explaining autosomal recessive inheritance patterns, such as cystic fibrosis, with realistic probability for future pregnancies.
- Prioritise empathetic listening as the child and family come to terms with the diagnosis.

Caring for families facing potentially fatal genetic disorders can be psychologically exhausting. Nurses must ensure they have their own support system to maintain resilience and well-being.

For more information on gene mutations, the National Human Genome Research Institute has a very good website (https://www.genome.gov/glossary).

The transference of genes

Introduction

Genetic information is passed both between cells and from parents to children. To support growth and replace dying cells without losing genetic information, cells must reproduce accurately. This occurs through two processes: mitosis and meiosis.

Mitosis

Cell reproduction takes place by mitosis, in which the number of chromosomes in the daughter cells has to be the same as in the original parent cell.

Mitosis can be divided into four stages:

- prophase
- metaphase
- anaphase
- telophase.

Before and after it has divided, the cell enters a stage known as interphase.

Interphase

Mitosis begins with interphase – during this period, the cell is actually very busy as it gets ready for replication (Fig. 2.7). During interphase, the cell is producing two of everything, not just DNA, but all the other organelles in the cell, such as the mitochondria. The cell obtains and digests nutrients so that it has the raw materials for this duplication and also for the energy that will power the various functions of the cell.

During interphase, the chromosomes in the nucleus of the cell are present in the form of long threads so that they can be duplicated. During the process of

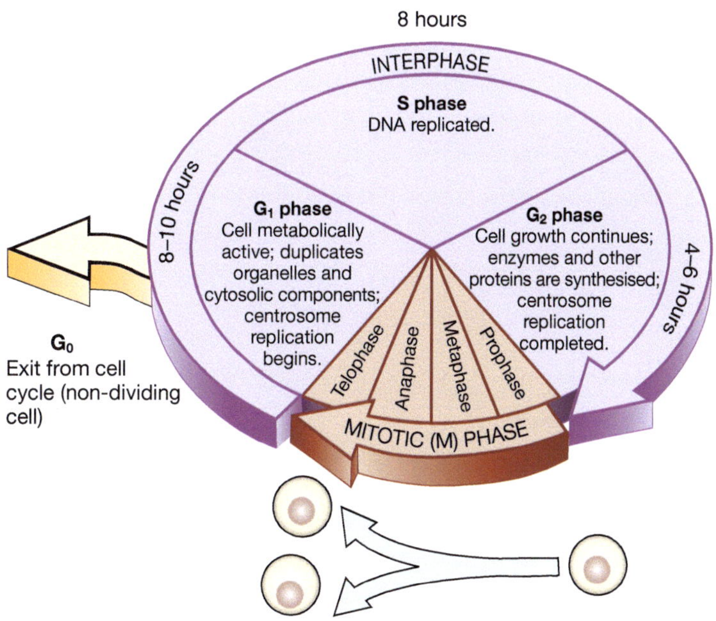

FIGURE 2.7 The cell cycle.
Source: Reproduced with permission of Peate & Gormley-Fleming (2015)/John Wiley & Sons.

duplication, the cells ensure that there will be sufficient genetic material for each of the two daughter cells. The strands of DNA separate and reattach to new strands of DNA. Because of the selectivity of the base-to-base necessary contact, an exact replication of the DNA will occur (Fig. 2.5).

In addition, extra cell organelles are manufactured by the replication of existing organelles, and the cell builds up a store of energy, which will be required for the process of division.

Prophase

The chromosomes become shorter, fatter and more easily visible. Each chromosome now consists of two chromatids, each containing the same genetic information. These two chromatids are joined together at the centromere. The two centrosomes move to opposite ends of the cell (the poles) and are joined together by the nuclear spindle, which stretches from pole to pole of the cell. Finally, the nucleolus and nuclear membrane disappear, leaving the chromosomes in the cytoplasm (Fig. 2.8).

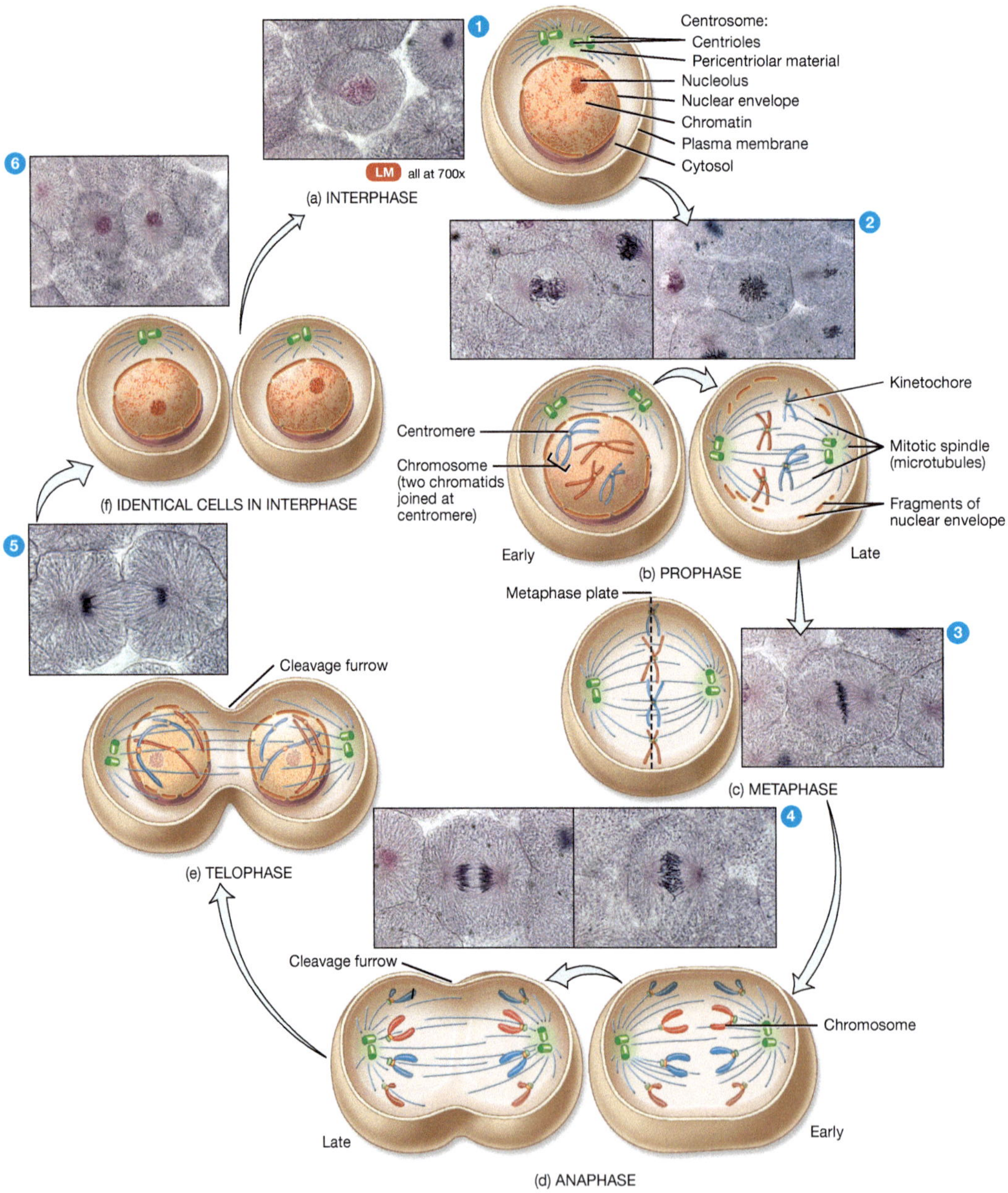

FIGURE 2.8 Mitosis.
Source: Reproduced with permission of Peate & Gormley-Fleming (2015)/John Wiley & Sons.

Metaphase

The 46 chromosomes (two of each of the 23 chromosomes), consisting of two chromatids, move to the centre of the nuclear spindle, and here they become attached to the spindle fibres (Fig. 2.8).

Anaphase

The chromatids in each chromosome are separated, and one chromatid from each chromosome then moves towards each pole (Fig. 2.8).

Telophase

There are now 46 chromatids at each pole, and these will form the chromosomes of the daughter cells. The cell divides to form two daughter cells. The nuclear spindle disappears, and a nuclear membrane forms around the chromosomes in each of the daughter cells. The chromosomes become long and threadlike again (Fig. 2.8).

Cell division

Cell division is now complete (Fig. 2.8), and the daughter cells themselves enter the interphase stage in order to prepare for their replication and division. This process of cell division explains how we grow by producing new cells as well as replacing old, damaged and dead cells.

Meiosis

Whilst mitosis is concerned with the reproduction of individual cells, meiosis is concerned with the development of whole organisms – for example, human beings.

The reproduction of humans depends upon the fusion of reproductive cells (known as gametes) from each of the parents. These gametes are:

- spermatozoa (sperm) from the male
- ova (eggs) from the female.

Each cell of the human body contains 23 pairs of chromosomes (i.e., 46 in total). It is very important that during the process of human reproduction, the cell formed when the gametes fuse has the correct number of chromosomes for a human being (23 pairs). Therefore, each gamete must possess only 23 single chromosomes because when gametes fuse during reproduction, all their chromosomes remain intact in the new life form. If each gamete had a full complement of 46 chromosomes, the resulting fused cell would possess 92 chromosomes – or four copies of each chromosome. To prevent this, the gametes only possess one copy of each chromosome so that the resulting cell would have 46 chromosomes.

- A diploid cell is a cell with a full complement of 46 chromosomes (23 pairs).
- A haploid cell is a cell with only half that number of chromosomes (23 single chromosomes).

Gametes are therefore haploid cells, because they only possess one copy of each chromosome, whilst all other cells of the body are diploid cells.

Gametes develop from cells with 46 chromosomes, and it is through the process of meiosis that they end up with just 23 chromosomes. During meiosis, the cells divide twice, without the replication of DNA occurring again before the second division.

Meiosis can be divided into eight stages (not four as in mitosis) and consists of two meiotic divisions, each with four stages. However, they have the same names, but are given either the number I or II. As with mitosis, these stages are continuous with one another.

First meiotic stage

- Prophase I
- Metaphase I
- Anaphase I
- Telophase I

Second meiotic stage

- Prophase II
- Metaphase II
- Anaphase II
- Telophase II

First meiotic division

Prophase I

Prophase I is similar to the stage of prophase in mitosis. However, instead of being scattered randomly, the chromosomes (consisting of two chromatids) are arranged in pairs – 23 in all. For example, the two chromosome 1s will pair up, as will the two chromosome 2s, and so on. Within each pair of chromosomes, genetic material may be exchanged between the two chromosomes, and it is these exchanges that are partly responsible for the differences between children of the same parents. This process is called 'gene crossover' (Fig. 2.9). Remember that the DNA is not replicated during the first meiotic division.

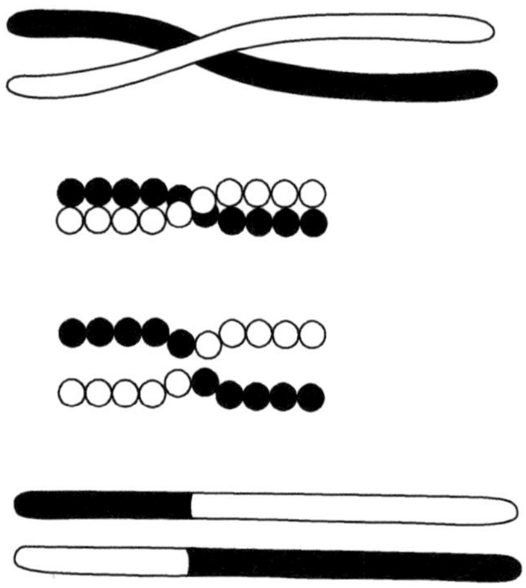

FIGURE 2.9 Gene crossover.
Source: Peate & Gormley-Fleming (2015)/with permission of John Wiley & Sons.

Metaphase I
The chromosomes become arranged on the spindles at the equator. However, they remain in pairs.

Anaphase I
One chromosome from each pair moves to each pole so that there are now 23 chromosomes at each end of the spindle.

Telophase I
The cell membrane now divides the cell into two halves. Each daughter cell now has half the number of chromosomes that each parent cell had.

Second meiotic division

During the second meiotic division, both of the cells produced by the first meiotic division now divide again.

Prophase II, metaphase II, anaphase II and telophase II are all similar to their equivalent stages in mitosis, with the exception that the chromosomes are not replicated before prophase II. So, there are only 23 single chromosomes in each of the 'granddaughter' cells. That way, when the gametes fuse during reproduction, there are still only 23 pairs of chromosomes per human cell.

Of the 23 pairs of chromosomes, 22 pairs are autosomal, and one pair consists of the sex chromosomes. Autosomal means 'self-body'. So, autosomal chromosomes are concerned with the body. On the other hand, the sex chromosomes determine the gender of a person. Male sex chromosomes are designated by the letter Y, and female chromosomes are designated by the letter X. A male will carry the chromosomes XY (an X chromosome from the mother and a Y chromosome from the father), whilst a female will carry the chromosomes XX (an X chromosome from both the father and the mother).

Mendelian genetics: the role of genetics in inheritance

There are two definitions:

1. **Genotype** = the actual genetic make-up of a person (full heredity information).
2. **Phenotype** = the actual observed characteristics, such as physical properties and development/behaviour (although environment also plays a large part in these). Mendel demonstrated that members of a pair of alleles separate clearly during meiosis. We all have a pair of genes (alleles) at each locus, but because of the process of meiosis, we can only pass one of those pairs of genes to our child.

This is further clarified in Fig. 2.10.

At the same locus on a chromosome, the father has the two alleles Aa, and the mother has the two alleles Bb. When they reproduce, the father can pass on either gene A or gene a (both are at the same locus and are therefore alleles), and the mother can pass on either gene B or gene b. However, each child can only inherit one of gene A or gene a from the father and one of gene B or gene b from the mother. Note that dominant genes are usually given capital letters, whilst recessive genes are usually given lower-case letters.

What the child cannot do is inherit both gene A and gene a or gene B and gene b. Only one allele from each parent can be inherited by a child. This is known as Mendel's first law.

What are the statistical chances of a child inheriting any one of those sets of genes from the parents AB, Ab, aB or ab? The answer is 1 in 4 (or 1 : 4). So, there is a 25%

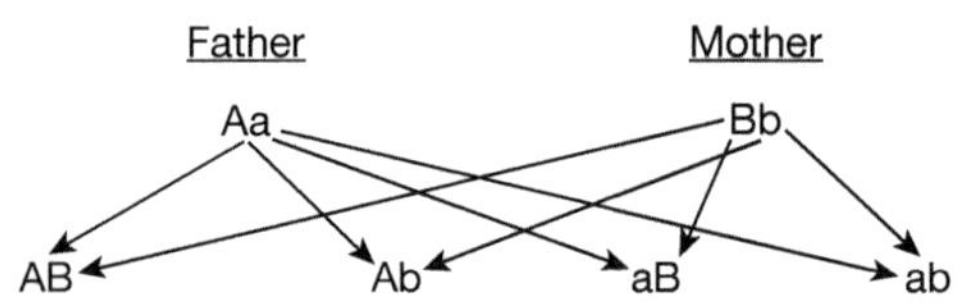

FIGURE 2.10 Genetic inheritance.
Source: Peate & Gormley-Fleming (2015)/with permission of John Wiley & Sons.

chance that any child will inherit one of those pairs of genes from its parents.

Mendel's second law states that different allele pairs segregate independently during gametogenesis. So, each allele can combine randomly with alleles from other pairs. Gametogenesis produces haploid sex cells carrying half of the parents' genetic material. This leads to the concept of dominant and recessive genes, which influence traits like eye and hair colour and play a role in many health conditions.

Dominant genes and recessive genes

Remember that at each locus, the two alleles can be either dominant or recessive.

Look again at Fig. 2.10. Suppose two parents had four children, and they all had different genotypes so that they each were represented by one of the pairs of genes. How many of the offspring would carry at least one dominant gene, and how many would carry only recessive genes at this locus?

The answer is that three out of the four children (75%) would carry at least one dominant gene, and one out of the four children (25%) would carry both recessive genes. Of course, in real life, all four children may inherit the same pair of genes at this locus, or maybe two will inherit the same genes. This means that there is a 1 in 4 chance at each pregnancy that the children will carry a certain genotype.

Example

A man with red hair married a woman with brown hair. As time goes by, they have several children, all of whom have brown hair. Which is the dominant gene for hair colour, and who carries it?

The gene for brown hair carried by the mother was the dominant gene in this instance.

Autosomal dominant inheritance and ill health

If the dominant gene of one of the parents is the one that causes a medical disorder, for example, Huntington's disease or neurofibromatosis, what will be the risk of any child of those parents having the disease?

The answer is 50% or a 1 in 2 risk of a child having an autosomal dominant disorder.

Why is this? Look back at Fig. 2.10, and assume that the father (genes **A** and **a**) carries the mutant gene on gene **A**. As a dominant gene is always expressed in the phenotype, then statistically there will be a 50% chance of any child having the disease, because the child could inherit gene **a**. Of course, any child who carries gene **A** will have a 100% chance of having the disease; there is no avoiding it.

Autosomal recessive inheritance and ill health

Autosomal recessive diseases occur when both parents are carrying the same defect on a recessive gene at the same locus. Both parents have to carry the defective gene; otherwise, the child cannot be affected by the disease.

In autosomal recessive diseases, a person with only one defective gene is a carrier and can pass it to their children. If two carriers have children, there is a risk that the child may inherit the disorder or become a carrier, a pattern that can persist across generations.

So, then, what are the risks of:

- a child being a carrier of the recessive gene?
- a child having the disease caused by this mutated/abnormal gene?

To work it out, look again at Fig. 2.10. In this case, the small-case letter '**a**' represents the abnormal recessive gene. In this scenario, both parents carry this abnormal gene, for example, for cystic fibrosis – this is a well-known disease that is inherited as an autosomal recessive disorder.

If one of the two recessive genes (a) that code for cystic fibrosis is carried by each of the parents, then the chances at each pregnancy of:

- having an affected child are 1 in 4 (or 25%)
- having a child who is a carrier are 2 in 4 (or 50%)
- having a child who is neither affected nor a carrier is 1 in 4 (or 25%).

Why is this so? Look at Fig. 2.10 again.

- Only one child possesses two affected genes (aa), and because both affected genes have to be present in order for the disease to appear, this is one child out of four, or 25%.

- Only one child does not possess an affected gene (a), and so the disease cannot occur, nor can the child be a carrier, because there is no affected gene to be carried. So, this is one child out of four, or 25%.
- Two children possess an affected gene, but they also contain an unaffected dominant gene. So, they are both carriers.

Whenever there is a dominant gene, then the affected recessive gene cannot be expressed in the phenotype – the dominant gene blocks the action of the affected recessive gene. So, two out of four children (or 50%) could be carriers. However, always remember that children who are carriers can pass the affected gene onto their children.

It is important to remember – and stress – that these odds occur for each pregnancy. So, you could have four children and have:

- 1 affected
- 2 carriers and 1 unaffected
- 4 carriers
- 3 affected and 1 carrier
- and so on.

Remember that the odds are the same for each child born to those parents!

Morbidity and mortality of dominant versus recessive disorders

Autosomal dominant disorders are usually less severe than recessive ones because carriers express the disorder. If dominant disorders were as severe as many recessive disorders, affected individuals would often die before reproducing, preventing the gene from being passed on.

An exception is Huntington's disease, which is a fatal autosomal dominant disorder, but it survives because the symptoms do not usually become apparent until the affected person is in their 30s, by which time they could have passed on the affected gene to their children.

X-linked recessive disorders

As well as autosomal inheritance, we can also inherit disorders via the sex chromosomes.

The main role of these chromosomes is to determine the gender of the baby.

- **XX = girl**
- **XY = boy**

First, look at the possibilities of having a boy or a girl when you decide to have a baby.

From Fig. 2.11, it can be seen that the chances for each pregnancy of a boy or a girl are 50%.

Some disorders are only passed on via the X chromosome. Examples are haemophilia and Duchenne muscular dystrophy. With these disorders, only the boys can be affected, and only girls may be carriers but unaffected.

If we assume that the small-case '**x**' is the affected gene for haemophilia, then what is going to happen with our family in Figure 2.11?

- The first child is a girl who does not carry the affected gene but rather two normal genes. So, she is neither a carrier nor affected.
- The second child carries a normal X and a Y. So, he is a boy who does not carry the abnormal gene – consequently, he is neither a carrier nor affected.

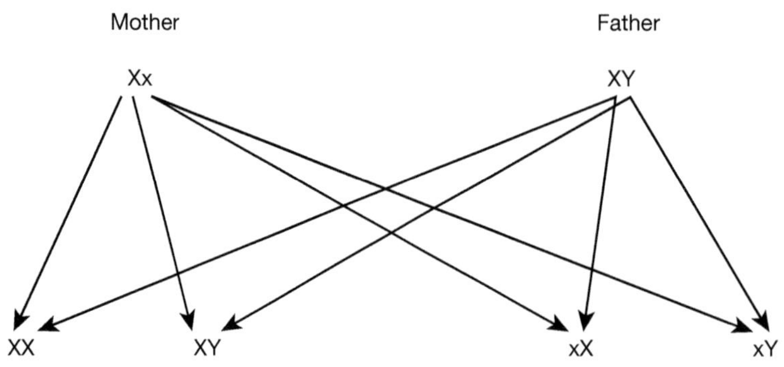

FIGURE 2.11 X-linked inheritance.

Source: Peate & Gormley-Fleming (2015)/with permission of John Wiley & Sons.

- The third child is a girl who carries the abnormal gene, but the action of that gene is blocked by the other normal X gene. So, she is not affected but is a carrier.
- The fourth child is a boy who carries an abnormal X gene and a normal Y gene. Unfortunately, the Y gene is unable to block the action of the abnormal gene. So, he is a carrier and is also affected.

Consequently, we can say that there is a chance that:

- 1 out of 2 girls (50%) will be a carrier.
- 1 out of 2 boys (50%) will be affected.

But remember that in real life, all or no girls could be carriers, and if no girl in a family is a carrier, then the abnormal gene cannot be inherited by future generations – the disease will 'die out' in that family.

Case study: sunburn

William, a 13-year-old fair-skinned boy, presented to the children's emergency admission unit with his mother, reporting severe pain affecting his face, arms, torso and legs, along with headache and nausea. His skin was extremely tender, preventing any contact or clothing.

Earlier that afternoon, William had been playing outdoors in a paddling pool wearing only swimming trunks. Although sunscreen had been applied after lunch, it was washed off during water play. He subsequently fell asleep on unshaded grass and, on waking, was acutely unwell, prompting urgent hospital attendance.

On initial assessment, the nurse measured William's vital signs and provided reassurance. Observations revealed a raised temperature and pulse, with low blood pressure (see PEWS, Fig. 2.12). These findings raised concern for potential heat-related illness in addition to sunburn. The nurse promptly escalated to the on-duty doctor.

The doctor confirmed the diagnosis of severe sunburn and initiated management with intravenous fluids and analgesia. Given the severity of his symptoms and systemic involvement, William was admitted to the ward for ongoing observation and supportive care, rather than being discharged home.

- Children with fair skin are at high risk of severe sunburn and heat-related illness.
- Exposure to sunlight without adequate protection, particularly during water play, can rapidly lead to significant injury.
- Vital signs provide crucial early warning: tachycardia, hyperthermia and hypotension may indicate systemic involvement.
- Prompt recognition, escalation and initiation of supportive care are essential to prevent complications.

When a young child is admitted to the hospital as an emergency, families often have little time to prepare. Nurses must consider the immediate and potential impact on the whole family, such as care for siblings if a parent stays with the hospitalised child. If a parent must leave, the nurse should reassure them that the child is well cared for and provide prompt updates on any changes in the child's condition.

Spontaneous mutation

Another way abnormal genes can arise and cause genetic disorders is through spontaneous mutation. During the rapid and precise processes of DNA replication in germ cells and protein synthesis, mistakes can occur, leading to mutations. Additionally, chemical- or trauma-induced mutations can also affect genes, potentially causing disorders such as cancer.

Conclusion

Understanding genetics is fundamental for nurses working with children and young people, as genetic factors shape identity, health risks, responses to treatment, and daily living. So, nurses must communicate complex genetic information clearly to both affected children and their families, who may struggle with guilt or distress.

Recent advances in gene therapy offer new treatment possibilities, particularly for primary immunodeficiency diseases. The first successful gene replacement for adenosine deaminase (ADA) deficiency in the early 2000s marked a milestone, and similar treatments continue to evolve. Scientists are now synthesising entire human genomes to develop targeted therapies and potential cures, highlighting the need for healthcare professionals to understand these breakthroughs for patient care, education and research involvement.

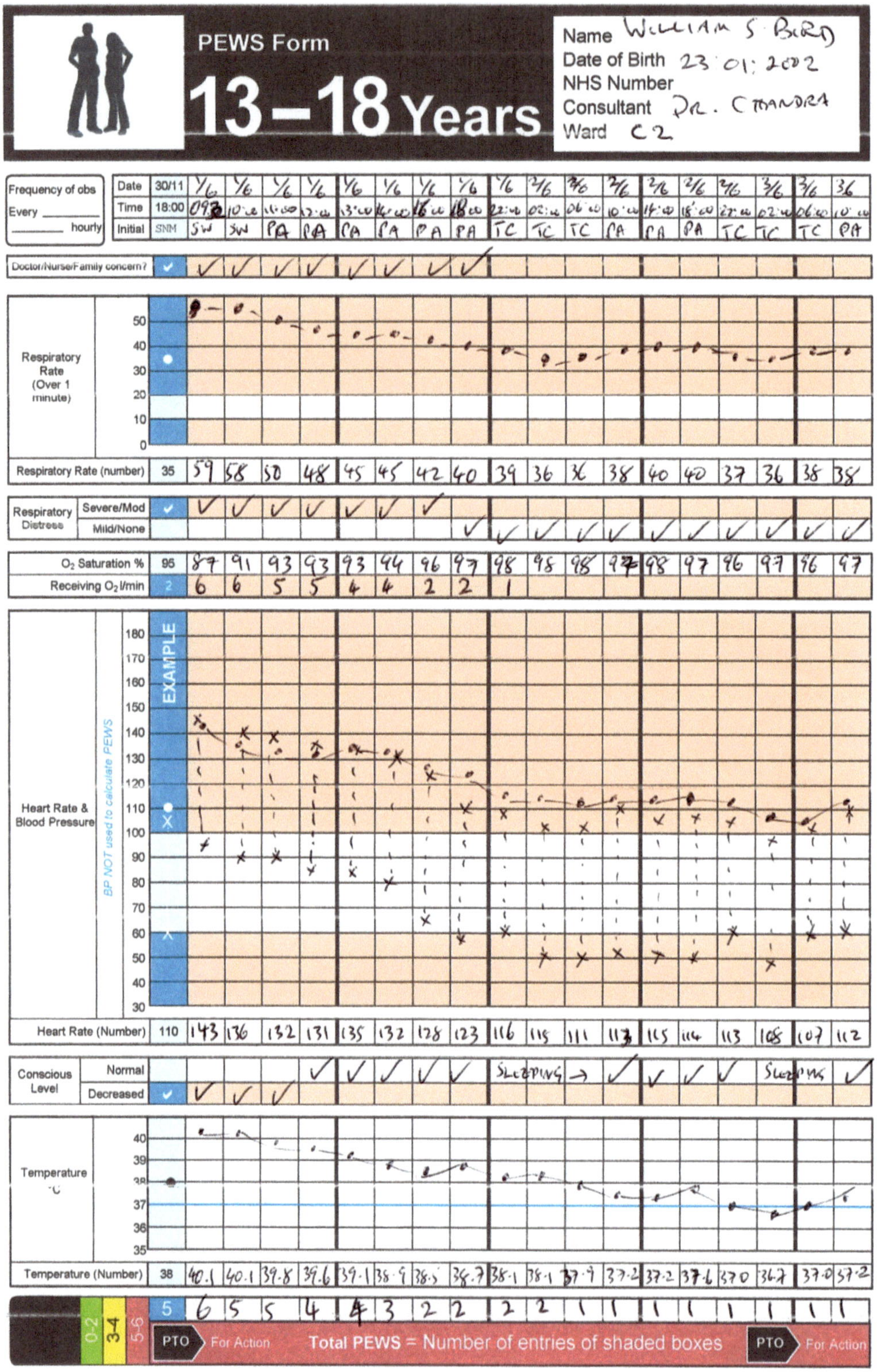

PEWS Form

13–18 Years

Name William S. Bird
Date of Birth 23:01:2002
NHS Number
Consultant Dr. Chandra
Ward C2

Frequency of obs Every ______ hourly

Date	30/11	1/6	1/6	1/6	1/6	1/6	1/6	1/6	1/6	1/6	2/6	2/6	2/6	2/6	2/6	2/6	3/6	3/6	3/6
Time	18:00	09:00	10:00	11:00	12:00	13:00	14:00	16:00	18:00	22:00	02:00	06:00	10:00	14:00	18:00	22:00	02:00	06:00	10:00
Initial	SNM	SW	SW	PA	PA	PA	PA	PA	PA	TC	TC	TC	PA	PA	PA	TC	TC	TC	PA
Doctor/Nurse/Family concern?	✓	✓	✓	✓	✓	✓	✓	✓	✓										
A Respiratory Rate (number)	35	59	58	50	48	45	45	42	40	39	36	36	38	40	40	37	36	38	38
B Respiratory Distress Severe/Mod	✓	✓	✓	✓	✓	✓	✓	✓											
Respiratory Distress Mild/None									✓	✓	✓	✓	✓	✓	✓	✓	✓	✓	✓
O_2 Saturation %	95	87	91	93	93	93	94	96	97	98	98	98	97	98	97	96	97	96	97
Receiving O_2 l/min	2	6	6	5	5	4	4	2	2	1									
C Heart Rate (Number)	110	143	136	132	131	135	132	128	123	116	115	111	113	115	114	113	108	107	112
Conscious Level Normal					✓	✓	✓	✓	✓	Sleeping	→	✓	✓	✓	✓	Sleeping		✓	
Conscious Level Decreased	✓	✓	✓	✓															
Temperature (Number)	38	40.1	40.1	39.8	39.6	39.1	38.9	38.5	38.7	38.1	38.1	37.9	37.2	37.2	37.6	37.0	36.7	37.0	37.2
Total PEWS	5	6	5	5	4	4	3	2	2	2	2	1	1	1	1	1	1	1	1

BP NOT used to calculate PEWS

EXAMPLE

0-2 3-4 5-6

PTO For Action Total PEWS = Number of entries of shaded boxes PTO For Action

FIGURE 2.12 PEWS chart for William.

Equally important are the ethical, legal and social considerations, including consent, unintended consequences and equitable access. Nurses must navigate these sensitively, supporting families while engaging in informed discussions about emerging therapies. A strong foundation in genetics enables nurses to provide safe, evidence-based care, explain procedures, offer emotional support, collaborate in multidisciplinary teams and advocate effectively for children undergoing gene therapy.

References

Bywater, R. (2025). Genetics. In: Peate, I. & Gormley-Fleming, E. (eds). *Fundamentals of Children and Young People's Anatomy and Physiology for Nursing and Healthcare Students*, 3rd edn. Oxford: Wiley, pp. 79–102.

Jorde, L.B., Carey, J.C., & Bamshad, M.J. (2019). *Medical Genetics*, 6th edn. Elsevier Health Sciences, Cambridge, MA.

Lister Hill National Center for Biomedical Communications (2010). John Wiley & Sons. Available at: http://ghr.nlm.nih.gov/handbook/basics/howmanychromosomes (accessed 16 September 2025).

National Library of Medicine (2025). Genetics. [online] Available at: https://ghr.nlm.nih.gov/ (accessed 16 September 2025).

NHS England (2023). 75 years of genetics and genomics in the NHS [online] Available at: www.genomicseducation.hee.nhs.uk/wp-content/uploads/2023/07/NHS75-Genomics-timeline.pdf (accessed 16 September 2025).

Patch, S., & Skirton, H. (2009). *Genetics for the Health Sciences*, 2nd edn. Scion Publishing, Banbury.

Peate, I. and Gormley-Fleming, E. (2015). *Fundamentals of Children's Anatomy and Physiology: A Textbook for Nursing and Healthcare Students*. John Wiley & Sons, Ltd, Oxford.

CHAPTER 3

Cancer

Simon Dean and Elizabeth Gormley-Fleming

AIM

The aim of this chapter is to introduce the reader to principles associated with cancer in children and young people.

LEARNING OUTCOMES

On completion of this chapter, the reader will be able to:

- Define cancer.
- Identify the most common childhood cancers and list different treatment approaches and potential side effects.
- Describe the common presenting symptoms of childhood cancer and what causes them.
- Discuss the psychological impact of childhood cancer on the child and family.

KEYWORDS

- cancer
- malignant
- tumour
- haematology
- oncology
- chemotherapy
- radiotherapy
- trials

Test your prior knowledge

1. Name three different treatment approaches for childhood cancer.
2. Name the most common form of childhood cancer.
3. What percentage of children with cancer are now cured? (a) more than 60%, (b) more than 70% or (c) more than 80%.
4. What is the difference between a malignant tumour and a benign tumour?
5. What are the differences between chemotherapy and radiotherapy?

Introduction

Approximately 1900 children are diagnosed with cancer per annum in the United Kingdom, with around 10 children and young people (CYP) diagnosed every day in the United Kingdom (Children with Cancer UK, 2021). The survival rate in childhood cancers has improved significantly in recent years, yet the diagnosis remains devastating for the child, their family/carers and communities.

The 5-year survival rate was 86% in 2020, and the 10-year survival rate was 82.5% (NHS Digital, 2023). Research

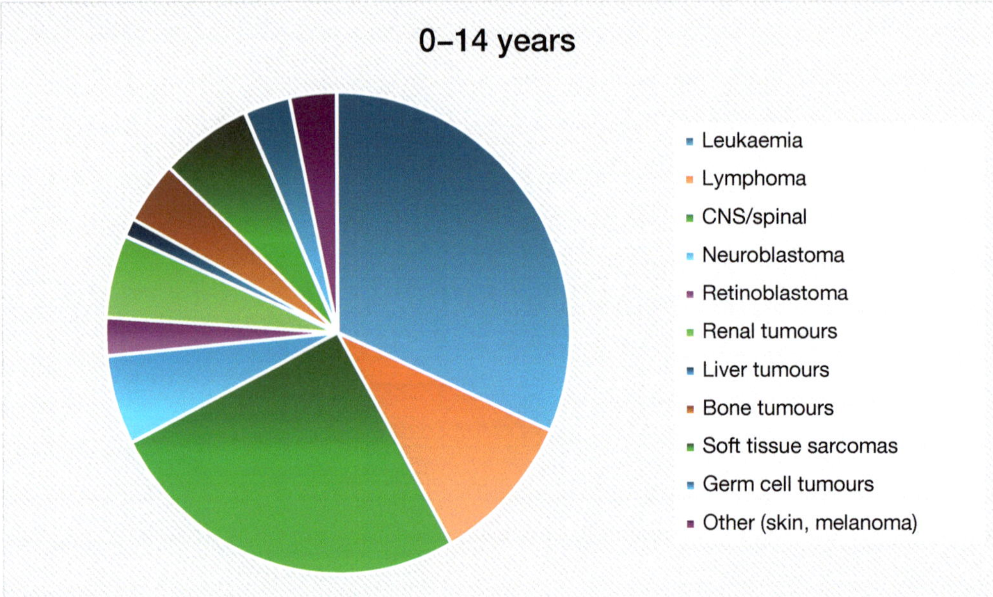

FIGURE 3.1 Incidence rates for childhood cancer.
Source: Adapted from Children with Cancer UK (2021).

through clinical trials continues to allow oncologists (solid tumours) and haematologists (blood cancers including leukaemia) to offer improved treatments that are improving cure rates and resulting in reduced side effects for the patients. Early detection and enhancements in services and treatments contribute to the survival rates.

Cancer remains the leading cause of death in CYP, with on average 240 deaths per year (Royal College of Paediatrics and Child Health [RCPCH], 2025). While it may be cured, a cure is not guaranteed. It is important that this is understood by all parties.

Despite being relatively rare, brain tumours are the most common cause of death in CYP after infancy (Clarke and Jacques, 2025).

Acute lymphoblastic leukaemia (ALL) is the most common form of childhood cancer, with approximately 400 new cases every year (CRUK, 2018; Children with Cancer UK, 2021; NHS, 2021). This is followed by tumours of the central nervous system (CNS) and lymphomas. Fig. 3.1 shows the incidence rates for childhood cancer.

Cancer at a cellular level

Cancer is caused by genetic changes that disrupt a cell's ability to control its growth. Normally, cells reproduce through mitosis, where DNA condenses into 23 pairs of chromosomes and replicates, and the cell divides into two daughter cells, each with identical chromosomes. This process is tightly regulated by master genes that signal cells to divide or stop. These genes are described later.

Cancer genes

There are three known major classes of cancer genes that control cell growth and that can lead to cancer development (American Cancer Society):

1. **Oncogenes:** Mutated genes that act dominantly, speeding up cell division and leading to cancer.
2. **Tumour suppressor genes:** Prevent the division of cancer cells and, therefore, cause cell death (or apoptosis). The most important tumour suppressor gene in human cells is *p53*, which is present in about 60% of cancer cases (Achatz *et al.*, 2025).
3. **Deoxyribonucleic acid (DNA) processing genes:** Normally regulate DNA replication in healthy cells and prevent uncontrolled growth. When these genes are mutated, they lose this control, allowing abnormal cells to multiply and potentially develop into blood cancers or solid tumours.

Current research has allowed scientists to have a much greater understanding of genes in cancer, with 50% of paediatric tumours having a specific genetic change that new targeted treatments can be used to treat more effectively (Achatz *et al.*, 2025). The more common gene mutations are listed as follows:

1. RAS – The most frequently mutated oncogene in cancer, particularly CNS tumours, bone and soft tissue sarcomas, neuroblastoma and leukaemia.
2. Amplification (or increasing the number of copies of) genes, e.g., MYCN – most commonly associated with neuroblastoma, with its presence linked with a poorer prognosis, changing the classification to 'high risk' in these patients. It is also less commonly present in other solid tumours such as rhabdomyosarcoma, Wilms tumour and retinoblastoma and also CNS tumours, including medulloblastoma.
3. Fusion genes such as BCR-ABL, RUNX1 or MLL cause cellular genetic changes in ALL, which reduce survival outcomes.

Genetic cancer predisposition

Some children are born with familial cancer syndromes that cause genetic changes called germline mutations that increase the probability of developing cancer. The most common of these is Li-Fraumeni syndrome, which affects the TP53 gene and increases the possibility of developing cancer by up to 50% (Achatz *et al.*, 2025). The affected relatives develop a diverse set of malignancies, including leukaemia, breast carcinomas, sarcomas (bone tumours) and brain tumours at unusually early ages (usually by 30 years of age).

Other known genetic predispositions include children with Down syndrome, who are known to have a higher risk of developing leukaemia (Siegel *et al.*, 2013). Furthermore, children who have hereditary retinoblastoma (RB) (a rare tumour of the eye) have an increased risk of developing a bone tumour called osteosarcoma. This is a classic example of a cancer resulting from an inherited genetic abnormality (Roganovic, 2024). Table 3.1 lists examples of congenital factors associated with childhood cancer.

TABLE 3.1 Examples of congenital factors associated with childhood cancer

Factor	Associated childhood cancer
Down syndrome (trisomy 21)	Acute myeloid leukaemia
Beckwith–Wiedemann (overgrowth) syndrome	Wilms tumour
Denys-Drash syndrome	Wilms tumour
Fanconi anaemia	AML, hepatoblastoma
Li-Fraumeni syndrome	Soft tissue carcinoma, adrenocortical carcinoma, osteosarcoma
Familial retinoblastoma	Retinoblastoma and osteosarcoma
Neurofibromatosis type 1 (NF1)	Astrocytoma, ALL and rhabdomyosarcoma

Other possible causes of cancer

Environmental factors

A link between pollution and pesticides with childhood cancer, specifically leukaemia, CNS tumours and Wilms tumour, has been suggested (Navarrete-Meneses *et al.*, 2024). However, further research does not fully support this, with limited evidence of these being firmly established as risk factors for childhood cancer (Roganovic, 2024). Air pollutants such as benzene fuels and proximity to areas of high traffic have shown an increase in ALL but not in all countries (Buser *et al.*, 2022). Contemporary research suggests that attention must be paid to climate change and the impact on childhood cancers going forward (Leffers, 2022).

Ionising radiation

Exposure to radiation delivered by previous radiotherapy treatment, X-rays and other scans, including CT scans and MRIs, has been a cause of concern and a possible link to leukaemia (Vora, 2016). Leaver *et al.* (2019) found only a very negligible risk of developing cancers from a cohort of children who required repeated radiological investigations for limb deformities. However, CYP who underwent cardiac catheterisation and had heart transplants were found to have a higher incidence of developing cancer (Harbon *et al.*, 2018). Apart from radiological investigations that utilise ionising radiation (IR), proximity to nuclear power plants must be considered in compiling the evidence base of the causal link between IR and incidences of childhood cancers. Until sound conclusions are known, protection and minimisation of IR will continue as best practice.

Viruses

There is an association with Epstein–Barr virus (EBV) and both Hodgkin and Burkitt lymphomas (Paola & Preciado, 2013). Congenital cytomegalovirus in newborns has a direct link to incidents of ALL (Francis *et al.*, 2017). The human papillomavirus is known to lead to carcinogenesis.

Summary table of the different types of cancer

Anatomical region of the body	Types of tumours that affect them
Adrenal gland	Neuroblastoma
Blood/bone marrow	Acute lymphoblastic leukaemia (ALL) Acute myeloid leukaemia Hodgkin lymphoma Non-Hodgkin lymphoma Anaplastic large cell lymphoma (ALCL)
Bone	Osteosarcoma Ewing sarcoma (also develops in soft tissue)
Brain and spinal cord	Ependymoma Medulloblastoma High-grade glioma Low-grade glioma Craniopharyngioma
Eye	Retinoblastoma
Kidneys	Wilms Clear cell sarcoma
Liver	Hepatoblastoma Hepatocellular carcinoma (HCC)

The difference between a 'solid tumour' and blood cancer?

Solid tumours form when cancerous cells cluster into a mass, which can be benign (non-growing and harmless) or malignant (growing and potentially harmful). Depending on their size and location, they may sometimes be felt during a physical examination.

Blood cancers, such as acute leukaemia, arise in the bone marrow (BM), which normally produces red blood cells, platelets and white blood cells. In leukaemia, a genetically altered white blood cell – called a blast, as in ALL – reproduces uncontrollably. Over time, the BM stops producing normal blood cells and fills with cancerous blasts, and these abnormal cells spill into the bloodstream, impairing normal blood function.

Signs and symptoms of cancer

There are no early warning signs or screening tests for cancer in children. Presenting symptoms vary widely depending on the type and site of the cancer, i.e., abdomen, bone, brain, kidney and blood. Commonly seen symptoms in blood cancers, including leukaemia and lymphoma, include:

- Tiredness, breathlessness and pale skin (due to anaemia as a consequence of the reduction in red blood cell production)
- Tiny red spots on the skin (petechiae) – due to the reduction in the production of platelets in the BM
- Abnormal bleeding of the gums and epistaxis – also due to the reduction in platelets
- Bone pain and muscle aches
- Abdominal pain due to an enlarged spleen and/or liver
- Swollen lymph glands in the groin, neck and under the arms
- Weight loss
- Night sweats (in CYP with Hodgkin lymphoma).

Solid tumours may present as a growing mass, pain or lethargy. Brain and spinal tumours can cause headaches, early-morning vomiting, vision changes or altered eye appearance. These general symptoms are often mistaken for more common childhood illnesses.

> A cancer diagnosis can have a major psychological impact on both the child and their family, who need support and opportunities to express their feelings. While psychologists and psychiatrists play a role, the support provided by nursing staff on the wards is equally vital.

Staging of cancers

The stage of a cancer is often used to describe its size and whether it is found in only one part of the body (localised disease) or has spread beyond its original site (metastatic disease). The higher the stage, the lower the prognosis (or likelihood of treating the cancer). Number staging is the most common method used, but the TNM system: Tumour, Nodes and Metastases may also be utilised (CRUK, 2023a).

Although cancer 'staging' is not applied in blood cancers, including acute leukaemia, the symptoms at diagnosis, genetic changes that are tested at diagnosis and early response to treatment are powerful predictors of cure. Combinations of these are used for risk stratification purposes to determine the intensity of treatment a particular patient should receive. Table 3.2 lists the current UK risk stratification approach as per the new Alltogether1 trial.

Patients who are slow to clear blast cells after initial treatment have a higher risk of relapse. Minimal residual disease (MRD) monitoring is a sensitive test that can detect relapse risk early in treatment.

Staging is performed after a cancer diagnosis to help indicate prognosis. It is determined using blood tests, imaging and biopsy. Knowing the cancer's type and stage guides decisions about the most appropriate treatment. The current standard classification scheme is the *International Classification of Diseases for Oncology*, third edition (ICD-O-3) (WHO, 2013).

Solid tumours are generally grouped as:

- Stage 1: Localised disease – often treated with surgery only, but not always the case.
- Stage 2/3: Spread into nearby tissues or lymph nodes.
- Stage 4: Distant metastases (or spread to other organs in the body) – often considered 'high risk' and requires more treatment to achieve remission (WHO, 2013).

Grading of a cancer describes how abnormal the cancers are compared to normal cells. It is this information that helps us understand how quickly the cancer will spread to other areas of the body.

TABLE 3.2 UK risk stratification for the treatment of ALL

Risk	Definition
Standard risk	Aged 1–9 White cell count (WCC) < 50×10^9/L
High risk	>10 years of age WCC > 50×10^9/L T-cell disease Any patient with high-risk genetic changes

Source: Adapted from Moppett (2020).

Brain tumours

Brain and spinal (or CNS) tumours in CYP are different from adult brain tumours as they are genetically different. As the brain is developing and growing quickly in the younger child, more aggressive treatment is required to prevent permanent damage (Clarke and Jacques, 2025). CNS tumours in CYP are now classified as low-grade (WHO grade 1 or 2) or high-grade (WHO grade 3 or 4) (Damodharan and Puccetti, 2023).

The most common CNS tumours in childhood are:

- Astrocytoma's
- Medulloblastoma
- Ependymoma.

These tumours make up about 75% of all CNS tumours in CYP, with half of these being diagnosed as astrocytoma (Stiller *et al.*, 2019). If a CNS tumour is found to have spread to different parts of the brain or spine or to the rest of the body, this is called metastatic disease. This is often referred to as the grade of the tumour and is described as follows:

Grade 1: Tumour is found in one part of the brain (sometimes called the 'primary site'), is slow-growing and less likely to spread

Grade 2: Similar to grade 1, but can spread into nearly all parts of the brain. Usually slow-growing. Sometimes called 'diffuse brain tumours'.

Grade 3: Tumour can be found in the brain and the spine. Cells are more aggressive (or malignant). Sometimes called 'anaplastic tumours'.

Grade 4: Very aggressive tumours that can be found in the brain or spine and in the rest of the body (CRUK, 2023a).

Treatment of cancer

Treatments of childhood cancer present unique challenges compared to adults, including the harsh side effects of chemotherapy and radiation, the higher likelihood of delayed diagnosis and the use of targeted therapies is working towards this (Agarwal, 2023). They are delivered with the following aims:

- Cure of the disease
- Management of symptoms in patients where cure is not achievable (palliative care).

Both of these are administered with the aim of minimising toxicity and preserving the patient's quality of life (Lee *et al.*, 2023).

The treatments themselves are often referred to as systematic anti-cancer treatment (or SACT) and are specific to the site, stage and type of cancer. A combination of treatment modalities is often used and will be described in greater detail as follows, including:

- Chemotherapy
- Radiotherapy
- Surgery
- Immunotherapy or 'targeted therapies'.

These SACT treatments are either used individually or in combination to improve the patient's chances of treatment success. They are commonly described in one of two ways:

1. Preoperative (neoadjuvant) therapy is given to a malignant tumour before surgery to shrink it, making removal easier, and to reduce the risk of spread. This approach is used in Wilms tumour, osteosarcoma and Ewing sarcoma.
2. Adjuvant therapy – The tumour is removed at diagnosis with chemotherapy, radiotherapy or immunotherapy administered post-operatively to 'mop up' any residual cancer cells that are remaining after the surgery. This approach is commonly used in the treatment of some brain tumours (Drechsel *et al.*, 2024).

If a child or their parents report frequent bleeding (e.g., nose or gums), increasing tiredness, pallor or excessive bruising, a thorough investigation is needed to rule out malignancy, particularly acute lymphoblastic leukaemia (ALL), even though other causes may exist

Chemotherapy

Chemotherapy agents are key in treating childhood cancer, working through various mechanisms to limit tumour cell growth and survival. Cells are most vulnerable and sensitive to chemotherapy while actively dividing. Some agents act at specific points in the cell cycle while others do not rely on a specific phase of a cycle (Dickens and Ahmed, 2018).

Chemotherapy works by either inducing cell death through apoptosis (cytotoxic) or preventing cell division (cytostatic). Thus, cytotoxic chemotherapy has the ability to shrink tumours, while cytostatic agents generally prevent further growth of the tumour. Chemotherapy is usually given in combinations and in cycles of treatment. These cycles are spaced depending on the diagnosis and treatment to allow for recovery of blood counts and healthy cells while preventing significant cancer cell regrowth (Aiuppa *et al.*, 2020).

Chemotherapy cannot distinguish between a cancerous and a normal cell, meaning both are damaged beyond repair (or apoptosis). This results in pancytopenia (pan = all, cyto = cells, penia = lack of/deficiency), which is a deficiency of all types of blood cells, including white blood cells, red blood cells and platelets. This is also referred to as the 'nadir' of the blood counts in a cycle of treatment and usually occurs approximately 7–10 days after the anti-cancer therapy is administered, with blood count recovery at between 14 and 21 days.

Chemotherapy is given at doses that maximise effect while minimising toxicity. Administration varies depending on whether a drug is cell-cycle-specific. Continuous infusions or prolonged maintenance therapy target slow-growing tumours by maximising tumour cell exposure at the appropriate cell-cycle phase.

Chemotherapy and supportive care (e.g., IV fluids and medications) must be administered by trained nurses, advanced practitioners or doctors. Intrathecal (IT) and intraventricular chemotherapy can only be given by a designated doctor on the hospital's IT register. A trained, competent nurse on the same register may second-check the procedure, verifying the doctor's registration beforehand.

Routes of chemotherapy administration

Intravenous chemotherapy

Intravenous chemotherapy must be given by trained, competent professionals via peripheral or central venous access, depending on the drug and administration time. The main risk with peripheral cannulae is extravasation, especially with vesicant agents such as vinca-alkaloids (e.g., vincristine and vinblastine).

> If these drugs are administered through a displaced device, extravasation occurs, delivering the medication into surrounding tissue, which can cause severe pain and potentially irreversible tissue damage.

Before giving vesicant chemotherapy, the device must bleed back and flush freely to confirm it is properly in the vein. Other agents, such as cisplatin and high-dose methotrexate, require a stable device for longer infusions.

To manage this, central venous access devices are inserted and can be either short-term devices, including peripherally inserted central catheters (PICCs), or longer-term devices, such as Hickman® lines (Fig. 3.2) or Portacath (port). The choice of central venous access depends on the diagnosis, treatment protocol and, where possible, the preference of the child or their parents.

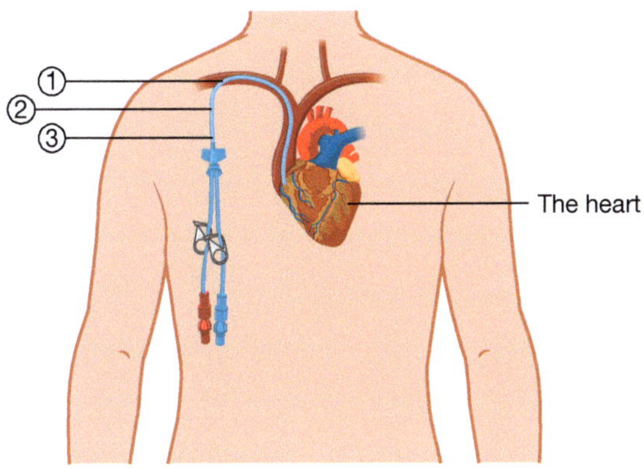

FIGURE 3.2 Hickman® line in situ.

Intramuscular route

Some non-chemotherapy agents that are used to treat CYP cancers (such as asparaginase in ALL) are administered via the intramuscular route.

Intrathecal chemotherapy

Intrathecal (IT) chemotherapy is administered directly into the cerebrospinal fluid (CSF), which surrounds the brain and spinal cord. It is commonly used in blood cancers such as ALL or any cancer that crosses the blood–brain barrier (BBB). This method bypasses the BBB, effectively preventing and treating CNS involvement. The drug is delivered via a lumbar puncture (LP), where a needle is inserted into the subarachnoid space (Fig. 3.3).

This procedure can only be performed in primary treatment centres (PTCs) (designated cancer treatment centres), and strict protocols must be adhered to. Each unit that administers IT chemotherapy must have designated medical staff (medical, nursing and pharmacy) who are on the hospital's IT register. Local policies must be strictly adhered to as this is an extremely high-risk procedure.

IT chemotherapy is administered under general anaesthetic (primarily for children and babies). Young people may opt for a local anaesthetic as long as they are fully informed and can lie still. Consent is essential in the administration of IT chemotherapy and can only be taken by a consultant or senior doctor. The drug will not be administered until consent has been confirmed and all other safety protocols followed.

National Patient Safety Alerts (NatPSAs) have dictated that all connections associated with LPs and the administration of IT drugs have different connectors to intravenous cannulas and adaptors. This is a safety mechanism to avoid incorrect medication being administered via an incorrect route. All equipment used to administer IT medication, including the chemotherapy prescription charts, medication packaging and labelling, should be distinctly different from all other packaging and colour coded.

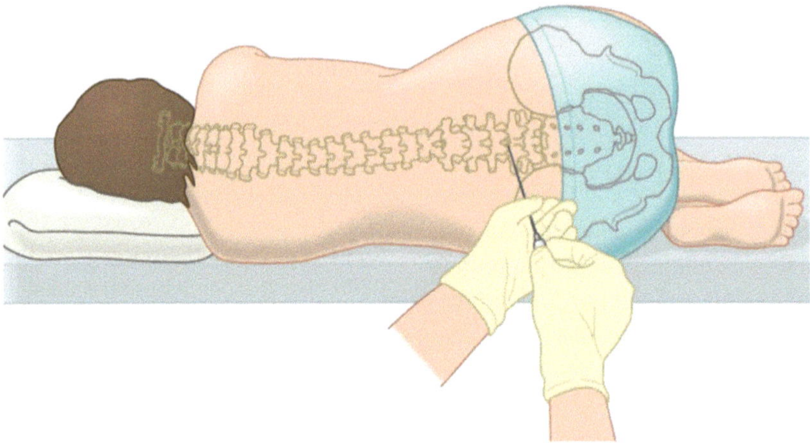

FIGURE 3.3 Lumbar puncture (LP) for IT administration of chemotherapy.

Oral chemotherapy

Some childhood cancer protocols use oral chemotherapy, either alongside other routes or as the sole treatment. A treatment protocol specifies the drugs, timing, required tests to confirm the child is fit for treatment and designated rest/recovery periods. Oral chemotherapy may be combined with intravenous therapy to improve survival outcomes or used alone to minimise treatment side effects.

Oral chemotherapy may be given alongside intravenous therapy to improve survival or used alone to reduce treatment side effects in selected patients. Examples of oral chemotherapy agents and their use in paediatric protocols are listed in Table 3.3.

Steroids

Corticosteroids are a type of steroid that is used to kill leukaemia cells, preventing them from coming back (Camire-Bernier *et al.*, 2021). They cause cell death by binding directly to a cell's DNA (Pourhassan *et al.*, 2024).

They are used in the following situations and diagnoses:

1. Treatment of disease: ALL (dexamethasone), non-Hodgkin lymphoma (NHL) (prednisolone). For cancers that are showing rapid rates of proliferation, such as NHL, steroids are particularly effective in reversing the process quickly.
2. Spinal cord compression: Immediate reduction of tumour growth in disease of the CNS, particularly the spinal cord. Dexamethasone is used to prevent spinal cord damage, potentially leading to lower limb paralysis if not treated.
3. Anti-emetic use: Dexamethasone is an effective drug in the prevention of chemotherapy-induced nausea and vomiting (CINV).

TABLE 3.3 Examples of oral chemotherapy agents

Chemotherapy agent	Diagnosis
6-mercaptopurine	ALL, Langerhans cell histiocytosis (LCH)
Methotrexate	ALL, LCH
Temozolamide	Some brain tumours, including medulloblastoma and diffuse midline glioma (DMG)

Source: Adapted from Moppett (2020).

When a child has received high-dose steroids for a prolonged period, they must be weaned gradually rather than stopped abruptly. Sudden cessation increases the risk of symptom flare-ups, including behavioural changes, aggression and adrenal insufficiency (Priya *et al.*, 2024).

Serious side effects of steroids are known to occur in prolonged use and in high doses (Camire-Bernier *et al.*, 2021). These include:

- Hyperglycaemia: High blood sugars may occur, requiring regular blood glucose monitoring and sometimes short-term insulin therapy, which rarely leads to lifelong diabetes.

- Adrenal suppression: This occurs when long-term steroid use reduces the body's stress response. Exogenous steroids suppress the hypothalamus and pituitary, lowering adrenocorticotropic hormone (ACTH) and cortisol production, which can be life-threatening. Severe cases may require hydrocortisone replacement to restore the stress response.
- Sleep disturbance.
- Severe changes in mood and behaviour: CYP become more emotional with more outbursts of anger.
- Hypertension: High blood pressure may require antihypertensive drugs.

Children on high-dose steroids should receive a Steroid Emergency Card to show any healthcare professional if they become ill. Steroids can cause adrenal insufficiency, reducing the ability to fight infection and increasing risk of allergic reactions. During sudden illness or severe injury, additional support or medications may be needed to help the child's nervous system respond.

Radiotherapy

There are two main types of radiotherapy administered to children: radiotherapy and proton beam therapy.

Radiotherapy uses high-energy gamma rays (IR) to damage cancer cells, preventing reproduction and inducing cell death (apoptosis). It is delivered in a specialist radiotherapy department over a series of short daily sessions, called fractions (# in medical notes), spanning several weeks.

Proton beam therapy is a type of radiotherapy that utilises beams of high-energy protons to treat specific cancers. The dose of high-energy protons precisely targets the tumour. It is only suitable for certain types of CYP cancers, such as complex brain tumours, head and neck tumours (e.g., craniopharyngiomas) and sarcomas (NHS England, 2020). This reduces damage to surrounding tissues and organs. Treatment normally takes place over five days for up to an hour per day. Proton beam therapy in the United Kingdom is relatively new, with an evolving evidence base.

It should be noted that children who receive proton beam therapy experience side effects similar to those who receive conventional radiotherapy (Chen *et al.*, 2023).

Growth and development

Previously, young children unable to stay still for radiotherapy required multiple general anaesthetics (GA), sometimes twice daily for several weeks. With the development of health play specialist (HPS) support, preparatory strategies now enable children as young as three to tolerate treatment awake. Techniques include custom moulds and masks, decorated with favourite characters, and simple reassurance methods, such as holding a ribbon with a parent during treatment (Cooper, 2015).

Radiotherapy can cause local tissue and organ swelling. Children receiving brain radiotherapy are usually inpatients for the first week for close monitoring of intracranial swelling, including 4-hourly neurological observations. Observations should also be closely tracked using the PEWS score to detect infection or sepsis, following local policy.

Surgery

The role of surgery in the management of childhood cancer is dependent on the type and the site of the cancer. Surgery may be required for biopsy in the diagnostic phase and also to enable treatment to commence for the insertion of an injectable device (Portacath or Hickman® line).

Bone cancers, such as osteosarcoma or Ewing sarcoma, require surgery alongside pre- and post-operative chemotherapy. Surgery may involve limb-sparing procedures or amputation. Pre-operative chemotherapy reduces tumour size, while post-operative chemotherapy, once wounds have healed and blood counts normalise, destroys any remaining cancerous cells.

Other solid tumours, including Wilms tumour, neuroblastoma, rhabdomyosarcoma and some brain tumours, may require surgical resection, but this depends on the tumour's response to chemotherapy. For brain tumours, the neurosurgeon plays a key role in diagnosis through surgical biopsy, and resection may be necessary depending on the tumour's location.

Surgery can be central to diagnosis when a biopsy is needed, allowing a pathologist to examine tissue under a microscope. Tissue samples can be obtained in several ways: fine needle biopsy (small sample), core needle biopsy (cylindrical tissue) or using endoscopy, laparoscopy or bronchoscopy. More invasive methods, such as excisional or incisional biopsy, laparotomy or thoracotomy, may also be required (CRUK, 2025).

Central venous access

Surgical intervention is required for the insertion of central venous catheters to facilitate the administration of treatment, supportive care and blood sampling. These long-term catheters can be made up of either one, two or three lumens, depending on the treatment required and can be either an implantable port as in a Poracath, or a Hickman® line. The benefit of a Portacath or a Hickman® line is that access is generally pain-free and avoids the need for repeated venepuncture. Extravasation is rare with implantable ports or Hickman® lines.

A PICC (a line is a temporary central line that may be used for CYP who have shortened treatment regimens or for supportive care). This does not require surgical insertion but is inserted by an experienced doctor or a clinical nurse specialist.

Hematopoietic stem cell transplantation

Hematopoietic stem cell transplantation (HSCT), formerly referred to as BM transplantation, has been used as a treatment for cancer since the late 1960s. HSCT involves the administration of chemotherapy and/or radiotherapy to eradicate the disease and render the BM empty. Harvested stem cells are then infused into the patient, allowing for recovery of healthy BM. These stem cells can be either:

the patient's own (autologous)
or
donated from another person (allogeneic): these could be from one of the following – brother or sister (sibling), parent (haplo) or an unrelated donor as long as that donor is matched genetically to the patient.

The harvests of somatic stem cells from donated umbilical cord blood can be used in HSCT. The mesenchymal stem cells from the umbilical cord tissue can be harvested and utilised in other tissue transplants (Nagamura-Inoue and Nagamura, 2023).

A number of donor registries exist in the United Kingdom (e.g., Anthony Nolan, NHS Stem Cell Donor). Donors are tissue-typed initially either through swab testing or through blood donation at a blood donor centre. Haematologists work with these registries when deciding which type of HSCT their patient requires. The BM is removed from the donor under general anaesthetic, then re-infusion intravenously via a central line or peripheral blood stem cell (PBSC) collection (more common method). The marrow can be stimulated prior to removal to produce more stem cells using granulocyte colony-stimulating factor (GCSF).

Autologous HSCT is now an established method in the treatment of solid tumours, including high-risk neuroblastoma and Ewing sarcoma (Elborai *et al.*, 2016). The patient's own stem cells are increased in number quickly using high-dose GCSF and then collected (harvested) via venous access. They are then frozen until required to act as a 'rescue' for the patient's BM following the administration of high-dose chemotherapy. This means the patient's immune system is severely reduced for a shorter amount of time, reducing the chances of severe infection or bleeding.

Immunotherapy (or targeted therapies)

Targeted therapies such as monoclonal antibody drugs (mAbs) are utilised in the treatment of CYP oncological and haematological malignancies. The benefit of these types of drugs is that they are targeted at specific tumours and therefore do not harm other healthy cells like chemotherapy does (Wedekind *et al.*, 2018) These mAbs can bind to an antigen on the tumour cell surface, and either mark that tumour cell for destruction by the patient's own immune system or carry a toxin that kills the cell directly. Examples of the more common immunotherapy drugs include:

Blinatumomab (relapsed ALL): This drug 'reprogrammes' the normal, non-cancerous T-cells (a type of white blood cell in the immune system that helps the body fight infection) by changing an antigen on its surface called CD3 to recognise a similar antigen on the surface of the leukaemic B-cell (also a type of white blood cell) called CD19 as a threat. This makes the T cell destroy the B cell and therefore treat the leukaemia. Blinatumumab is helping improve survival rates in those patients whose leukaemia has not been treated by their first-line treatment (Gupta *et al.*, 2025).

Dinutuximab (high-risk neuroblastoma): This drug targets the GD2 antibody that is present on most neuroblastoma cells, meaning the body's immune system targets and destroys the cancer cells. It also targets some normal cells in the peripheral nervous system, causing severe nerve pain when it is administered, and this is a well-documented side effect. Dinutuximab is improving the overall survival rates of high-risk neuroblastoma (Balaguer *et al.*, 2023). Personalised immunotherapy to treat blood cancers in CYP is recommended best practice (NICE, 2024).

Supportive care

Managing the toxicities and side effects of cancer treatment is just as important as the delivery of the treatment itself. These toxicities are often reversible (Ruggiero *et al.*, 2021). Each systemic anti-cancer treatment (SACT) agent has its own recognised side effects that can be managed through the delivery of additional medications following strict protocols. The most common side effects include:

- Chemotherapy-induced nausea and vomiting (CINV): The severity is ranked from low to very high depending on the chemotherapy agent, with national guidance on the choice of drugs that prevent nausea and vomiting (often referred to as 'anti-emetic' drugs) available (Hooke and Linder, 2019).
- Alopecia (or hair loss): This is short-term, and the hair will grow back once the BM has recovered from the chemotherapy or radiotherapy.
- Haemorrhagic cystitis: Certain types of chemotherapy (e.g., cyclophosphamide) cause bleeding of the bladder lining, which causes abdominal pain and haematuria. IV fluids are used to flush the bladder alongside the administration of Mesna (British National Formula for Children, 2025) are part of the treatment plan to prevent this.
- Kidney damage: IV fluids are administered alongside some chemotherapy agents to protect the kidneys and prevent irreversible damage. However, caution is required in case of known renal impairment.
- Liver damage: Liver function is monitored through a liver function test (LFT).
- Pain (acute): Mucositis (see herewith for a definition) can cause severe pain. Dinutuximab causes acute nerve pain while the infusion is running and can be managed with nerve-based analgesia, including gabapentin (Balaguer *et al.*, 2023).

Following the administration of the SACT agents, the patient is then at risk of the following effects on the body that require additional support from the healthcare professional caring for them to manage:

- Mucositis is irritation of the thin, vascular lining of the digestive tract, causing bleeding, ulcers, pain, vomiting and diarrhoea. Symptoms can range from a sore mouth and difficulty swallowing to severe pain requiring intravenous analgesia and fluids until recovery.
- BM suppression damages normal blood cells as well as cancerous ones, sometimes requiring red blood cell or platelet transfusions. Low neutrophil levels (neutropenia) increase the child's risk of infection until BM recovery.
- Febrile neutropenia: The immunocompromised child receiving SACT is at greater risk of infection when the neutrophil count is below 0.5×10^9/L and requires immediate review and antibiotic cover to prevent sepsis. Recent advances have shown that not all patients require hospitalisation and intravenous antibiotics, and a scoring system called the Australian-UK-Swiss (AUS) score is now available that acts as a severity 'predictor' system with regard to the likelihood of sepsis and potential intensive care admission (Jackson *et al.*, 2023).
- Tumour lysis syndrome: Cancers that grow quickly, like ALL or NHL, are often described as 'highly proliferative' diseases. Once treatment is started, the cancerous cells respond quickly to treatment and break down. These necrosed cancer cells are removed from the body through the urine. If the volume being filtered through the kidneys at once becomes excessive, the renal tubules within the kidneys can become occluded, leading to renal failure. This is treated with IV fluids and medication, including allopurinol (Adeyinka *et al.*, 2024).

Children receiving cytotoxic drugs are at risk of infection, particularly bacterial. The risk is greatest in children undergoing intensive treatment such as HSCT, high-dose chemotherapy with stem cell support or during leukaemia induction and delayed intensification treatment. Children with solid malignancies can also become severely pancytopenic. Blood count nadir usually occurs 1–14 days after a course of treatment and recovery by day 21.

Health promotion is essential for children and families during and after cancer treatment. This includes diet, lifestyle choices (smoking, vaping and alcohol), exercise and encouraging immunisations, particularly the HPV vaccine for 12- to 13-year-olds, which protects against HPV-related cancers (Szymonowicz & Chen, 2020).

Prophylactic antibiotics are given to children who are expected to have a prolonged period of neutropenia. Neutropenia is classed as an actual neutrophil count (ANC) $\leq 0.5 \times 10^9$/L. Febrile neutropenia is classed as a single temperature $\geq$38.0 or >37.5 °C on two occasions more than 1 hour apart. If the neutrophils are between 0.5 and $<1.0 \times 10^9$/L, management is determined by the overall condition of the child and also whether the WCC is likely to still be falling or is expected to rise soon. Any child receiving chemotherapy who appears unwell but is not febrile or neutropenic may still require treatment with antibiotics. If in any doubt about whether antibiotics are needed, it is preferable to err on the side of caution and give them. Always refer to local policy and discuss with a senior colleague (Jackson *et al.*, 2023).

Prevention of childhood cancers

Unlike adult cancers, the cause of most childhood cancers is not yet known. Few cancers in children are due to lifestyle or environmental factors. Certain risk factors, such as chronic infection, have been identified, e.g., malaria, HIV and EBV (WHO, 2025). It is estimated that 10% of all childhood cancers are as a result of genetic factors (Steliarova *et al.*, 2017).

Promoting healthy lifestyles to children and families is important, particularly to instil healthy behaviours to prevent certain types of cancers. Targeting teenagers and young adults regarding the risks of developing cancer from smoking, vaping and sexual behaviours is important.

Case study: acute lymphoblastic leukaemia

You are working on a children's ward at a District General Hospital and are assigned to Nathan, a 5-year-old transferred from the Children's Emergency Department with suspected acute lymphoblastic leukaemia (ALL). He initially presented to his GP with malaise, nosebleeds, fever and widespread bruising, and has had recurrent viral infections over the past few months. His GP referred him to the hospital for further review and investigations, which included:

Full blood count (FBC) including blood film, urea and electrolytes (U&Es), LFTs and chest X-ray. The FBC (detailed herewith) shows a low haemoglobin (Hb), high WCC, low platelets, low neutrophils (neutropenia) and leukaemia blast cells. This raises suspicion of a blood cancer, and he will need further investigation in a specialist children's hospital with a PTC for paediatric cancer. The nearest PTC is 2 hours away and is currently trying to arrange a bed to transfer him over to them.

Initial assessment: Nathan is asleep, appears pale, mother reports overnight headaches unrelieved by paracetamol and ongoing nosebleeds. Nathan is febrile with a temperature of 38.5 °C. He has a cannula in his right hand but is not currently receiving IV fluids or antibiotics.

Investigation	Results	Reference range
Hb g/dL	56 g/L	130–160
White cell count 10^9/L	120	4.5–14.5
Platelets 10^9/L	18	150–450
Neutrophils 10^9/L	0.4	1.8–8.0
Blasts	70%	0

Think about the information presented, particularly your initial assessment of Nathan and then consider the following points:

- Are there any aspects of his care that you might want to talk to a senior colleague about (for example, any treatment or medications that he might need to start)?
- What symptoms suggest that Nathan might need a blood product transfusion?
- What support could you give (or find) Nathan and his family?

Follow-up to this case study and the treatment of ALL:

Nathan is transferred that evening to the PTC via ambulance and receives further diagnostic testing, including a BM aspirate under general anaesthetic. He recovers well from the anaesthetic, but he continues to ooze blood from his iliac crest, where the bilateral BM aspirates were performed. **The BM confirms a diagnosis of B-cell ALL**. He has no poor-risk cytogenetics identified from his BM.

The family receives a specific plan of treatment from Nathan's treating consultant haematologist. They are aware that the treatment is approximately two and a half years long as per the ALLTogether01 trial. The treatment on this trial is made up of at least 5 courses of SACT treatment that includes different types of chemotherapy and steroids. The first 28 days of treatment are called induction and includes high-dose steroids, vincristine and PEG asparaginase. The treatment's aim is to destroy all of the leukemic cells in the body. The remainder of the treatment is aimed at mopping up the rest of any remaining leukemic cells and preventing them from re-developing in the BM. This treatment is a mix of inpatient- and outpatient-based care. Treatment is oral chemotherapy and steroids, intravenous chemotherapy, intramuscular injections and IT chemotherapy.

Now you have this additional treatment information and reflecting back to your earlier reading in this chapter:

- Consider and add to your earlier list new factors that will have an impact on Nathan and his family.
- What treatment risk group will Nathan have been risk-stratified into? Why?
- Thinking about Nathan's age, what other aspects of his care should be considered by the multi-professional team?
- What further surgical procedures will Nathan require?
- What are some of the short-term side effects or toxicity effects Nathan may experience from his cancer treatments?

Live vaccines should never be given to children receiving chemotherapy or within 6 months of completing treatment, as chemotherapy suppresses immune responses and may reduce vaccine effectiveness. The exception is the inactivated influenza vaccine, which can be given during treatment or within 6 months post-chemotherapy, unless the child is under 6 months, has an egg allergy or has a known vaccine-specific allergy (Patel *et al.*, 2023).

Outcomes and survivorship

One in 1000 adults in the United Kingdom is a survivor of childhood cancer, with 5-year childhood cancer survival rates of 86% in 2020 (NHS Digital, 2023). This unfortunately does mean that 14% of CYP do not survive to 5 years after completing their treatment, and childhood cancer continues to be the leading cause of death among CYP in the United Kingdom, which is a sobering fact (Royal College of Paediatrics and Child Health, RCPCH 2020). ALL in children, for example, has an overall survival rate of over 90% if the disease is controlled with first-line therapy. However, this rate falls to 20–50% with disease relapse (Bartram *et al.*, 2020).

Late effects

Not all effects on the body caused by chemotherapy or radiotherapy are considered short-term and wear off a few weeks after the treatment is given. Some effects only become apparent when the CYP have become adults, and these 'late effects' can present a significant risk to health and well-being (Chang *et al.*, 2022). A late effect is the term used to describe any physical, psychological or social consequence of the disease or treatment.

The most common late effects of SACT treatments are:

- Growth hormone deficiency
- Cognitive deficits
- Endocrine function
- Infertility
- Heart damage

- Reduced lung function
- Hearing loss
- Secondary cancers.

(Roganovic, 2025)

At least two-thirds of childhood cancer survivors will experience at least one late effect, and the endocrine system is commonly involved. At least 20% of patients will develop two or more late effects, which may be severe or life-threatening (Roganovic, 2025). Among CYP who survive CNS tumour, 62% have at least one impairment, including motor and visual impairments and epilepsy (Clarke and Jacques, 2025). To monitor these effects, most units now offer a long-term follow-up (LTFU) service that starts to see patients once they are 5 years after they completed their SACT. They use a combination of radiological imaging, bloods and other necessary tests to achieve this (Hudson *et al.* 2021).

Conclusion

Childhood cancer presents many challenges for the child, family and healthcare team. This chapter has outlined some types of childhood cancers, their treatments and associated side effects, highlighting the importance of safe, effective and interdisciplinary care.

References

Achatz, M.I., Villani, A., Bertuch., A.A., *et al.* (2025). Update on cancer screening recommendations for individuals with Li–Fraumeni syndrome. *Clinical Cancer Research* 31(10), 1831–1840.

Adeyinka, A., Kaur, A., & Bashir, K. (2024). Tumour lysis syndrome. *Stat pearls.* Available at: https://www.ncbi.nlm.nih.gov/books/NBK518985/ (accesses 25 September 2025).

Agarwal, S. (2023). Pediatric cancers: Insights and novel therapeutic approaches. *Cancers (Basel)* 15(14), 3537.

Aiuppa, L., Cartaxo, T., Spicer, C.M., *et al.* (2020). *Childhood Cancer and Functional Impacts Across the Care Continuum Treatment Modalities for Childhood Cancers*, 3rd edn. National Academies Press, US.

Balaguer, J., Hidalgo, L.G., Hladun, R., *et al.* (2023). Recent evidence-based clinical guide for the use of dinutuximab beta in pediatric patients with neuroblastoma. *Targeted Oncology* 18, 77–93.

Bartram, J., Veys, P., & Vora, A. (2020). Improvements in outcome of childhood acute lymphoblastic leukaemia (ALL) in the UK – A success story of modern medicine through successive UKALL trials and international collaboration. *British Journal of Haematology* 191(4), 562–567.

British National Formula for Children (2025). Mesna. Available at: https://bnfc.nice.org.uk/drugs/mesna/ https://bnf.nice.org.uk/drugs/mesna/ (accessed 23 September 2025).

Buser, J.M., Lake, K., & Ginier, E. (2022). Environmental risk factors for childhood cancer in an era of global climate change: A scoping review. *Journal of Pediatric Health Care* 36(1), 46–46.

Camire-Bernier, E., Nidelet, E., Baghdadli, A., *et al.* (2021). Parents' experiences with home-based oral chemotherapy prescribed to a child diagnosed with acute lymphoblastic leukemia: A qualitative study. *Current Oncology* 28(6), 4377–4391.

Cancer Research UK [CRUK] (2018). Cancer statistics for the UK. [online] Available at: http://www.cancerresearchuk.org/health-professional/cancer-statistics (accessed March 2025).

Chang, W., Katsoulis, M., Tan, Y.Y., *et al.* (2022). Late effects of cancer in children, teenagers and young adults: Population-based study on the burden of 183 conditions, in-patient and critical care admissions and years of life lost. *The Lancet Regional Health – Europe* 2022, 12.

Chen, Z., *et al.* (2023). Proton versus photon radiation therapy: A clinical review. *Frontiers in Oncology* 13.

Children with Cancer UK (2021). Children cancer facts and statistics. Available at: https://www.childrenwithcancer.org.uk/?gad_source=1&gad_campaignid=1730378794&gbraid=0AAAAAC08FEgeDaoXXoUXOf2gmz_6rgDZW&gclid=EAIaIQobChMI6qa6kMXzjwMVtpFQBh0Y6hokEAAYASAAEgLVwfD_BwE (accessed 23 September 2025).

Clarke, M. & Jacques, T. (2025). The frontline of paediatric brain tumour diagnostics: Advances challenges and opportunities. *The Royal College of Pathologists.* Available at: The frontline of paediatric brain tumour diagnostics: Advances, challenges and opportunities (accessed 23 March 2025).

Cooper, C. (2015). Play works. Empowering children undergoing radiotherapy treatment at Sheffield Children's Hospital. *The Journal of the National Association of Health Play Specialists* 2(56), 8–12.

CRUK (2023a). Staging of cancer. Available at: https://www.cancerresearchuk.org/about-cancer/what-is-cancer/stages-of-cancer (accessed 22 September 2025).

CRUK (2023b). Grades of brain tumours. Available at: https://www.cancerresearchuk.org/about-cancer/brain-tumours/grades (accessed 19 September 2025).

CRUK (2025). What is a biopsy. Available at https://www.cancerresearchuk.org/about-cancer/tests-and-scans/biopsy?_gl=1*1*1*1mr31*1rl*_gcl_au*MTgyNTA4MDI2OS4xNzUxMjk0NTg2*_ga*MTI0Mzc1*1NzY4Ny4xNzUxMjk0NTg2*_ga_58736Z2GNN*czE3NTgyNjk0ODEkbzEwJGcxJHQxNzU4MjY5NTA5JGozMiRsMCRoMA (accessed 19 September 2025).

Damodharan, S., & Puccetti, D. (2023). Pediatric central nervous system tumor overview and emerging treatment considerations. *Brain Sciences* 13, 1106.

Dickens, E., & Ahmed, S. (2018). Principles of cancer treatment by chemotherapy. *Surgery (Oxford)* 36(3), 134–138.

Drechsel, K.C.E., Broer, S.L., Stoutjesdijk, F.S., *et al.* (2024). The impact of treatment for childhood classical Hodgkin lymphoma according to the EuroNet-PHL-C2 protocol on serum anti-Müllerian Hormone. *Human Reproduction* 39(8), 1701–1711.

Elborai, Y., Hafez, H., Moussa, E.A., *et al.* (2016). Comparison of toxicity following different conditioning regimens for advanced stage neuroblastoma: Experience of two transplant centers. *Pediatric Transplantation* 20, 284–289.

Francis, S.S., Wallace, A.D., Wendt, G., *et al.* (2017). In utero cytomegalovirus infection and development of childhood acute lymphoblastic leukemia. *Blood* 129(12).

Gupta, S., *et al.* (2025). Blinatumomab in standard-risk B-cell acute lymphoblastic leukemia in children. *The New England Journal of Medicine* 392, 875–891.

Harbron, R.W., Chapple, C.L., O'Sullivan, J.J., *et al.* (2018). Cancer incidence among children and young adults who have undergone x-ray guided cardiac catheterization procedures. *European Journal of Epidemiology* 33(2018), 393–401.

Hooke, M., & Linder, L. (2019). Symptoms in children receiving treatment for cancer-part I: Fatigue, sleep disturbance, and nausea/vomiting. *Journal of Pediatric Oncology Nursing* 36(4), 244–261.

Hudson, M., Bhatia, S., Casillas, J., *et al.* (2021). Long-term follow-up care for childhood, adolescent, and young adult cancer survivors. *Pediatrics* 148(3).

Jackson, T.J., Napper, R., Haeusler, G.M., *et al.* (2023). Can I go home now? The safety and efficacy of a new UK paediatric febrile neutropenia protocol for risk-stratified early discharge on oral antibiotics. *Archives of Disease in Childhood* 108, 192–197.

Leaver, T., Johnson, B., Lampard, J., *et al.* (2019). The risks following the exposure to radiation associated with the surgical correction of limb deformities in children are minimal. *Bone and Joint Journal* 101-B, 241–245.

Lee, E., Jiménez-Fonseca, P., Galán-Moral, R., *et al.* (2023). Toxicities and quality of life during cancer treatment in advanced solid tumors. *Current Oncology* 30(10), 9205–9216.

Leffers, J.M. (2022). Climate change and health of children: Our borrowed future. *Journal of Pediatric Health Care* 36(1), 12–19.

Moppett, J. (2020). ALLTogether1– A Treatment study protocol of the ALLTogether Consortium for children and young adults (0-45 years of age) with newly diagnosed acute lymphoblastic leukaemia (ALL). Available at: https://www.cclg.org.uk/magazine-articles/alltogether-1-trial-finding-more-effective-leukaemia-treatments-children (accessed 23 September 2025).

Nagamura-Inoue, T., & Nagamura, F. (2023). Umbilical cord blood and cord tissue banking as somatic stem cell resources to support medical cell modalities. *Inflamm Regener* 43, 59.

NHS England (2020). Clinical Commissioning Policy: Proton Beam Therapy for Children, Teenagers and Young Adults in the treatment of malignant and non-malignant tumours. Available at: https://www.england.nhs.uk/wp-content/uploads/2020/10/proton-beam-therapy-clinical-commissioning-policy.pdf (accessed 22 September 2024).

National Institute for Health and Care Excellence (2024). NICE recommended personalised immunotherapy to treat blood cancer in children and young adults to be made routinely available on the NHS. Innovative CAR-T therapy recommended to treat an aggressive form of leukaemia. Available at: https://www.nice.org.uk/news/articles/nice-recommended-personalised-immunotherapy-to-treat-blood-cancer-in-children-and-young-adults-to-be-made-routinely-available-on-the-nhs (accessed 22 September 2024).

Navarrete-Meneses, M., Salas-Labadía, C., Gómez-Chávez, F., & Pérez-Vera, P. (2024). Environmental pollution and risk of childhood cancer: A scoping review of evidence from the last decade. *International Journal of Molecular Sciences* 25(6), 3284.

NHS Digital (2023). Cancer survival in England, cancers diagnosed 2018 to 2020 followed up top 2021.

Childhood Cancer Survival (2023.). Available at: https://digital.nhs.uk/data-and-information/publications/statistical/cancer-survival-in-england/cancers-diagnosed-2016-to-2020-followed-up-to-2021/childhood-cancer-survival (accessed 22 September 2024).

NHS England (2021). Children, teenagers and young adults UK cancer statistics report. https://www.cancerresearchuk.org/health-professional/cancer-statistics/childrens-cancers/incidence#heading-zero (accessed March 2025).

Paola, A.C., & Preciado, M.V. (2013). EBV primary infection in childhood and its relation to B-cell lymphoma development: a mini-review from a developing region. *International Journal of Cancer* 133, 1286–1292.

Patel, S., Skinner, R., & Heath, P. (2023). Vaccinations for paediatric patients treated with standard-dose chemotherapy and haemopoietic stem cell transplantation (HSCT) recipients. CCLG. Available at: https://www.cclg.org.uk/sites/default/files/2025-03/vaccinationcclgsep2023.pdf (accessed 23 September 2025).

Pourhassan, H., Murphy, L., & Aldoss, I. (2024). Glucocorticoid therapy in acute lymphoblastic leukemia: Navigating short-term and long-term effects and optimal regimen selection. *Current Hematologic Malignancy Reports* 19(4), 175–185.

Priya, G., Laway, B.A., Ayyagari, M., *et al.* (2024). The glucocorticoid taper: A primer for the clinicians. *Indian Journal of Endocrinology and Metabolism* 28(4), 350–362.

Royal College of Paediatrics and Child Health (RCPCH) (2020). State of child health. London. www.stateofchildhealth.rcpch.ac.uk. (accessed 16 February 2025).

Royal College of Paediatrics and Child Health (RCPCH) (2025). Cancer. Available at: https://stateofchildhealth.rcpch.ac.uk/evidence/long-term-conditions/cancer/ (accessed 23 September 2025).

Roganovic, J. (2024). Genetic predisposition to childhood cancer. *World Journal of Clinical Pediatrics* 13(3), 95010.

Roganovic, J. (2025). Late effects of the treatment of childhood cancer. *World Journal of Clinical Cases* 13, 7, 98000.

Ruggiero, A., Skinner, R., & Zekri, W.Z.D. (2021). Editorial: Adverse and toxic effects of childhood cancer treatment. *Frontiers in Oncology* 11.

Siegel, R., Naishadham, D., & Jemal, A. (2013). Cancer statistics 2013. *Cancer Journal for Clinicians* 63, 71–81.

Steliarova-Foucher, E., Colombet, M., Ries, L.A.G., *et al.* (2017). International incidence of childhood cancer, 2001-10: A population-based registry study. *The Lancet Oncology* 18(6), 719–731.

Stiller, C., Bayne, A.M., Chakrabarty, A., *et al.* (2019). Incidence of childhood CNS tumours in Britain and variation in rates by definition of malignant behaviour: population-based study. *BMC Cancer* 19(139).

Szymonowicz, K., & Chen, J. (2020). Biological and clinical aspects of HPV-related cancers. *Cancer, Biology & Medicine 17*(4), 864–878.

Vora, A. (2016). Childhood acute lymphoblastic leukaemia. In: Hoffbrand, V., Higgs, D., Keeling, D., & Mehta, A. (eds). *Postgraduate Haematology*, 7th edn. Oxford: Wiley.

Wedekind, M.F., Denton, N.L., Chen, C.Y., & Cripe, T.P. (2018). Pediatric cancer immunotherapy: Opportunities and challenges. *Paediatric Drugs* 20(5), 395–408.

World Health Organization (2025). Childhood cancer. Available at: https://www.who.int/news-room/fact-sheets/detail/cancer-in-children (accessed 19 September 2025).

World Health Organization (2013). *International Classification of Diseases for Oncology*, 3rd edn [online] Available at: http://apps.who.int/iris/bitstream/10665/96612/1/9789241548496_eng.pdf?ua=1 (accessed January 2017).

CHAPTER 4

Homeostasis

Mary Brady

AIM

The aim of this chapter is to further develop and apply your understanding of homeostatic mechanisms within the body related to children and young people.

This chapter will build on the learning gained in various chapters in Peate and Gormley-Fleming (2025).

LEARNING OUTCOMES

On completion of this chapter, the reader will be able to describe the impact of:

- Dehydration on homeostasis.
- Respiratory illness on homeostasis.
- Renal disease on homeostasis.
- Diabetes on homeostasis.

KEYWORDS

- internal and external environments
- metabolism
- hormones
- pituitary gland
- hypothalamus
- nervous system
- electrolytes
- feedback systems
- compensatory systems
- homeostatic regulation of disorders

Test your prior knowledge

1. What is homeostasis?
2. How do acute and chronic respiratory illnesses affect the body?
3. How do acute and chronic renal illnesses affect the body?
4. What effect does diabetes have on homeostasis?
5. How should the nurse escalate concerns to senior staff?

Introduction

Despite significant improvements in childhood mortality over the past 30–40 years, statistics from the World Health Organization (WHO, 2024) demonstrate that there are still approximately 6300 newborn deaths every day, which globally amounts to nearly 47% of all child deaths under the age of 5 years. Causes for these deaths include acute respiratory infections, diarrhoea and malaria, along with pre-term birth complications, birth asphyxia and trauma and congenital anomalies. Many of these deaths are preventable with appropriate access to skilled delivery at birth, during the postnatal period, including health education relating to breastfeeding, nutrition, vaccinations and treatment for common childhood diseases.

The WHO (2024) identified sub-Saharan Africa and southern Asia as areas that account for more than 80% of the 4.9 million deaths of children under 5 years of age. In addition, Sub-Saharan Africa had the highest neonatal mortality rate in 2022 at 27 deaths per 1000 live births, followed by Central and Southern Asia with 21 deaths per 1000 live births.

> Children's nurses must ensure that they understand the benefits of breastfeeding for mother and child and have the knowledge and skills to assist new mothers who would like to breastfeed but are experiencing difficulties due to their child's prematurity or illness.

The human body functions within a narrow range of parameters, maintained by multiple homeostatic mechanisms (Brady, 2025). This chapter focuses on pathophysiological disruptions that impair normal homeostasis.

Children's nurses often care for patients whose ability to maintain homeostasis is severely compromised. In such cases, nurses must detect subtle changes, initiate emergency care, escalate concerns to the multidisciplinary team and communicate clearly with families about the child's condition and any treatments provided.

This chapter uses the term 'child' to refer to those in the 0- to 18-year age range, except where specific information is provided for neonates and premature infants.

> As a children's nurse, you work in partnership with parents and carers and must appreciate their knowledge of their child's behaviours when well and unwell.
>
> 1. It is fundamental to the child's care that you build a rapport with the child, their parents or carers so that they can communicate their concerns.
> 2. It is often the subtle 'not quite right' observations by parents/carers that provide vital data for clinical staff.

Dehydration

Children are more prone to dehydration due to their large surface area-to-volume ratio and higher percentage of water volume ranging between 60% and 80% (Gormley-Fleming and Haviland (2021)), depending on their age. Fluid loss due to acute gastroenteritis accounts for about 1.7 million cases globally each year, of which 443 832 deaths occurred in children under 5 years old (WHO, 2024) and an additional 50 851 children aged 5–9 years.

Dehydration due to gastrointestinal fluid loss

Outerridge (2025) discusses gastrointestinal anatomy and physiology further.

Babies under one year are particularly susceptible to dehydration because of their large surface area and immature kidneys that are unable to concentrate urine (Gormley-Fleming, 2025). In addition, they are more susceptible to gastrointestinal infections that cause diarrhoea and vomiting because of a reduced amount of hydrochloric acid in their stomach and an immature immune system, especially if the baby was born prematurely. At birth, the stomach contents are less acidic with a neutral pH of 7 due to the amniotic fluid that has been swallowed while in utero. Gradually, with the introduction of feeding, especially breastfeeding, the bacteria that make up the microbiota in the gastrointestinal tract begin to develop and are inherited from the mother (Cook *et al.*, 2021). *Lactobacillus bifidus* proliferates, and this helps increase the acidity within the stomach. Furthermore, Shandler *et al.* (2023) support the beneficial effects of breastfeeding due to its non-nutritive components such as *Streptococcus*, *Staphylococcus*, *Bifidobacterium*, *Lactobacillus*, *Enterococcus* and *Propionibacterium*, which suppress the growth of potentially pathogenic bacteria. Furthermore, the World Health Organization (2025) clearly endorses the value of exclusive breastfeeding for the first 6 months of life to maximise these benefits.

By about 10 years of age, gastric secretions have reached adult levels; thus, children are vulnerable to gastrointestinal infections during the early part of their life, and this is a relatively common problem seen in both the developed and developing world.

Fluid loss from vomiting or diarrhoea can quickly cause dehydration and shock, where circulating volume is insufficient to perfuse organs. Normally, the anterior hypothalamus detects changes in fluid osmolality and volume, triggering thirst. Very young children cannot verbalise this, relying on crying to alert caregivers to provide fluids.

An unwell child has a reduced blood volume that leads to a decrease in blood pressure, although it is important to note that hypotension is a late sign in children due to their ability to compensate for fluid loss. The reduced circulating blood volume stimulates the kidneys to release the enzyme renin, which acts on angiotensin, converting it to angiotensin I, which is converted into angiotensin II by the angiotensin-converting enzyme (ACE) produced by the lungs and nephrons. Angiotensin II causes aldosterone to be produced by the adrenal cortex, which leads to vasoconstriction of the arterioles, which subsequently helps increase the blood pressure (Fig. 4.1).

Fluid loss causes weight loss, so children should be accurately weighed to guide rehydration – children under 2 years should be weighed naked. Nurses should also record vital signs (temperature, pulse, respiratory rate, blood pressure, oxygen saturation and capillary refill) and assess skin and eye turgor, fontanelle depression and urine output.

Signs of dehydration and medical shock vary depending on the age of the child or young person, as noted by Gormley-Fleming and Haviland (2021). For instance, the fontanelle in infants under 18 months is a useful indicator of their state of hydration, with a depressed fontanelle indicating dehydration. Other early signs of medical shock include restlessness and tachycardia with a weak pulse, pallor and a widening core-peripheral temperature gap (Table 4.1). These observations become even more crucial as the child's condition worsens and they become quiet and lethargic. Furthermore, the amount of urine produced will reduce as the body strives to conserve fluid, and kidney perfusion will reduce due to hypotension.

To gain a more accurate clinical picture, blood samples (Table 4.2) are taken, such as blood gas analysis, urea and electrolytes and blood glucose, to identify the cause and initiate treatment.

About 70% of dehydrated children have isonatraemic dehydration with plasma sodium levels between 135 and 145 mmol/L and normal plasma osmolality of 275–295 mOsm/kg H_2O. This is usually due to diarrhoea and vomiting, and in this situation, the amount of sodium and water loss is equal, and the kidneys facilitate equilibrium by compensating; however, the extracellular fluid in the blood vessels and interstitial space is reduced with the ensuing hypotension.

About 10% of dehydration is hyponatraemic where more sodium is lost via micturition and usually arises due

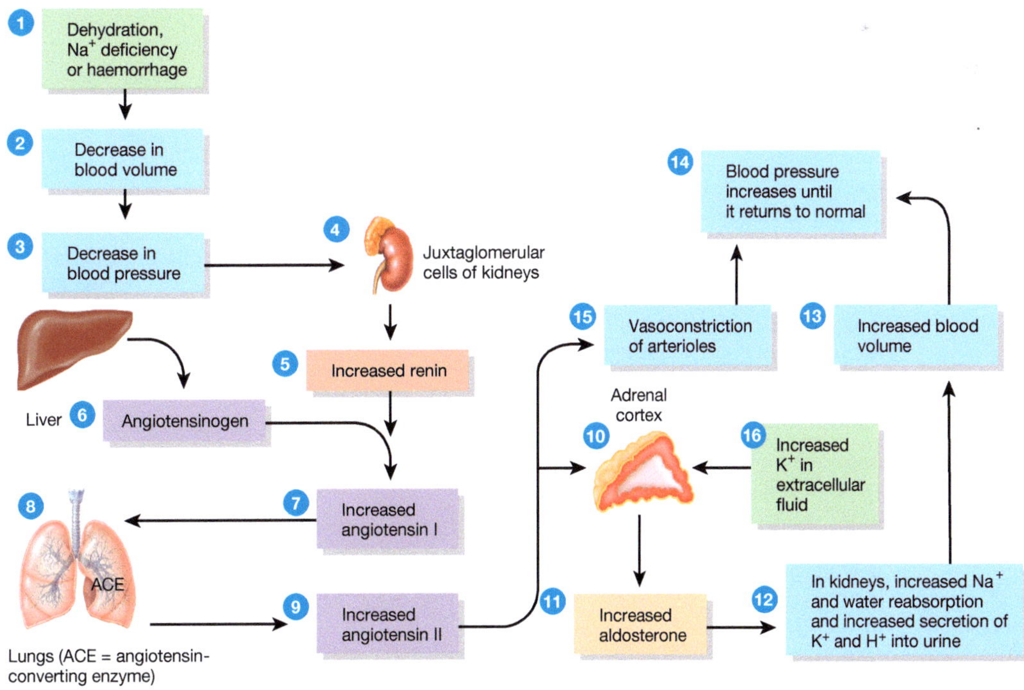

FIGURE 4.1 Regulation of aldosterone by the renin–angiotensin–aldosterone pathway.
Source: Reproduced with permission of Peate & Gormley-Fleming (2015)/John Wiley & Sons.

TABLE 4.1 Signs and symptoms of medical shock

Observation	Finding
Temperature	Depends on the underlying cause, which may be raised due to infection
Heart rate	Tachycardic
Respiratory rate	Tachypnoea
Colour	Pallor with peripheral mottling or cyanosis
Blood pressure	May be normal or low
Level of consciousness	Restless, confused
Oxygen saturations	May be normal or low, depending on the cause
Capillary refill	More than 2 seconds

TABLE 4.2 Blood tests and other investigations used in dehydration

Test	Finding
Blood gas	Anaerobic tissue metabolism
Haemoglobin (Hb)	Reduced due to haemorrhage
Packed cell volume (PCV)	Decreased due to haemorrhage Raised if less than 55% plasma due to hypovolaemia
Urea	Raised urea indicating reduced GFR and kidney excretory capacity due to hypovolaemia
Sodium	Raised if the fluid volume in the blood vessels and cells is reduced, giving a higher concentration of solute
Plasma osmolality	Raised if there is less fluid in the blood vessels, giving a concentrated plasma
Blood glucose	Hypoglycaemia
Electrocardiogram	Cardiac arrhythmia due to abnormal potassium levels
Central venous pressure (CVP)	Low in severe dehydration. A CVP line will monitor fluid replacement

to severe burns or vomiting and diarrhoea. Hypotonic intravenous fluids may be given, or the child could be encouraged, if well enough, to drink large quantities of sugary drinks, thereby counteracting the fluid loss as the cells take in the glucose and leave the water in the extracellular spaces. Careful monitoring is required to ensure the correct diagnosis, since the imbalance could be due to water intoxication where too much water has been consumed or where the cause is due to inappropriate antidiuretic hormone (ADH) syndrome.

Twenty per cent of children will have hypernatraemic dehydration with plasma sodium levels greater than 145 mmol/L and plasma osmolality greater than 295 mOsm/kg H_2O. In this situation, more water is lost than sodium, and it is a manifestation of conditions such as diabetes insipidus, hyperpyrexia and hyperventilation with loss of fluids due to increased insensible loss. Another reason could be the accidental administration of hypertonic intravenous fluids, leading to fluid in the cells passing into the circulatory system to dilute the plasma. A similar situation arises with diabetes mellitus, where there is hyperglycaemia instead of hypernatraemia, resulting in a reduced volume in the circulatory system and in the interstitial spaces.

The RCPCH (2025a) online learning resource 'Spotting the sick child' provides useful information to help early identification of the sick and deteriorating child.

Dehydration due to blood loss

Children may haemorrhage following surgery or trauma; the cause needs to be ascertained promptly, and investigations commenced as per Table 4.2, in addition to obtaining a full blood count (FBC) since the haemoglobin (Hb) and packed cell volume (PCV) levels will be decreased due to haemorrhage. As well as administering intravenous fluids (0.9% saline), a blood transfusion may also be given depending on the severity of the blood loss. Drugs to strengthen cardiac function (inotropes) may also be required.

The child requiring surgery

In the past, concern has been raised regarding the possibility of regurgitation and aspiration of acidic gastric contents for all patients undergoing surgery, and to reduce this incidence, all patients requiring surgery were fasted overnight prior to undergoing surgery. However, with children, this is recognised as dangerous because of the risk of dehydration and impact on their different physiology, haemodynamic stability. Consideration also needs to be given to the variety of food given from breast milk, formula feed and solid food. It is also necessary to understand their different physiology; for instance, babies have faster stomach emptying times, especially if fed breast milk.

Cognisant of this, the amount of time that a child should be fasted prior to surgery has been investigated over several years. Pattrick (2024) highlighted that when prolonged unplanned fasting occurs due to delayed operations, the child can experience adverse physiological symptoms such as hypoglycaemia, dehydration and headaches. Recent guidance (RCN, 2020) states that solid foods and milk can be given 6 hours pre-surgery, breast milk up to 4 hours and clear fluid up to 2 hours. Additionally, Disma *et al.* (2021), who debated the fasting times for children, concluded that providing clear fluids up to 1 hour pre-operatively resulted in significant benefits for the child with no increased risk of aspiration.

Sometimes, a child's surgery may have to be delayed due to another child's need for emergency surgery; this can result in a child being fasted for longer than originally planned. The nurse must advocate for the child and insist on intravenous fluids being commenced to avoid hypoglycaemia and dehydration.

The child with respiratory impairment

Respiratory problems are common in childhood (Lissauer & Carroll, 2022). Although these illnesses can range from upper respiratory tract infections to bronchiolitis, chest infections, asthma and many more, some of which may become life-threatening or have a debilitating impact on the child's quality of life.

When a child's ability to breathe is compromised, the amount of oxygen circulating falls (hypoxia) and carbon dioxide (CO_2) levels increase (hypercapnia). This reaction stimulates chemoreceptors within the aorta and carotid arteries. Information is then transmitted via the glossopharyngeal and vagus nerves, stimulating the diaphragm and intercostal muscles to contract, thereby increasing the intake of oxygen and exhalation of CO_2. These muscles also receive further impulses via the phrenic and intercostal nerves, as the rising level of CO_2 within the cerebrospinal fluid is detected by chemoreceptors within the medulla oblongata (Figs. 4.2 and 4.3). So, the child or young person's respiratory rate becomes faster and deeper to remove the excess CO_2. If the situation continues, the CO_2 combines with water to form carbonic acid ($^-HCO_3$), which alters the pH of the circulating blood, as demonstrated in the reversible equation herewith:

$$CO_2 + H_2O \leftrightarrow H_2CO_3 \leftrightarrow H^+ + {}^-HCO_3$$

Since the reason for the shift in pH is due to an accumulation of acid and the origin is respiratory, the child or young person is described as having a respiratory acidosis.

Children and young people who have chronic respiratory or cardiac problems, such as cystic fibrosis, tend to tolerate higher than normal CO_2 levels, so their physiology differs, in that the stimulus to breathe depends on a low level of oxygen. It follows that when administering oxygen to a child with a chronic respiratory or cardiac problem and using a pulse oximeter to titrate the amount of oxygen required, it is possible to impede the stimulus to breathe, so agreement needs to be reached between the medical and nursing staff caring for the child/young person regarding acceptable oxygen saturation levels, for example, to keep saturations at 85% rather than above 94%.

The child with renal impairment

Gormley-Fleming (2025) provides a discussion of the anatomy and physiology of the renal system.

Rainey (2023) noted that globally, chronic kidney disease is a common long-term condition that affects about 9% of adults. Furthermore, the renal impairment may have been acquired in childhood or due to a congenital abnormality. Nowadays, with antenatal screening, congenital abnormalities are detected in 1 in 200–400 births, enabling damage limitation interventions to prevent renal

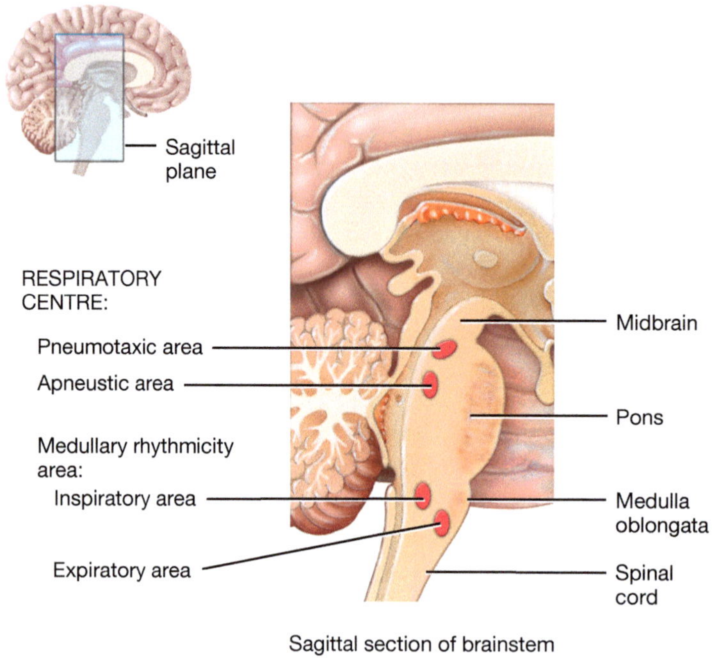

FIGURE 4.2 Locations of areas of the respiratory centre.
Source: Peate & Gormley-Fleming (2025)/with permission of John Wiley & Sons.

scarring that would otherwise affect kidney function (Lissauer & Carroll, 2022). Antenatal screening can detect:

- absent kidney (renal agenesis)
- multicystic dysplastic kidney
- horseshoe kidney
- duplex kidney
- bladder exstrophy
- pelvi-ureteric junction obstruction
- vesico-ureteric junction obstruction
- urethral valves (male infant).

Acquired renal conditions include urinary tract infections and conditions considered to be due to an autoimmune reaction following a bacterial or viral infection, such as nephrotic syndrome and glomerulonephritis.

Inflammation of the nephron at the glomerular region results in a disruption to filtration, which allows protein to leak out of the circulatory system with ensuing water loss and hypoalbuminaemia. Hypoalbuminaemia reduces oncotic pressure that counterbalances hydrostatic pressure, causing hypotension leading to oedema, as fluid accumulates outside the circulatory system in the interstitial space. The child, although oedematous, is hypovolaemic due to the shift in fluid location, which leads to sodium retention either by triggering the renin–angiotensin response (Brady, 2025) or, in nephrotic syndrome, the renal tubule may be affected, which is thought to cause sodium retention (Bailey & Tosh, 2021).

A further complication of hypoalbuminaemia affects the pleural and peritoneal membranes, resulting in the movement of fluid into the pleural space, resulting in a pleural effusion and into the peritoneal space resulting in ascites, which will have an additional negative impact on breathing (Bailey & Tosh, 2021).

Glomerulonephritis may result in a reduction of the glomerular filtration rate (GFR), which leads to a reduced urine output and the retention of sodium and water with ensuing oedema and hypertension as the water is redistributed.

When hypovolaemia is detected by baroreceptors in the aortic arch and carotid sinus with ensuing slight reduction in blood pressure, the child's body initially compensates by increasing the heart rate and respiratory rate to maximise oxygen transportation around the body. Additionally, the peripheral circulation vasoconstricts and fluid moves from the interstitial spaces into the intravascular compartments to increase the circulating blood volume, and the pulse pressure (difference between systolic and diastolic pressures) reduces, as does the capillary refill time. The renin–angiotensin–aldosterone is also activated, which results in an increase in blood pressure (Brady, 2025). However, the situation is temporary because

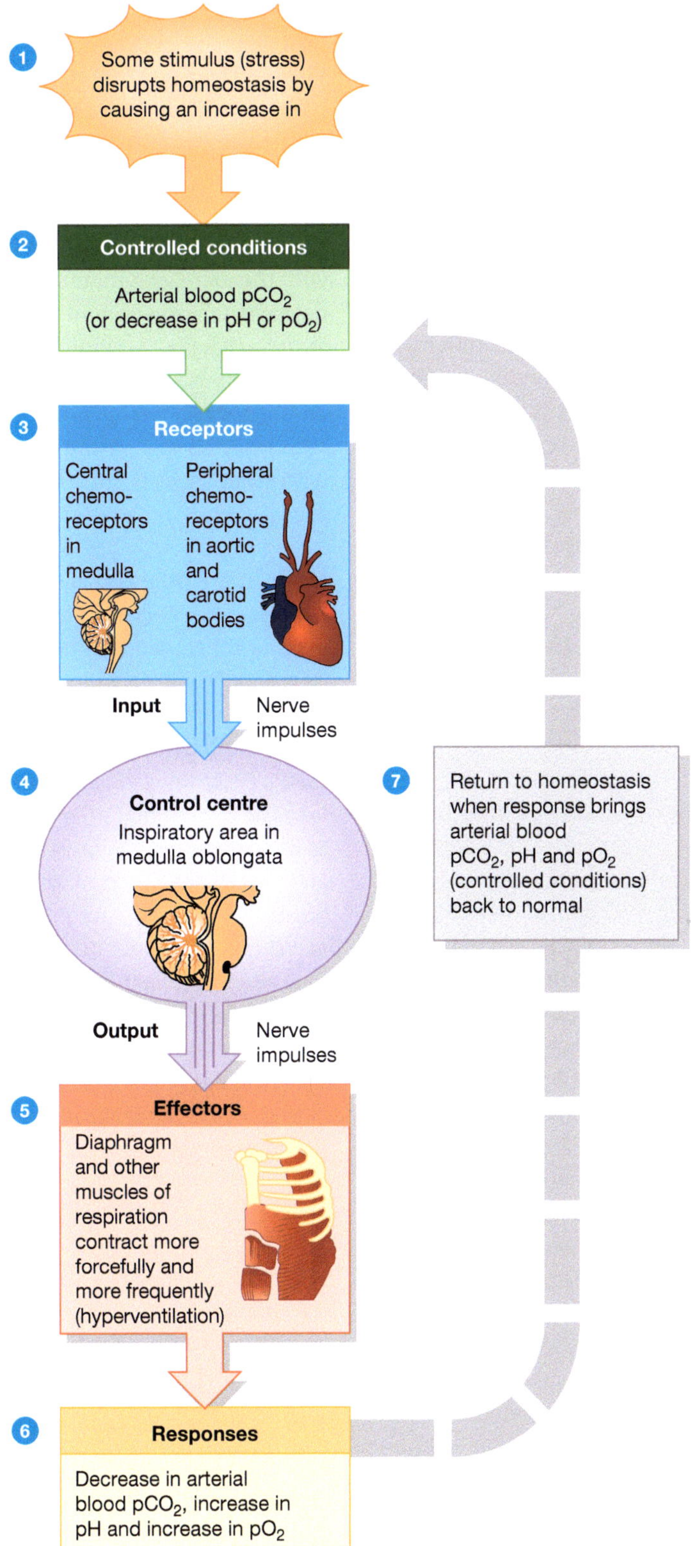

FIGURE 4.3 Regulation of breathing in response to changes in blood pCO_2, pO_2 and pH (H^+ concentration) via negative feedback control.

Source: Tortora and Grabowski (2003)/with permission of John Wiley & Sons.

children can withstand a loss of 20–25% of their circulating volume (McNee & Davey, 2021) and require correction of the fluid loss to avoid hypotension and cell necrosis.

The child with an infection

Mosenthal (2025) describes and discusses inflammation and infection in further detail.

Infections remain a common aspect of childhood, with data from the National Childhood Mortality Database (2023) highlighting that infection accounted for 9978 childhood deaths in England between 2019 and 2022. Worldwide, although some improvement has occurred with a reduction from 12.6 million in 1990 to 5 million in 2020 (WHO, 2025), it remains a major area of concern, with many of the illnesses being preventable with appropriate healthcare provision.

At birth, the term baby possesses an immature immune system consisting of immunoglobulins acquired from the mother transplacentally. This innate immune system consists of barriers (such as the skin and mucous membranes), cell-mediated mechanisms and antimicrobial proteins, which provide a humoral defence mechanism (Fig. 4.4).

Over the ensuing few months, these reduce, increasing the baby's vulnerability to infection, and at the same time, the body develops an immune response as it becomes exposed to a variety of pathogens.

If the baby has no immunity to a specific bacterium or virus and this microorganism gains access to the tissues, where they rapidly reproduce, plasma proteins known as complement are activated, initiating phagocytosis, where the invading microorganism is engulfed to destroy the infection. The macrophages are derived from monocytes and neutrophils (formed from the bone marrow); however, the neutrophils are short-lived but do have a fast response and ability to create anti-bactericidal enzymes known as lysozymes, which destroy the bacteria.

Inflammation also occurs and is seen as redness, swelling, heat and pain, for example, with inflamed skin, tonsils and breathing difficulties due to reduced airway lumen. Histamine and serotonin are released, causing vasodilation, which enables a greater flow of blood (with plasma proteins) to the affected area to trap and destroy the invading microorganisms. The accumulated dead cells and microorganisms form pus, which may be visible at the site of infection, such as in tonsillitis with red, inflamed, pus-producing tonsils (Fig. 4.5).

Prostaglandin and leukotrienes are produced by the cell walls of the affected tissue and are responsible for the pain associated with inflammation. The body temperature increases after the release of cytokines by macrophages, which act on the hypothalamus, causing a resetting of thermoregulation. The hypothalamus stimulates the sympathetic nervous system to cause vasoconstriction, raising the metabolic rate. To deal with the increased metabolic rate, there is an increased demand for oxygen and energy release from glycogen stores. Usually, a higher temperature indicates more pathogens in the body; however, children under 5 have an immature nervous system and thereby immune response, so temperature does not always correlate with the severity of the infection (Sahib El-Radhi *et al.*, 2019).

Furthermore, the steep rise in temperature may result in a febrile convulsion as the body reacts to the hyperpyrexia. This is an alarming event for parents who may be concerned that their child will develop epilepsy. However, febrile convulsions are usually benign and due to a viral infection, but if focal, prolonged or repeated, they should be investigated for an underlying pathology (Sahib El-Radhi *et al.*, 2019).

The pyrexia that accompanies an infection is thought to be therapeutic, in that it reduces the availability of iron and zinc in the blood, which are needed by bacteria for growth. In addition, according to Moon *et al.* (2023), the elevated core temperature affects the RNA within the cell and alters the lipid composition of the cell membrane, thus rendering the bacteria inert. However, the pyrexia-related sweating may cause dehydration, especially since small children have relatively large heads in comparison to their bodies and may lose significant heat and water by evaporation through their heads.

- A young child's temperature may not indicate the severity of their illness.
- It is important to be alert for the often-subtle signs of sepsis and attend to the parents'/carers' concerns.
- Use an age-appropriate Paediatric Early Warning System (PEWS) chart to document observations. Although most clinical areas will have incorporated these electronically, printed copies may exist.
- Escalate concerns to appropriate senior staff as advised, using the score generated from the PEWS data and using a communication tool such as Identify, Situation, Background, Assessment, Recommendation, Decision and Read back (ISBARD) (RCPCH, 2025b).

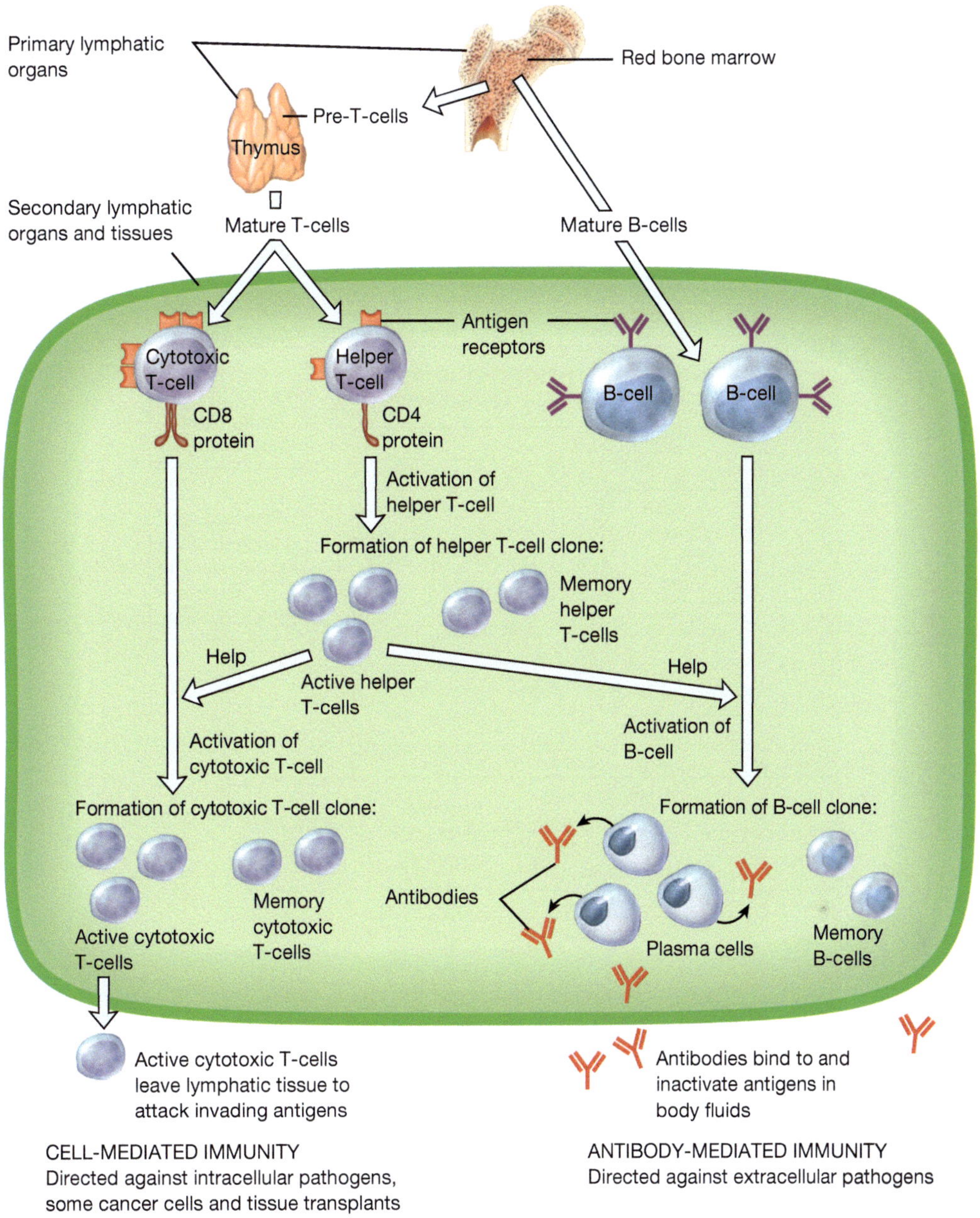

FIGURE 4.4 Cellular and humoral immune responses.
Source: Reproduced with permission of Peate & Gormley-Fleming (2025)/with permission of John Wiley & Sons.

The diabetic child

See also Brady (2025), where additional information concerning homeostasis can be located.

Diabetes is a condition where the body's ability to metabolise glucose is impaired, resulting in hyperglycaemia. The incidence of diabetes continues to increase, and according to NHS England (2024), there were 75 180 people aged 0–25 years with diabetes in England in 2022/23. Of those, 79.8% had Type 1 diabetes, 14.9% had Type 2 diabetes and 5.3% had other types of diabetes.

The exact cause of Type 1 diabetes is unclear; possibilities include a post-viral response that elicits an autoimmune disease, a genetic predisposition and environmental triggers (The British Diabetic Association, 2025), whereas Type 2 diabetes is related to obesity and appears to be increasing in children/young people.

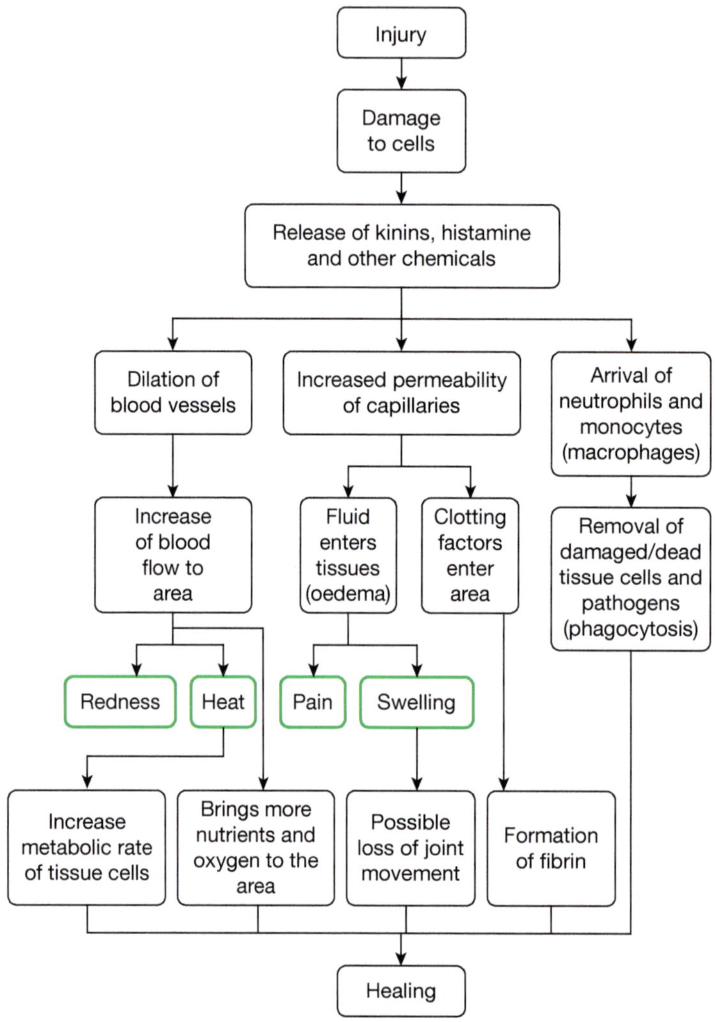

FIGURE 4.5 Flowchart of inflammatory events.
Source: Adapted from Marieb and Keller (2021).

In diabetes, the autoimmune response leads to the destruction of beta cells, with the resultant inability to respond adequately to the need for insulin to release glucose for energy, thus seriously impairing homeostasis.

Insulin and glucagon are hormones that are secreted by the pancreas. Insulin is secreted by beta cells and glucagon by alpha cells. When blood glucose levels rise, insulin is secreted and acts on the cell membranes, enabling the conversion of glucose into glycogen for storage in the liver and muscles (by glycogenesis) and the storage of fats within adipose tissue. When blood glucose levels fall, glucagon is secreted, which acts on the liver enzyme phosphorylase that enables glycogen to be converted to glucose for release into the blood circulation.

Newly diagnosed children/young people have usually exhibited the symptoms of lethargy, thirst, weight loss and polyuria in the preceding weeks. Their blood results will indicate above-normal blood glucose levels and metabolic acidosis. Depending on their blood results, the child may need rehydration with 0.9% saline intravenously and correction of acidosis.

Overall management of this challenging condition involves good glycaemic control, measured by frequent blood glucose tests and titration of insulin accordingly, as well as 2–3-monthly glycated haemoglobin A_{1c} (HbA_{1c} levels) to reduce the development of microvascular complications such as retinopathy, nephropathy and neuropathy (NICE, 2023). Technological developments over

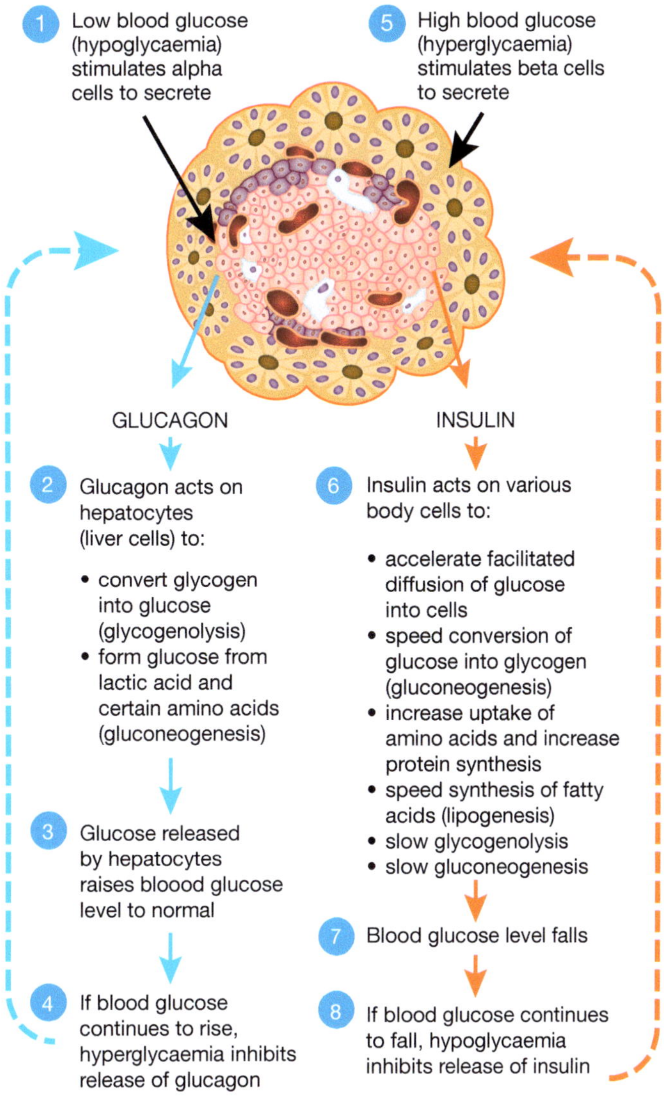

FIGURE 4.6 Negative feedback regulation of the secretion of glucagon (blue arrows) and insulin (orange arrows).
Source: Tortora and Derrickson (2011)/with permission of CABI Publishing.

recent years have enabled improved control with the use of continuous infusion pumps that enable a basal rate of insulin to be infused and additional boluses to be given as required. Home blood testing is also more accessible with user-friendly devices that enable the transfer of data to a computer, which enables tracking of glycaemic control (Fig. 4.6).

At times, extreme levels of hyperglycaemia arise, resulting in the potentially fatal condition called diabetic ketoacidosis (DKA). This may be due to illness or non-compliance with insulin injections, resulting in glycosuria and metabolic acidosis caused by the metabolism of fats and proteins into glucose. The hyperosmolar effect of glycosuria causes the excretion of vast amounts of urine with ensuing dehydration.

An electrolyte imbalance also occurs as potassium is lost in the urine, and the higher levels of sodium within the body lead to an accumulation of water within the cells, with an associated risk of cerebral oedema as fluid enters the brain cells (Gormley-Fleming, 2021). Careful fluid rehydration is commenced with 0.9% saline and added glucose plus potassium chloride to correct any potassium deficit with an insulin infusion that is titrated to blood glucose levels. In addition to the usual observations, neurological observations are required to detect any cerebral oedema and subsequent neurological deficit.

Hypoglycaemia is another complication and can be due to a discrepancy between the amount of insulin given, food consumed and exercise. It occurs when more insulin has been given in comparison to the intake of food. Correction is by addressing the hypoglycaemia with sufficient carbohydrate and adjustment of insulin dosage. The cause needs to be ascertained, for example, concurrent infection or growth spurt and involvement from a Diabetic Specialist Nurse to help address any underlying reasons and educational requirements regarding therapeutic management.

During puberty, hormonal changes that result in increased growth (and increased insulin requirements), and changes due to cognitive development and the transition towards independence have an impact on diabetic control, where glycaemic control may be erratic.

Illness and infection also have a negative impact on glycaemic control; as the body responds to the stress, the adrenal glands produce adrenaline and noradrenaline. The production of adrenaline results in an increased need for glucose with associated need for insulin; however, the diabetic person is unable to respond and will therefore rely on the administration of extra insulin via injection or pump mechanism. It follows that during times of illness, the need for vigilance of blood glucose and ketone levels is imperative in ensuring that homeostasis is maintained. Increasing ketone levels indicate that the body has had to metabolise fat and amino acids to facilitate glucose availability.

Escalating your concerns as a nurse

As a nurse, you should be observing for pyrexia, tachycardia, tachypnoea, low saturations, hypotension, pallor, anorexia, tiredness and widening peripheral-core temperature gap. The frequency of these observations will depend on the child's condition and potential for deterioration. Your recordings will be noted on an age-appropriate PEWS chart to enable monitoring for trends, illustrate deterioration and the calculation of a score. As a nurse, it is important that you also take note of any concerns that parents/carers may have, in that their child is not behaving as they normally would. Prompt escalation of the PEWS score to senior staff is imperative, using a clear and succinct communication tool such as Identify, Situation, Background, Assessment, Recommendation, Decision and Read back (ISBARD) and Concern, Uncomfortable, unSafe, Stop (CUSS) are vital (RCPCH, 2025b). The CUSS tool can be useful when seeking clarity regarding an instruction or plan of care. Paediatric early warning score charts, alongside the ISBARD tool, should be used to escalate concerns promptly and with all the relevant information. However, your interpretation and synthesis of data as a nurse are crucial to this activity. As always, accurate documentation of your findings and subsequent actions is fundamental.

Conclusion

During illness, the body's homeostasis is disrupted, and this chapter has explored common conditions that affect it. It has also covered recording and interpreting patient observations and analysing the underlying pathophysiology.

Prompt escalation of concerns is highlighted as a crucial part of the nurse's role.

To help consolidate learning, some activities have been included. The answers are at the end of this chapter. To assist with your analysis of the case studies, please use the PEWS charts available at:

NHS England (2023) National Paediatric Early Warning System (PEWS) observation and escalation charts [Online]. Available at: https://www.england.nhs.uk/publication/national-pews-observation-and-escalation-charts/

Case study 4.1

Solape is 8 months old. She was previously well, but has started to experience diarrhoea and vomiting. So, she has been admitted to the emergency department with a 3-day history of his illness. Solape has a sunken fontanelle, looks pale and is rather drowsy, and last had a wet nappy about 6 hours previously. Her parents are concerned and think she has lost weight and is difficult to rouse. It is estimated that she has lost about 10% of her body weight, which has now been recorded as 7 kg.

- Her observations are:
- Heart rate: 160/minute
- Respiratory rate: 60/minute
- Blood pressure: 90/45
- Temperature: 36.5 °C
- Oxygen saturation in air: 91%
- Capillary refill: 4 seconds

1. Access the PEWS chart for 0–11-month-olds and plot her observations. Also, calculate her PEWS score.
2. What actions will you take as a nurse?
3. Using the ISBARD tool, document how you would cascade this data to a senior person.
4. What possible treatment will she require?

Case study 4.2

Abdul is a 5-year-old child who has been admitted to the ward. In the Emergency Department, he received a bronchodilating nebuliser, but remains pale with an audible wheeze, tracheal tug and use of intercostal accessory muscles. He is barely able to talk but says he does not have asthma. His mother is with him and visibly worried and upset; she does not appear to speak much English and has not been able to contact her husband. On admission, his observations are:

- Heart rate: 124
- Respiratory rate: 30/minute with an audible wheeze
- Temperature: 37 °C
- Oxygen saturations in air: 91%
- Capillary refill: 3–4 seconds
- Blood pressure: 88/94

1. Access the PEWS chart for 5–12-year-olds and plot Abdul's observations.
2. Calculate his PEWS score.
3. What actions will you take as a nurse?
4. Using the ISBARD tool, document how you would cascade this data to a senior person.
5. What possible treatment will he require?

References

Brady, M. (2025). Homeostasis. In: Peate, I. & Gormley-Fleming, E. (eds). *Fundamentals of Children's Anatomy and Physiology*, 3rd edn. Oxford: Wiley, Chapter 2.

Cook, N., Shepherd, A., & Boore, J. (2021). *Essentials of anatomy and physiology for nursing practice*, 2nd edn. Sage Publications Ltd, London.

Disma, N., Fryholm, P., Cook-Sather, S.D., & Lerman, J. (2021). Pro-con debate: 1- vs 2-hour fast for clear liquids before anaesthesia in children. *Anaesthesia and Analgesia* 133(3), 581–591.

Gormley-Fleming, E. (2021). Caring for children with diabetes and other endocrine disorders. In: Glasper, A., Richardson, J., & Randall, D. (eds). *A Textbook of Children and Young People's Nursing*, 3rd edn. London: Churchill Livingstone Elsevier, pp. 340–364.

Gormley-Fleming, E. (2025). The renal system. In: Peate, I. & Gormley-Fleming, E. (eds). *Fundamentals of Children's Anatomy and Physiology*, 3rd edn. Oxford: Wiley, Chapter 13.

Gormley-Fleming, E., & Haviland, A. (2021). Homeostasis and the deteriorating child. In: Glasper, A., Richardson, J., & Randall, D. (eds). *A Textbook of Children and Young People's Nursing*, 3rd edn. London: Churchill Livingstone Elsevier, pp. 164–181.

Lissauer, T., & Carroll, W. (eds) (2022). *Illustrated Textbook of Paediatrics*, 6th edn. Elsevier, London.

Marieb, E.N., & Keller, S.M. (2021). *Essentials of Human Anatomy and Physiology*, 13th edn. Pearson Education Ltd, Harlow.

McNee, P., & Davey, P. (2021). Caring for children with critical illness. In: Glasper, A., Richardson, J., & Randall, D. (eds). *A Textbook of Children and Young People's Nursing*, 3rd edn. Edinburgh: Churchill Livingstone Elsevier, pp. 553–582.

Moon, S., Ham, S., Jeong, J., *et al.* (2023). Temperature matters: bacterial response in temperature change. *Journal of Microbiology*, 343–357.

Mosenthal, A. (2025). The immune system. In: Peate, I. & Nair, M. (eds). *Fundamentals of Anatomy and Physiology for Student Nurses*. Oxford: Wiley, Chapter 7.

National Childhood Mortality Database (2023). Infection related deaths of children and young people in England National Child Mortality Database Programme Thematic Report Data from April 2019 to March 2022 [Online] Available at: https://www.ncmd.info/wp-content/uploads/2023/12/Infection-related-deaths-of-children-and-young-people-in-England.pdf (accessed 27 March 2025).

National Institute for Health and Care Excellence (NICE) (2023). Diabetes (type 1 and type 2) in children and young people: diagnosis and management. NICE Guideline [NG18]. Methods, evidence and recommendations. [online]. Available at: https://www.nice.org.uk/guidance/ng18/resources/diabetes-type-1-and-type-2-in-children-and-young-people-diagnosis-and-management-1837278149317 (accessed 29 March 2025).

NHS England (2023). National paediatric early warning system (PEWS) observation and escalation charts [Online] Available at: https://www.england.nhs.uk/publication/national-pews-observation-and-escalation-charts/ (accessed 29 March 2025).

NHS England (2024). Right care children & young people diabetes toolkit [Online] Available at: https://www.england.nhs.uk/wp-content/uploads/2024/07/children-and-young-people-diabetes-toolkit.pdf (accessed 15 March 2025).

Outerridge, J. (2025). The digestive system and nutrition. In: Peate, I. & Gormley-Fleming, E. (eds). *Fundamentals of Children's Anatomy and Physiology*, 2nd edn. Oxford: Wiley, Chapter 12.

Pattrick, K. (2024). Care of children and young people in the peri-and-post operative recovery period. In: Price, J., McAlinden, O., & Veal, Z. (eds). *Essentials of nursing children and young people*, 2nd edn. London: SAGE, pp. 254–267.

Peate, I., & Gormley-Fleming, E. (eds) (2015). *Fundamental of Children's Anatomy and physiology*. John Wiley & Son, Oxford.

Peate, I., & Gormley-Fleming, E. (eds) (2025). *Fundamentals of Children's Anatomy and Physiology*, 3rd edn. Wiley, Oxford.

Rainey, H. (2023). Chronic kidney disease: understanding its association with other long-term conditions. *Nursing Standard* https://doi.org/10.7748/ns.2023.e12081 (accessed 13 April 2025).

Royal College of Nursing (2020). *Day Surgery for Children and Young People: RCN Guidance*. Royal College of Nursing. Available at: https://rcn.access.preservica.com/uncategorized/IO_fe1dbe70-6920-435e-9e48-e196226e6719/, London (accessed 18 March 2025).

Royal College of Paediatrics and Child Health (2025a). Spotting the sick child. [Online] Available at: https://www.rcpch.ac.uk/resources/spotting-sick-child-online-learning (accessed 26 March 2025).

Royal College of Paediatrics and Child Health (2025b). UK Paediatric Early Warning Systems (PEWS) [Online] Available at: https://www.rcpch.ac.uk/resources/UK-paediatric-early-warning-systems (accessed 29 March 2025).

Sahib, E.-R.A., Carroll, J., & Klein, N. (2019). *Clinical Manual of Fever in Children*, 2nd edn. Springer, Cham (accessed 27 March 2025).

Schanler, R., Feldman-Winter, L., Younger Meek, J., *et al.* (2023). *Breastfeeding Handbook for Physicians*. American Academy of Pediatrics.

The British Diabetic Association (2025). Diabetes Uk' Available at : https://www.diabetes.org.uk/ (accessed 15 March 2025).

Tortora, G.J., & Derrickson, B.H. (2011). *Principles of Anatomy and Physiology*, 13th edn. Wiley, Hoboken, NJ.

Tortora, G.J., & Grabowski, S.R. (2003). *Principles of Anatomy and Physiology*, 10th edn. Wiley, Hoboken, NJ.

World Health Organization (2024). Diarrhoeal disease. Fact sheet. [online]. Available at: https://www.who.int/news-room/fact-sheets/detail/diarrhoeal-disease (accessed 13 March 2025).

World Health Organization (2025). *Breast feeding*. [online]. Available at: https://www.who.int/health-topics/breastfeeding#tab=tab_1 (accessed 15 March 2025).

Bailey, K., & Tosh, K. (2021). Renal conditions in childhood. In: Glasper, A., Richardson, J., & Randall, D. (eds). *A Textbook of Children and Young People's Nursing*, 3rd edn. London: Churchill Livingstone Elsevier, pp. 239–248.

CHAPTER 5

Inflammation, immune response and healing

Alison Mosenthal

AIM

This chapter provides the reader with an understanding of the complexities associated with inflammation and the immune response.

LEARNING OUTCOMES

On completion of this chapter, the reader will be able to:

- Describe how the body responds to infection.
- Discuss the features of the inflammatory response.
- Describe the processes involved in wound healing.
- Discuss normal and abnormal pathophysiological changes occurring during the immune response.

KEYWORDS

- immune system
- white blood cells
- pathogens and infection
- inflammatory process
- innate immunity
- acquired immunity
- hypersensitivity reaction
- immunodeficiency

Test your prior knowledge

1. List the blood cells, tissues and organs of the immune system.
2. Discuss what is meant by innate and adaptive immunity.
3. Describe the systemic signs of inflammation.
4. Discuss what factors might contribute to impaired immune function in the infant and child.
5. Describe the features of anaphylaxis.

Introduction

From birth, individuals are exposed to harmful microbes and the immune system, comprising cells and tissues, coordinates a response to eliminate them. This defence involves the innate and adaptive immune systems.

This chapter explores their roles in non-specific and specific immunity, including the inflammatory response in wound healing and acute or chronic inflammation. It also covers how the immune system distinguishes 'self' from 'non-self', responds to known antigens (relevant to vaccination and transplantation) and how immune defects or deficiencies alter normal function.

The immune system

Host defence is the body's ability to fight infection (Macpherson & Austyn, 2012) and involves the innate and adaptive immune systems. Innate immunity is non-specific, rapid and provides the first line of defence, often acting within minutes or hours. Adaptive immunity responds more slowly, usually over days, but is specific to known antigens and retains immunological memory for faster responses upon re-exposure. Both systems are essential, with the innate system activating the adaptive response.

The immune system is made up of organs, tissues, cells and molecules that are connected by the blood and lymphatic systems. The coordinated reaction of these cells to infectious microbes is known as the immune response (Abbas *et al.*, 2024), see Fig. 5.1.

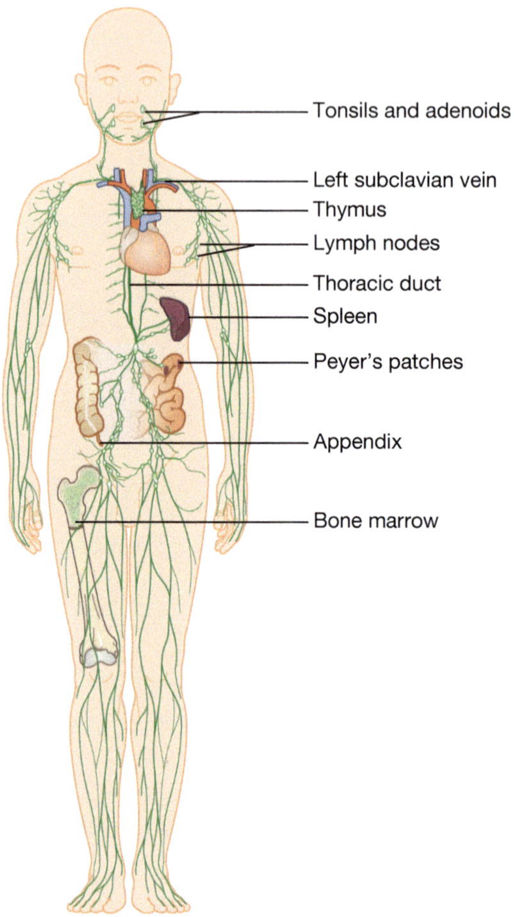

FIGURE 5.1 Distribution of lymph vessels and nodes.
Source: Reproduced with permission of Peate and Gormley-Fleming (2025)/John Wiley & Sons.

The blood cells primarily involved in immune function are the white blood cells (leukocytes), specialised to perform different functions. Figure 5.2 shows the development of the blood cells.

The white cells involved within the innate response are:

- neutrophils
- eosinophils
- basophils
- tissue macrophages and monocytes.

Further details regarding the roles of these cells are discussed in Peate and Gormley-Fleming (2025).

The other group of cells that play an important part in the innate response are the natural killer (NK) cells. These are able to detect the presence of virally infected cells and are described as cytotoxic (cell-killing) cells, and play an important part in the destruction of virally infected cells.

The white blood cells involved in the adaptive immune response are the lymphocytes, divided into two main groups:
B lymphocytes
T lymphocytes.

Both B and T lymphocytes are produced in the bone marrow, with B cells maturing there before entering the blood. B cells have specific receptors for antigens; exposure stimulates rapid growth and multiplication. Mature B cells include plasma cells, which secrete antibodies, and memory cells, which respond rapidly upon re-exposure to the same antigen by producing new plasma cells.

T lymphocytes migrate to the thymus to mature, differentiating into regulator/coordinator cells for adaptive immunity and cytotoxic cells that kill infected cells via apoptosis. Unlike NK cells, cytotoxic T cells require exposure to an antigen-presenting cell before responding. T cells also learn to distinguish self from non-self and develop antigen-specific recognition (see Table 5.1).

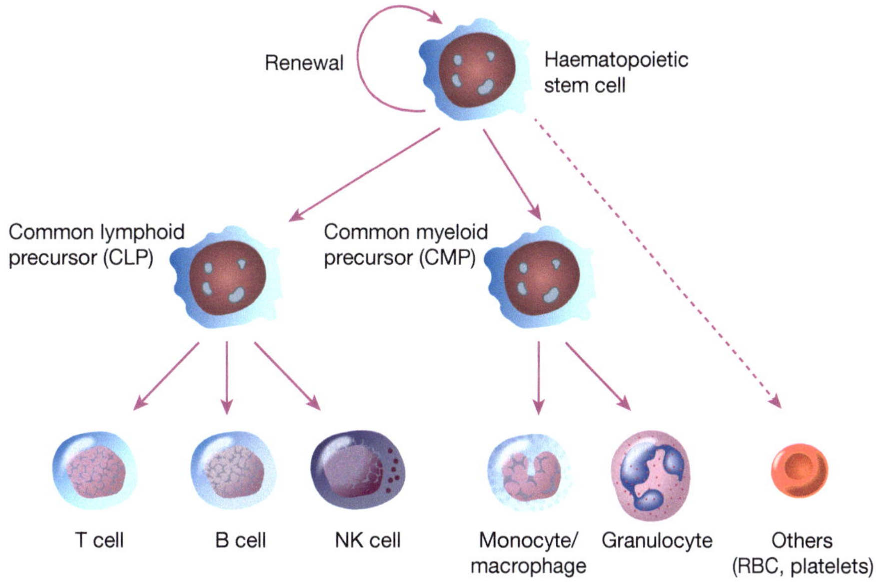

FIGURE 5.2 Diagram showing development of blood cells.
Source: Peate and Gormley-Fleming (2025)/John Wiley & Sons.

TABLE 5.1 Different types of cells involved in the innate and adaptive immunity

Innate immune system	Function
Neutrophil	Phagocytosis
Macrophage	Phagocytosis, antigen presentation
Tissue mast cells	Release of histamine and other inflammatory mediators
Natural killer cells	Apoptosis of virally infected cells
Adaptive immune system	
B lymphocytes	Produce plasma cells which secrete immunoglobulin
T lymphocytes	Apoptosis of virally infected cells, activated cells release cytokines

Defence against infection

Our bodies are constantly exposed to microorganisms, most of which are harmless, but some cause serious disease and are called pathogens. Major classes include viruses, bacteria, protozoa and worms, which invade the host, reproduce and spread to others. Pathogens use different strategies: some, like viruses and certain bacteria or fungi, live inside cells, while others exist extracellularly, and some protozoa and worms inhabit body cavities (Macpherson & Austyn, 2012). Pathogen invasion triggers an immune response, beginning with the innate system and inflammation, followed by adaptive immunity.

Innate immune system

The innate immune system consists of a range of non-specific defence mechanisms to try and prevent entry by these pathogens and further infection. However, there are natural barriers, which provide a first line of defence before these systems are activated, and these are demonstrated in Figure 5.3. The skin and the mucosal surfaces of the respiratory, gastrointestinal and urogenital tracts are the first areas of contact for invading microbes and have specialised protective functions.

The skin

The skin is a major barrier against pathogens, with mast cells, macrophages and dendritic cells initiating immune responses in the epidermis and dermis. Although sterile at birth, the skin quickly becomes colonised by mostly harmless commensal microbes that help prevent pathogenic colonisation. However, hospital-acquired infections can be transmitted from healthcare workers' skin, making

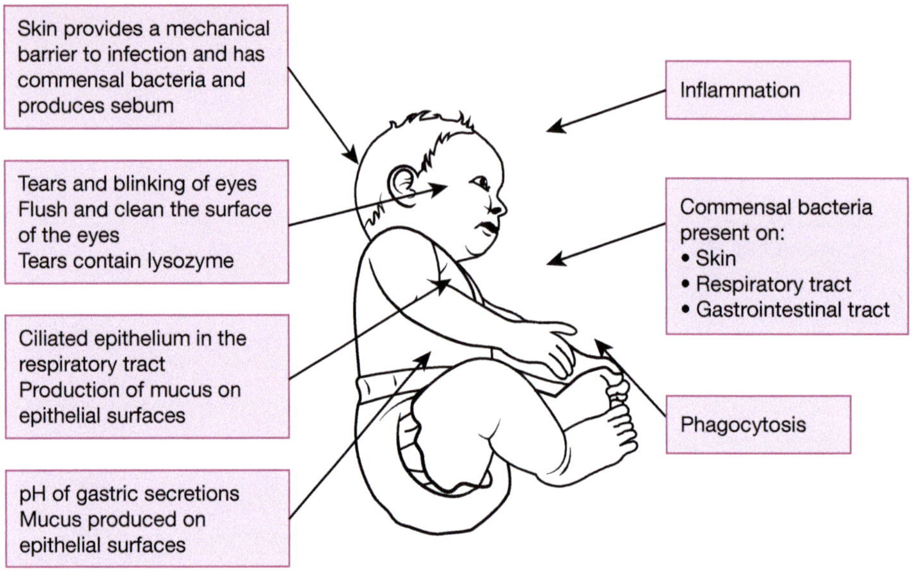

FIGURE 5.3 Features of the innate immune system.

good hand hygiene essential for infection control (NICE, 2017). Peate and Gormley-Fleming (2025) provide further detail on the anatomy and physiology of the skin.

The preterm infant's skin has a thinner epidermis and immature stratum corneum, reducing its barrier function and increasing susceptibility to infection.

Special consideration

The preterm infant's skin is fragile and prone to tears, so careful handling and the use of appropriate equipment and dressings are essential to maintain skin integrity.

Mucosal surfaces of the body

Epithelial membranes in the respiratory, gastrointestinal and urogenital tracts contain goblet cells that produce mucus to trap pathogens. In the respiratory tract, cilia move mucus towards the mouth and nose for removal via sneezing and coughing. Children with cystic fibrosis struggle to expel microbes and need nebulised mucolytics and daily physiotherapy to aid mucus clearance.

Mucosal surfaces produce antimicrobial substances. Lysozyme in tears, sweat and saliva breaks down bacterial cell walls, and secretions create an acidic environment that inhibits bacterial growth. In the stomach, hydrochloric acid, bile salts and digestive enzymes destroy pathogens. Individuals unable to secrete gastric acid are more susceptible to gastrointestinal infections such as *Salmonella* (Macpherson & Austyn, 2012; Helbert, 2017).

Commensal bacteria on the skin and mucosal surfaces of the gastrointestinal, respiratory and vaginal tracts act as a barrier against pathogens. Antibiotics can disrupt this barrier, allowing pathogenic bacteria to invade and cause disease.

Growth and development

At birth, the gut is relatively sterile but rapidly becomes colonised with bacteria, and the early introduction of maternal breast milk to the preterm infant provides immunological and growth factors to prevent infections such as necrotising enterocolitis (Brown *et al.*, 2019).

Phagocytosis

Phagocytosis is the process by which neutrophils and macrophages engulf and destroy invading organisms, providing the first line of cellular defence. This mechanism removes small extracellular pathogens, including bacteria, protozoa, fungi and dead or damaged cells (Helbert, 2017), preventing them from becoming pathogenic (see Fig. 5.4).

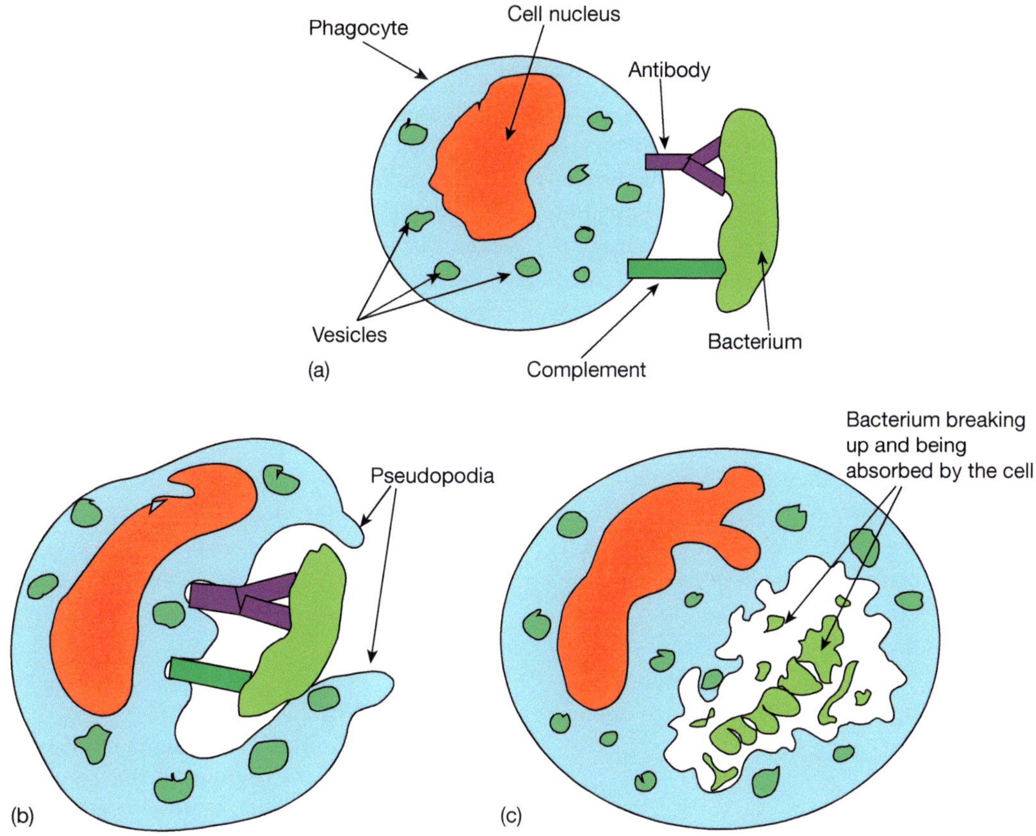

FIGURE 5.4 Stages of phagocytosis: (a) stage 1, (b) stage 2 and (c) stage 3.
Source: Peate and Gormley Fleming (2025)/with permission of John Wiley & Sons.

Neutrophils and monocyte-derived macrophages are produced in the bone marrow from the same stem cells, with more neutrophils made daily. Neutrophils have a short lifespan (1–2 days) and are usually absent from tissues, but migrate rapidly to infection sites via chemotaxis, guided by chemicals from invading bacteria and local proteins.

The neutrophils have receptors that recognise bacteria and other pathogens (Helbert, 2017). They are essential for the defence against pyogenic (pus-forming) bacteria such as *Staphylococcus* and *Streptococcus*. During an infection, the number of neutrophils will increase rapidly and the blood levels of neutrophils will increase. The rapid production of neutrophils by the bone marrow is further stimulated by colony-stimulating factors released by the tissue macrophages. Neutrophils are highly phagocytic and once they have engulfed the invading microbe, antibacterial enzymes such as lysozyme contained within the cytoplasmic granules are released to destroy it.

Medicine management

Neutrophils have a short lifespan, so conditions affecting bone marrow production – such as ionising radiation, chemotherapy, stem cell transplant or congenital neutropenia – can rapidly cause neutropenia, increasing vulnerability to bacterial and fungal infections.

Treatment may include subcutaneous recombinant human granulocyte colony-stimulating factor (filgrastim), which accelerates neutrophil production and helps protect against life-threatening infections. Common injection sites are the arms, thighs and abdomen, and sites should be rotated with each dose.

Monocytes enter tissues and differentiate into macrophages, which are found throughout the body and are key components of the innate immune system. Their surface receptors recognise different infectious agents, including viruses, bacteria and fungi. Some receptors trigger phagocytosis of the pathogen, while others stimulate the release of cytokines, small, hormone-like molecules that attract neutrophils and activate the adaptive immune response.

During infection, large numbers of monocytes migrate with neutrophils to the affected site and develop into macrophages with enhanced phagocytic abilities, known as inflammatory macrophages. After phagocytosis, further enzyme pathways are activated in an oxidative burst that generates toxic molecules to destroy pathogens.

In chronic granulomatous disease, a rare immune deficiency, this oxidative process cannot occur. Affected children have normal neutrophil numbers and can initiate phagocytosis, but cannot kill the ingested bacteria. They experience recurrent fungal and pyogenic (staphylococcal and streptococcal) infections, such as abscesses, ENT infections and pneumonia and may develop granulomas due to persistent infection (Helbert, 2017).

When phagocytes die at the inflammatory site, they undergo lysis, releasing enzymes into surrounding tissues and contributing to the tissue damage seen in inflammation.

Inflammation

If microbes succeed in getting across these barriers, the innate immune system responds rapidly in an attempt to eliminate them by the process of inflammation and by antiviral mechanisms (Abbas *et al.*, 2024).

Inflammation is the body's non-specific response to tissue damage or injury and forms an essential part of the innate immune system. The role of inflammation is to localise and minimise the tissue damage and to ensure that the specialised cells and molecules that are required to deal with the infectious agent are transported to the correct place to allow healing to take place (Macpherson & Austyn, 2012).

Causes of inflammation

Any type of tissue damage will stimulate the inflammatory response, even if infection is not present. This could be:

- trauma (this includes a cut with a sterile scalpel)
- irritation with chemicals, including extremes of pH
- extreme heat
- infection by pathogens.

Recognition of infection at a peripheral site triggers local inflammation, characterised by redness, heat, swelling and pain. When the infection is short-lived, and the pathogen is quickly eliminated, the process is termed acute inflammation, as seen in conditions such as skin abscesses, otitis media, meningitis and pneumonia.

When infection persists and microbes remain in the tissues, inflammation continues and causes more extensive damage; this is termed chronic inflammation. It occurs in wound and bone infections and in deep-seated infections of internal organs, such as a liver abscess, which can be life-threatening. In some cases, the body cannot eliminate the pathogen, as in tuberculosis. Mycobacterium tuberculosis may survive for months or years, leading to granuloma formation, where specialised macrophages cluster around the organism to contain it.

Inflammation at the site of infection can also affect more distant sites, and this is known as the systemic effects of infection. This leads to the rise in temperature (pyrexia), loss of appetite and malaise associated with an infection.

The inflammatory process

When an injury, either from trauma or infection, occurs, mast cells that are present in the connective tissue release the inflammatory mediators histamine and serotonin. These substances act on the blood vessels, causing vasodilatation (an increase in the diameter), which increases the blood flow to the affected area, providing oxygen and nutrients for the cellular activity that takes place. There are also changes within the endothelial cells of the blood vessels where the adhesiveness is increased. This allows the increased number of leukocytes that have been recruited to the area as part of the inflammatory response to enter the inflamed area (Murphy *et al.*, 2022). The increased blood flow causes the heat and redness associated with the inflammatory response.

The inflammatory mediators also make the blood vessels more permeable and, in conjunction with the increased blood flow, allow fluid from the plasma in the blood to leak out of the capillaries into the surrounding tissues. The fluid contains plasma proteins, including antibodies and clotting factors. This increases the osmotic pressure within tissues, drawing more fluid out of the blood vessels, which forms swelling within the tissue called oedema.

Other plasma proteins are activated during the inflammatory process; these include the kinins and the complement system, as well as the antibodies and clotting factors. Kinins affect the dilation and permeability of the blood vessels and also form bradykinin, which, with prostaglandins, stimulates pain nerve fibres. The complement system consists of soluble proteins circulating in blood, becoming activated when in contact with foreign cells such as bacteria and fungi. They also cause vasodilation and attract the phagocytic cells (neutrophils and macrophages) to the affected areas by chemotaxis (release of chemicals to attract them). Another function of the complement is to enhance the process of phagocytosis by opsonisation, where the microbes are coated with complement and are directed to specialised receptors on the phagocytes, which increases their uptake and elimination by the phagocytes. Complement seems to be particularly effective against pyogenic (pus-forming) bacteria such as *Streptococcus pyogenes* and *Staphylococcus aureus,* and children who have a genetic defect in their ability to produce complement are very susceptible to these infections. Complement deficiency may also contribute to autoimmune diseases such as systemic lupus erythematosus and other immune deficiencies (Abbas *et al.*, 2024; Helbert, 2017).

The clotting factors are stimulated to arrive at the site of inflammation and migrate through the permeable cell walls of the blood vessels, where they start to produce fibrin. This forms an insoluble mesh within the tissue space, which helps to localise the infected area and trap the invading bacteria and prevent the spread of infection. See Figs. 5.5 and 5.6.

Wound healing and abscess formation

Acute inflammation causes tissue damage; an important part of inflammation is to stimulate the process of repair and healing (Macpherson & Austyn, 2012). Where there has been minimal destruction of tissue (e.g., when there has been a cut in a surgical incision), healing takes place by primary healing (also called first intention). Wounds heal by tissue regeneration and repair. Generally, in children, wounds will heal quickly and require minimal intervention (Jonas *et al.*, 2012).

Platelets adhere to the cut surfaces; a blood clot is formed and stabilised by the fibrin laid down with cell

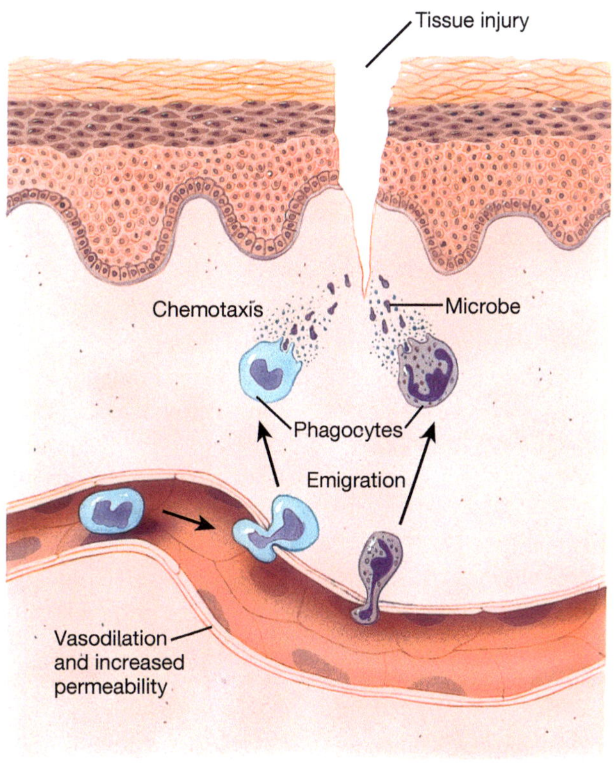

FIGURE 5.5 Inflammation and the stages that occur.
Source: Reproduced with permission of Peate and Gormley-Fleming (2025)/John Wiley & Sons.

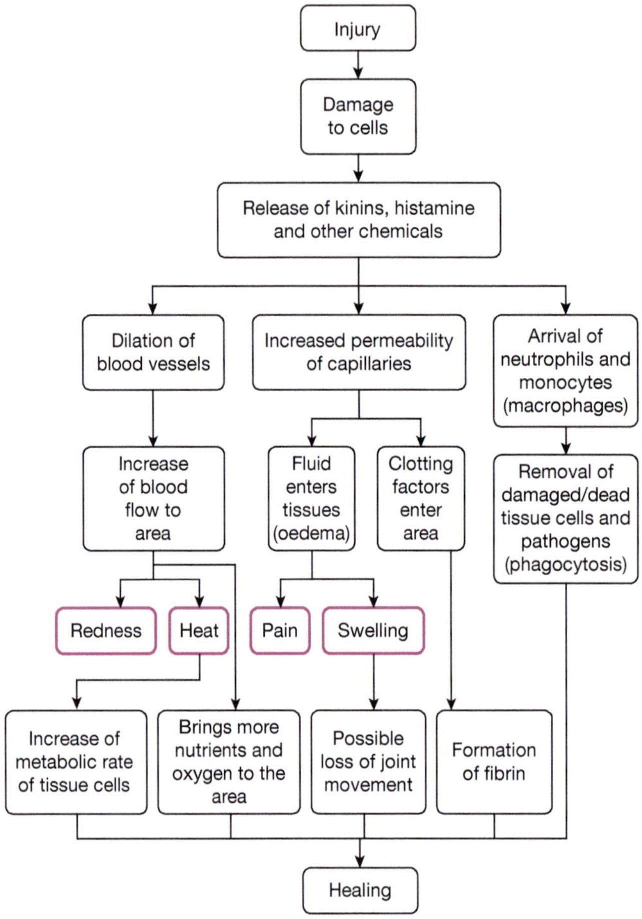

FIGURE 5.6 Flowchart of inflammatory events.
Source: Peate and Gormley-Fleming (2025)/John Wiley & Sons.

debris filling other spaces. Monocytes move into the area and differentiate into inflammatory macrophages, and they begin to remove the cell debris by ingesting and digesting the damaged cells (Marieb and Keller 2022). They also stimulate the production of fibroblasts, which form collagen and other connective tissue within the inflamed area, bringing wound margins together.

If the inflammation is caused by infection, the tissue damage is more extensive with increased recruitment of neutrophils and macrophages. The healing of the affected area may be delayed with increased formation of collagen and scarring of the tissue, known as healing by second intention. As part of the inflammatory process, there may be separation of necrotic (dead) tissue from healthy tissue due to the action of phagocytes within the inflammatory exudate, which is known as slough. Fig. 5.7 demonstrates the stages of wound healing.

Acute inflammatory reactions to extracellular bacteria result in the formation of pus. These extracellular bacteria are known as pyogenic (pus-forming) and exist and multiply in extracellular tissues and fluids. Some of these bacteria include: *Staphylococcus aureus,* which causes skin abscesses; *Streptococcus pyogenes,* which causes throat infections; *Haemophilus influenzae* and *Streptococcus pneumoniae,* which cause respiratory infections.

A collection of pus within a cavity is called an abscess. Superficial abscesses often form under the skin – for example, a boil is pus within an infected hair follicle. These superficial abscesses may rupture spontaneously and discharge pus onto the skin surface. Deeper abscesses may also rupture but release only part of the pus, leaving an open, infected channel or sinus. Figure 5.8 shows a pilonidal sinus.

Abscesses can rupture into adjacent organs, forming a channel open at both ends called a fistula. In some

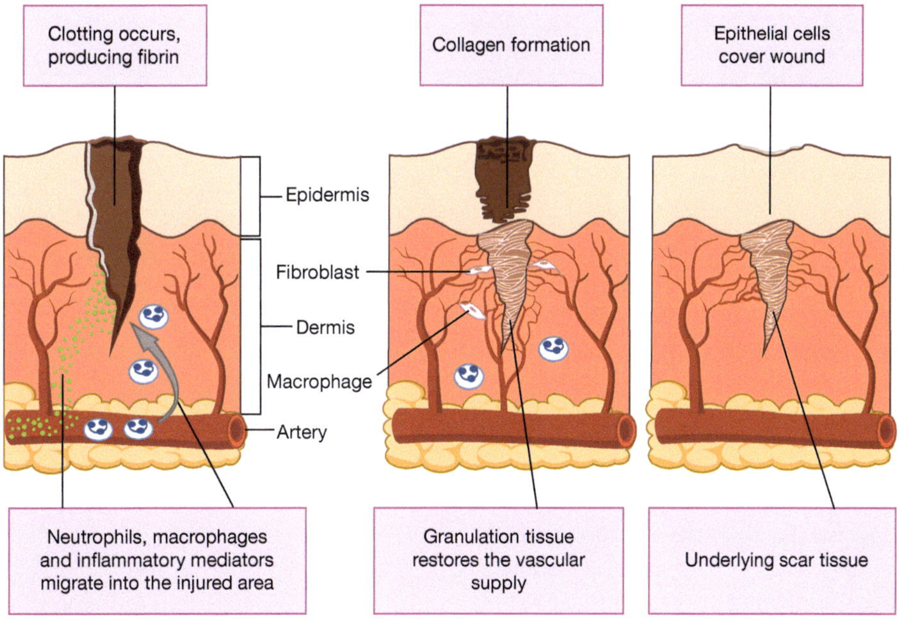

FIGURE 5.7 Stages of wound healing.

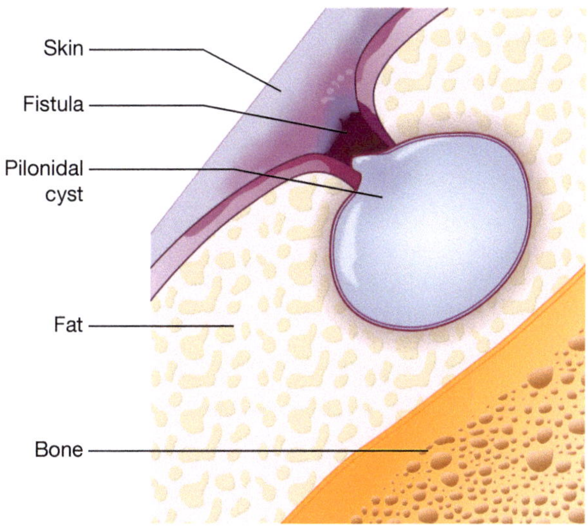

FIGURE 5.8 Diagram to show pilonidal abscess.
Source: Google images/Unknown.

chronic infections, abscesses may be encased in fibrous tissue, forming granulomas that contain live pathogens, as seen in tuberculosis.

Wounds

Jonas *et al.* (2012) describe the following types of wounds commonly seen in children:

- Cuts from accidental and non-accidental injuries
- Animal bites
- Burns and scalds
- Surgical wounds
- Pressure-related, which can be from equipment (e.g., saturation probe) or in relation to a child's immobility
- Extravasation following intravenous fluid and drug administration
- Congenital abnormalities, e.g., epidermis bullosa.

When assessing a child's wound, the nurse should consider its size, location and underlying cause. Other factors include the stage of healing and any exudate, infection, slough or necrosis. The child's pain should be assessed, and analgesia given before dressing changes as needed.

Systemic effects of inflammation

Generally, the inflammatory process will contain the infection within the local area. The effects of this response may also be felt systemically, and the child who has an infection can feel unwell with a fever, headache, muscle pains and loss of appetite. This response is due to the release of cytokines, which are proteins that act as chemical messengers affecting the functions of the immune cells (Murphy, Weaver & Berg, 2022). Some of these will stimulate the inflammatory response and affect the endothelial cell changes, resulting in increased permeability of the blood vessels and the recruitment of neutrophils and macrophages discussed earlier. Others affect wound healing and tissue repair, and some cytokines enter the bloodstream and act on distant tissues, such as the bone marrow, the liver and the hypothalamus in the brain.

The main cytokines involved in these systemic effects are interleukin (IL)-1 and IL-6 and tissue necrosis factor (TNF). Their effects are summarised in Fig. 5.9. They affect the hypothalamus in the brain, resetting the temperature-regulating centre to cause the rise in temperature associated with a fever (Helbert, 2017). These cytokines are sometimes called endogenous pyrogens. The increased temperature inhibits the action of the invading pathogens and also enhances the adaptive immune response (Murphy *et al.*, 2022).

Feverish illness is very common in young children, particularly in the under-5 age group, and it is the most common reason for parents to seek medical advice. In most cases, the fever is due to a self-limiting viral infection, but it may also be indicative of a more serious bacterial infection, such as meningitis, pneumonia or a urinary tract infection (NICE, 2021). It is important that children are assessed rapidly and receive the appropriate treatment. Recent guidelines from NICE provide a traffic light system to assist health professionals in this assessment.

Recording temperature in children

For children aged 4 weeks to 5 years, NICE guidance (2021) recommends measuring temperature using:

- Electronic thermometer in the axilla
- Chemical dot thermometer in the axilla
- Infrared tympanic thermometer

For infants under 4 weeks, an electronic axillary thermometer is preferred. Parental reports of fever should always be taken seriously. Routine assessment of a febrile child should also include heart rate, respiratory rate and capillary refill time (NICE, 2021; RCN, 2013).

When assessing a child, other considerations include:

- **Age:** Infants under 3 months may present with non-specific signs such as poor feeding, drowsiness or irritability, and may have bacterial infections not detectable on examination.

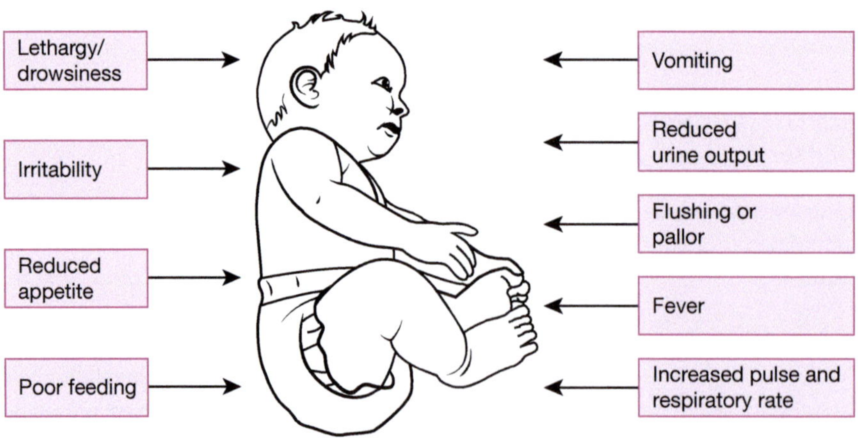

FIGURE 5.9 Diagram to show systemic signs of infection.

- Illness in family members
- Immunisation status
- Recent travel abroad
- History of recent infections, which may suggest immunodeficiency
- Rashes, which may accompany fever or indicate specific conditions (e.g., meningococcal meningitis)
- Evidence of a focus of infection, such as otitis media or abscess.

Investigations for a febrile child with a suspected infection include:

- **Blood tests:** Full blood count with differential and inflammatory markers (CRP and ESR)
- Blood cultures to identify the infecting organism
- Urine sample
- Other investigations as indicated by symptoms, such as chest X-ray, lumbar puncture or wound swabs

The effect of the cytokines on the bone marrow is the increased production of white blood cells (leucocytosis) to produce neutrophils and macrophages, which migrate to the site of infection.

Sepsis and septic shock

In severe infections, bacterial toxins are released into the blood, and the activation of the innate immune system can cause an overwhelming response leading to septic shock. Activation of the cytokines and other inflammatory mediators in high concentrations can cause vasodilation, increased permeability of the capillaries, affecting the venous flow to the heart. This results in hypotension and multi-organ failure and is life-threatening.

Sepsis leading to septic shock is a medical emergency and is recognised as the leading cause of death in all age groups (NICE, 2024a). The importance of rapid assessment of a child with suspected sepsis cannot be overemphasised. Guidance from NICE (2024a) ensures that health professionals use the traffic light system in the assessment of the acutely ill child and have protocols in place for the management of patients with meningitis and meningococcal septicaemia, neonatal infection and neutropaenic sepsis (see also NICE, 2020).

Risk factors contributing to the onset of sepsis and septic shock are:

- Age: Preterm infants and children under 1 year due to immature immunity
- Impaired immune function: e.g., neutropenia after cytotoxic therapy or immunodeficiency
- Critical illness or injury
- Indwelling central venous catheters for fluids or parenteral nutrition
- Invasive procedures, such as cannulation
- Surgical incisions and wounds
- Burns
- Long-term antibiotic therapy
- Chronic illness

Acquired immunity

The innate immune system provides an immediate response to any invading organism and often is sufficient to eliminate it. However, the immune system is also able to respond to specific organisms and destroy them. This specific immunity involves the B and T lymphocytes and their ability to recognise an antigen. Antigens are foreign molecules found on the surfaces of pathogenic organisms, toxins, cancer cells, transfused blood cells, transplanted tissues, foods and pollens. Receptors on the lymphocytes recognise these antigens, and the cells of the adaptive immune system are activated. Specialised antigen-presenting cells (APCs) found in the epithelia of the skin (dendritic cells), gastrointestinal, respiratory and genitourinary tracts capture the antigens, transport them to the lymph tissue and organs and present them to the lymphocytes (Abbas *et al.*, 2024).

B and T lymphocytes are found in the lymphoid organs, which consist of the lymph nodes, the spleen and the specialised mucosal lymphoid tissue found in the gastrointestinal and respiratory tracts. Examples include Peyer's patches, the appendix and adenoids and tonsils (see Fig. 5.1).

T lymphocytes

Immature T lymphocytes undergo a maturation process within the thymus gland prior to their migration to the lymph tissue. The thymus is situated in the chest area in the upper anterior thorax, just above the heart. It is a relatively large organ in babies and grows until puberty, when it begins to atrophy; by adulthood, there is only a very small amount of tissue left (Helbert, 2017).

During this process, the T lymphocytes learn to recognise the body's own cells and differentiate self from non-self. Non-self cells include cancer cells, transplanted cells and pathogens. Lymphocytes need to be exposed initially to the foreign proteins on the cell membrane to recognise the antigen. Once the T lymphocytes have matured, they migrate to the lymph nodes and spleen, and will activate when exposed to that specific antigen by the antigen-presenting cells that have been activated during the innate immune response. This is known as cell-mediated immunity. A summary of the T-cell functions is shown in Table 5.2.

The B lymphocytes, like the T lymphocytes, are initially produced by the bone marrow, but unlike the T cells, they mature in the bone marrow before being released into the blood. The B cells have specialised surface receptors to antigens, and when exposed to that antigen with the help of an activated helper T cell, they stimulate the B cells to grow and multiply rapidly by a process called cloning. Two types of mature B cells are produced – plasma cells secreting antibodies and memory cells circulating in the blood – and when they meet the antigen again, they can rapidly start to produce plasma cells.

Antibodies are soluble proteins that circulate in the blood and are produced as a response to a specific antigen; using a lock and key analogy, the structure of the antibody matches that of the antigen (Tortora & Derrickson, 2017). The functions of the antibodies are summarised in Table 5.3.

TABLE 5.2 T-cell functions

Cytotoxic T cells	Destroy and kill abnormal cells, e.g., virus-infected cells, cancer cells and cells of transplanted tissue. Bind to foreign cells, release enzymes, causing the cell to be destroyed by apoptosis.
Helper T cells	When activated, act on innate and adaptive immune system. Release cytokines which stimulate the production of B lymphocytes and cytotoxic T cells. Recruit neutrophils and phagocytic cells to the site of the infection.
Regulatory T cells	Suppress activity of B and T lymphocytes, which stops the immune response once the antigen is destroyed. Prevents overactivity of the immune system.
Memory T cells	Antigen-specific memory cells that reactivate rapidly when exposed to the same antigen.

TABLE 5.3 Functions of antibodies

Antibody	Function
IgA	Present in body secretions and mucosal surfaces, e.g., saliva, tears, sweat, nasal secretions and breast milk. Provides localised protection from bacteria and viruses. Provides protection in the neonatal period from gastrointestinal infections.
IgD	Found on the surface of B cells and activates B cells.
IgE	Found on the surfaces of mast cells and basophils. Activation of mast cells when an antigen binding to IgE triggers the release of histamine and initiates the inflammatory response. Responsible for allergic reactions when present in excess.
IgG	Most prevalent antibody in serum. Can pass through placenta, providing maternal protection to the newborn infant. Neutralises bacterial toxins and prevents attachment of some viruses to body cells. Activates the complement system. Opsonisation of antigen for phagocytosis.
IgM	Most predominate immunoglobulin in early phase of the immune response. Causes agglutination of bacteria and activation of complement.

Primary and secondary responses to infection

The immune response following the first encounter with an antigen is the *primary response*. This initial exposure results in a delay in the production of antibodies known as the lag phase, as the T lymphocytes are activated and stimulate the production of the B lymphocytes. One of the special features of the adaptive immune system is its ability to respond to future encounters with a known antigen, known as immunological memory, as a result of the newly formed memory B cells. On subsequent exposure to the antigen, the immune response is much faster and more powerful, ensuring that the antigen is destroyed effectively, known as the *secondary response* to infection (see Fig. 5.10).

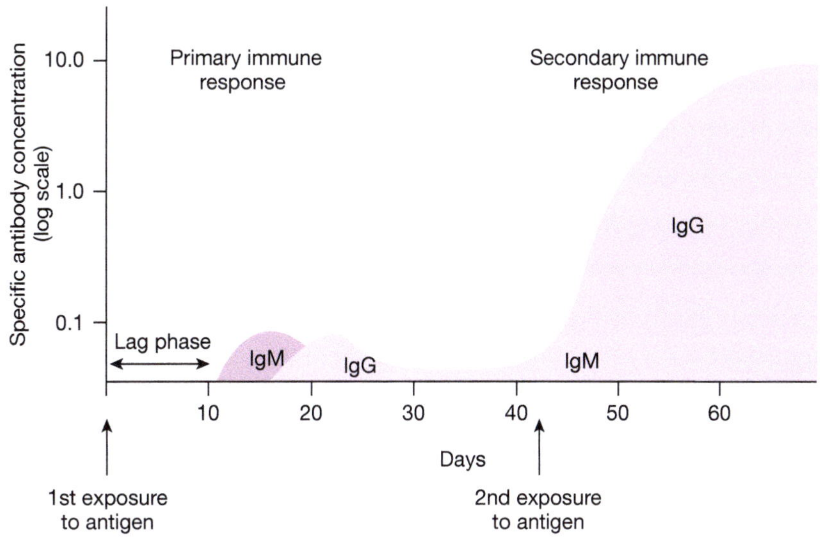

FIGURE 5.10 Primary and secondary responses to infection.
Source: Peate and Gormley-Fleming (2025)/with permission of John Wiley & Sons.

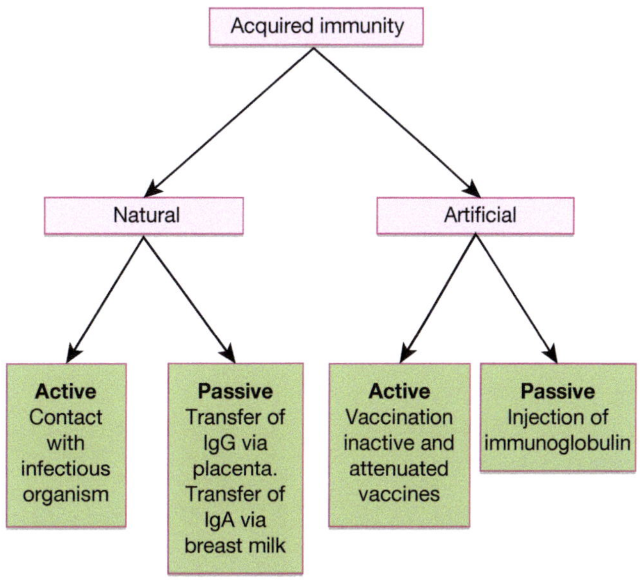

FIGURE 5.11 Acquired (specific) immunity.
Source: Reproduced with permission of Peate and Gormley-Fleming (2025)/John Wiley & Sons.

Immunity can be acquired actively by the individual's response to an antigen and production of antibodies, or passively by the transfer of antibodies to the host. In both types of immunity, this can be acquired naturally or artificially.

A newborn baby acquires passive immunity naturally by the transfer of maternal IgG through the placenta and IgA in the colostrum of breast milk. A child with immunodeficiency who receives an infusion or injection of antibodies will acquire immunity artificially by passive immunisation (see Fig. 5.11).

Natural active immunity is acquired by the body's response to infection. Immunisation with vaccines provides artificially acquired active immunity by allowing immunological memory to develop without a primary infection (Helbert, 2017). Vaccines contain small amounts of the infective organism that are inactivated (killed) or attenuated (weakened) live organisms; this is sufficient to stimulate an immune response without causing disease. Vaccination against communicable diseases is an essential part of public health programmes, and children will receive their vaccinations as part of the current vaccination schedule (United Kingdom Health Security Agency, 2025).

Routine childhood immunisation uptake has declined in the United Kingdom, with some areas falling well below the WHO target of 95% needed for herd immunity. This has contributed to recent measles outbreaks (UK Health Security Agency, 2024).

Alterations in immunity and inflammation

The immune system provides a complex network of mechanisms to protect the individual from foreign antigens, particularly infectious agents. However, at times, this ability to protect the individual is compromised, and there may be an inappropriate immune response. These can include reactions to environmental antigens such as pollen (allergy), against the body's own cells (autoimmunity), against foreign tissue and cells in transplantation and blood transfusion, and deficiency or abnormal function of the immune system (Brashers, 2023). The result of these reactions can be serious or life-threatening, as demonstrated in the COVID-19 pandemic in 2019, where the inflammatory responses to the virus were the cause of the significant morbidity rather than the damage caused by the virus itself (Abbas *et al.*, 2024).

An excessive immune response is described as a hypersensitivity reaction (Helbert, 2017). This is further categorised by the types of immune response involved (Table 5.4). In each type of hypersensitivity reaction, the response is made by the adaptive immune system and previous exposure to the antigen (sensitisation) is required

TABLE 5.4 Types of hypersensitivity reaction

Type of hypersensitivity	Antigen	Onset	Immune response	Characteristics of reaction
Type I Immediate hypersensitivity	Pollen, house dust mite, foods, e.g., cow's milk protein, peanut, insect venom	Rapid – can occur within seconds of exposure	IgE-mediated Degranulation of mast cells and eosinophils, resulting in release of immune mediators such as histamine	Allergy Hay fever Eczema Asthma Anaphylaxis (severe reaction)
Type II Tissue-specific hypersensitivity	Cell expressing foreign antigen	Rapid onset	IgG reacts with antigen and interacts with complement and phagocytes	Autoimmunity, e.g., rheumatoid arthritis Haemolytic disease of the newborn Blood transfusion reactions
Type III Immune complex hypersensitivity	Formation of immune complex with antigen and antibody	Onset within hours	Immune complexes deposited at site of production or circulated interacting with complement and neutrophils, causing tissue damage	Glomerulonephritis Vasculitis Penicillin allergy
Type IV Delayed hypersensitivity	Pathogen, e.g., hepatitis B virus, *Mycobacterium tuberculosis* Environmental allergen, chemicals, plant extracts, e.g., poison ivy	Days	T-cell response to antigen in conjunction with macrophages can also be associated with presentation of human leukocyte antigen (HLA)	Tuberculin skin testing Contact dermatitis, e.g., nickel allergy Graft and transplant rejection

for the reaction to occur. The reactions can be immediate (minutes or a few hours), as seen in allergies, or delayed (up to several days), depending on the time of re-exposure to the antigen.

Allergy (type I hypersensitivity)

The incidence of allergy is increasing, with approximately 1 in 4 individuals affected in the United Kingdom; half are children (Allergy UK, 2025). There is a familial association and individuals who are susceptible are said to be atopic. A child can develop an allergy in isolation, but there is also evidence that children who are predisposed to allergy can develop allergic disorders at different times. For example, an infant can develop atopic eczema, then develop food allergies as a toddler and rhinitis and asthma may then develop in early childhood. This is referred to as the allergic march (Helbert, 2017) (see Fig. 5.12).

Allergy is an immediate IgE-mediated hypersensitivity reaction, triggered by antigens called allergens. Allergens enter the body through ingestion, inhalation, drugs or insect bites. Exposure rapidly increases IgE, which binds to mast cells in tissues – mainly the gastrointestinal tract, respiratory tract and skin. Symptoms depend on the route of entry. Histamine release causes smooth muscle constriction, vasodilation and increased vascular permeability, leading to fluid and protein exudation. Table 5.5 lists allergic diseases affecting children.

Fig. 5.13 describes a range of allergic symptoms.

Care of a child with allergy

Once a child has been diagnosed with an allergy, a written individualised care plan must be provided for the child and their family. This outlines the symptoms of mild, moderate and severe reactions, and the appropriate treatment (see British Society for Allergy & Clinical Immunology; www.bsaci.org).

Avoiding allergens can help minimise allergic reactions. For children with asthma triggered by house dust mites, allergen-proof covers on mattresses, pillows and duvets; washing bedding at 60 °C; removing carpets and vacuuming with a high-filtration vacuum can reduce exposure.

Children with a food allergy should avoid the trigger and may need supervision by a paediatric dietician. Early recognition and treatment of symptoms can prevent more severe reactions.

> **Growth and development**
>
> Guidance on the introduction of foods when weaning an infant that may cause allergy is to introduce foods one at a time in small quantities, and if tolerated, to continue these foods as part of the normal diet to minimise the risk of an allergy developing. In addition, the introduction of egg and peanut should not be delayed beyond 6–12 months, as there is evidence that this increases the risk of an allergy developing (Anaphylaxis UK, 2020; NHS, 2025).

The plan should also include details of any medication, any emergency treatment in the event of a further reaction, together with advice and support for the child's nursery and school. Drugs that are used in the treatment of allergy include

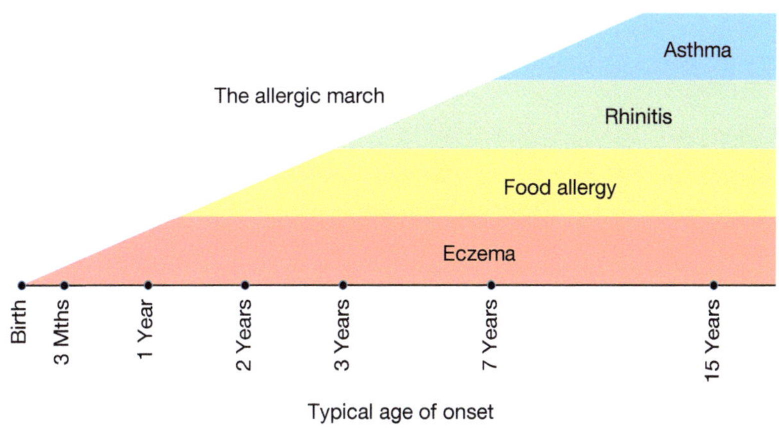

FIGURE 5.12 Diagram of the allergic march.

TABLE 5.5 Allergic diseases that affect children

Allergic diseases	Allergen	Symptoms
Food allergy	Peanuts, tree nuts, cow's milk, eggs, fish, shellfish, legumes, wheat, seeds and fruits	Increased peristalsis causes diarrhoea and vomiting May also be associated with urticaria, angioedema and anaphylaxis (see later)
Allergic rhinitis and conjunctivitis associated with hay fever	Pollens from trees and grasses Fungal spores and moulds House dust mite	Inflammation of mucous membranes of nasal passages and eyes, and production of excessive mucus Sneezing, discharge and nasal obstruction
Asthma	Tree, grass and weed pollens House dust mite Fungal spores and moulds Animal dander	Constriction of the bronchi with excessive production of mucus, oedema and swelling of the respiratory mucosa causing wheezing, coughing and breathlessness
Urticaria or hives	Food and drug reactions Also associated with exposure to temperature, stress and other systemic diseases	Localised release of histamine and increased vascular permeability result in the formation of fluid-filled blisters (wheals) surrounded by areas of redness (flares)
Atopic eczema	Associated with food allergies such as egg, and family history of atopy	Atopic eczema is associated with IgE antibodies to allergens. A genetic defect in the skin barrier increases susceptibility to inflammation and allows allergens and bacteria to interact with the immune system
Insect sting hypersensitivity	Insect venom	Mild to moderate reactions involve swelling and urticaria Severe reactions can be systemic with wheeze and anaphylaxis

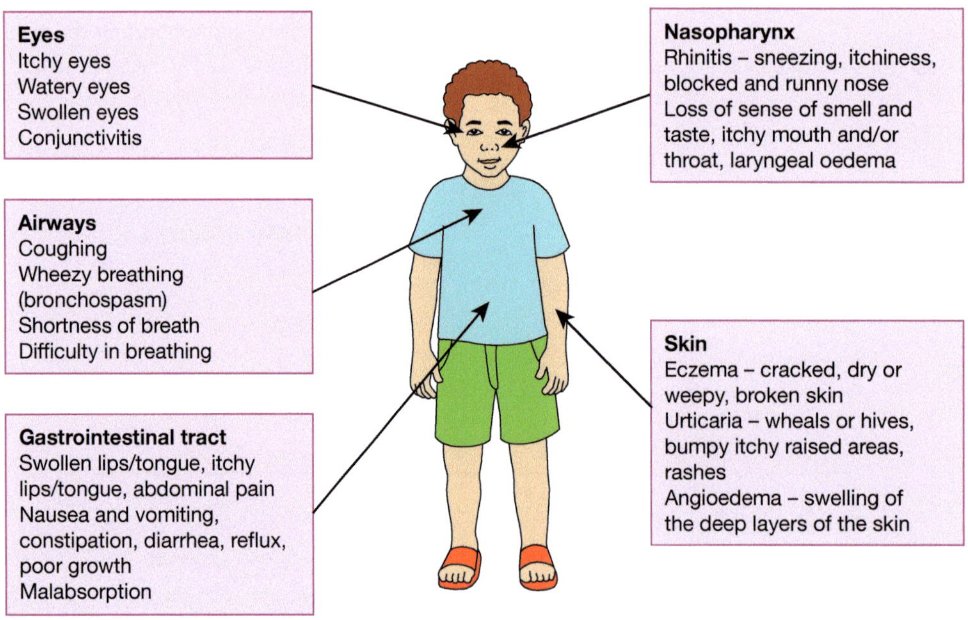

FIGURE 5.13 An overview of allergic symptoms.

antihistamines that block specific histamine receptors. Non-sedating antihistamines are the treatment of choice. Oral histamines are effective in the treatment of nasal allergies and hay fever, and for mild to moderate allergic reactions to food. Corticosteroids are effective in allergic reactions and can prevent the immediate hypersensitivity reaction and also help prevent chronic allergic inflammation (Helbert, 2017). They are used topically, for example, hydrocortisone cream in eczema, and inhaled in the treatment of asthma. Sodium cromoglycate can also be used topically as eye drops and nasal cream in the treatment of allergic rhinitis. For those children who have a severe allergic reaction with respiratory and cardiovascular involvement (anaphylaxis), intramuscular epinephrine (adrenaline) should be administered.

Anaphylaxis

Anaphylaxis is the most severe form of type I hypersensitivity with a systemic reaction resulting in angioedema, affecting the larynx, causing airway obstruction and hypoxia, bronchoconstriction, vasodilation and a decrease in blood pressure. This can be life-threatening without prompt treatment and is a result of widespread mast cell degranulation due to the systemic presentation of the allergen. The most common allergens to cause anaphylaxis in children are foods, but other triggers include insect stings, drugs and latex, and it can also be exercise-induced. The majority of anaphylaxis in children occurs in those under the age of 5 years and is linked to food allergy. However, there is an increased incidence of anaphylaxis fatality in adolescence associated with nut allergy and asthma (Tanno & Demoly, 2020). A child who experiences anaphylaxis may present with facial swelling and symptoms of difficulty in swallowing or speaking, severe asthma, abdominal pain, nausea and vomiting, feeling dizzy due to the drop in blood pressure, which can rapidly progress to loss of consciousness (see Anaphylaxis Campaign; www.anaphylaxis.org.uk/).

Care of a child with anaphylaxis

Management of suspected anaphylaxis in a child is an emergency. It may occur at home, in community settings (e.g., nurseries, schools and immunisation clinics), or during drug administration, such as intravenous antibiotics. Early recognition is essential. Children's community nurses administering medication at home should carry an anaphylaxis pack, and all staff in clinical areas should know the location of emergency resuscitation equipment and medications.

It is important to recognise that the child is seriously unwell and seek emergency medical treatment urgently. Early treatment with the administration of intramuscular epinephrine is the treatment of choice for anyone experiencing anaphylaxis (Resuscitation Council, 2021), and if it is available, parents and carers should use it prior to seeking emergency help (Fig. 5.13). Epinephrine stimulates both α and β adrenergic receptors, and this decreases vascular permeability, increases blood pressure and helps to reverse airway obstruction (Helbert, 2017).

On admission to the emergency unit, assessment of the child should follow the **A**irway, **B**reathing, **C**irculation, **D**isability, **E**xposure (ABCDE) approach to recognise potential problems and treat the child. Following administration of the epinephrine, assessment of the child's breathing and circulation should be monitored closely (pulse rate, blood pressure and pulse oximetry) to assess the child's response to the drug. In addition to intramuscular epinephrine, the child may require supportive therapy with oxygen and intravenous fluids and also treatment with antihistamine and steroids. These drugs can assist with the treatment of urticaria and also reduce the chance of further reactions. As discussed earlier, children with allergies may also have asthma, and this should be treated in line with emergency treatment for asthma with bronchodilator therapy (NICE, 2024b) (Fig. 5.14).

A detailed history should identify the allergen causing the anaphylactic reaction. After emergency treatment, the child should be observed for at least 6 hours or admitted if there is a risk of recurrence, history of asthma or asthma symptoms during the reaction. Before discharge, parents should receive advice on allergen avoidance and a written emergency plan. The child may be prescribed an epinephrine autoinjector, with training provided to the family. Follow-up in an allergy clinic is essential to confirm the diagnosis and develop a personalised care plan. Families should also be directed to allergy and anaphylaxis support groups for guidance and support.

An adrenaline autoinjector is a pre-filled, disposable syringe and should be carried at all times. Families need to be reminded to check the expiry date, as the shelf-life of these devices is 1–2 years. It is important to monitor the child's weight as there are two doses of epinephrine: 0.15 mg (for children who are 15–30 kg) and 0.3 mg (over 30 kg). Patients may be prescribed two autoinjectors with advice to administer a second dose after 5 minutes (British National Formulary for Children, 2017).

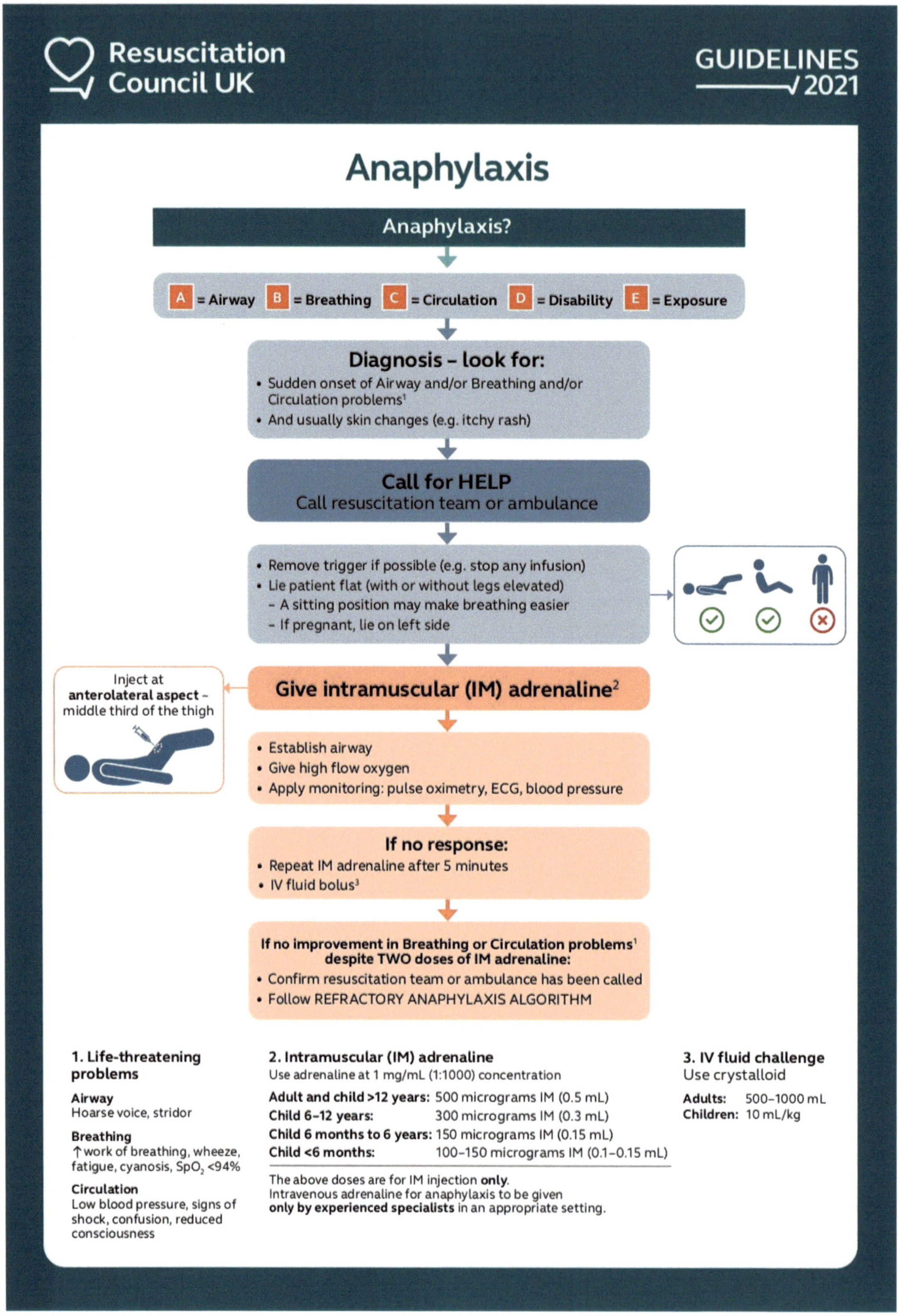

FIGURE 5.14 Emergency treatment of anaphylaxis.

Source: Resuscitation Council UK: 'Emergency treatment of anaphylactic reactions/Resuscitation Council (UK).

Case study: a child with anaphylaxis

A 2-year-old boy is brought into the emergency department by his parents with a history of swelling of the face and eyes and generalised itching with a rash on his chest. His parents have also noted that he has started to wheeze during the journey to the hospital. His parents report that he had taken a bite of his father's peanut butter sandwich and they noticed the facial swelling within minutes.

The paediatric team urgently reviews the child and a suspected diagnosis of a severe allergic reaction is made. He receives intra-muscular epinephrine 0.15 mg and has oxygen administered via a face mask. He is also prescribed chlorphenamine and hydrocortisone and is monitored closely in the emergency department.

His vital signs on admission are:

Vital sign	Observation	Normal range
Temperature	37.2 °C	36.5–37.2 °C
Pulse	135 beats per minute	90–140
Respiratory rate	42 breaths per minute	20–40 breaths per minute
Blood pressure	75/40 mmHg	80–95 mmHg (systolic)
CRT	2 seconds	<2 seconds
Oxygen saturation	100% in oxygen	98–100%
Level of consciousness	Drowsy and responding to voice on the AVPU scale	Alert on the AVPU scale

His PEWS score is 4, his respiratory rate is above the normal range, he has required oxygen and has an inspiratory wheeze and is drowsy.

What explanation can you give for this?

What is the possible significance of his blood pressure recording and why is this not included within the PEWS score?

Following treatment with the epinephrine his condition stabilises quite quickly but he is monitored closely by the nursing staff and is admitted to the paediatric ward as he has had asthma-type symptoms.

What advice and support should the child and family receive prior to discharge the following day?

Autoimmune disease

Autoimmune disease occurs when the adaptive immune system loses its ability to distinguish self from non-self, and the immune cells start to attack the body's own cells, causing tissue damage through hypersensitivity reactions (types II–IV). Factors that are thought to contribute to the development of autoimmunity are:

- **genetic** – autoimmune conditions are often found in members of the same family, e.g., type 1 diabetes mellitus and coeliac disease;
- **environmental triggers** – the disease may not be evident until it is triggered by something, e.g., ultraviolet light in systemic lupus erythematosus and gluten in the diet in coeliac disease;
- **infection** is thought to also play a significant part, and it may be a connection with some or all of these factors that precipitates the inflammatory response associated with these conditions (Helbert, 2017; Abbas *et al.*, 2024);
- **hormones** – there seems to be an increased incidence of autoimmune disease in adolescent girls and young women.

Autoimmune conditions can be either organ-specific, affecting one organ or a specific type of tissue, or systemic (non-organ-specific), where there is widespread tissue damage.

Diagnosis and management of autoimmune disorders

Autoimmune conditions are rare in children and can be difficult to diagnose. Some cause organ-specific symptoms, such as those seen in diabetes or hyperthyroidism, but often children present with non-specific signs like recurring fevers, rashes, fatigue, joint pain and weight loss, requiring further investigation. These conditions may have periods of remission and flare-ups, which can significantly affect the child's school attendance and social activities.

Investigations will include blood tests for full blood count and inflammatory markers – CRP and ESR, and further diagnostic tests to include identification of the presence of autoantibodies and rheumatoid factor. CRP and ESR are abnormal proteins which the body can make when attacking itself, and are serological markers for autoimmune disease. However, these tests must be interpreted in conjunction with the child's presenting symptoms. Other investigations may include magnetic resonance imaging (MRI) and ultrasound in order to examine the organs and tissues more closely. In some cases, biopsy of the affected tissue may assist with diagnosis.

Treatment for autoimmune disease depends on the specific condition and aims to control and suppress disease activity. Organ-specific conditions may be managed with metabolic control, such as insulin for type 1 diabetes or thyroxine for hypothyroidism. In conditions like rheumatoid arthritis, biological therapies using monoclonal antibodies have proven highly effective (Isenberg & Mahto, 2021).

Transfusion reactions

Red blood cells have antigens expressed on the surface of their cells and form the basis of the ABO blood groups (see Peate & Gormley-Fleming, 2025). IgM antibodies against the red cell antigens are produced as natural antibodies and are present in the plasma. This means that an individual with blood group A has anti-B antibodies, group B has anti-A antibodies, group AB has no antibodies and group O has both anti-A and anti-B antibodies. If a child who is group A receives blood from a group B donor, the donor erythrocytes will be destroyed by activation of complement and opsonisation of the donor cell. This occurs extremely rapidly and is a type II hypersensitivity reaction; the resulting cytokine release can cause severe shock and is potentially fatal. Prior to a transfusion, a sample of the child's blood should be cross-matched with the donor blood to ensure compatibility.

The other consideration is the rhesus (Rh) D factor, where individuals are classified as Rh positive or negative depending on whether they express the Rh system antigen on the erythrocytes. Unlike the ABO group natural antibodies, Rh antigens are not normally produced, but a Rh-negative mother and a Rh-positive father may produce a Rh-positive foetus. This does not cause problems during a first pregnancy, but during delivery, there may be mixing of foetal and maternal blood so that exposure occurs to a foreign antigen for the mother, and IgG anti-Rh antibody is formed. In a subsequent pregnancy with another Rh-positive foetus, the IgG antibody will cross the placenta into the foetal circulation causing destruction of the foetal red blood cells. This can cause death in utero or haemolytic disease of the newborn (Macpherson & Austyn, 2012). Treatment for haemolytic disease of the newborn is an exchange transfusion with blood that is cross-matched with that of the mother. This condition can be prevented by giving the mother anti-D antibody, which destroys the Rh-positive foetal cells before the mother can make her own before and after delivery (Helbert, 2017).

Immune responses against transplantation

Transplanting tissue or cells from one person to another has greatly improved outcomes for children with cancer, primary immune deficiencies and organ failure. However, foreign tissue can trigger an immune response, leading to transplant rejection. This is a normal reaction when a transplant takes place between genetically non-identical individuals of the same species and is known as allogenic. It occurs when the T lymphocytes of the recipient react against the antigens on the donor cells, which are called transplant antigens. The most significant of these are the major histocompatibility complex molecules (MHC), which are crucial for the presentation of antigen to T cells in the adaptive immune response. The MHC molecules in humans are known as human leukocyte antigens (HLAs).

In order to minimise the possibility of rejection during transplantation of tissue, for example, solid organ transplantation such as kidney or cells (stem cell transplant), the donor and recipient should be tissue typed for ABO compatibility and also for HLA, as matching the donor and recipient will increase the chances of a successful acceptance of the graft (Brashers, 2023). Ideally, a sibling donor will provide the greatest chance of a compatible donor, and there is a 1:4 chance that a sibling will be an identical match on tissue typing. One of the major complications of stem cell transplantation is graft-versus-host disease (GVHD), which occurs when the T cells of the donor respond to antigens of the recipient. This can result in effects on the skin (skin rashes), the gastrointestinal tract (diarrhoea and vomiting), the liver (jaundice) and the lungs.

To maximise the success of organ or stem cell transplantation, children require immunosuppressive treatment. This increases their risk of infection, so they should be nursed in a single room in the hospital, avoid contact with infected individuals at home, and steer clear of crowded places and public transport. Parents should seek urgent medical advice if the child develops a fever or has been exposed to measles or chickenpox, as specific immunoglobulin may be needed. Live vaccines should be avoided during immunosuppressive treatment.

Immune deficiency

Immune deficiencies result from defects in the immune system, leading to increased susceptibility to infection. Young children normally have an immature immune system and may experience several infections. However, severe, persistent, unusual or recurrent infections should prompt investigation for immune deficiency. These can be:

- Primary immunodeficiency (PID) where one or more components of the immune system are not working due to a genetic abnormality. These are rare conditions that can result in severe, life-threatening infections.
- Secondary immunodeficiency where the immune deficiency is acquired as a result of other factors, such as infection, medical treatments, nutritional defects and exposure to environmental toxins. These are much more common than primary immunodeficiency.

Primary immunodeficiency

Primary immunodeficiency conditions are caused by genetic defects and can be inherited as X-linked or autosomal recessive disorders. There may also be a history of parental consanguinity and a family history of unexplained death of children – usually boys (Helbert, 2017) (see Fig. 5.15). However, in many cases, the genetic cause may not be inherited but a result of a sporadic genetic mutation. There are over 450 different PID conditions, and they can present with a wide range of symptoms that can vary in their severity (Immunodeficiency UK, 2025).

Care and management of a child with primary immunodeficiency

The diagnosis of PID can take place after admission to hospital with a serious life-threatening infection or following recurrent infections that are persistent or severe or caused by unusual microorganisms. A full history from the child's parents is important to establish the history of infections, family history and presentation of symptoms. A physical examination is also carried out, including a record of the child's weight and height, as the child may often present with a failure to gain weight or grow normally (Immunodeficiency UK, 2025).

Investigations include blood tests that help to identify the immune deficiency. These include:

- full blood count – gives total number of red cells, white blood cells and platelets;
- white cell differentiation – quantifies number of lymphocytes, granulocytes and monocytes;

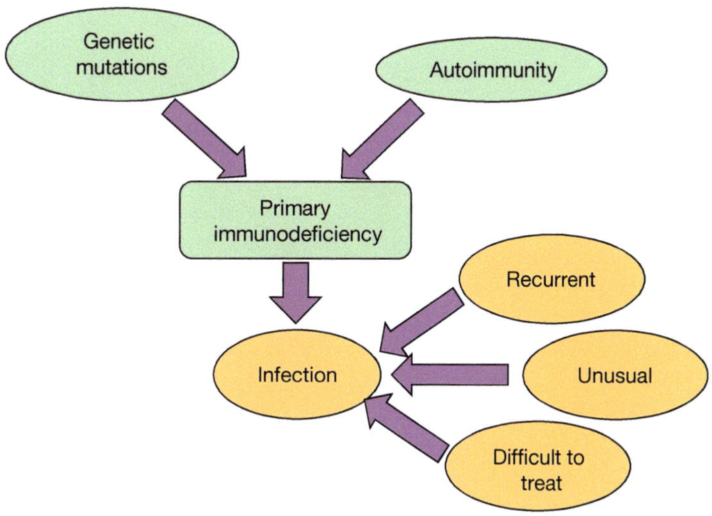

FIGURE 5.15 Features of primary immunodeficiency.
Source: Helbert (2017)/with permission of Elsevier.

- lymphocyte subsets – quantifies number of T and B lymphocytes, which can identify whether the defect is in B or T lymphocyte;
- serum immunoglobulin levels – quantifies the amount of circulating antibody (IgG, IgA and IgM);
- specific antibody reactions – antibody reactions to vaccines (pneumococcus, *Haemophilus influenzae*, tetanus and measles), which can determine the IgG response by B lymphocytes;
- other blood tests may be carried out for phagocyte function, complement and genetic testing for known mutations in PID, and to exclude secondary immunodeficiency.

The severity and type of antibody deficiency will determine the treatment for children diagnosed with PID. Children who have mild antibody deficiency may receive prophylactic antibiotic therapy; they also receive an early intervention of an alternative antibiotic therapy in the event of an infection. For those children who have a more severe antibody deficiency, replacement immunoglobulin treatment is needed. The immunoglobulin provides antibodies against a wide range of pathogens and is obtained from pooled plasma donations (Helbert, 2017). This is known as artificially acquired passive immunity. Replacement immunoglobulin can be administered intravenously or subcutaneously and is normally a lifelong treatment. Diagnosis and treatment may take place in specialist centres, which can add to the stress encountered by the families if they have long distances to travel. Once treatment is established, home therapy treatment for the child under the supervision of a specialist nurse can be initiated.

Consideration

The dosage of immunoglobulin replacement treatment is prescribed according to the weight of the child, so it is important to monitor the weight and height of the child during outpatient visits to ensure optimum dosage.

Secondary immunodeficiency

Immunodeficiencies that are not caused by a genetic defect are secondary or acquired (Macpherson & Austyn, 2012). Secondary immunodeficiencies can cause the same types of infections as PID, depending on which part of the immune system is affected. They are more common than PID and can be related to many factors, such as age of the child, cancer, drugs, nutrition, infection and surgery (see Fig. 5.16).

Special consideration

Stigma around HIV remains significant, and many parents find it difficult to discuss the diagnosis with their child. Children and families receive medical, psychological and social support in specialist multidisciplinary clinics. It is important that children and young people understand their condition to make informed decisions about treatment and safer sex as they mature. Patient support groups, such as CHIVA, provide information and guidance for children, young people and families.

Case study: a child with appendicitis

An 8-year-old girl, Renuka, was admitted to the emergency department with 12 hours of abdominal pain and vomiting. Examination revealed tenderness in the right iliac fossa. Her vital signs on admission were:

Vital sign	Observation	Normal range
Temperature	37.5 °C	36.5–37.2 °C
Pulse	110 beats per minute	70–120
Respiratory rate	36 breaths per minute	20–30 breaths per minute
Blood pressure	85/50 mmHg	80–100 mmHg (systolic)
CRT	2 seconds	<2 seconds
Oxygen saturation	98% in air	98–100%
Level of consciousness	Alert on the AVPU scale	Alert on the AVPU scale
Pain score	4	1 (no pain)

Renuka's PEWS score is 2, her respiratory rate is elevated and her pulse rate is at the upper end of the normal range.

What explanation can you give for this?

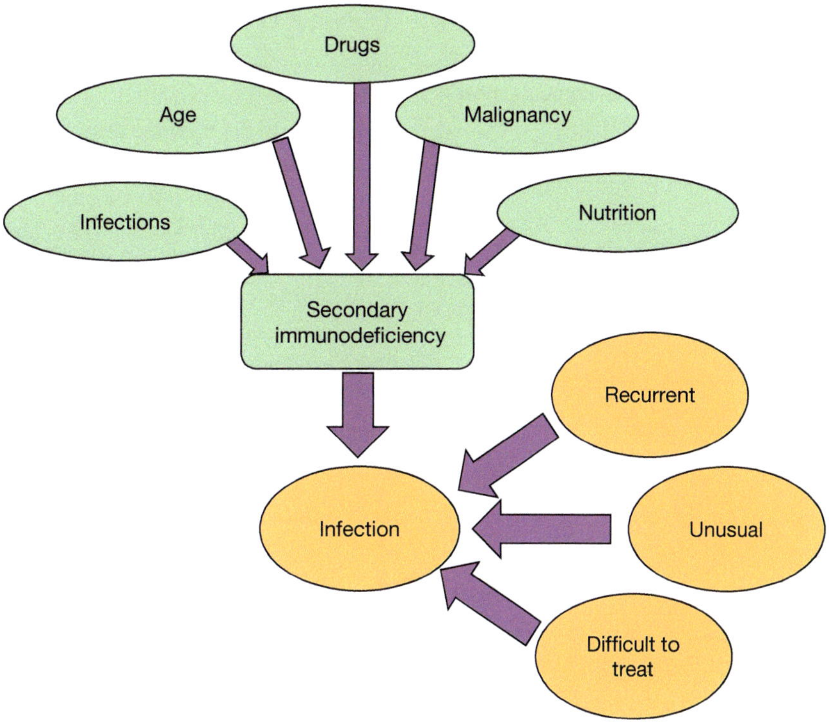

FIGURE 5.16 Features of secondary immunodeficiency.
Source: Helbert (2017)/with permission of Elsevier.

Blood test and urinalysis indicate:

Blood test	Result	Normal range
Haemoglobin	125 g/L	115–155 g/L
White blood cells	13.2×10^9/L	$4.5–13.5 \times 10^9$/L
Neutrophils	8.5×10^9/L	$1.5–8.0 \times 10^9$/L
Lymphocytes	6.6×10^9/L	$1.5–7.0 \times 10^9$/L
Platelets	420×10^9/L	$150–450 \times 10^9$/L
C-reactive protein	42 mg/L	0–10 mg/L
Urinalysis	+ve nitrites and leucocytes on testing	

Renuka's white blood cell count is at the upper end of the normal range, and she has an elevated neutrophil count and raised C-reactive protein.

What do you think the significance of this might be?

She is admitted to the paediatric ward and following administration of analgesia and starting intravenous fluids, Renuka is monitored closely with hourly recordings of her vital signs. Six hours later, she is still complaining of abdominal pain and her recordings are now as follows:

Vital sign	Observation	Normal range
Temperature	38.5 °C	36.5–37.2 °C
Pulse	125 beats per minute	70–120
Respiratory rate	34 breaths per minute	20–30 breaths per minute
Blood pressure	80/55 mmHg	80–100 mmHg (systolic)
CRT	3 seconds	<2 seconds
Oxygen saturation	98% in air	98–100%
Level of consciousness	Lethargic and responding to voice on the AVPU scale	Alert on the AVPU scale
Pain score	4	1 (no pain)

Her PEWS score is now 4, and Renuka is reviewed by the paediatric surgeon. On examination, her abdomen is tense. Blood tests indicate that the neutrophil count is now 12.2×10^9/L and the C-reactive protein is 110 mg/L.

What explanation can you give for this?

What care and support will Renuka and family need at this time?

Renuka underwent appendicectomy for a perforated appendix and received intravenous antibiotics postoperatively. She recovered well and was discharged home after four days, with follow-up from the children's nursing team for wound care. She completed her antibiotic course orally.

Conclusion

This chapter has provided insight into the anatomy and physiology of the immune response and inflammation, and has discussed how the pathophysiology of the altered effects of these can affect a child and his/her family. The focus in this chapter has been to present an overview of the interplay between the innate and adaptive immune systems and to consider how the inflammatory process can manifest locally and systemically within the body. Emphasis has been given on how alterations in immunity can affect the infant and child, and the implications of providing care for the child and the family have been discussed.

References

Abbas, A.K., Lichtman, A.H., & Pillai, S. (2024). *Basic Immunology*, 7th edn. Elsevier, Philadelphia.

Allergy UK (2025). *What is an allergy?* [online] Available at: https://www.allergyuk.org/about-allergy/what-is-an-allergy/ (accessed 31 March 2025).

Anaphylaxis UK (2020). *Infant Weaning Guidance*. Available at: https://www.anaphylaxis.org.uk/wp-content/uploads/2022/07/Infant-weaning-compressed.pdf?x66701 (accessed 31 March 2025).

Brashers, V.L. (2023). Alterations in immunity. In: Rogers, J., Brashers, V., McCance, K.L., & Huether, S.E. (eds). *McCance and Huether's Pathophysiology: The Biological Basis for Disease in Adults and Children*, 9th edn. Philadelphia: Elsevier, pp. 255–280.

British National Formulary (2017). BNF for children. [online] Available at: https://bnfc.nice.org.uk/drugs/adrenaline-epinephrine/#prescribing-and-dispensing-information (accessed 31 March 2025).

Brown, J.V.E., Walsh, V., & McQuire, W. (2019). Formula versus maternal breast milk for feeding preterm or low birth weight infants (Review). *Cochrane Database of Systematic Reviews 2019* (8). Art. No.: CD002972. https://doi.org/10.1002/14651858.CD002972.

Helbert, M. (2017). *Immunology for Medical Students*, 3rd edn. Elsevier, Philadelphia.

Immunodeficiency UK. (2025) *Immunodeficiency*. Available at: https://www.immunodeficiencyuk.org/immunodeficiency/ (accessed 31 March 2025)

Isenberg, D., & Mahto, A. (2021). Autoimmunity and immunosuppression. In: Male, D., Stokes Peebles, R., & Male, V. (eds). *Immunology*, 9th edn. Philadelphia: Elsevier, pp. 287–305.

Jonas, D., Muldowney, Y., Byrne, I., & Southern, H. (2012). Essential care. In: Coyne, I., Neill, F., & Timmins, F. (eds). *Clinical Skills in Children's Nursing*. Oxford: Oxford University Press, pp. 115–145.

Macpherson, G., & Austyn, J.M. (2012). *Exploring Immunology Concepts and Evidence*. Wiley-VCH, Weinheim.

Marieb, E.N., & Keller, S. (2022). *Essentials of Human Anatomy and Physiology*, 13th edn. Pearson Education Ltd, Harlow.

Murphy, K., Weaver, C., & Berg, L. (2022). *Janeway's Immunobiology*, 10th edn. W.W Norton & Company, New York.

National Health Service (NHS) (2025). *Food Allergies in Babies and Young Children*. Available at: https://www.nhs.uk/conditions/baby/weaning-and-feeding/food-allergies-in-babies-and-young-children/ (accessed 31 March 2025)

National Institute for Health and Care Excellence (NICE) (2017), *Health care-associated infections: prevention and control in primary and community care*. Clinical guideline [CG 139]. Available at: https://www.nice.org.uk/guidance/cg139 (accessed 23 March 2025).

National Institute for Health and Care Excellence (NICE) (2020). *Neutropaenic sepsis: prevention and management in people with cancer*. Clinical guideline [CG151]. Available at: https://www.nice.org.uk/guidance/cg151 (accessed 26 March 2025).

National Institute for Health and Care Excellence (NICE) (2021). *Fever in under 5s: assessment and initial assessment*. NICE guideline [NG 143]. Available at: Recommendations | Fever in under 5s: assessment and initial management | Guidance | NICE (accessed 17 March 2025).

National Institute for Health and Care Excellence (NICE) (2024a). *Sepsis: recognition diagnosis and early management*. NICE guideline [NG51]. Available at: https://www.nice.org.uk/guidance/ng51 (accessed 17 March 2025).

National Institute for Health and Care Excellence (NICE) (2024b). *Asthma Pathway (BTS, NICE, SIGN)*. NICE guideline [NG 244].

Available at: https://www.nice.org.uk/guidance/ng244 (accessed 31 March 2025)

Peate, I., & Gormley-Fleming, E. (2025). *Fundamentals of Children's Anatomy and Physiology*, 3rd edn. Wiley, Oxford.

Resuscitation Council (2021). *Emergency treatment of anaphylactic reactions: guidelines for healthcare providers*. Resuscitation Council UK, London. Available at: https://www.resus.org.uk/library/additional-guidance/guidance-anaphylaxis/emergency-treatment (accessed 17th March 2025).

Royal College of Nursing (RCN) (2013). *Caring for children with fever. RCN good practice guidance for nurses working with infants, children and young people*. Royal College of Nursing, London.

Tanno, L.K., & Demoly, P. (2020). Anaphylaxis in children. *Paediatric Allergy and Immunology* 31(26), 8–10.

Tortora, G.J., & Derrickson, B.H. (2017). *Principles of Anatomy and Physiology*, Global edn. Wiley, Hoboken, NJ.

UK Health Security Agency (2024). *Quarterly vaccination coverage statistics for children aged up to 5 years in the UK (Cover Programme): October to December 2023*. Available at: https://www.gov.uk/government/statistics/cover-of-vaccination-evaluated-rapidly-cover-programme-2023-to-2024-quarterly-data/quarterly-vaccination-coverage-statistics-for-children-aged-up-to-5-years-in-the-uk-cover-programme-october-to-december-2023. (accessed 27 March 2025)

UK Health Security Agency (2025). *The complete routine immunisation schedule from 1 February 2025*. Available at: https://www.gov.uk/government/publications/the-complete-routine-immunisation-schedule/the-complete-routine-immunisation-schedule-from-february-2022 (accessed 27 March 2025)

CHAPTER 6

Shock

Karen Roberts-Edema and Michelle White

AIM

The aim of this chapter is to offer an introduction to shock, which can develop into a life-threatening condition.

LEARNING OUTCOMES

On completion of this chapter, the reader will be able to:

- Understand the basic physiology of shock states in children and young people.
- Know the classification and recognition of clinical shock states.
- Understand the pathophysiology of septic shock and explain changes that occur in a child or young person's vital signs.
- Discuss the pathophysiological changes occurring in anaphylactic shock and articulate the immediate care required.
- Discuss the initial management of shock in children and young people.

KEYWORDS

- cardiac output
- hypovolaemic
- cardiogenic
- stroke volume
- hypotension
- compensatory shock
- anaphylaxis
- hypoperfusion
- distributive
- preload
- afterload

Test your prior knowledge

1. Explain compensatory shock and its mechanisms.
2. List the clinical features of warm shock.
3. Identify four clinical conditions that can lead to left ventricular failure (LVF) and cardiogenic shock.
4. Identify three causes of distributive shock.
5. Discuss the diagnosis and pathophysiological changes that occur with anaphylactic shock.

Introduction

Shock contributes to approximately 2% of paediatric hospital admissions globally, with an estimated 10 million child fatalities attributed to shock each year (Gobinathan & Suresh Kannan, 2018). The predominant types of shock observed in children include distributive, hypovolaemic and cardiogenic shock (Waltzman, 2015), with sepsis being one of the most frequently encountered forms. Sepsis is responsible for 10–20% of paediatric mortality, with 30–50% of these deaths occurring within the initial days following diagnosis (Miura *et al.*, 2023). Sinniah (2012) found that out of 147 cases of paediatric shock with the highest mortality, 57% were septic shock, 24% hypovolaemic shock, 14% had distributive shock and 5% cardiogenic shock. Given its high mortality if not promptly recognised and treated, understanding the various forms of shock is vital in caring for children and young people.

Shock is a life-threatening condition caused by acute circulatory failure, leading to inadequate tissue perfusion, oxygenation and impaired clearance of metabolic waste (Stephenson, 2020). It is a complex syndrome affecting nearly every organ system. Recognising shock in a child is crucial, as failure to do so can be life-threatening or result in serious long-term consequences.

This chapter explains the pathophysiology of shock and its initial management. Effective circulation in children depends on three key components: the blood, which carries oxygen and removes waste; the heart, which pumps fluid; and the blood vessels, which distribute fluid throughout the body.

Normal metabolism depends on oxygen delivery and waste removal, which require effective cardiac, pulmonary and circulatory function. Adequate blood flow, circulating volume, cardiac efficiency and vascular autoregulation are essential to maintain perfusion pressure and organ function. Dysfunction in any of these areas can lead to shock, defined as acute circulatory failure.

Shock can be defined at the cellular and clinical levels. Cellularly, it is an inadequate substrate for aerobic respiration, causing tissue hypoperfusion, poor oxygen delivery and toxic waste accumulation. Clinically, it presents as changes in heart rate (HR) and rhythm, deranged capillary refill, altered mental state and muscle tone (floppiness), changes in skin colour and temperature and complications such as reduced kidney perfusion and low urine output.

Shock is classified according to the cause or abnormality that occurs. Table 6.1 illustrates different types of shock depending on their pathophysiology.

Distributive shock

Distributive shock is associated with dysfunctional blood flow and intravascular volume. As blood vessels lose tone and become larger, this causes a relative hypovolaemia, and blood does not flow efficiently. For various reasons, for example, toxins and inflammatory proteins (in septic shock) or allergens (in anaphylactic shock), the blood vessels widen to such an extent that they lose their tone and blood pools in the vessels rather than circulating normally. This manifests in symptoms of early shock as the body tries to compensate by increasing the HR. Three different types of distributive shock are described in the following sections. These are: sepsis and septic shock, neurogenic shock and anaphylactic shock (Blumlein & Griffiths, 2022).

TABLE 6.1 Classification of shock

• **Hypovolaemic shock:** Due to a reduction in circulating volume from intravascular losses (e.g., burns), haemorrhage (e.g., trauma and surgery) or interstitial losses (e.g., burns, ascites and other third spacing or sepsis). Haemorrhagic shock and severe dehydration fall into this category.
• **Cardiogenic shock:** Due to cardiac pump failure or dysfunction. Pump failure can be due to right or left heart or both right and left heart failure. Cardiogenic shock causes impairment of cardiac contractility.
• **Distributive shock:** This is due to a relative hypovolaemia caused by vasodilation (poor vascular/vasomotor tone) and low total systemic vascular resistance (SVR). Sepsis mediators, anaphylaxis or autonomic dysfunction from head and/or spinal injury can cause this type of shock.
• **Obstructive shock:** Due to impaired blood flow, such as pulmonary embolism (rare in children), cardiac tamponade, tension pneumothorax or pulmonary hypertension. In neonates, coarctation of aorta, interrupted aortic arch and aortic valvular disease can cause obstructive shock. Obstructive shock results in cardiogenic shock and death if left untreated.

Septic shock

Sepsis/septic shock is a serious type of distributive shock caused by a dysregulated and overwhelming host response to infection (Singer *et al.*, 2016). In this type of shock, pathogens such as gram-negative bacteria and their microbial products, for example, lipopolysaccharides (LPS), cause a highly immunogenic and toxic molecule to activate the inflammatory system – the body's natural response to injury (in this case, injury to the endothelial system). However, microbial toxins and activated inflammatory cytokines from the inflammatory pathway cause vasodilatation and low SVR, i.e., poor vessel tone, which increases vessel permeability, causing fluid to leak out of the circulatory system. SVR refers to the resistance offered by all blood vessels to the aortic valve when it opens to eject blood. Low SVR can be caused by the host (child's) own response to inflammation – the systemic inflammatory response syndrome (SIRS). Inflammatory mediators (e.g., cytokines, interleukins) and bacterial toxins (e.g., LPS) cause dilatation of blood vessels and lead to low SVR, also known as warm shock.

In septic shock, patients will be admitted to the hospital with compensated shock, also known as warm shock. Other features of warm shock are tachycardia, bounding peripheral pulses and warm skin. Warm shock results in high cardiac output (CO) and low SVR. These children will require a detailed Airway, Breathing, Circulation, Disability, Exposure (A–E) approach to a systematic assessment and documentation of their vital signs on a Paediatric Early Warning Score (PEWS) chart, to aid the decision-making process and monitoring of the child's condition as the child may decompensate into shock with hypotension secondary to low SVR. Alternatively, they may quickly decompensate into cold shock, which is more difficult to treat. Children in septic shock sometimes present with features of cold (or late) shock. In cold shock, the child becomes excessively vasoconstricted; skin is pale, cool or cold to touch with mottling as blood is shunted away; and capillary refill time is prolonged. However, in children with darker skin tones, clinical signs such as mottling may not be readily observable. In such cases, nurses should consider alternative assessment strategies, including evaluating the child's behaviour, closely monitoring vital signs and consulting with parents regarding any noticeable changes in the child's skin appearance compared to when the child is in a well state. In cold shock, the sympathetically mediated response maintains the child's blood pressure for a while until there is decompensation and the child collapses. By this stage, capillary blood flow becomes sluggish, capillaries become leaky and permeable and there is third-spacing of fluid, further exacerbating the hypovolaemic state and metabolic acidosis. Cold shock is associated with low CO, high SVR and poor outcome. Refractory shock is defined by irreversible shock, multi-organ failure and death (Stephenson, 2020). Initially, as a compensatory mechanism, blood vessels try to maintain tone, which is one of the major differences between adults and children, as children will maintain their SVR and blood pressure until the pre-terminal stage. See Figure 6.1 for an overview of life-threatening conditions associated with septic shock. 97

In the compensatory phase of shock, diastolic blood pressure may rise slightly, and pulse pressure may narrow, keeping systolic blood pressure normal. Monitoring

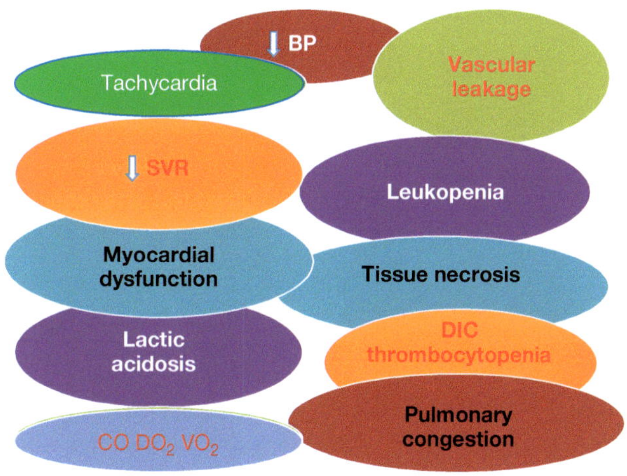

FIGURE 6.1 Life-threatening complications of septic shock.

blood pressure trends is essential for nurses during A–E assessment, and accurate documentation on admission establishes a baseline. Early tachycardia is a key sign, as the sympathetic nervous system releases catecholamines (adrenaline and noradrenaline) to maintain CO and circulating volume. Other early signs include warm and flushed skin, flash capillary refill and bounding pulses, indicating hyperdynamic circulation. Fluid resuscitation at this stage can reverse symptoms. In children with darker skin, changes in pallor may be less obvious. So, assessment should include skin temperature, texture and moisture, and parents can provide useful observations of skin changes.

In cases where a child presents with distributive shock or sepsis and is assessed as requiring fluid resuscitation, the Resuscitation Council UK (2021) recommends the prompt administration of intravenous (IV) or intraosseous (IO) fluids at an initial volume of 30 mL/kg. Crystalloids or 0.9% sodium chloride should be used for initial volume resuscitation. If the child remains hypotensive during or following fluid administration, vasopressors (medication to increase the blood pressure) should be initiated to maintain a mean arterial pressure of ≥65 mmHg. At this stage, referral to the paediatric intensive care unit (PICU) is necessary for advanced management.

This life-threatening emergency typically presents with clinical features of cold shock, including cool or cold extremities, cyanosis or mottled skin, prolonged capillary refill time, reduced urine output (oligo-anuria), metabolic acidosis, tachycardia and hypotension. Children in this condition are critically ill and are at risk of developing disseminated intravascular coagulation (DIC), a serious complication associated with severe sepsis.

Children can present with more than one type of shock. For example, a child in a road traffic collision with a head injury may develop distributive shock from loss of vascular control and hypovolaemic shock from blood loss (Stephenson, 2020). In some cases of sepsis, such as neutropenic or neonatal sepsis, the compensatory phase may be very brief or absent, leading to rapid decompensation.

Children generally return to their pre-illness levels and functioning due to their brain plasticity.

DIC is an over-activation of the inflammatory and clotting systems (Fig. 6.1). Injuries, including endothelial damage in shock, trigger these systems: inflammation protects the body and clotting seals injured vessels. In DIC, extensive microvascular injury, as in sepsis, causes rapid consumption of clotting factors, leading to deranged clotting that is difficult to correct.

Another complication of DIC is not only the resulting coagulopathy but also the microvascular clotting and fibrin deposits that occur in the small blood vessels, which then occlude tissues from extracting oxygen. As aerobic metabolism requires oxygen, tissue dysoxia initially leads to anaerobic metabolism, metabolic acidosis and a rise in lactate – the by-product of anaerobic metabolism – all of which will eventually lead to cell death. That is why DIC is a marker of poor prognosis and is associated with the mnemonic **D**eath **I**s **C**oming (Moore *et al.*, 2016). Thus, DIC is both a clotting and bleeding disorder that is difficult to treat. The underlying condition, i.e., the stimulus for DIC, in this case sepsis, must instead be treated and controlled. Treatment of DIC is therefore only symptomatic, and patients will require many blood and blood product transfusions. These patients are usually cared for in the PICU. The majority of children with sepsis and septic shock do recover to lead normal lives. International efforts such as the Surviving Sepsis Campaign and Sepsis 6 (National Institute for Health and Care Excellence [NICE], 2024) aim to improve diagnosis and survival rates of children with sepsis through early recognition and timely treatment. Thus, nurses and other healthcare professionals play a vital role in recognising and reporting the signs and symptoms of sepsis early so that children are given the best chance of survival.

While early signs of compensated shock may be brief, decompensated shock has obvious clinical features. Vasoconstriction maintains circulating volume and shunts blood to vital organs, causing cold, clammy and mottled skin, poor muscle tone or floppiness in infants and young children and persistent tachycardia.

If a child with suspected or proven infection has at least two of the criteria set out in Fig. 6.2, then it should be assumed that sepsis is present and full screening should proceed.

Tachycardia will decompensate further into bradycardia, a pre-terminal sign, if this stage is not adequately or promptly managed. In decompensated shock, capillary refill time is prolonged, and there may be low rather than high core temperature. Unlike adults who become hypotensive at an early stage, children will remain normotensive but significantly tachycardic until they become pre-terminal. As blood flow is diverted from the kidneys to more vital organs, there may be oliguria or anuria and poor perfusion to other non-vital organs, for example, the gut. Urine output ≤ 2 mL/kg/h in young children and ≤ 1 mL/kg in older adolescents must be reported in a timely manner, as this is a very serious but early feature of poor kidney blood flow and perfusion (Stephenson, 2020). Monitoring urine output and maintaining an accurate fluid balance chart is, therefore, a vital part of the nurse's role.

Cold shock from any cause is a more severe type of shock and is more difficult to treat. It is a life-threatening condition that requires invasive monitoring and intensive care drugs, only possible in PICU. Regardless of the type of shock, however, all patients suspected of being septic must have appropriate antibiotics administered without delay, as this can be lifesaving (Dellinger *et al.*, 2013).

The clinical features of warm and cold shock are highlighted in Table 6.2.

A sepsis 6 flow chart is highlighted in Fig. 6.2.

Fig. 6.3 demonstrates the Resuscitation Council UK algorithm for Septic Shock.

Case study 6.1

Winston is a 5-year-old boy who presented to the emergency department with abdominal pain in the right iliac fossa in the lower right quadrant. Winston's father advises that there has been a 3-day history of abdominal pain, reduced appetite and vomiting. He has had a temperature of 37.5 °C for the last 24 hours. Winston is very quiet on presentation and does not answer any questions. Winston's father states that he appears pale, and you observe that he is lethargic and sleepy.

Vital sign	Observation	Normal range
Temperature	37.5 °C	36.5–37.2 °C
Pulse	130 beats per minute	70–120 beats per minute
Respiratory rate	32 breaths per minute	20–30 breaths per minute
Blood pressure	88/45 mmHg	80–100 mmHg (systolic)
Capillary Refill Time (CRT)	2 seconds	< 2 seconds
Oxygen saturation	96% in air	98–100% in air
Level of consciousness	Alert on the AVPU scale	Alert on the AVPU scale
Pain score	6	1 (no pain) – 10 (severe pain)

Winston's PEWS score is 3, his pulse and respiratory rate are slightly elevated and his pain score is 6 out of 10.

What explanation can you give for this?
What management does Winston need?

Blood test and urinalysis indicate:

Blood test	Result	Normal range
Haemoglobin	125 g/L	115–155 g/L
White blood cells	20.2×10^9/L	$4.5–13.5 \times 10^9$/L
Neutrophils	10×10^9/L	$1.5–8.0 \times 10^9$/L
Lymphocytes	8.1×10^9/L	$1.5–7.0 \times 10^9$/L
Platelets	420×10^9/L	$150–450 \times 10^9$/L
C-reactive protein (CRP)	330 mg/L	0–10 mg/L
Urinalysis	Unable to get a sample	

Winston's white blood cell count is high, and he has an elevated neutrophil count and raised CRP.

What do you think the significance of this might be?
What ongoing management does Winston need?

He is admitted to the paediatric ward; the nurse carries out admission observations. See herewith.

Vital sign	Observation	Normal range
Temperature	38.8 °C	36.5–37.2 °C
Pulse	153 beats per minute	70–120 beats per minute
Respiratory rate	38 breaths per minute	20–30 breaths per minute
Blood pressure	78/35 mmHg	80–100 mmHg (systolic)
CRT	3 seconds	< 2 seconds
Oxygen saturation	96% in air	98–100% in air
Level of consciousness	Alert on the AVPU scale	Alert on the AVPU scale
Pain score	8	1 (no pain) – 10 (severe pain)

Now Winston's observations have deteriorated, and his temperature has increased, pulse and respiratory rates elevated and blood pressure decreased.

What do you know about a patient who has low blood pressure? What do you need to do to manage Winston's condition?

Investigations and fluid resuscitation:

- Give high-flow oxygen
- Obtain IV/IO access and take blood
  - Blood, full blood count (FBC), urea and electrolytes (U&E), CRP, lactate, blood cultures and blood glucose
- Give IV antibiotics
- Consider fluid resuscitation
  - Give up to 30 mL/kg of crystalloids or 0.9% sodium chloride.

Source: Resuscitation Council UK (2021)

Winston will be taken to PICU for further management.

TABLE 6.2 **The clinical features of warm and cold shocks**

Warm shock	Cold shock
Increased respiratory rate	Increased respiratory rate
Tachycardia	Tachycardia
Vasodilation	Capillary refill > 2 seconds
Widening pulse pressure	Narrowing pulse pressure
Low peripheral vascular resistance	Mottles, cool extremities
Warm skin	Decreased urine output
Flushed skin	Hypothermia
Decreased urine output	
Hyperthermia	

Neurogenic shock

Another type of distributive shock is neurogenic shock. Neurogenic shock is caused by the sudden loss of autonomic control and impairment of autoregulation resulting from injury to the spinal cord (SCI) – especially above T6. Here, disruption to the descending pathways of the sympathetic nervous system results in unopposed vagal (parasympathetic) tone. Loss of tone and dilatation of vascular smooth muscles and an increased venous capacitance result in a decreased SVR. There will be a relative hypovolaemia, meaning that the circulating volume is unchanged. However, as the blood vessel capacity enlarges, the existing circulating volume becomes inadequate to fill it. The relative hypovolaemia and the disruption to vessel autoregulation result in hypotension.

At 15% to 20%, spinal cord injuries are the most common cause of neurogenic shock. However, surgical intervention in the lumbar region, cerebral ischaemia, subarachnoid haemorrhage, meningitis or rapid onset of Guillain–Barré syndrome (Standl *et al.*, 2018) can also be causes. Although rare, children and young people with Guillain-Barré syndrome (GBS) can develop neurogenic shock due to the body's

Child unwell, parental concern, elevated Paediatric Early Warning Scores (PEWs)
Think Sepsis

Sepsis risk

Does the child have an infection or any of the following:

- Temperature ≤ 36 or ≥ 38 degrees
- Tachycardia
- Altered mental state
    - Floppiness, sleepy, irritability, lethargy.
- Prolonged capillary refill ≥ 2 seconds
- Elevated PEWS

Red flags

- Hypotension
- Lactate ≥ 2 mmol/L
- Extreme tachycardia/tachypnoea
- Saturations ≤ 90% grunting/cyanosis/apnoea
- P or U on AVPU
- Immunocompromised
- Non-blanching rash

Contact a senior doctor

Document evidence

Consider sepsis or septic shock

Sepsis bundle within 1 hour

- Give high-flow oxygen
- Obtain IV/IO access and take blood
    - Bloods, full blood count, urea & electrolytes C-reactive protein, lactate, blood cultures and blood glucose
- Give IV antibiotics
- Consider fluid resuscitation
    - Give up to 30 mL/kg of crystalloids or 0.9% sodium chloride.

FIGURE 6.2 Sepsis 6.
Source: Adapted from Great Ormond Street Hospital Sepsis 6 protocol (2015).

Resuscitation Council UK

GUIDELINES 2021

Septic shock and sepsis-associated organ dysfunction in children

RECOGNITION

Assess with ABCDE approach

A, B assessment

- Airway, RR, work of breathing, oxygen saturations, breath sounds, recognition respiratory distress/failure.
- Open airway and start high-flow oxygen via non-rebreather mask with reservoir or BMV as appropriate.

C assessment

- HR, CRT, BP, peripheral and central perfusion, rhythm recognition; recognition circulatory failure/shock.
- Establish IV/IO access (take blood cultures, full blood count, blood glucose, urea and electrolytes, lactate*, blood gas and other bloods as indicated**) and give fluid resuscitation as below.

D assessment

- AVPU score; recognition of altered mental status secondary to poor perfusion.

E assessment

- Rash, temperature (high or low).

Sepsis is diagnosed if there is evidence of infection as cause of the acute illness (suspected or proven) plus at least two of the following: core temperature < 36°C or > 38.5°C; white cell count elevated or depressed for age; inappropriate tachycardia; altered mental state; reduced peripheral perfusion.

10–15 MIN

Initial resuscitation

- If no signs fluid overload (hepatomegaly, crackles at lung bases) then give 10 mL kg^{-1} balanced crystalloids*** IV bolus over 5–10 min and re-assess after each bolus up to 40–60 mL kg^{-1} or until perfusion improved.
- Therapeutic end points: CRT < 2 s; normal BP for age; UO > 1 mL kg^{-1} h^{-1}, normal pulses, normal mental state.
- Watch for signs of fluid overload; if present stop bolus therapy and start inotropic support.
- Correct hypoglycaemia and hypocalcaemia.
- Start broad-spectrum antibiotics; seek and aggressively control any infection source.
- Call for more senior help and an anaesthetist urgently; call PICU for bed +/- PICU transfer team.
- If mechanical ventilation is required, then cardiovascular instability during intubation is less likely after appropriate cardiovascular resuscitation.

15–60 MIN

Fluid refractory shock?

Start IV/IO inotrope infusion; central (preferable) or peripheral IV (clinical signs unreliable at differentiating 'warm' and 'cold' shock in children).

Adrenaline 0.05–0.3 mcg kg^{-1} min^{-1} (use more dilute infusion if peripheral)

and/or

Noradrenaline via central IV or IO, starting infusion rate 0.05 mcg kg^{-1} min^{-1}

Titrate inotropes upwards according to clinical response and haemodynamic effects using haemodynamic monitoring (where possible)****

Use ketamine +/- atropine IV/IO/IM to gain central access and airway if needed.

Fluid and catecholamine-resistant shock?

Further management as per Paediatric Intensive Care/retrieval service advice.

Warm shock – high cardiac output with low systemic vascular resistance.	**Cold shock** – low cardiac output with high systemic vascular resistance.	**Fluid in mL kg^{-1} should be dosed for ideal body weight (max bolus 500 mL)**

* lactate measurements are useful if available as they have prognostic ability if measured serially.

** Other bloods that may be indicated: coagulation studies, liver function tests, magnesium levels or any others indicated by the child's clinical picture.

*** Balanced (buffered) fluids are used in preference to 0.9% sodium chloride, but if not available, 0.9% sodium chloride should be used.

**** These are starting dose ranges for these inotropes, and increases may be necessary but should be guided by PICU retrieval team/senior clinicians. Choice of inotropes is dictated by clinician preference, response to treatment and monitored parameters, and again decisions should be made in conjunction with PICU teams.

EPALS Resuscitation Council UK

FIGURE 6.3 Septic shock algorithm Resuscitation Council UK Guidelines (2024).

autonomic nervous system malfunctioning, which in turn leads to a decrease in blood pressure and HR.

Initial management of neurogenic shock in children is to prioritise haemodynamic stability through IV fluid resuscitation. Initial fluid resuscitation with 10–20 mL/kg should be adequate to replace the relative hypovolaemia.

Patients receiving treatment for neurogenic shock should be treated in an ICU where fluids should be given cautiously as excessive administration can lead to complications such as pulmonary oedema (Dave *et al.*, 2023). Measurement of central venous pressure may be required to guide fluid replacement in patients where hypotension persists. Vasopressors and inotropes can also be used in cases where hypotension continues despite euvolemia. The treatment should support blood pressure until the patient overcomes and the body has time to adapt to the changed system due to the SCI. Bradycardia, another consequence of neurochemical derangement and autonomic dysregulation in SCI, should be managed with medication such as atropine or glycopyrrolate. These drugs can be given prophylactically prior to suctioning or turning the patient if they are particularly sensitive to these interventions, which may cause a vagal response. Patients experiencing neurogenic shock may present with warm, flushed-looking skin, contrasting with cool and pallid skin often seen in patients experiencing hypovolaemic shock. Other dysrhythmias are also possible in severe conditions and should be controlled, as cardiac dysrhythmias can result in poor ejection of blood out of the heart (Hobson and Chima, 2013). Efficient bowel and bladder management is crucial in SCI patients as constipation, urinary retention, a distended abdomen and pain have the potential to trigger an episode of neurogenic shock.

Neurogenic shock can occur anytime following injury up to 6 weeks post-injury (Kripa & Khanal, 2021). There is no diagnostic test for this condition. So, history, the nature of SCI and exclusion of other causes for hypotension and bradycardia contribute to the diagnosis of neurogenic shock. Bradycardia in these patients is exacerbated by any condition that increases intracranial pressure, such as suctioning, defaecation, coughing, turning the patient and hypoxia. Initially, the skin can be warm and flushed in this condition, but heat loss from profound vasodilatation has the potential to cause hypothermia.

> Neurogenic shock should not be confused with spinal shock. Spinal shock is the reversible dysfunction of the spinal cord associated with injury, which can exist alone or in combination with permanent cord injury.

> It is important to signpost patients and their families to support groups, counselling and mental health services to help them cope with neurogenic shock and the ongoing challenges of living with a spinal cord injury.

Anaphylactic shock

Anaphylaxis is a state of immediate hypersensitivity resulting in distributive shock due to loss of vasomotor tone and massive vasodilatation. The most frequent trigger for anaphylaxis is exposure to food allergens and medications such as antibiotics (e.g., penicillin allergy). The condition is caused by the release of mediators, especially histamine, from mast cells and basophils. Histamine has a vasodilatory effect and increases blood vessel permeability. Typical signs of anaphylaxis are stridor, swelling around the mouth and face, wheezing, respiratory distress, vomiting and urticaria.

> Diagnosis may be difficult due to inconsistent clinical manifestations. So, it is essential that a rational approach, ABCDE, is taken.

Stridor, indicating partial airway obstruction, and wheeze from narrowed airways can progress to complete airway obstruction with respiratory and cardiac arrest. Reduced circulating volume due to vasodilatation and increased permeability can also cause cardiac arrest. Intramuscular epinephrine dampens the anaphylactic response and reverses symptoms, with systemic corticosteroids and anti-histamines often required. See Fig. 6.4 for the Resuscitation Council UK anaphylaxis algorithm.

Hypovolaemic shock

Hypovolaemic shock is caused by a significant reduction in circulating blood volume (CBV) (Blumlein & Griffiths, 2022). Hypovolaemic shock is one of the most common forms of shock and is characterised by an insufficient intravascular volume resulting from significant blood and/or fluid loss. It occurs when the reduction in circulating volume is severe enough that the body's metabolic demands can no longer be adequately

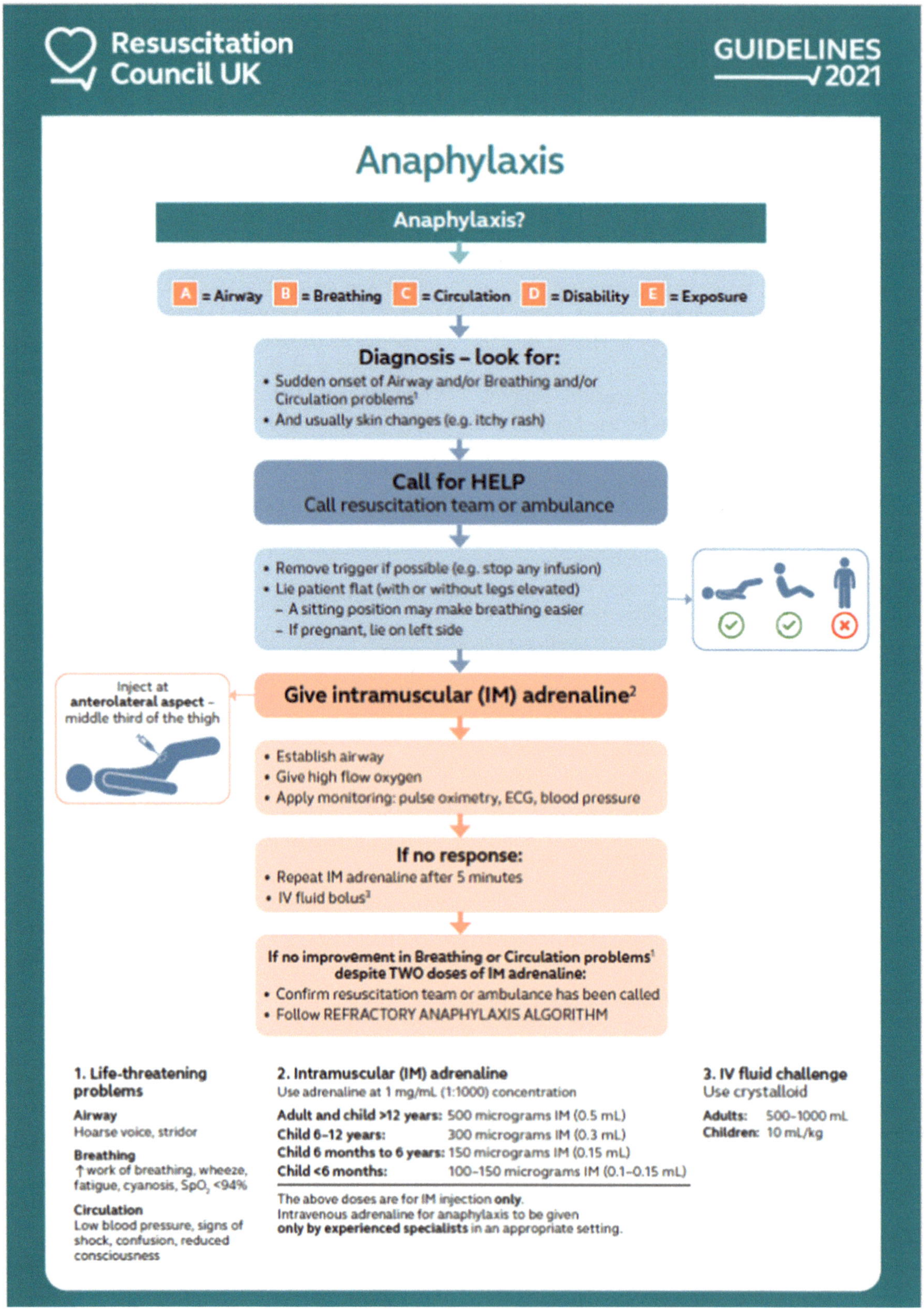

FIGURE 6.4 Anaphylaxis algorithm Resuscitation Council UK Guidelines (2024).

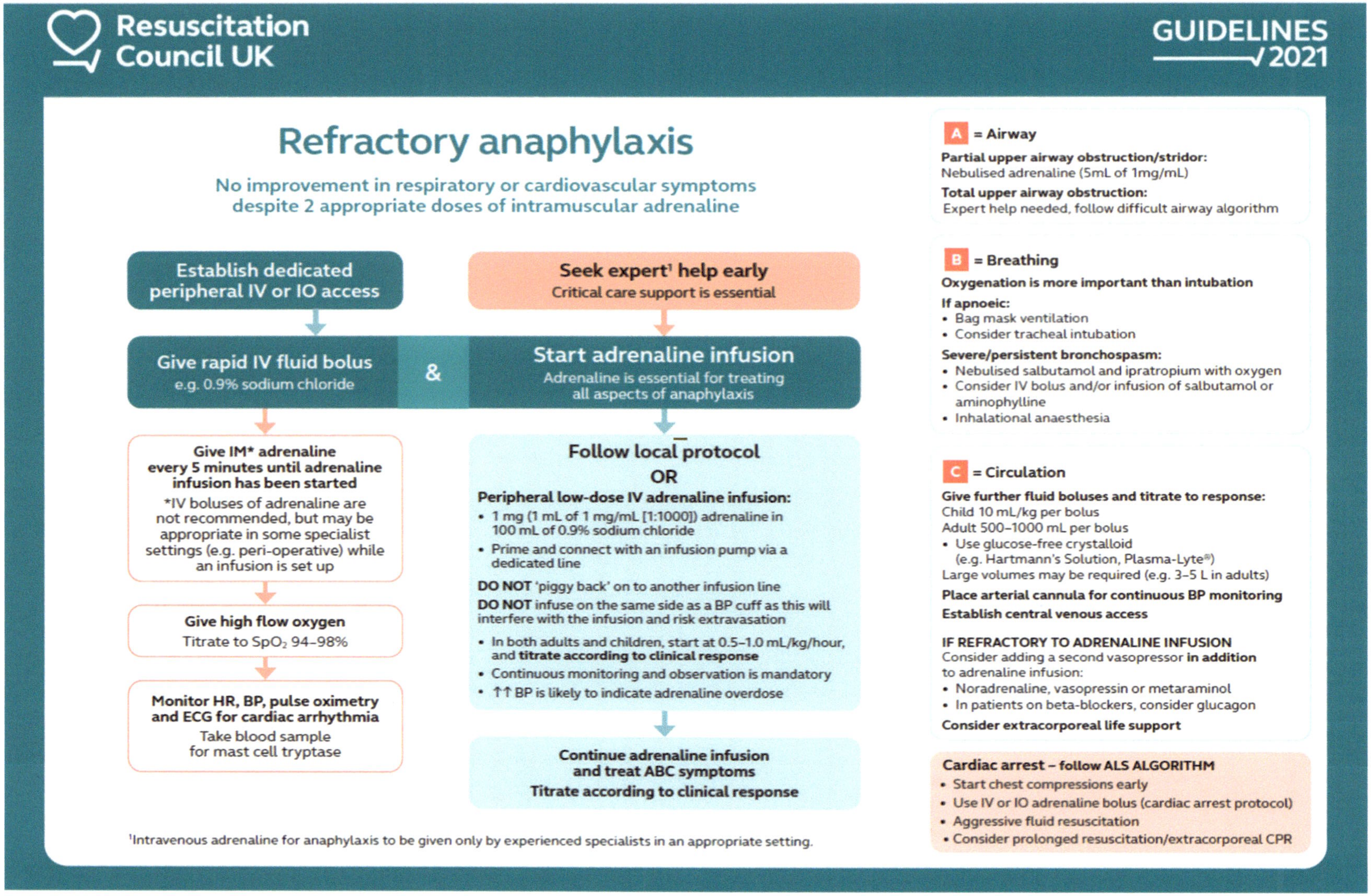

FIGURE 6.4 *(Continued)*

met (Blumlein & Griffiths, 2022). Hypovolaemic shock in children and young people is primarily caused by a reduction in CBV, which can occur due to various factors, such as gastroenteritis, diarrhoea and vomiting, or diabetes insipidus caused by pituitary dysfunction, which results in excessive urinary loss. Haemorrhage also causes direct loss of fluid, in this case, loss of whole blood.

Relative hypovolaemia, as seen in distributive shock, occurs when increased capillary permeability causes fluid to leak from the circulation, as in sepsis. Other causes of 'third-spacing' include burns, liver failure, pancreatitis and bowel obstruction. For example, ascites in liver failure represents fluid lost from the circulation. Without adequate fluid replacement, patients risk severe dehydration and hypovolaemic shock. This section discusses two types of hypovolaemic shock: dehydration-induced shock and haemorrhagic shock.

Extreme/severe dehydration

In hypovolaemic shock, fluid loss (e.g., from diarrhoea and vomiting) or inadequate intake causes dehydration and shock. Compensatory mechanisms, including the renin-angiotensin-aldosterone system and anti-diuretic hormone (ADH) release, work to conserve circulating volume and maintain blood pressure. These responses reduce urine output, an important observation for nurses to monitor and report.

Vasopressin (ADH) also causes vasoconstriction and shunting of blood to vital organs, leading to weak, thready peripheral pulses and prolonged capillary refill in hypovolaemic shock. However, in conditions like diabetic ketoacidosis (DKA), these signs can be misleading. Hyperosmolar, hyperglycaemic blood draws fluid from cells. So, despite severe cellular dehydration, capillary refill may remain normal, and polyuria occurs instead of oliguria. Capillary refill must be interpreted cautiously in DKA, highlighting the importance of understanding different shock pathophysiologies. Figure 6.5 shows the Resuscitation Council UK DKA algorithm.

Hypovolaemic shock can also be classified according to serum sodium levels. In hyponatraemic hypovolaemia, serum sodium is less than 130 mmol/L. Serum sodium is within 130–150 mmol/L in isonatraemic hypovolaemia, while in hypernatraemic hypovolaemia, serum sodium is over 150 mmol/L. The rapid correction of sodium levels with aggressive fluid resuscitation is dangerous and will risk cerebral oedema, brain herniation and brainstem death (Advanced Life Support Group, 2021).

Haemorrhagic shock

Haemorrhagic shock, a type of hypovolaemic shock, occurs when severe blood loss impairs oxygen delivery to tissues. Causes include blunt or penetrating trauma and post-operative bleeding (Cannon, 2018). Loss of red blood cells reduces the blood's oxygen-carrying capacity. The first 6 hours post-trauma are critical, as most deaths from haemorrhagic shock occur then. Children with traumatic or post-operative injuries who show tachycardia and poor peripheral pulses require urgent assessment for bleeding. Due to their smaller blood volume, children are at higher risk of significant blood loss leading to haemorrhagic shock.

A child's physiological response to trauma differs from that of an adult. Children can maintain a normal arterial blood pressure even with approximately 25–30% blood loss. This is maintained through HR and SVR changes (Lin *et al.*, 2024).

The definitive treatment for haemorrhagic shock is haemostasis and replacement of RBC via blood transfusions (Barratt & Curry, 2025). Although crystalloid boluses may be given, these must be kept to a minimum as fluid overload should be avoided (Resuscitation Council UK, 2021).

As with all types of shock in children, tachycardia is a very early symptom of haemorrhagic shock, which should be reported promptly. Other symptoms may include tachypnoea and oliguria, and narrowing pulse pressure may be the initial sign. Cool extremities, pallor and delayed capillary refill are signs of peripheral vasoconstriction (Hooper & Armstrong, 2022).

In the initial stage of shock, the body prioritises oxygenated blood flow to essential organs, the brain, heart and lungs through physiological compensatory mechanisms.

Therefore, in the early stages of haemorrhagic shock, tachycardia is the most common early sign of impending shock as other clinical parameters such as blood pressure may remain within normal range. With a class I haemorrhage, i.e., 10–15% blood loss, the child will compensate with a 10–20% increase in HR while blood pressure and capillary refill time remain unchanged. Even with 15–30% blood loss (class II haemorrhage), there is little change apart from tachycardia, tachypnoea and perhaps a prolonged capillary refill.

Resuscitation Council UK

GUIDELINES 2021

Early management of diabetic ketoacidosis (DKA) in children

adapted from NICE NG18 (updated 2020) & BSPED Guideline for the Management of Children & Young People under the age of 18 years DKA 2021

Recognition

History of polyuria, polydipsia and weight loss.
May have confusion, abdominal pain and hyperventilation.

- Blood glucose > 11 mmol L^{-1}
- pH < 7.3
- Blood bicarbonate < 15 mmol L^{-1}
- Ketones: blood beta-hydroxybutyrate > 3 mmol L^{-1} or urine ketonuria ++ and above

Note: Usually not vomiting, acidotic or drowsy unless more than 5% dehydrated

Severity of DKA and degree of dehydration	
Mild: 5% dehydration	Venous pH 7.2–7.29 or Bicarbonate < 15 mmol L^{-1}
Moderate: 5% dehydration	Venous pH 7.1–7.19 or Bicarbonate < 10 mmol L^{-1}
Severe: 10% dehydration	Venous pH < 7.1 or Bicarbonate < 5 mmol L^{-1}

Management

Resuscitation

A ensure airway patency, insert NG tube if reduced conscious level or vomiting to decrease gastric distension

B 100% oxygen via a face mask with reservoir bag + titrate to oxygen saturations 94–98%; avoid intubation unless respiratory arrest or respiratory failure when anaesthetic assistance urgently required

C establish IV access, take venous bloods (pH, $PaCO_2$, bicarbonate, sodium, potassium, urea, creatinine, beta-hydroxybutyrate levels, glucose), monitor ECG, identify shock

- Give a fluid bolus 10 mL kg^{-1} of balanced isotonic crystalloid or 0.9% sodium chloride over 30 min to children with NO shock
- Give a fluid bolus 10 mL kg^{-1} of balanced isotonic crystalloid or 0.9% sodium chloride over 5–10 min and re-assess; repeat to a maximum of 40 mL kg^{-1}; inform PICU if shock is persists

D seek and identify signs and symptoms of raised intracranial pressure – headache, confusion, irritability, posturing, falling GCS, rising BP with bradycardia. Treat with 3% sodium chloride or mannitol, seek PICU advice and call an anaesthetist. Consider CT brain to determine the cause.

E Consider sepsis if fever, hypothermia, hypotension, lactic acidosis, refractory acidosis

Intravenous therapy: fluids and insulin

For children with dehydration, nausea and vomiting:

Calculate fluid requirements (FR) for each child

Aim: to correct fluid deficit over 48 h

FR = Maintenance fluids for 48 h + fluid deficit

Subtract 10 mL kg^{-1} from fluid requirement for children who did not present with shock

Do not subtract resuscitation fluid volumes from fluid requirements for children who presented in shock

Isotonic balanced crystalloids or 0.9% sodium chloride initial fluid of choice - add potassium once passing urine and serum potassium is in normal range (usually < 5.5 mmol L^{-1}); add 5% dextrose to fluid when glucose less than 14 mmol L^{-1}

1–2 h after intravenous fluids commenced, start insulin infusion at 0.05–0.1 units kg^{-1} h^{-1} (0.05 units kg^{-1} h^{-1} for children < 5 years old recommended)

Monitor serum potassium and treat hypokalaemia

Do not give intravenous bicarbonate to correct acidosis

Observations

Strict fluid balance

Hourly capillary blood gas and blood glucose measurements

Capillary blood ketone levels 1–2 h (ideally point of care testing)

Initially two-hourly U+E's

Hourly BP, HR, RR, temperature

Hourly assessment of level of consciousness

Half hourly neuro observations including level of consciousness in children with severe DKA and children < 2 years old.

Urgently escalate symptoms of headache, bradycardia, changes in level of consciousness or changes in ECG (ST and T wave changes may indicate hypokalaemia)

Maintenance fluids calculation
4 mL kg^{-1} h^{-1} for first 10 kg of body weight
2 mL kg^{-1} h^{-1} for second 10 kg of body weight (11–20 kg)
1 mL kg^{-1} h^{-1} for each kg of body weight above 20 kg (up to max of 75 kg)

Fluid deficit (mL) = % dehydration x weight (kg) x 10
Fluid requirement (FR) over 48 h for a 10 kg child = maintenance requirement for 48 h + (fluid deficit – initial fluid given) (if no shock) (Note: max FR allowance for 5% dehydration = 3750 mL, 10% dehydration = 7500 mL)
Example: 5% dehydrated, no shock at presentation, given 10 mL kg^{-1} 0.9% saline = (4 x 10 x 48) + (5 x 10 x 10) – (10 x 10) = 1920 + 500 – 100 = 2320 mL over 48 h = 48 mL h^{-1}

Updated January 2023

FIGURE 6.5 Early management of DKA Resuscitation Council UK Guidelines (2024).

However, there may be diminished pulse pressure (difference between systolic and diastolic blood pressure) and an anxious demeanour. Tachycardia, tachypnoea, hypotension, oliguria and mental state changes become very evident at class III haemorrhage (30–40% blood loss). Class IV haemorrhage results in over 40% blood loss and the child becomes hypotensive and anuric and loses consciousness. In the United Kingdom, a protocol is initiated (sometimes known as a 'code red') when a massive haemorrhage is suspected, alerting the blood bank to ensure effective treatment is provided. In cases where bleeding persists, a surgical review is mandatory. If an injured child continues to deteriorate despite achieving haemostasis, other causes of shock must be investigated, for example, tension pneumothorax (a type of obstructive shock) or spinal shock (a type of distributive shock).

In haemorrhagic shock, red blood cell loss reduces oxygen delivery. Supplementary oxygen and RBC transfusion are important to restore oxygen-carrying capacity. Nurses must ensure supplemental oxygen is given when appropriate and monitor oxygen saturation (SpO_2) in any child in shock.

A child's CBV is higher than that of an adult. In infants, it is around 85–90 mL/kg of body weight; in younger children, 75–80 mL/kg; and in older children, 70–75 mL/kg. It is good practice to calculate a patient's CBV, especially post-surgery. So, you can monitor the percentage of blood loss.

Coordination between the multi-disciplinary teams (emergency, surgical, critical care and paediatrics) ensures optimal outcomes.

Case study 6.2

Timmy, a 10-year-old boy, arrives in the emergency department with his mother after a bicycle accident in which he fell onto a fence post, striking his abdomen. He was initially conscious and talking, but became pale and lethargic en route. There is no obvious external bleeding, though he is groaning in pain.

Vital signs	Observation	Normal Range
Temperature	36.8 °C	36.5–37.2 °C
Pulse	135 beats per minute	65–110 beats per minute
Respiratory rate	32 breaths per minute	18–30 breaths per minute
Blood pressure	85/50 mmHg	90–120 mmHg (diastolic)
CRT	3.5 seconds	Less than 2 seconds
Oxygen saturation	96% in air	95–100% in air
Level of consciousness	GCS 14 – slightly drowsy	GCS 15 – Alert on the AVPU scoring tool
Pain score	8/10	1/10 (no pain)

Timmy's PEWS is scoring at 5 due to his tachycardia, tachypnoea, reduced capillary refill time and level of consciousness. Skin is pale and his peripheral pulses are weak.

What are your immediate concerns regarding Timmy?
What management does Timmy need?

Investigations and fluid resuscitation

IV access – Two large-bore cannulas inserted
Full bloods, including crossmatch
Blood products
Fluid resuscitation – Initial 20 mL/kg of crystalloid solution
Oxygen therapy – 10/L via nonrebreather mask
Analgesia administered

It is recommended that blood products take priority over crystalloid fluid when significant blood loss may have occurred. Why do you think this is?

Timmy has a CT of his abdomen, and there is a laceration to his liver and active bleeding noted.

He is transferred to the operating theatre where haemostasis is achieved and then transferred to PICU.

Cardiogenic shock

Whilst all other types of shock are defined by poor intravascular volume, cardiogenic shock is defined as low CO with tissue hypoxia in the presence of adequate intravascular volume (Puri *et al.*, 2024). In other words, there is adequate circulating volume, but the heart is unable to pump this out efficiently or effectively. Thus, Sachdev *et al.* (2012) define cardiogenic shock as: sustained hypotension for a minimum of 30 minutes (systolic blood pressure for less than two standard deviations (2SD) for age, a reduced cardiac index <2.2 L/min in the presence of elevated pulmonary occlusion pressure (pressure measured in the left heart during cardiac catheterisation in the cardiac lab or during cardiac surgery).

Cardiogenic shock can have cardiac or non-cardiac causes. In aortic stenosis, adequate circulating volume exists, but a narrowed aorta obstructs blood flow from the left ventricle, causing poor tissue perfusion. In newborns, a patent ductus arteriosus initially maintains perfusion, but as it closes, critical obstruction develops; prostaglandin E_1 is used to keep it open until emergency treatment. This illustrates both cardiogenic shock and obstructive shock. Cardiac tamponade, where fluid compresses the heart, is another life-threatening cause. Septic shock can also lead to cardiogenic shock if heart contractility is impaired, with no element of obstruction.

Cardiac conditions that cause cardiogenic shock can be both congenital and/or acquired. Table 6.3 outlines the causes of cardiogenic shock in children. Specialist children's cardiac ICU with specially trained personnel and equipment are required to care for children with congenital or acquired cardiac conditions because they are at high risk of developing cardiogenic shock.

Cardiogenic shock can be differentiated into right and left ventricular failures. Table 6.4 shows causes of right ventricular failure (RVF). Table 6.5 highlights causes of left ventricular failure (LVF). It is important to appreciate these differences as treatment strategies can differ.

Table 6.6 provides an overview of the pathophysiology of the signs and symptoms of cardiogenic shock.

Early markers of compensation in shock include tachycardia and tachypnoea. Signs of decompensation include reduced urine output, cyanosis, cold extremities, altered

TABLE 6.4 Cardiogenic shock related to right ventricular failure (RVF)

- **Systolic dysfunction (decreased contractility)**
- RV infarction
- Ischaemia
- Hypoxia
- Acidosis
- **Increased afterload**
- Pulmonary embolism
- Pulmonary vascular disease
- Hypoxic pulmonary vasoconstriction
- Positive pressure ventilation with PEEP
- High alveolar pressures
- Acute respiratory distress syndrome
- Pulmonary fibrosis
- Sleep-disordered breathing
- Chronic obstructive pulmonary disease
- **Arrhythmias**

Source: Sachdev *et al.* (2012)/Manvinder Sachdev.

TABLE 6.3 Causes of cardiogenic shock in children

Congenital heart disease	Dysrhythmias	Metabolic	Ischaemia	Trauma
Hypoplastic left heart syndrome	Supraventricular Tachycardia	Acidosis	Myocarditis	Tension pneumothorax
Coarctation of the aorta	Ventricular tachycardia	Hyperkalaemia	Chemotherapy toxicity	Haemo-pericardium
Interrupted aorta	Atrioventricular block	Hypercalcaemia	Anaemia	Myocardial contusion
Transposition of the great arteries		Inborn errors of metabolism	Myocardial infarction	Cardiac aneurysm
Aortic stenosis		Drug toxicity	Kawasaki disease	
Tricuspid/mitral atresia			Calcium-channel blockers	
Mitral stenosis				
Atrial septal defect				
Ventricular septal defect				
Atrioventricular septal defect				

Source: Smith and Bigham (2013), Kar (2015) and Kosaraju *et al.* (2023).

TABLE 6.5 Cardiogenic shock related to left ventricular failure (LVF)

- **Systolic dysfunction (decreased contractility)**
- Ischaemia/infarction
- Global hypoxaemia
- Valvular disease
- Myocardial depressant drugs (beta-blockers, calcium-channel blockers and anti-arrhythmics)
- Myocardial contusion
- Respiratory acidosis
- Metabolic derangements
- **Diastolic dysfunction**
- Ischaemia
- Ventricular hypertrophy
- Restrictive cardiomyopathy
- Prolonged hypovolaemic or septic shock
- Ventricular interdependence
- Pericardial tamponade
- **Increased afterload**
- Aortic stenosis
- Hypertrophic cardiomyopathy
- Dynamic aortic outflow tract obstruction
- Coarctation of aorta
- Malignant hypertension
- **Valvular or structural anomaly**
- Mitral stenosis
- Endocarditis
- Mitral aortic regurgitation
- Obstruction
- Papillary muscle dysfunction or rupture
- Ruptured septum
- **Arrhythmias**

Source: Sachdev *et al.* (2012)/Manvinder Sachdev.

mental status or behaviour and hypotension. Persisting hypotension despite correction of hypovolaemia, arrhythmias, hypoxia and acidosis requires urgent treatment. Table 6.7 outlines treatment goals for children with cardiogenic shock.

Treatment strategies aim to increase stroke volume (SV) and cardiac contractility and reduce afterload. These may include cautious fluid resuscitation to minimise overload, drugs to support offload and/or support the heart (diuretics, inotropes, chronotropes and inodilators) and, in extreme cases, mechanical support such as extracorporeal membrane oxygenation (ECMO), which helps support the heart and lung functions in patients with severe cardiac and/or respiratory failure.

TABLE 6.6 Pathophysiology of the signs and symptoms of cardiogenic shock

Sign/symptom	Pathophysiology
Tachypnoea	Reflex response to rise in pulmonary venous pressure, LV volume and pressure
Dyspnoea	Pulmonary congestion, compression of bronchi by dilated pulmonary arteries or atria and pulmonary oedema
Feeding difficulty	Lack of energy to suck and tire quickly
Faltering weight	Inadequate calories due to feeding difficulty and extra work of breathing cause increased metabolic demand
Irritability	Reduced oxygen transport to the brain
Oliguria	Impaired renal perfusion
Diaphoresis	Increased sympathetic activity
Increased precordial activity	Chamber dilatation
Tachycardia	Increased sympathetic activity as a compensatory mechanism to increase oxygen delivery to tissues
Gallop sounds	Increased afterload, decreased compliance
Hepatomegaly, oedema	Systemic venous congestion
Reduced capillary filling	Reduced tissue perfusion
Lung crackles	Alveolar oedema

Source: Sachdev *et al.* (2012)/Manvinder Sachdev.

TABLE 6.7 The goals of treatment of children with cardiogenic shock

- General supportive care to maintain systemic perfusion
- Relieve systemic and pulmonary congestion
- Improve myocardial performance
- Optimise afterload
- Treat and manage the underlying cause

Source: Sachdev *et al.* (2012)/Manvinder Sachdev.

A common pathway to the pathophysiology of shock

Shock is characterised by poor circulating volume, hypoperfusion, organ dysfunction and organ failure. Reduced blood flow forces cells to use anaerobic metabolism, which is inefficient and produces lactic acid. Lactic acid creates an acidic environment that disrupts enzyme function. Lactate, normally cleared by the liver, can be measured at the bedside and serves as a marker of organ perfusion. Elevated lactate helps determine the need for fluid resuscitation or drugs to support vascular tone and cardiac function. Rising lactate increases morbidity and mortality in cardiogenic shock (Jentzer *et al.*, 2022).

The goal of shock treatment is to improve cardiac function and circulating volume to enhance oxygen delivery. Initial fluid resuscitation involves rapid boluses of 5–20 mL/kg to restore volume in hyperdynamic states. In cardiogenic shock or renal failure, fluids are given cautiously to avoid overload, which impairs cardiac contraction. Fluid resuscitation optimises preload and end-diastolic pressure, stretching cardiac muscle fibres to enhance SV without over- or under-stretching.

Fluid overload is harmful, causing respiratory congestion, impaired gas exchange and ventilation/perfusion mismatch. Diuretics or drugs to reduce cardiac load may be needed. Non-invasive ventilation can help manage pulmonary oedema, but positive pressure ventilation may worsen venous return and cause haemodynamic instability.

Fluid overload can be assessed by observing peripheral and pulmonary oedema, hepatomegaly, basal lung crackles, pink frothy sputum and jugular venous distension in older children. A chest X-ray can show pulmonary oedema and pleural effusions, and an ECG may also be useful.

An adequate circulatory system is required to deliver oxygenated blood to tissues to maintain their integrity. This requires a good venous return, adequate preload and end-diastolic pressure. Without good venous return, there will be poor ejection of systemic blood, which will cause poor flow and organ perfusion. Additionally, there must be a clear and patent pathway for blood to flow to the lungs so that haemoglobin can be oxygenated. Any obstruction to blood flow, inefficient or failing pulmonary function, low haemoglobin levels or structurally poor haemoglobin (e.g., in sickle cell disease) and poor oxygen saturation will all affect the oxygen content of arterial blood (CaO_2) and, in turn, oxygen delivery to the tissues. Heart and pulmonary diseases, such as asthma or bronchiolitis, which lead to excessive gas-trapping and increased transpulmonary pressure, plus positive pressure ventilation for respiratory failure, can impede venous return and thus preload.

The ultimate aim in managing shock is to restore circulating volume and oxygen delivery to tissues. Several key variables are fundamental to achieving this:

1. cardiac output (to deliver oxygen to tissues)
2. oxygen content in the blood
3. haemoglobin to bind oxygen.

CO is dependent on two variables, as shown in Fig. 6.6.

SV (Fig. 6.7) is the volume of blood ejected by the heart in one beat. SV depends on preload, afterload and cardiac contractility.

Cardiac output = heart rate × stroke volume

FIGURE 6.6 Cardiac output and its variables.

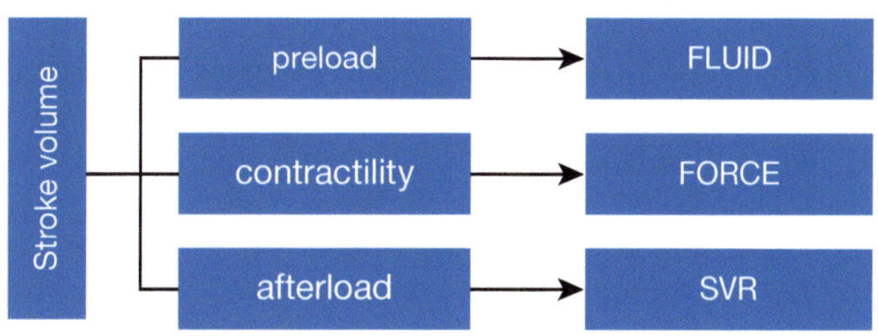

FIGURE 6.7 Stroke volume and its variables.

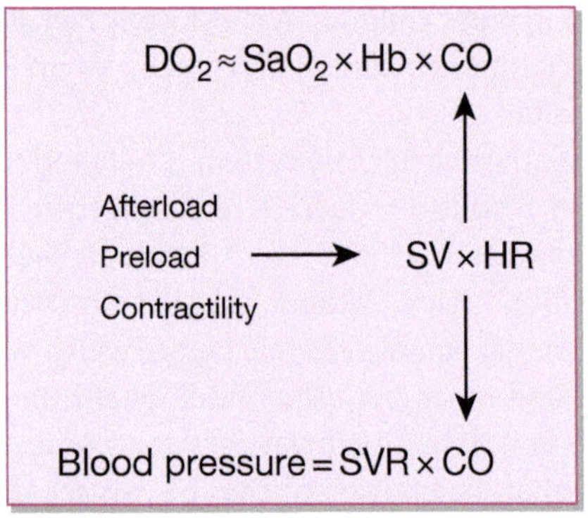

FIGURE 6.8 Oxygen delivery, blood pressure and its variables.
Source: Reproduced with permission.

It is essential to understand these principles to appreciate the pathophysiology of shock and its management.

The variables for oxygen delivery (DO_2) are highlighted in Fig. 6.8. Management focuses on the manipulation of one or more of these variables to reinstate oxygen delivery to tissues.

As identified in Fig. 6.6, CO is one of the variables associated with oxygen delivery, but CO is dependent on SV and HR. Older children can augment their CO by increasing both SV and HR but SV is relatively fixed in young children who cannot increase their SV to any great extent. This is because young hearts are less compliant and cannot stretch easily enough to accommodate an increasing SV. Thus, in young children, sympathetic stimulation leads to tachycardia very quickly and is one of the early signs of compensatory shock. Changes in HR are therefore very significant in unwell or sick children and must be closely monitored.

Extreme or prolonged fast HR (tachycardia), however, is dysfunctional. Extreme tachycardia shortens the diastolic phase of the cardiac cycle. As perfusion to cardiac muscle occurs during diastole, a shortened diastolic phase will affect cardiac perfusion. A very rapid HR will also increase myocardial oxygen consumption. This can cause the heart to become ischaemic. Children who are monitored using an electrocardiogram (ECG) will show an S-T depression on their ECG complex if the heart is ischaemic or under strain. Observing for this sign is an important duty for nurses who monitor children's ECGs. Bradycardia is a pre-terminal event.

In older children, extreme or prolonged tachycardia can lead to loss of the 'atrial kick', the final volume of blood ejected from the atria into the ventricles before atrial diastole. Atrial kick contributes to end-diastolic volume and pressure, influencing cardiac contractility, SV and CO according to the Frank–Starling principle. It helps prevent cardiac and pulmonary congestion and ensures efficient systolic contraction. Fluids or drugs may be given to normalise HR and should be closely monitored.

Strategies for caring for and managing the child or young person in shock

Early recognition and prompt treatment are fundamental in managing shock. The goals are to improve circulating volume, CO and blood pressure and reduce the risk of organ failure. While protocols vary, the aim is to restore circulating volume and perfusion pressure, which depends on blood pressure and SV. Strategies include fluid resuscitation, afterload manipulation, vasopressors and surgical intervention when needed. In extreme cases, mechanical support such as extracorporeal membrane oxygenation (ECMO) or extracorporeal life support (ECLS) may be required. Family involvement can aid early recognition, as they often notice subtle changes before medical staff (Hazinski 2013).

Monitoring end-organ perfusion

Monitoring end-organ perfusion is one of the most important and fundamental functions of the nurse and healthcare team. Poor end-organ perfusion is an early sign of shock. Poor end-organ perfusion includes changes to mental state and behaviour like confusion, agitation or lethargy. A prolonged capillary refill time of longer than 2 seconds, a skin temperature gradient, cool peripheries, pale, mottled skin and poor urine output are also very clear features of poor perfusion, which nurses should monitor closely. The PEWS, a track and trigger tool for identifying and recognising children at risk, is a useful tool for monitoring end-organ perfusion for children in shock states. Recovering patients show improvements in behaviour and mental status and recover a normalised capillary refill of less than 2 seconds, normal skin colour and temperature, moist mucous membranes and a good urine output.

The Paediatric Early Warning Tool does not score blood pressure, but baseline measurements should be taken and monitored in children with suspected shock to detect deterioration.

A systematic approach to assessing the patient in shock

The ABCDE(F) approach is a systematic approach to assessing the patient in shock.

Airway (A): The patient's airway may be at risk for several reasons. The moribund, obtunded patient, floppy and with a low coma score or unconsciousness, will be unable to protect their own airway. Patients requiring large volumes of fluid boluses (>60 mL/kg) will also be at risk due to possible oedema or soft tissue swelling. Patients undergoing invasive procedures require sedation, which may compromise their airway. A good GCS, cough and gag reflex are part of the airway assessment.

Breathing (B): Patients who are shocked require oxygen therapy, but this must be balanced against oxygen toxicity in neonates in particular, and in cardiac patients with cyanotic conditions and duct dependency. Central and peripheral cyanosis must be reported. Oxygen must be prescribed and titrated to condition, need, saturations and blood gases. Respiratory rate and effort, work of breathing and use of accessory muscles, chest wall expansion, the efficiency and effect of breathing are important parameters. Sputum must be analysed for appearance, volume, consistency, colour and smell. Fine crackles on auscultation may indicate pulmonary oedema. Coarse crackles may suggest sputum/secretions from infection or aspiration. Wheezing and stridor may be due to anaphylaxis. A chest X-ray may be required.

Circulation (C): Colour, skin temperature and central and peripheral capillary refill time are assessed to determine perfusion status. Core temperature, HR and rhythm, pulse rate, volume, character and rhythm are assessed. Central and peripheral pulses are palpated and compared. ECG monitoring may be in situ. Blood pressure trends are monitored and reported. Central venous pressure may be monitored, and a central venous gas may be required to determine volume status. Septic screens, FBC, clotting and coagulation profiles and U&E will be monitored. An echocardiogram may be performed.

Disability (D): Glasgow coma score is assessed and managed. A floppy patient is seriously unwell. Blood glucose level is monitored.

Exposure (E): The patient must be fully exposed and assessed. There may be obvious bleeding. A distended abdomen may suggest internal bleeding. Bruises may indicate low platelets or a clotting disorder. Rashes must be carefully assessed. A petechial rash may point to meningococcal septicaemia. An urticarial rash may be a sign of anaphylaxis. Other discolouration or anomalies give clues to the reason for the shocked state and response to treatment.

Family (F): The family will also require support during this time.

As the patient begins to recover, a more holistic approach, such as Roper's activities of living model, can be taken. In the unfortunate situation that the patient is in irretractable shock, then a dignified approach to end-of-life care is required.

In darker skin, cyanosis may appear greyish or whitish. Assess subtle signs in the mucous membranes, nail beds and eyes rather than relying on skin tone alone.

Conclusion

Shock is a life-threatening condition. This chapter has outlined its types, management and key concepts, including oxygen delivery, fluid resuscitation, perfusion, end-organ assessment and systematic patient monitoring. Nurses must understand the pathophysiology and apply these principles to provide effective care. With timely and appropriate treatment, most patients recover and can lead normal lives.

References

Advanced Life Support Group (2021) Advanced Paediatric Life Support: A Practical Approach to Emergencies: 7th ed. Chichester: Wiley-Blackwell

Barrett, L., & Curry, N. (2025). Transfusion in trauma: empiric or guided therapy? *Research and Practice in Thrombosis and Haemostasis* 9(1), 102663.

Blumlein, D., & Griffiths, I. (2022). Shock: aetiology, pathophysiology and management. *British Journal of Nursing* 31(8), 422–428.

Cannon, J.W. (2018). Hemorrhagic shock. *The New England Journal of Medicine* 378(4), 370–379.

Dave, S., Dahlstrom, D., & Weisbrod, L. (2023). *Neurogenic Shock.* StatPearls Publishing LLC.

Dellinger, R.P., Levy, M.M., Rhodes, A., *et al.* (2013). Surviving sepsis campaign: international guidelines for management of severe sepsis. *Intensive Care Medicine* 39(2), 165–228.

Gobinathan, S., & Suresh Kannan, K. (2018). Study of prevalence, eitology, response to treatment and outcome of paediatric shock in tertiary care hospital Internation. *Journal of Contemporary Paediatrics* 5(3), 1104.

Great Ormond Street Hospital for Children (2015). *Paediatric Sepsis 6 Protocol* Great Ormond Street Hospital [retrieved on April, 25th, 2025] chrome-extension://efaidnbmnnnibpcajpcglclefindmkaj/https://cats.nhs.uk/wp-content/uploads/guideline-sepsis.pdf.

Hazinski, M.F. (2013). *Nursing Care of the Critically Ill Child*, 3rd edn. Elsevier Mosby, St. Louis.

Hobson, J.H., & Chima, S.R. (2013). Pediatric hypovolemic shock. *The Open Pediatric Medicine Journal* 7, 10–15.

Hooper, N., & Armstrong, T.J. (2022). Hemorrhagic shock. In: *StatsPearl.* StatsPearls publishing https://www.ncbi.nlm.nih.gov/books/NBK470382/.

Jentzer, J.C., Schrage, B., Patel, P.C., *et al.* (2022). Association between the acidemia, lactic acidosis, and shock severity with outcomes in patients with cardiogenic shock. *Journal of the American Heart Association* 11(9), e024932–e024932.

Kar, S.S. (2015). Pediatric cardiogenic shock: current perspectives. *Archives of Medicine and Health Sciences* 3(2), 252–265.

Kosaraju, A., Pendela, V.S., Hai, O. (2023) Cardiogenic Shock. In StatPearls [Internet]. Treasure Island (FL): StatPearls Publishing; 2025 Jan-. Available from: https://www.ncbi.nlm.nih.gov/sites/books/NBK482255/

Kripa, K.C., & Khanal, S. (2021). Use of midodrine and fludrocortisone in neurogenic shock: a case report. *Annals of Medicine and Surgery* 70, 102811.

Lin, N., Jin, J., Yang, S., *et al.* (2024). A nomogram for predicting hemorrhagic shock in pediatric patients with multiple trauma. *Scientific Reports* 14(1), 13308–13309.

Miura, S., Michihata, N., Hashimoto, Y., *et al.* (2023). Descriptive statistics and risk factors analysis of children with community-acquired septic shock. *Journal of Intensive Care* 11(6).

Moore, G., Knight, G., & Blann, A. (2016). *Haematology*, 2nd edn. Oxford University Press, Oxford.

National Institute for Health and Care Excellence (NICE) (2024). Sepsis: recognition, diagnosis and early management. NICE guideline [NG51]. NICE, UK.

Puri, K., Jentzer, J., Spinner, J., *et al.* (2024). Clinical presentation, classification, and outcomes of cardiogenic shock in children. *Journal of the American College of Cardiology* 83(5), 595–608.

Resuscitation Council UK Guidelines (2021). Special Circumstances Guidelines Resuscitation Council UK [retrieved on April, 25th, 2025] https://www.resus.org.uk/library/2021-resuscitation-guidelines/special-circumstances-guidelines.

Resuscitation Council UK Guidelines (2024). *Paediatric emergency algorithms and resources version 3* Resuscitation Council UK [retrieved on April, 28th 2025] chrome-extension://efaidnbmnnnibpcajpcglclefindmkaj/https://www.resus.org.uk/sites/default/files/2024-07/RCUK%20Paediatric%20emergency%20algortihms%20and%20resources%20Jun%2024%20V3.pdf.

Sachdev, M.S., Aggarwal, N., Joshi, R.K. & Joshi, R. (2012). Cardiogenic shock in children. [Review article] [online] Available at: https://www.researchgate.net/publication/278021324 (accessed 15 March 2016).

Singer, M., Deutschman, C.S., Seymour, C.W., *et al.* (2016). The third international consensus definitions for sepsis and septic shock (Sepsis-3). *JAMA* 315(8), 801–810.

Sinniah, D. (2012). Shock in children. IeJSME 6(Suppl 1), S129–S136. https://pdfs.semanticscholar.org/8485/636ffb90f8816b31f2061538a1481484770e.pdf (accessed April 2018).

Smith, K., & Bigham, M.T. (2013). Cardiogenic shock. *The Open Pediatric Medicine Journal* 7(1: M5), 19–27.

Standl, T., Annecke, T., Cascorbi, I., *et al.* (2018). The nomenclature, definition and distinction of types of shock. *Deutsches Ärzteblatt International* 115(45), 757–768.

Stephenson, M. (2020). Understanding shock in children. *British Journal of Nursing* 29(6), 350–352.

Waltzman, M.L. (2015). Pediatric shock. *Journal of Emergency Nursing.* 41(2), 113–118 https://doi.org/10.1016/j.jen.2014.12.015.

CHAPTER 7

Trauma and rehabilitation

Louise McLaughlin

AIM

The aim of this chapter is to develop an insight into how trauma affects children and young people within the four domains of health.

LEARNING OUTCOMES

On completion of this chapter, the reader will be able to:

- Explain the C-ABCDE mnemonic in relation to trauma.
- Discuss the implications of safeguarding for children and young people who suffer non-accidental injuries.
- Describe the lethal triad of death and the implications for the child or young person.
- Discuss how trauma affects the child and young person's mental health and how nursing staff can support the child or young person when delivering care.

KEYWORDS

- trauma
- haemorrhage
- acidosis
- hypothermia
- trauma-informed care
- pre-hospital care
- receiving care
- rehabilitation
- shock
- stress

Test your knowledge

1. Hypothermia is associated with what range of temperatures?
2. What is the function of the meninges?
3. What may cause trauma to children and young people?
4. What may cause trauma to the neonate or foetus?
5. What four stages make up the major trauma pathway?

Introduction

Trauma care is unplanned and involves treating and rehabilitating patients who have been injured in unexpected events such as falls, road traffic collisions or sporting accidents. Any body structure can be affected, so trauma care occurs in a range of settings, including the children's emergency department, paediatric intensive care unit (PICU) and orthopaedic trauma unit (Santy-Tomlinson *et al.*, 2023).

This chapter will examine the major trauma pathway and the settings in which a child or young person may receive care, from the scene of injury to trauma units and wards. It will also consider the ways children and young people may experience trauma, associated pathophysiological changes and the social and psychological impacts.

National Institute for Health and Care Excellence (NICE) guidance

NICE published guidance in 2016 on managing major trauma in both pre-hospital and hospital settings, aiming to reduce mortality and disability in people with serious injuries. Two key documents are relevant. The first document, *Major Trauma: Service Delivery* (NG40), provides recommendations on pre-hospital triage, determining the most appropriate destination for major trauma patients, organising hospital trauma services, supporting families and ensuring effective documentation and audit (NICE, 2016a). It also highlights the anatomical, pathophysiological and psychosocial needs of children, with specific guidance on paediatric trauma teams, safeguarding, minimising radiation exposure from imaging and supporting distressed families and carers.

The companion guidance, *Major Trauma: Assessment and Initial Management* (NICE, 2016b), focuses on the rapid identification and treatment of major trauma in both pre-hospital and hospital settings. Like the service delivery guidance, it emphasises the specific needs of children and young people. It recommends X-ray and ultrasound as first-line imaging for chest trauma in those under 16, owing to the radiation risks of CT. The document also provides clear advice on referral and management of active bleeding and major haemorrhage. Venous access is addressed as well, with intraosseous (IO) access recommended as first line when peripheral access is likely to be difficult.

Trauma in the child and young person

Trauma can be associated with significant mortality and morbidity. It is one of the leading causes of death in children and is a cause of disability (RCPCH, 2020). In England, moderate to severe trauma is often a result of falls, traffic incidents and direct blows (Jones *et al.*, 2019). Whilst penetration injuries are relatively low, there is a worrying trend of knife crime.

TABLE 7.1 Common causes of trauma by age

Age (years)	Cause of trauma
0–1 years	Non-accidental injury (NAI), choking, burns, drowning, falls
2–4 years	Road traffic incidents, burns drowning
5–14 years	Road traffic incidents, road traffic incidents as a pedestrian, bicycle injuries, burns, drowning.

Source: Fisher *et al.* (2017).

Table 7.1 breaks down the common causes of trauma by age. It is particularly worth noting the non-accidental injury (NAI) in the 0–1-year group.

Injury causes vascular and tissue damage, leading to bleeding and loss of circulating volume. Trauma also triggers local inflammatory responses, with endothelial damage allowing intravascular fluid to shift into the extravascular space. Together, these effects result in hypovolaemia, which becomes problematic as compensatory mechanisms become less effective (Clews *et al.*, 2022).

Major trauma pathway

The major trauma pathway can be divided into four stages: pre-hospital care, reception, definitive care and rehabilitation (Bramley *et al.*, 2022). This ensures that the patient receives the correct care and treatment at the correct time.

Pre-hospital care

This may include transferring the child or young person to a major trauma centre (MTC) with the appropriate pre-hospital care. The MTCs have the appropriate resources to treat the trauma population within the region and are required to have the specialist facilities to treat patients with any type of injury combinations (Lucena-Amaro and Zolfaghari, 2022).

Within the hospital setting, the usual assessment of ABCDE (airway, breathing, circulation, disability, exposure) is recommended; within the pre-hospital setting, it is important to consider catastrophic bleeding ahead of

TABLE 7.2 C-ABCDE assessment

Recognise	Assess for	Management
Catastrophic bleeding	Life-threatening haemorrhage	Apply direct pressure, compression bandage or tourniquet
Airway compromise	Patent airway	Protect airway with adjuncts. Consider cervical spine protection
Breathing difficulty	Poor respiratory effort Pneumothorax	Administer oxygen. Chest decompression
Circulation (haemorrhagic shock)	Cool skin Tachycardia Bleeding	Apply compression bandage. Administer tranexamic acid. Blood transfusion if available
Disability (head injury)	Reduced consciousness	Protect airway
Exposure	Hypoglycaemia Hypothermia	Maintain normothermia.

Source: Adapted from Mercer (2018).

bleeding (C-ABCDE) (Table 7.2). This is because haemorrhage is the cause of over 50% of deaths from major trauma (Spahn *et al.*, 2019). It is important to stop bleeding quickly due to the limited blood volume.

Catastrophic bleeding

This is time-critical for all, but even more so for babies whose blood volume is much smaller than that of older children. According to Hunt *et al.* (2015), catastrophic bleeding may be defined as 20% blood loss in less than one hour or 50% blood volume loss in less than 3 hours (infant blood volume 90 mL/kg and older child 80 mL/kg).

Airway

Airway patency with cervical spine control is the priority, as respiratory function can deteriorate rapidly in children (Chapter 12). Children's smaller airways make them more prone to obstruction from swelling, and loose teeth in younger children may dislodge during injury or airway manoeuvres (Riccio & Parikh, 2021). Observing airway sounds helps identify problems: stridor may indicate upper airway trauma, gurgling suggests blood or secretions pooling and grunting, snorting or choking may signal obstruction (Bramley *et al.*, 2022; Mininder & Newman, 2021). The head should be kept neutral, with a jaw thrust if needed. Oral or nasopharyngeal airway adjuncts may be used, unless a basal skull fracture is suspected, and a supraglottic airway may be required if these measures fail (Grice *et al.*, 2022; NICE, 2016b).

Breathing

As discussed in Chapter 12, children have specific anatomical and physiological considerations. Breathing should be assessed by inspection, auscultation, percussion and palpation. Breath sounds should be equal in both lungs; diminished or absent sounds may indicate pneumothorax, haemothorax or a displaced endotracheal tube (Mininder & Newman, 2021). The thorax should be examined for penetrating injuries, tracheal deviation (suggesting tension pneumothorax on the opposite side) and subcutaneous emphysema in the chest or neck, which may also indicate tension pneumothorax.

Circulation

Circulatory compromise may present as an elevated heart rate, falling blood pressure, delayed capillary refill or cool, mottled extremities. Importantly, children can compensate for significant blood loss before becoming hypotensive or showing other signs of hypovolaemic shock (Minder & Newman, 2021).

Disability

The Glasgow Coma Scale (GCS) is used to assess neurological function, measuring eye opening, verbal response and motor response (Teasdale & Jennett, 1974), aiding assessment and clinical decision-making. AVPU (Alert, Voice, Pain, Unresponsive) (American College of Surgeons Committee on Trauma, 1989) is a simpler, rapid alternative for assessing consciousness. Pupil assessment is also important in head trauma: oval or sluggish pupils, or a deviated pupil, may indicate herniation or raised intracranial pressure, while bilaterally small pupils may suggest opioid toxicity.

Exposure

Clothing should be removed for inspection, while maintaining the child's dignity, and the patient should be kept warm with blankets. Visible injuries, including lacerations, abrasions and fractures, should be examined, with fractures assessed for bruising, swelling, deformity, immobility and pain. Bladder trauma may occur after blunt or penetrating abdominal injury; significant pain, suprapubic tenderness or bleeding at the urethral meatus warrants further investigation (Kang & Geube, 2022). Body temperature should also be noted, as hypothermia contributes to the lethal triad in haemorrhage.

Reception – receiving team

The trauma team prepares for the patient's arrival, prioritising the identification and treatment of immediately life-threatening conditions in a rapid assessment, usually under one minute (Lucena-Amaro & Zolfaghari, 2022). Once stabilised, a full examination identifies injuries and medical conditions, allowing a definitive care plan to be developed (Bramley *et al.*, 2022).

Interventions

Early imaging is essential in the trauma pathway to identify life-threatening injuries. For children under 16, X-ray or ultrasound is recommended first-line due to radiation risks (NICE, 2016b). CT, offering rapid, high-resolution imaging, is commonly used in patients over 16 (Lauder & Driscoll, 2022). Indications for CT include:

- Any haemodynamic instability
- Significant injuries, including head and/or spine
- Any severe injuries that cannot be excluded by clinical examination, with consideration of the mechanism of injury and presentation
- Any X-rays that suggest any significant injury such as a pneumothorax

Arterial blood gas analysis may be required, particularly with thoracic trauma or intubation, providing information on oxygenation, carbon dioxide, haemoglobin and lactate, which indicates tissue perfusion and oxygenation (Goode *et al.*, 2022).

Definitive care

Definitive care is consultant-led and multidisciplinary, involving physical and psychological support if the patient is fit for discharge (Bramley *et al.*, 2022). Transfer or retrieval to areas such as PICU may be necessary, so local transfer guidelines should be followed to ensure safe and efficient movement of the child with major trauma.

Rehabilitation

Lockey (2018) notes that improved survival from major trauma, thanks to trauma networks and MTCs, has increased the demand for services supporting children and young people to regain their pre-injury quality of life. This support may occur in hospital or community settings.

Rehabilitation involves assessment, treatment and management to help the child achieve independence and a good quality of life (Graham, 2022). The multidisciplinary team works with the child and family to meet these goals. Children's rehabilitation needs differ from adults', reflecting their functional priorities. Key considerations include (Grice *et al.*, 2022):

- Supporting return to previous functional levels, including nursery, school or college
- Emotional, psychological and psychosocial support
- Provision of equipment and adaptations
- Ongoing recovery from injury
- Further surgery or hospital readmissions

NICE (2016a) recommends that children meeting major trauma criteria have a rehabilitation assessment and plan within 72 hours of admission. The plan should:

- Involve the patient and/or their family in its development
- Be administered by a specialist in children's rehabilitation
- Include a clear rehabilitation plan
- Be shared with the child, family, GP and next care provider, if applicable

The rehabilitation plan should meet the following minimum standards:

- Patient demographics
- Safeguarding assessment related to the injury circumstances, even if no concerns exist
- Actions for community teams, including GP and parents/carers
- Management plan for each injury

- Ongoing rehabilitation needs
- Any referrals made
- Educational plan
- Safety-netting guidance
- Section for the child and family to record comments

The triad of death – hypothermia, acidosis and coagulopathy – can be fatal following major trauma. Although rare, trauma patients often present with significant bleeding, creating a vicious cycle that is difficult to reverse (Credland, 2016).

Lethal triad of death

Hypothermia can result from issues such as fluid resuscitation, central nervous system injuries related to unstable thermoregulation or exposure of the skin/body to the surrounding environment (Dyer & Neal, 2017). Hypothermia is defined as a core body temperature below 35°C (Azarkane *et al.*, 2024). Hypothermia is associated with a poor outcome, such as death, particularly in those whose core body temperature falls below 32°C. Wolberg *et al.* (2004) discovered that during the coagulation cascade, enzyme function, platelet adhesion and aggregation were impaired below 33°C. Clots are able to form in the hypothermic patient, but this was at a much slower rate in patients with temperatures between 33 and 33.9°C. Rewarming measures should be taken in hypothermic trauma patients to counteract the contribution hypothermia adds to coagulopathy.

Trauma patients often develop acidosis, usually from hypoperfusion due to severe haemorrhage. Reduced blood flow shifts cellular metabolism from aerobic to anaerobic, leading to lactate accumulation and poor outcomes, including death (Dyer & Neal, 2017). Acidosis also worsens coagulopathy, as blood pH below 7.2 directly impairs clotting factors and haemostasis (Dyer & Neal, 2017).

The third component of the triad of death is coagulopathy, which can be worsened by hypothermia and acidosis. Impaired coagulation leads to further blood loss, intensifying hypothermia and acidosis. Haemorrhage depletes platelets, clotting factors and fibrinogen, while local inflammation may reduce the function of some coagulation factors. The triad of death is summarised in Fig. 7.1.

Intraosseous/peripheral access

Circulatory access is essential for delivering fluids and medications to trauma patients. Access may be peripheral, or, if difficult, IO access should be used (NICE, 2016a). Vascular access can be challenging due to blood loss, collapsed veins, trauma or factors such as obesity (Qasim & Joseph, 2024). IO access delivers fluids and medications

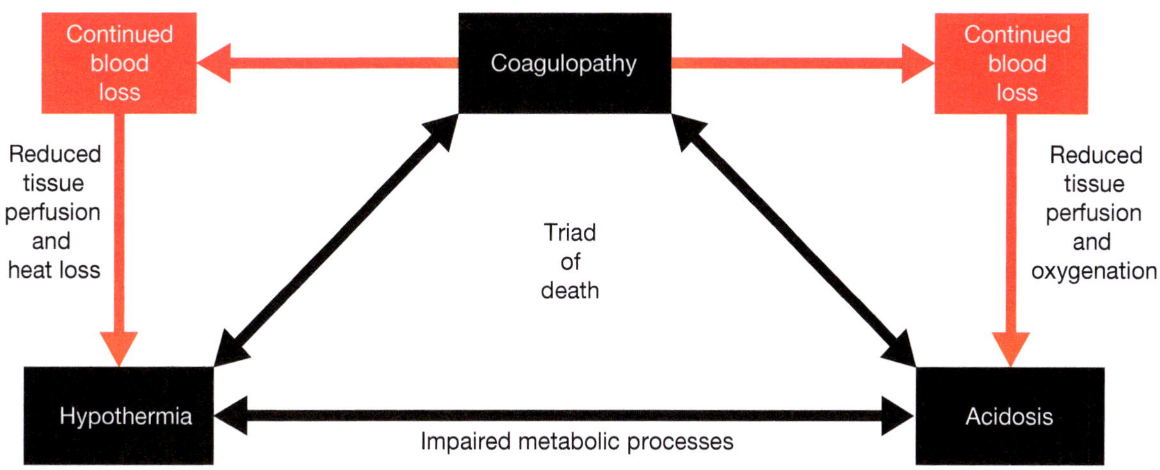

FIGURE 7.1 The triad of death.
Source: Reproduced from Clews *et al.* (2022)/John Wiley & Sons.

directly to the bone marrow. Site selection depends on the child's age, clinical situation and clinician preference: the proximal tibia is preferred for all ages, the distal femur for children under six, and the proximal humerus for children over six (SORT, 2022). IO access is contraindicated if these sites are unidentifiable, fractured or infected or have had an IO insertion within the past 48 hours.

Non-accidental injuries

Local policy must be followed when managing suspected non-accidental injury (NAI). Suspicious injuries include long bone fractures in non-mobile children, metaphyseal or epiphyseal injuries, spiral fractures, rib fractures in young infants, burns in unexpected areas and injuries inconsistent with the reported cause. Other warning signs include delayed presentation, incompatible histories or changing accounts over time. Further guidance is provided by NICE (2017).

Special considerations

Children with complex needs or developmental delays may rely entirely on carers for daily needs. When assessing injuries, it is important to consider the child's abilities in relation to the reported mechanism, for example, a burn on the leg of a non-mobile teenager.

Head trauma

Traumatic brain injury is a leading cause of death and disability in children and young people. Those from lower socioeconomic backgrounds are at higher risk of falls (Lawrence *et al.*, 2016), highlighting the importance of targeted prevention, such as home safety and cycle safety measures.

'Secondary injury' refers to the ongoing cascade following the initial trauma, involving inflammatory mediators, continued brain cell death and metabolic disturbances. Early, aggressive management of respiratory and cardiovascular status is crucial, as hypoxia can worsen brain injury. Secondary injury causes greater morbidity in children than adults due to higher brain metabolic demand and limited substrate availability.

A history should be taken for any head injury, including the date and time, mechanism (including fall height) and witnesses. Symptoms may include loss of consciousness, headache, confusion, agitation, drowsiness, vomiting or post-injury seizures (Davis *et al.*, 2017). Assessment depends on the injury mechanism, with consideration of the cervical spine. Neurological evaluation should include GCS and pupil assessment (see Chapter 10). Scalp signs such as haematomas or lacerations should be noted; large 'boggy' haematomas (>5 cm or over the parietal/occipital bones) may indicate an underlying fracture (Davis *et al.*, 2017).

Investigations

Majority of head injuries require minimal investigations. A CT scan may be required to exclude significant intracerebral injury. NICE (2023) provides guidance for the use of CT imaging. Some of the risk factors identified by NICE are:

- Post-traumatic seizure
- A GCS less than 14 or 15 2 hours after injury
- Suspected open or depressed skull fracture
- Any sign of basal skull fracture, such as panda eyes, Battle's sign or any cerebrospinal fluid leakage from the nose or ears
- Suspicion of non-accidental injury

Non-accidental head injury (shaken baby syndrome)

The term 'non-accidental head injury' is preferred, as it emphasises the deliberate nature of the trauma rather than the action itself, helping healthcare professionals focus on the cause rather than the mechanism.

The brain is encased in three meninges whose function is to protect the brain (see Fig. 7.2, the meninges).

The pia mater closely encases the brain, followed by the arachnoid, with the subarachnoid space between them. The outermost membrane, the dura, surrounds the brain and extends down the spinal cord. Between the dura and arachnoid lies the subdural space, which contains bridging veins.

Non-accidental head injury in infants often presents with the triad of encephalopathy, subdural haemorrhage

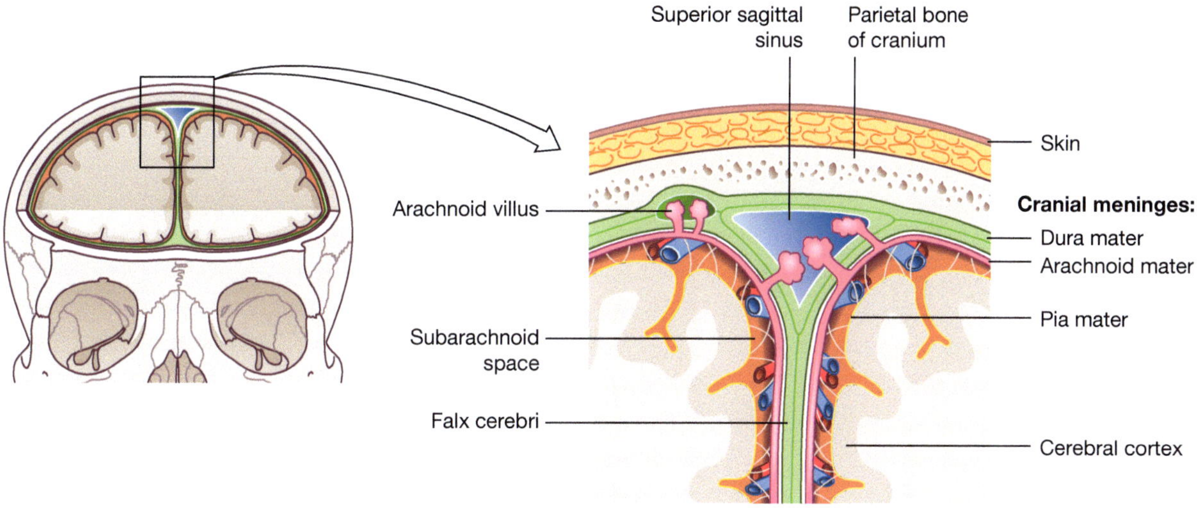

FIGURE 7.2 The coverings of the brain.

and retinal haemorrhage. These injuries are thought to result from shaking, with or without impact, causing the brain to move within the skull. Acceleration and deceleration forces can move the vitreous gel in the eyes, leading to retinal haemorrhage from traction and shearing; severe cases may cause traumatic retinoschisis (Shouldice *et al.*, 2018). Fontanelle fullness may indicate raised intracranial pressure. Periorbital ecchymosis (raccoon eyes) and ecchymosis behind the ears (Battle's sign) suggest a basal skull fracture (Titchner *et al.*, 2016). These signs are rare without major head injury and may take time to appear.

Infants are vulnerable to non-accidental head injury due to their size and portability, dependency on their caretakers and their inability to report abuse.

Acquired brain injury in the foetus and newborn

> *In utero*, a foetus receives nutrients and oxygen via the umbilical cord. In the United Kingdom, pregnant people are offered regular scans and midwife assessments to monitor foetal development. Any concerns identified during these checks prompt referrals to appropriate specialist teams.

Preterm neonates have a higher risk of neurological injury due to an immature germinal matrix in the ventricles and an underdeveloped cerebral blood supply before 34 weeks' gestation (Mangahis *et al.*, 2024). This increases the risk of bleeding and ischaemic brain damage, which can lead to cerebral palsy and other adverse neurodevelopmental outcomes (Leijser & de Vries, 2024).

During labour, interruptions to a foetus's oxygen and nutrient supply – due to cord complications, placental abruption or infection – can impair brain function, potentially causing hypoxic-ischaemic encephalopathy (HIE) (Martinez-Biarge & Cowan, 2024). In preterm neonates, HIE can be difficult to detect due to naturally low muscle tone, ventilation and assisted feeding needs, with signs appearing 12–24 hours after the event in both preterm and term infants. There is no specific treatment for preterm HIE, as they are vulnerable to hyperglycaemia and haemorrhage. Term infants may receive therapeutic hypothermia, but this is unsuitable for preterm neonates due to risks to haemodynamic and physiological stability (Herrera *et al.*, 2018). Prognosis is poorer in preterm infants, often involving central grey matter and brainstem injury, multiorgan failure and developmental impairment in survivors.

Head injuries may occur during delivery or from assisted interventions and can be classified as extracranial or intracranial. Fig. 7.3 shows the brain regions at risk. These injuries are discussed in detail further.

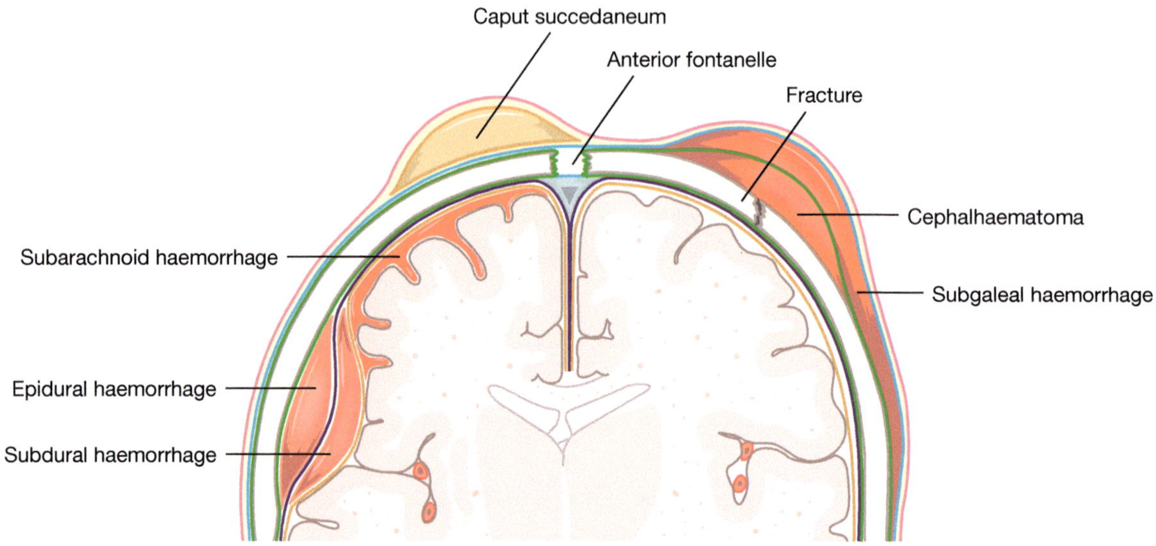

FIGURE 7.3 Neonatal brain injury.
Source: Gerda et al. (2025)/Springer International Publishing AG.

Extracranial injuries

Extracranial injuries that occur outside the cranium are as follows:

- Caput succedaneum: Oedema over the presenting part during vaginal birth, which forms due to the pressure against the vaginal wall while the head is passing through the birth canal. Serosanguineous fluid may leak from subcutaneous tissue, causing oedema. It is usually asymptomatic and subsides over time.
- Cephalohaematoma: It is a collection of blood or serosanguinous fluid caused by the skull compressing against the pelvic bone during birth. This shearing bleeds into the subperiosteal layer, lifting the periosteum, but is contained by ligaments at cranial suture lines, so it does not cross sutures. It usually enlarges in the first days after birth and resolves by 6–7 weeks. Cephalohaematoma can increase the risk of jaundice and secondary infection, and may be associated with skull fractures. Surgical intervention may be required for ossified lesions.
- Subgaleal haemorrhage: It is a potentially life-threatening emergency, often linked to perinatal asphyxia. Signs include diffuse scalp swelling, displaced earlobes, swollen eyelids, increased head circumference, pallor, poor perfusion, lethargy, poor feeding, tachypnoea, laboured breathing, tachycardia (more than 160 beats per minute), apnoea and seizures (Mohammed *et al.*, 2024). Neonates with a history of traumatic birth or vacuum-/forceps-assisted delivery should be closely monitored and assessed using a strict protocol.

Intracranial injuries

Intracranial injuries that occur within the cranium are as follows:

- Subdural haemorrhage: This can be common in term infants and can be an incidental finding on brain magnetic resonance imaging (MRI). Risk factors are similar to those of other mechanical birth injuries, such as instrumental delivery and foetal distress. A subdural haemorrhage is usually small and asymptomatic, but can present with seizures and/or episodes of apnoea if substantial. If asymptomatic, no interventions are usually required, but emergency neurosurgical drainage or aspiration may be necessary if the bleed is large and symptomatic. Subdural haemorrhage can be associated with poor outcome, especially with associated perinatal asphyxia (Hong & Lee, 2018).

- Subarachnoid haemorrhage: Larger subarachnoid haemorrhages can be associated with seizures and/or apnoeas and bradycardia. Prognosis is usually favourable unless comorbidities such as HIE and hydrocephalus exist. Treatment is usually supportive and symptomatic (Mohammed *et al.*, 2024).

Case study 7.1

Pawel, aged 6, was struck by a car mounting the pavement while walking home from school, being thrown approximately 6 m. Witnesses called 999. On ambulance arrival, he was unresponsive with a large, actively bleeding laceration on the right forehead. He was immobilised, received fluids via an IO in the left tibia, and was transferred to a children's emergency department.

On arrival, his observations are recorded as:

Vital sign	Observation	Normal range
Temperature	36.8 °C	36.5–37.5 °C
Pulse	64 beats per minute	75–115 beats per minute
Respiratory rate	10 breaths per minute	18–24 breaths per minute
Blood pressure	85/42 mmHg (systolic)	82–115 mmHg (systolic)
CRT	4 seconds	<2 seconds
Oxygen saturation	92%	98–100%
Level of consciousness	Voice on AVPU scale	Alert on AVPU scale
Pain score	10	No pain

A CT is indicated in accordance with NICE guidance. This suggests a large subdural haematoma, which needs to be surgically drained. He goes straight into surgery for this and is then admitted into PICU. He makes a full recovery with assistance from the MDT team, including speech and language therapists (SALT), physiotherapists, doctors and nurses, only to name a few.

Orthopaedic trauma care

Orthopaedic trauma care is specifically focused on trauma to the musculoskeletal system. Fractures are common in children due to factors such as play, sports and a curious nature. Most fractures occur outdoors, with a quarter of fractures occurring in the radius, and boys are more likely to sustain a fracture than girls (Diab & Staheli, 2015). Trauma to the bones can affect the growth, causing the metaphysis and epiphysis to unite, or on the other hand, it may stimulate the growth plate to overdevelop (Diab & Staheli, 2015).

Healthy bone development in children requires a diet rich in calcium and vitamin D, along with outdoor time for sun exposure to boost vitamin D levels. However, socio-economic factors such as housing and finances can limit access to a nutritious diet and outdoor activities.

Spinal injury

Typically, those who sustain a new spinal cord injury (SCI) in the United Kingdom may develop neurological consequences such as paraplegia, quadriplegia and even death (Todd, 2022). Following the trauma, the spinal cord function must be preserved to prevent any neurological damage. Therefore, any vertebral column or spinal cord movement must be stopped and optimal cord perfusion maintained.

Spinal cord injury (SCI) is irreversible, but secondary mechanical, hypoxic and hypotensive damage can be prevented. Most secondary neurological deterioration results from abnormal movement of an unstable vertebral column (Todd *et al.*, 2015). Strategies should therefore be used to prevent avoidable neurological harm until spinal injuries are confirmed or excluded, especially in children with concerning trauma mechanisms, reduced consciousness or significant distracting injuries (Grice *et al.*, 2022).

The head, and particularly the occipital region, is much larger in babies and children than it is in adolescents. Therefore, when assessing the child with a potential SCI, care must be taken not to hyperextend the neck as this could result in further spinal cord damage as well as airway obstruction. According to Grice *et al.* (2022), SCI in children under 8 years of age most commonly occurs in the first three vertebrae, increasing the likelihood of SCI due to abnormal movement of the vertebrae.

Ballistic trauma

Within recent years, gang violence, including knife and gun crime involving children and young people, has increased (Deucher *et al.*, 2022). Whilst trauma is generally categorised as blunt or penetrating, gunshot wounds have features of both. As a bullet penetrates the body, it converts its kinetic energy into injury as it passes through the tissues that it directly contacts, creating what is known as the permanent cavity. As the bullet expands its kinetic energy, a 'shock wave' known as the secondary or temporary cavity occurs around the permanent cavity. This temporary cavity is the result of tissues stretching before going back to their normal configuration. It is when the elasticity of tissue reaches its limit, injuries occur. Therefore, tissues with high elasticity such as the bowel and the lung are more resistant to temporary cavity-related injury as opposed to relatively inelastic tissues such as the liver (Ditkofsky *et al.*, 2023).

Exit wounds are usually larger and irregular in shape than the entry wound. Determining the exit site may be difficult if the bullet has become fragmented or ricocheted off dense material, such as bone (Baum *et al.*, 2022). While soft tissues respond to impact by 'crushing and stretching', bone reacts to similar trauma by fracturing. The way the bone fractures will be dependent on the impact energy and location (Baum *et al.*, 2022).

Shock and hypovolemia following trauma

Shock occurs when there is a circulatory collapse in which the blood supply to tissues is inadequate and so does not provide the oxygen and nutrients required for normal cellular metabolism (Driscoll *et al.*, 2023). More information on shock can be found in Chapter 7 of this book.

Burns

Severe burns can result in clinically significant morbidity and may lead to severe scarring. Major burns initiate a profound systemic response that has significant long-term effects, which may lead to rapid development of organ failure and death (Greenhalgh, 2019). As with the assessment discussed earlier in this chapter, a C-ABCDE assessment should be undertaken. However, there are some specific considerations for burns, such as management of their airway. Children who have suffered massive burns are at risk of their airway swelling and obstructing, so endotracheal intubation is required before the airway is lost. The threshold for intubation should be around 30 to 40% of the patient's total body surface area (TBSA) (Greenhalgh, 2019). It is also important to note any thermal injury from inhalation of hot vapours and chemicals to the respiratory tract (Pape & Sollars, 2022).

Assessment of the size and depth of the burn forms part of the secondary survey and guides both fluid resuscitation and the location of ongoing care, so accuracy is imperative. Overestimation of the burn can have serious implications due to the excessive resuscitation the patient may have received (Dries, 2019). The depth of the burn is determined by identifying the damage to the layers of the skin (Fig. 7.4). Burns range from superficial to partial thickness and full thickness. This assessment helps establish the likely timescale for healing.

The TBSA is usually assessed using the Lund and Browder burns chart. This indicates the percentage of body surface and changes with the age of the child (Fig. 7.5).

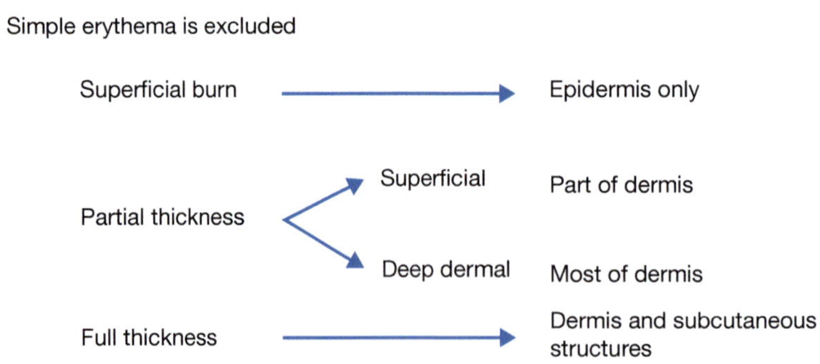

FIGURE 7.4 Burn thickness.
Source: Suman and Owen (2020)/with permission of Elsevier.

Lund and browder charts

Ignore
Simple erythema

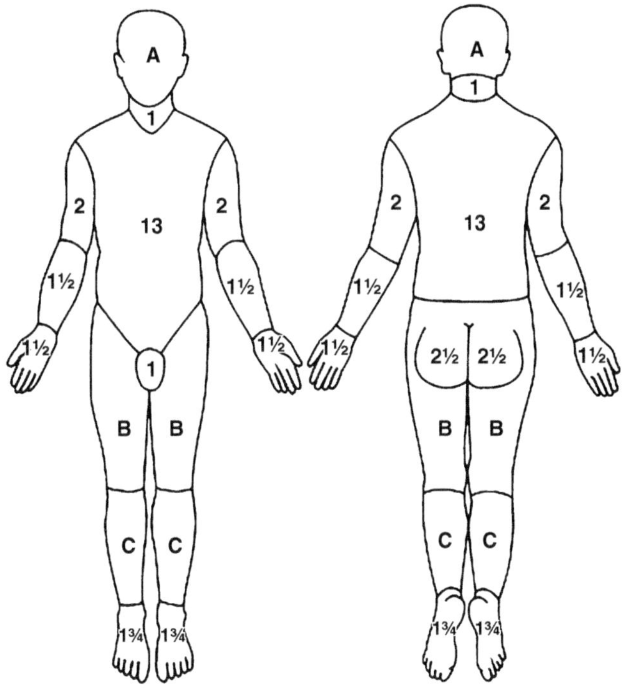

Superficial

Deep

Region	%
Head	
Neck	
Ant.trunk	
Post.trunk	
Right arm	
Left arm	
Buttocks	
Genitalia	
Right leg	
Left leg	
Total burn	

Relative percentage of body surface area affected by growth

Area	Age 0	1	5	10	15	Adult
A = ½ of head	9½	8½	6½	5½	4½	3½
B = ½ of one thigh	2¾	3¼	4	4½	4½	4¾
C = ½ of one leg	2½	2½	2¾	3	3¼	3½

FIGURE 7.5 Lund and Browder – total body surface area.
Source: Suman and Owen (2020)/with permission of Elsevier.

Fluid management

Fluid management in paediatric burns is important because of fluid shift due to increased vascular permeability. This shift results in an intravascular volume depletion. In general, the loss of circulating volume after burn injury is proportional to the severity of the burns; for minor burns, oral hydration may be acceptable.

Patients may experience systemic inflammatory response syndrome, which may lead to myocardial depression. Additionally, systemic oedema may occur, which develops at 4 hours and continues until 36 hours after injury (Suman and Owen, 2020). Such changes will reduce cardiac output and ultimately cause hypoperfusion and circulatory shock in severe cases. Therefore, fluid resuscitation is essential.

Any paediatric burn with greater than 10% TBSA requires fluid replacement via the IV route. One of the most commonly used formulas for calculating the fluid required is the Parkland Formula (Baxter & Shires, 1968). This is 3–4 mL/kg multiplied by the TBSA percentage burns over a 24-hour period. Half the total is given over the first 8 hours from the time of the burn injury, and the other half over the next 16 hours. The resuscitation fluid should be crystalloid, such as Hartmann's, due to increased capillary permeability (Guilabert *et al.*, 2016).

Over-resuscitation can harm children, causing acute respiratory distress syndrome, multi-organ dysfunction, cerebral oedema and compartment syndrome (Suman & Owen, 2020). Fluid volumes, including medications and electrolytes, should be carefully monitored. A urinary catheter should be placed to monitor urine output (Pape & Sollars, 2022).

TABLE 7.3 Drugs used in pain management in burns: routes, frequency and rationale

Drug	Route	Rationale
Paracetamol	Oral, intravenously or rectally	Suitable for all patients. For mild to moderate pain. Can be used alongside opioids
NSAIDS	Oral or rectally	Suitable for mild to moderate pain. Contraindicated in children with renal issues
50:50 nitrous oxide/oxygen (Entonox)	Inhaled	For conscious and co-operative patients. Can be self-administered and quick-acting.
Opioids	Oral, intranasal, rectal, IV	Can be titrated to the patient's response.

Medicine management – pain relief for children with burns.

Analgesia should be administered promptly. All burns are painful, though pain type varies with burn type, and the child may feel frightened. Drug choice, route and frequency should be tailored to the patient's needs. Table 7.3 outlines the rationale for commonly used medications.

Special considerations

Culture can influence a child's perception and expression of pain. Language barriers, cultural norms, beliefs and socioeconomic factors may affect their ability to communicate pain (Miller & Abu-Alhaija, 2019). Culturally sensitive pain assessment tools and individualised pain management strategies should be used.

Non-accidental injury should always be considered in children presenting with burns. Suspicion increases with inconsistent history, unusual burn patterns, delayed presentation or the child's age and mobility. Any concerns must be reported to the local safeguarding team.

The psychological effects on patients with burns

Burns, regardless of their size, can lead to mental trauma for the person experiencing the burn and their families. There may be feelings of guilt and anger, as well as body image difficulties and flashbacks. With the appropriate support and rehabilitation, patients can minimise the psychological effects and go back to leading a good-quality life both socially and vocationally.

Rehabilitation of the child or young person with burns

There are several goals for patients who have suffered a burn due to the physical and psychological effects. According to Pape and Sollars (2022), these are:

- Maintaining an active range of movement
- Minimising physical scarring and any contracture development
- Enhancing quality of life
- Psychological well-being
- Facilitating self-management

To achieve these goals, a specialist multi-disciplinary team should be involved in the child or young person's care. Professionals such as physiotherapists, occupational therapists, dieticians, psychologists, as well as nurses, doctors and surgeons should be involved. Other specialities such as clinical nurse specialists and surgeons may also be involved. Rehabilitation is important for the child and young person (CYP) as well as their family, so it is important that they understand what the rehabilitation will consist of and the importance of it.

Rehabilitation

Psychological well-being is crucial for successful rehabilitation in children and young people (Pape & Sollars, 2022). Each individual experiences losses differently, such as bereavement, disruption to education or work, loss of independence and changes to daily routines. Poorly managed losses during rehabilitation can negatively impact recovery.

Children may exhibit a wide range of emotional responses following trauma, influenced by factors such as personality. Some may be expressive, while others withdraw. Absence of an immediate reaction does not indicate resolution, as emotional responses can be delayed or triggered by later events.

Case study 7.2

Dinah, a 15-year-old girl with cerebral palsy, attended a local fancy dress party with her younger sister when her costume caught fire. The flames were quickly extinguished by adults, and an ambulance was called. On arrival, Dinah was anxious and emotional, with some open and some intact blisters on her legs, hands and abdomen. She was transferred to the emergency department on IV fluids with her wounds covered and received analgesia. On admission, her observations were:

Vital sign	Observation	Normal range
Temperature	39 °C	36.5–37.5 °C
Pulse	140 beats per minute	60–100 beats per minute
Respiratory rate	35 breaths per minute	16–20 breaths per minute
Blood pressure	85/40 mmHg (systolic)	92–130 mmHg (systolic)
CRT	Unable to complete	<2 seconds
Oxygen saturation	94%	98–100%
Level of consciousness	Voice on AVPU scale	Alert on AVPU scale
Pain score	7	No pain

Dinah had a 40% TBSA 3rd degree burns and so was transferred to a burn's unit for further management. She remained an inpatient for 3 months, where she received further surgery and rehabilitation. She worked alongside physiotherapists who were able to support her in gaining her normal range of mobility. She worked alongside physiotherapists who were able to support her gaining her normal range of mobility, as well as a number of specialists who were able to support her psychological recovery. She continues to receive ongoing psychological support due to her anxieties around entering public spaces.

Post-traumatic stress disorder

Post-traumatic stress disorder (PTSD) is a common and disabling condition that can occur as a result of trauma. Children can have similar symptoms to adults, particularly nightmares and avoidance. They may also experience physiological symptoms such as stomach aches and headaches. Children will often re-enact the traumatic event through play.

PTSD causes significant changes within the brain. Reduced volume and activity within the hippocampus may cause memory issues. The amygdala is also affected and so there may be an exaggerated stress response. There may also be a reduced ability to regulate emotions, causing fear when the child is faced with a stimulus connected to the trauma. It is the chronic dysregulation of the hypothalamic–pituitary–adrenal axis (HPA axis) that is thought to ensure the body's response to the perceived threat that underpins the child's PTSD (Kelmendi *et al.*, 2016; Bae *et al.*, 2020). Children and young people who experience PTSD are more likely to make negative life-course decisions, such as completing and succeeding academically. This can affect the course of the CYP's life as employment may be affected, as well as being able to maintain personal relationships.

Ethical and legal issues

Ethics refers to how people conduct themselves in morally acceptable or unacceptable ways (Wheeler, 2012). It can be learned through observation or adherence to behavioural codes, distinct from formal codes of conduct such as the NMC (2018), which provide frameworks for ethical decision-making. 'An ethic' can also describe the morals of a group, such as nursing (Thompson *et al.*, 2006). In trauma scenarios, ethical decisions are influenced by the multidisciplinary team, family involvement and cultural or religious considerations. As the child is usually unknown to the care team, rapid decisions must be made in the patient's best interests, often assuming consent to provide lifesaving care (McLaughlin, 2023). In cases where survival is impossible, organ recovery may be considered, but in the United Kingdom, family consent is required for any organ donation in children and young people.

Trauma-informed care and adverse childhood experiences

Adverse childhood experiences (ACEs) are the umbrella term used to describe traumatic events a child may have endured, such as abuse, neglect, violence and serious injury before the age of 18 years. This chapter has so far examined the physiological responses to trauma. However, it would be important to note how the stress response endured during trauma can affect how the body responds after the traumatic event. During a traumatic event, it is a normal response for the body to activate the HPA axis. When danger is sensed, the part of the brain that is responsible for the processing of images and sounds – the amygdala sends a signal to the hypothalamus. Consequently, heart rate, respiratory rate and blood pressure are raised. Activation of the HPA axis stimulates cortisol, putting the body into a heightened state of alert. Usually, once the stress has passed, the cortisol levels decrease, and the parasympathetic nervous system stops this process. However, when chronic or toxic stress has occurred, cortisol levels remain elevated, and epinephrine continues to be released into the body. The long-term HPA axis activation can cause long-term poor health outcomes, particularly in adulthood, such as obesity, diabetes, cardiovascular disease, cancer and obstructive pulmonary disease (Hornor, 2015; Goddard, 2021).

Chronic and toxic stress can significantly affect a child's developing brain. Elevated cortisol levels may cause auditory and visual delays and reduce hippocampal function, impairing memory and potentially leading to learning difficulties and maladaptive behaviours (Shonkoff & Garner, 2012).

A child or young person's trauma should be considered throughout care, from the initial episode through recovery, and integrated holistically rather than treated separately (Cleary *et al.*, 2020). Trauma-informed care recognises the trauma, its manifestations and the individual's needs, supporting them psychologically while minimising the risk of re-traumatisation (Cleary *et al.*, 2018).

The Office for Health Improvement and Disparities (2022) provides 6 key principles of trauma-informed practice (see Table 7.4).

TABLE 7.4 Principles of trauma-informed practice

Safety	The CYP will feel physically, psychologically and emotionally safe by: • Staff caring for the CYP having an understanding of what makes them feel safe • They are free from threat or harm as reasonably possible • Policies, practices and safeguarding arrangements in place
Trustworthiness	Staff will build trustworthiness with the CYP through: • Explaining any procedures and interventions • Expectations of the staff made clear
Choice	CYPs are supported in shared decision-making by: • Listening to the needs and wishes of the CYP • Choices explained clearly and transparently • Acknowledging the trauma and the lack of safety and control the CYP may be experiencing
Collaboration	The CYP and staff will work together to overcome challenges by: • Asking the CYP what they need and collaboratively considering how these can be met • Actively involve the CYP in the delivery of care
Empowerment	The CYP should be given a voice at individual and organisational levels by: • Validating feelings • Listening to the CYP's wants and needs • Acknowledging the trauma and possible isolation
Cultural consideration	Stereotypes and biases should be shelved and individualised care given by: • Offering access to gender-responsive services • Acknowledging the healing value of traditional cultural connections • Policies, protocols and processes should be responsive to the needs of the CYP

However, as Cleary *et al.* (2020) study highlighted, there are many barriers to delivering trauma-informed care. These can be due to a lack of awareness or acceptance of trauma-informed care in the organisational culture. Nurses may focus on a bio-medically focused approach or may not feel they have the skills or knowledge to provide trauma-informed care. Bruce *et al.* (2018) and McNally *et al.* (2023) also highlighted that the lack of knowledge and training was an issue for nurses delivering trauma-informed care, with time constraints also being highlighted as a barrier. As some individuals may not always share that they have suffered a previous trauma, it is important that all patients are treated with the recognition that, as caregivers, the nursing staff do not always know what previous trauma they may have experienced (Stokes *et al.*, 2024). Consequently, the lack of training and awareness can have a profound impact on the child or young person. Nursing staff should be able to identify victims of trauma, advocate for patient safety, improve patient outcomes and work together with the multidisciplinary team (Guest, 2021).

Conclusion

This chapter has explored trauma and rehabilitation across the foetus, neonate, child and young person. It has outlined the major trauma pathway, highlighted relevant NICE guidance and described assessments from initial injury to definitive care and rehabilitation. While not exhaustive, it has discussed various ways children may experience trauma and emphasised the multidisciplinary team's role in addressing physical, psychological and social needs during rehabilitation.

References

American College of Surgeons Committee on Trauma (1989). Advanced trauma life support course for physicians.

Azarkane, M., Rijnhout, T.W.H., van Merwijk, I.A.L., *et al.* (2024). Impact of accidental hypothermia in trauma patients: a retrospective cohort study. *Injury.* 55(1), 110973 https://doi.org/10.1016/j.injury.2023.110973.

Bae, S., Sheth, C., Legarretta, M., *et al.* (2020). Volume and shape analysis of the Hippocampus and Amygdala in veterans with traumatic brain injury and post traumatic stress disorder. *Brain Imaging and Behaviour* 14, 1850–1864.

Baum, G.R., Baum, J.T., Hayward, D., & MacKay, B.J. (2022). Gunshot wounds: ballistics, pathology, and treatment recommendations, with a focus on retained bullets. *Orthopedic Research and Reviews* 14, 293–317 https://doi.org/10.2147/ORR.S378278.

Baxter, C.R., & Shires, T. (1968). *Physiological response to crystalloid resuscitation of severe burns. Annals of the New York Academy of Sciences* 1968(150), 874–894.

Bramley, D., Goode, P.N., Hupfl, M., & Burns, B. (2022). In: Driscoll, P.A. *et al.* (eds). *ABC of Major Trauma: Rescue, Resuscitation with Imaging, and Rehabilitation.* John Wiley & Sons, Incorporated. *ProQuest Ebook Central*, https://ebookcentral.proquest.com/lib/herts/detail.action?docID=7069529.

Bruce, M., Kassam-Adams, N., Rogers, M., *et al.* (2018). Trauma providers' knowledge, views, and practice of trauma-informed care. *Journal of Trauma Nursing* 25(2), 131–138.

Cleary, M., West, S., McLean, L., *et al.* (2018). Connecting past and present: Nurses' role in identifying signs of child sexual abuse in adults and supporting survivors. *International Journal of Mental Health Nursing* 27, 1587–1591 https://doi.org/10.1111/inm.12495.

Cleary, M., West, S., Kornhaber, R., *et al.* (2020). Moving the lenses of trauma — Trauma-informed care in the burns care setting. *Burns* 46(6), 2020,1365–2020,1372 https://doi.org/10.1016/j.burns.2020.01.011.

Clews, A., Lecky, F., & Driscoll, P.A. (2022). Shock and Hypovolemia following trauma. In: Driscoll, P.A., Skinner, D.V., & Goode, P.N. (eds). *ABC of Major Trauma: Rescue, Resuscitation with Imaging and Rehabilitation.* Oxford: Wiley and Blackwell.

Credland, N. (2016). Managing the trauma patient presenting with the lethal triad. *International Journal of Orthopaedic and Trauma Nursing* 20, 45–53 https://doi.org/10.1016/j.ijotn.2015.09.003.

Davies, F., *et al.* (2017). *Emergency Care of Minor Trauma in Children.* Taylor & Francis Group. *ProQuest Ebook Central*, https://ebookcentral.proquest.com/lib/herts/detail.action?docID=5143941.

Deuchar, Ross, McLean, Robert, Holligan, Chris, Densley, James. (2022). Introduction: Gangs and Violence in the UK. https://doi.org/10.1332/policypress/9781529210569.003.0001.

Deucher, R., McLean, R., Holligan, C., & Densley, J. (2022). Introduction: gangs and violence in the UK. *Youth Justice*, 1–8 https://doi.org/10.1332/policypress/9781529210569.003.0001.

Diab, M., & Staheli, L.T. (2015). *Practice of Paediatric Orthopaedics.* Wolters Kluwer. *ProQuest Ebook Central*, https://ebookcentral.proquest.com/lib/herts/detail.action?docID=4786240.

Ditkofsky, N., Nair, J.R., Frank, Y., *et al.* (2023). Understanding ballistic injuries. *Radiologic Clinics of North America* 61(1), 119–128 https://doi.org/10.1016/j.rcl.2022.08.005.

Dries, D.J. (2019). Resuscitation Part 2: trauma and burn injury. *Air Medical Journal* 38(6), 400–403 https://doi.org/10.1016/j.amj.2019.05.012.

Driscoll, P.A., Skinner, D.V., & Goode, P.N. (eds) (2022). *Abc of major trauma : Rescue, resuscitation with imaging, and rehabilitation.* John Wiley & Sons, Incorporated.

Drsicoll, P.A., Skinner, D.V., & Goode, P.N. (2022). *ABC of Major Trauma: Rescue, Resuscitation with Imaging and Rehabilitation*, 5th edn. Wiley and Sons.

Dyer, M., & Neal, M.D. (2017). Defining the lethal triad. In: Pape, H., Peitzman, A.B., Rotondo, M.F., & Giannoudis, P.V. (eds). *Damage control management in the polytrauma patient.* Springer International Publishing AG.

Fisher, R., Roland, D., Coats, T., *et al.* (2017). *Severe Injury in Children: England and Wales January 2015 – December 2016.* TARN, Salford.

Goddard, A. (2021). Adverse childhood experiences and trauma-informed care. *Journal of Pediatric Health Care* 35(2), 145–155, ISSN 0891-5245, https://doi.org/10.1016/j.pedhc.2020.09.001.

Goddard, A. (2021). Adverse childhood experiences and trauma-informed care. *Journal of Pediatric Health Care.* 35(2), 145–155.

Goode, P.N., Arbid, D., Driscoll, P.A., *et al.* (2022). In: Driscoll, P.A., Skinner, D.V., & Goode, P.N. (eds) (2022). *ABC of Major Trauma: Rescue, Resuscitation with Imaging, and Rehabilitation*, 5th edn. John Wiley & Sons, Incorporated.

Graham, L. (2022). Rehabilitation of patients with major trauma. In: Driscoll, P.A., Skinner, D.V., & Goode, P.N. (eds) (2022). *ABC of Major Trauma: Rescue, Resuscitation with Imaging, and Rehabilitation*, 5th edn. John Wiley & Sons, Incorporated.

Greenhalgh, D.G. (2019). Management of Burns. *The New England Journal of Medicine* 380(24), 2349–2359.

Grice, J., Hardcastle, J., Stibbards, S., & Schofield, M. (2022). Paediatric trauma. In: Driscoll, P.A., Skinner, D.V., & Goode, P.N. (eds) (2022). *ABC of Major Trauma: Rescue, Resuscitation with Imaging, and Rehabilitation*, 5th edn. John Wiley & Sons, Incorporated.

Guest, H. (2021). A concept analysis of trauma-informed care. *Nursing Forum* (Hillsdale) 56(4), 1000–1007.

Guilabert, P., Usua, G., Martin, N., *et al.* (2016). Fluid resuscitation management in patients with burns: update. *British Journal of Anaesthesia* 117, 284–296.

Herrera, T.I., Edwards, L., Malcolm, W.F., *et al.* (2018). Outcomes of preterm infants treated with hypothermia for hypoxic-ischemic encephalopathy. *Early Human Development* 125, 1–7 https://doi.org/10.1016/j.earlhumdev.2018.08.003.

Hong, H.S., & Lee, J.Y. (2018). Intracranial haemorrhage in term neonates. *Child's Nervous System* 34(6), 1135–1143.

Hong, H.S., & Lee, J.Y. (2018). Intracranial hemorrhage in term neonates. *Childs Nerv Syst.* 34(6), 1135–1143.

Horner, G. (2015). Childhood trauma exposure and toxic stress: what the PNP needs to know. *Journal of Pediatric Health Care* 29(2), 191–198.

Hunt, B.J., Allard, S., Keeling, D., *et al.* (2015). A practical guideline for the haematological management of major haemorrhage. *British Journal of Haematology* 170, 788–803 https://doi.org/10.1111/bjh.13580.

Jones, S., Tyson, S., Young, M., *et al.* (2019). Patterns of moderate and severe injury in children after the induction of major trauma Networks. *Archives of Disease in Childhood* 104, 366–371.

Kang, L. and Geube, A. (2022). *Bladder Trauma.*

Kelmendi, B., Adams, T.G., Yarnell, s., *et al.* (2016). *Ptsd: from neurobiology to pharmacological treatments. European Journal of Psychotraumatology* 7, 31858.

Lauder, J., & Driscoll, P.A. (2022). In: Driscoll, P.A., Skinner, D.V., & Goode, P.N. (eds). *ABC of Major Trauma: Rescue, Resuscitation with Imaging, and Rehabilitation (5).* John Wiley & Sons, Incorporated.

Lawrence, T., Helmy, A., Bouamra, O., *et al.* (2016). Traumatic brain injury in England and Wales: prospective audit of epidemiology, complications and standardised mortality. *BMJ Open* 6, e012197.

Leijser, & de Vries (2024). Intraventricular Haemorrhage and Post Haemorrhagic Ventricular Dilation in *Neonatal Brain Injury : An Illustrated Guide for Clinicians Counselling Parents and Caregivers.* In: Meijler, G. & Mohammad, K. (eds). Springer, 2025 *ProQuest Ebook Central*, https://ebookcentral.proquest.com/lib/herts/detail.action?docID=31879504.

Lockey, D.J. (2018). Improved trauma outcomes after the introduction of a trauma system in England. *EClinicalMedicine* 2–3, 3–4.

Lucena-Amaro, S., & Zolfaghari, P. (2022). Trauma nursing 1: an overview of major trauma and the care pathway. *Nursing Times* [online] 118, 11.

Managhis, *et al.* (2024). Altered anatomy and physiology in the neonate. In: Petty, J. *et al.* (eds). *A Guide to Neonatal Care : Handbook for Health Professionals.* Taylor & Francis Group. *ProQuest Ebook Central*, https://ebookcentral.proquest.com/lib/herts/detail.action?docID=7116540.

Martinez-Biarge, M., & Cowan, F.M. (2024). Magnetic Resonance Imaging (MRI). In: Meijler, G. & Mohammad, K. (eds). *Neonatal Brain Injury.* Cham: Springer https://doi.org/10.1007/978-3-031-55972-3_15.

McLaughlin, M. (2023). Ethical challenges in the care of the trauma patient. *Critical Care Nursing Clinics* 35(2), 145–149.

McNally, K., Ragan, K., Varese, F., & Lovell, K. (2023). The ongoing importance of the routine enquiry into trauma and abuse and trauma-informed care within mental health trusts in England. *Journal of Psychiatric and Mental Health Nursing* 30(6), 1130–1136.

Meijler, G., & Mohammad, K. (eds) (2025). *Neonatal brain injury : An illustrated guide for clinicians counselling parents and caregivers.* Springer.

Mercer, J.M. (2018). The trauma call. *British Medical Journal* 361, k2272.

Miller, E., Abu-Alhaija, D.M., & Miller, E.T. (2019). *Cultural Influences on Pain Perception and Management. Pain Management Nursing* 20(3), 183–184.

Mininder, K., & Noonan, K. (2021). *Pediatric Musculoskeletal Physical Diagnosis: A Video-Enhanced Guide*. Wolters Kluwer Health. ProQuest Ebook Central, https://ebookcentral.proquest.com/lib/herts/detail.action?docID=6882215.

Mohammed, K., de Vries, L. S., Meijer, G., and Cowan, F.M. (2024) Hypoxic-Ischemic Encephalopothy (HIE) in Term and Near term Infants In G. Meijler, K. Mohammad (eds.), Neonatal Brain Injury, https://doi.org/10.1007/978-3-031-55972-3_8

National Institute for Health and Care Excellence (2016a). *Major Trauma: Assessment and Initial Management.* NICE guideline NG39

National Institute for Health and Care Excellence (2016b). Major trauma: Service Delivery. NICE guideline NG40. London: NICE

National Institute for Health and Care Excellence (2017). *Child Maltreatment: When to suspect Maltreatment in under 18s.* Clinical Guideline CG89. London: NICE.

National Institute for Health and Care Excellence (2023). *Head Injury: Assessment and Early Management.* Clinical guidance ng232. London: NICE.

Nursing and Midwifery Council (2018). *The Code: Professional Standards of Practice and Behaviour for Nurses, Midwives and Nursing Associates.* Nursing and Midwifery, London.

Brimble, M., & McNee, P. (eds) (2021). *Nursing Care of Children and Young People with Long-Term Conditions.* John Wiley & Sons, Incorporated. *ProQuest Ebook Central*, http://ebookcentral.proquest.com/lib/herts/detail.action?docID=6448948.

Office for Health Improvement and Disparities (2022). *Working definition of trauma informed practice.*

Pape, S., & Sollars, A. (2022). Management of severe burns. In: Driscoll, P.A., Skinner, D.V., & Goode, P.N. (eds). *ABC of Major Trauma: Rescue, Resuscitation with Imaging, and Rehabilitation*, 5th edn. John Wiley & Sons, Incorporated.

Qasim, Z.A., & Joseph, B. (2024). Intraosseous access in the resuscitation of patients with trauma: the good, the bad, the future. *Trauma Surgery & Acute Care Open* 9(Suppl 2), e001369 https://doi.org/10.1136/tsaco-2024-001369.

Rao, R., Trivedi, S., Vesoulis, Z., *et al.* (2017). Safety and short-term outcomes of therapeutic hypothermia in preterm neonates 34-35 weeks gestational age with hypoxic-ischemic encephalopathy. *The Journal of Pediatrics* 183, 37–42.

Riccio A.I., and Parikh, S.N., (2021) In Noonan, K. and Kocher, M. Pediatric musculosketal physical diagnosis: a video enhanced guide ProQuest Ebook Central - Reader

Royal College of Pediatrics' and Child Health (2020). *State of Child Health.* RCPCH, London. Available at: stateofchildhealth.rcpch.ac.uk.

Santy-Tomlinson, J., Clarke, S., & Droza, M. (2023). An introduction to orthopaedic trauma care. In: Clarke, S. & Drozd, M. (eds). *Orthopaedic and Trauma Nursing: An Evidence-Based Approach to Musculoskeletal Care.* John Wiley & Sons, Incorporated.

Shonkoff, J.P., & Garner, A.S. (2012). Committee on psychosocial aspects of child and family health, committee on early childhood, adoption, and dependent care, section on developmental and behavioural pediatrics. the lifelong effects of early childhood adversity and toxic stress. *Pediatrics* 129(1), e232–e246.

Shonkoff, J.P., Garner, A.S., Committee on Psychosocial Aspects of Child and Family Health, & Committee on Early Childhood, Adoption, and Dependent Care (2012). Section on Developmental and Behavioural Pediatrics. The lifelong effects of early childhood adversity and toxic stress. *Pediatrics* 129(1), e232–e246.

Shouldice, M., Al-Khattabi, F., Thau, A., *et al.* (2018). Traumatic macular retinoschisis in infants and children. *Journal of the American Association for Pediatric Ophthalmology and Strabismus (JAAPOS)* 22(6), 433–437.e2.

Southampton Oxford Retrieval Team (SORT). Paediatric Intraosseous insertion at a glance. 2022.

Spahn, D.R., Bouillon, B., Cerny, V., *et al.* (2019). The european guideline on management of major bleeding and coagulopathy following trauma: fifth edition. *Critical Care* 23, 98.

Stokes, Y., Cloutier, P., Aggarwal, D., *et al.* (2024). Youth, caregiver and healthcare professional perspectives on planning the implementation of a trauma-informed care programme: a qualitative study. *Journal of Advanced Nursing* 81(10), 6602–6624.

Suman, A., & Owen, J. Update on the management of burns in paediatrics. *BJA Education* 20(3), 103–110.

Teasdale, G., & Jennett, B. (1974). Assessment of coma and impaired consciousness: A practical scale. *Lancet* 304, 81–84.

Thompson, I., Melia, K., Boyd, K., *et al.* (2006). In: Brimble, M. & McNee, P. (eds). *Nursing Ethics (fifth edition). Edinburgh, Churchill Livingstone. Nursing Care of Children and Young People with Long-Term Conditions.* John Wiley & Sons, Incorporated, 2021. *ProQuest Ebook Central*, http://ebookcentral.proquest.com/lib/herts/detail.action?docID=6448948.

Titchener, T., Aloi, M., & Gupta, P. (2016). Pediatric head trauma. In: MD, FAAP, FACEP & Dietrich, A. (eds). *Pediatric Trauma: Essential Care and Practical Application.* Relias Learning. *ProQuest Ebook Central*, https://ebookcentral.proquest.com/lib/herts/detail.action?docID=5145812.

Todd, N. (2022). Acute spinal injury. In: Driscoll, P.A. *et al.* (eds). *ABC of Major Trauma : Rescue, Resuscitation with Imaging, and Rehabilitation.* John Wiley & Sons, Incorporated, 2022. *ProQuest Ebook Central*, http://ebookcentral.proquest.com/lib/herts/detail.action?docID=7069529 (Created from herts on 2026-02-12 21:28:19).

Todd, N., Skinner, D., & Wilson-MacDonald, J. (2015). Secondary neurological deterioration in traumatic spinal injury: data from medicolegal cases. *Bone Joint J* 97, 527–531.

Wheeler, H. (2012). *Law, Ethics and Professional Issues for Nursing: A Reflective and Portfolio Building Approach.* Routledge, Abingdon.

Wolberg, A.S., Meng, Z.H., & Monroe.D.M. and Hoffman M. (2004). A systematic evaluation of the effect of temperature on coagulation enzyme activity and platelet function. *Journal of Trauma* 56(6), 1221–1228.

CHAPTER 8

Pain and pain management

Helen Monks, Kate Heaton-Stockton, and Sarah McDonald

AIM

This chapter provides an overview of mechanisms of pain and pain management.

LEARNING OUTCOMES

On completion of this chapter, the reader will be able to:

- Outline the pathophysiology of children's pain.
- Discuss common myths relating to pain in infants, children and young people.
- Describe common approaches to pain assessment.
- Describe common pharmacological and non-pharmacological pain management interventions.

KEYWORDS

- nociceptive pain
- gate control theory
- neuropathic pain
- cognitive development
- neurodiversity
- pain perception
- behavioural cues
- pharmacological/non-pharmacological
- opioids/non-opioids
- distraction

Test your prior knowledge

1. Identify the body system and any anatomy and physiology involved in transmission, sensation and perception of pain.
2. What do you understand by acute, chronic and neuropathic pain?
3. How would you assess a child's pain?
4. Name five non-pharmacological techniques used in treating pain in a child.
5. Discuss one of the pharmacological methods used to manage acute pain.

Introduction

In July 2020, for the first time since 1979, the International Association for the Study of Pain (IASP) revised its definition of pain and included 6 keynotes to add further context to the definition (IASP, 2020).

Pain does not always result from tissue damage. It may arise from ordinary stimuli, such as touch, or even from absent tissue, as in phantom limb pain. Pain is therefore a complex phenomenon.

The definition from IASP (2020) is especially important for children and young people (CYP) because:

- it relates to the physiology of pain
- it relates to how pain is perceived by a child
- it relates to the experience of pain during childhood and the effect this has on the way pain is experienced in adulthood.

Therefore, while general anatomical and physiological explanations of children's pain are possible, the definition suggests that much of a child's pain experience is individual and depends on biopsychosocial factors (Table 8.1).

Given these biopsychosocial influences, it becomes clear why the pain experience is unique to each individual. Pain involves both perception and response. Although some people are described as having a high or low pain threshold, it is likely that while physiological factors may be broadly similar, psychological and other factors vary and can markedly shape the pain experience. The IASP (2023) supports this, noting that the threshold is often defined as the lowest stimulus intensity at which pain is perceived, meaning the true threshold is the patient's internal experience, whereas the measured intensity is an external event. In contrast, Tortora and Derrickson (2021) describe the pain threshold as the first point at which pain is felt and argue that this is consistent across people; what differs is pain tolerance, the maximum intensity an individual can endure.

TABLE 8.1 Biopsychosocial factors affecting pain experience in children and young people

Biological factors	Age
	Cognitive development
	Genes
	Temperament
Psychological factors	Fear
	Previous experiences of pain
Social factors	Culture
	Family learning
	Gender

Source: Twycross *et al.* (2014)/John Wiley & Sons.

For children, some biopsychosocial factors carry even greater significance. A child's age and developmental stage shape how they understand pain. For example, younger children may interpret pain as a punishment, whereas older children may associate it with more serious concepts such as death or dying (Twycross *et al.*, 2014).

In children, early experiences and responses to pain can have profound effects both immediately and later in life. Pain also serves as an important developmental learning tool: children learn to avoid certain actions because they discover that pain signals danger (Franck *et al.*, 2000). Tortora and Derrickson (2021, p.575) emphasise that 'pain is indispensable for survival' due to its protective function in signalling harmful, tissue-damaging conditions. For this reason, such pain is often termed protective pain.

> Some children cannot feel pain due to altered physiology, such as nerve damage, so pain fails to serve as a warning. Others may feel pain but cannot respond to it, for example, immobile children who cannot withdraw from a painful stimulus.

Webb and Steeds (2022) suggest that pain results from a complex interplay between nociception, neural pathways transmitting noxious stimuli to the brain, signalling systems, modulation and the individual's unique perception.

Anatomy and physiology of pain in children

To provide safe and effective care for individuals in pain, nurses must understand the anatomy and physiology of pain transmission and sensation, as well as the key characteristics of nociceptive and neuropathic pain. The nervous system is divided into:

1. **Peripheral nervous system (PNS):** comprising cranial nerves, spinal nerves and the autonomic nervous system.
2. **Central nervous system (CNS):** comprising the brain and spinal cord.

Although much is known about pain mechanisms, research continues to reveal new insights into its anatomy and physiology. Pain is broadly classified into two types: nociceptive and neuropathic.

Nociceptive pain

Four stages

1. Pain receptors (nociceptors) in the skin are stimulated.
2. Message travels to the spinal cord.
3. Neurotransmitters within the dorsal horn of the spinal cord communicate with nerves and pass the message to the brain.
4. The thalamus 'unravels' the message, sending it to various parts of the brain to be analysed and interpreted.

Stages 1 and 2 are within the PNS.

Stages 3 and 4 are within the CNS.

See Fig. 8.1.

McCaffery and Pasero (1999) describe the processes involved for nociceptive pain as:

- transduction
- transmission
- perception
- modulation.

Transduction

A noxious stimulus is detected by nociceptors, transforming it into an electrical signal. In simple terms, **transduction** is the conversion of one type of energy into another, in this case, into an electrical impulse (Mears & Mears, 2023). Noxious stimuli are generally categorised into three main types (Wheeldon, 2021).

1. mechanical, e.g., laceration
2. thermal, e.g., burn
3. chemical, e.g., inflammation caused by release of histamines.

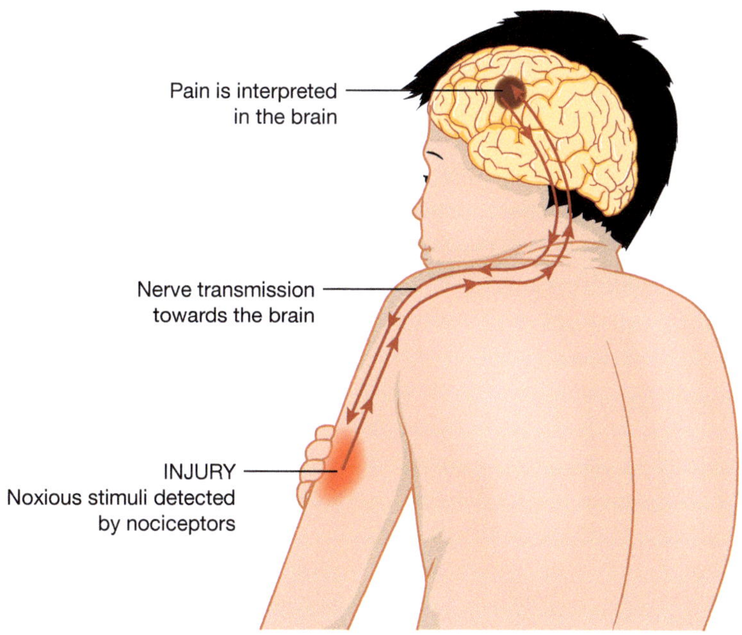

FIGURE 8.1 Pathway of pain transmission and interpretation.

Nociceptors are free nerve endings of nerve fibres found in almost every tissue, responding to painful stimuli resulting from physical or chemical damage to skin and tissue (Tortora & Derrickson, 2021).

Transmission

During this phase, information is sent via nerve fibres (A and C, see later) to the dorsal horn in the spinal cord and ultimately to the thalamus in the brain. This is known as the ascending pain pathway. Transmission of a signal or impulse is an electrochemical event (Marieb & Keller, 2018).

Perception

This is when pain is felt. Pain is perceived when the thalamus sends signals to the brain for processing. The somatosensory cortex identifies and locates pain, the limbic system triggers an emotional response and aids pain memory for future avoidance, and the reticular system initiates appropriate action (Melzack & Wall, 1996; Godfrey, 2005).

Modulation

The body modulates pain through descending pathways that can increase or decrease pain signals. Analgesic neuropeptides – endorphins, enkephalins and dynorphins – play a key role, and individual differences in their production may explain why people experience pain differently (Wheeldon, 2021; Briggs, 2010). Activities such as distraction can inhibit pain signals, a strategy widely used in children during painful procedures, including self-distraction through play (Melzack & Wall, 1965; Twycross *et al.*, 2014; McCaffery & Beebe, 1989). This is described by the gate control theory, discussed later.

Ascending pain pathways

The ascending pain pathways (Fig. 8.2) originate from the spinal cord and are primarily responsible for sending information to the brain. This pathway is divided into three tracts. Two are specifically involved in the transmission of pain impulses to the brain: the spinothalamic tract and the spinoreticular tract (Twycross *et al.*, 2009).

When nociceptors are stimulated, a pain impulse travels along the ascending pathway to the thalamus, where it is analysed and interpreted. The pathway involves first-, second-, and third-order neurones transmitting the signal sequentially:

- First-order neurones travel from nociceptors to the spine.
- Second-order neurones travel from the spine to the thalamus.
- Third-order neurones travel between various parts of the brain.

Neurotransmitters transmit pain signals between neurones. First-order sensory fibres – A-delta and C fibres – carry the initial message. Conduction speed depends on fibre diameter and myelination: A-delta fibres are larger and myelinated, conducting signals quickly, while smaller, unmyelinated C fibres conduct more slowly (Wheeldon, 2021). Myelination also explains the distinction between white (myelinated axons) and grey matter (cell bodies and dendrites) (Colbert *et al.*, 2020). This underlies the two-wave perception of pain: fast, sharp pain followed by slower, dull pain (Fig. 8.3), as experienced when stubbing a toe (Tortora & Derrickson, 2021) (Tables 8.2).

Reflex arc

Pain messages are processed rapidly to produce protective motor responses, such as quickly lifting a foot from a sharp object. A reflex – specifically a flexor or withdrawal reflex – uses a three-neurone arc, involving synapses with interneurones in the CNS. This reflex arc consists of five elements:

- **Sensory receptor**, for example, picking up stimulus of sharp object under the foot
- **Sensory afferent neurone** sends information to the
- **Interneurone** in the brain to be analysed and interpreted, also transmits the information to a
- **Motor efferent neurone** which in turn produces the
- **Effector organ** (lifts foot up)
  (Marieb & Keller, 2018)

Descending pain pathways

Descending pain pathways originate within the brain and can inhibit ascending nerve signals. Therefore, it is within the descending nerve pathway that modulations occur, and it is here that Melzack and Wall's gate control theory (1965) can be illustrated.

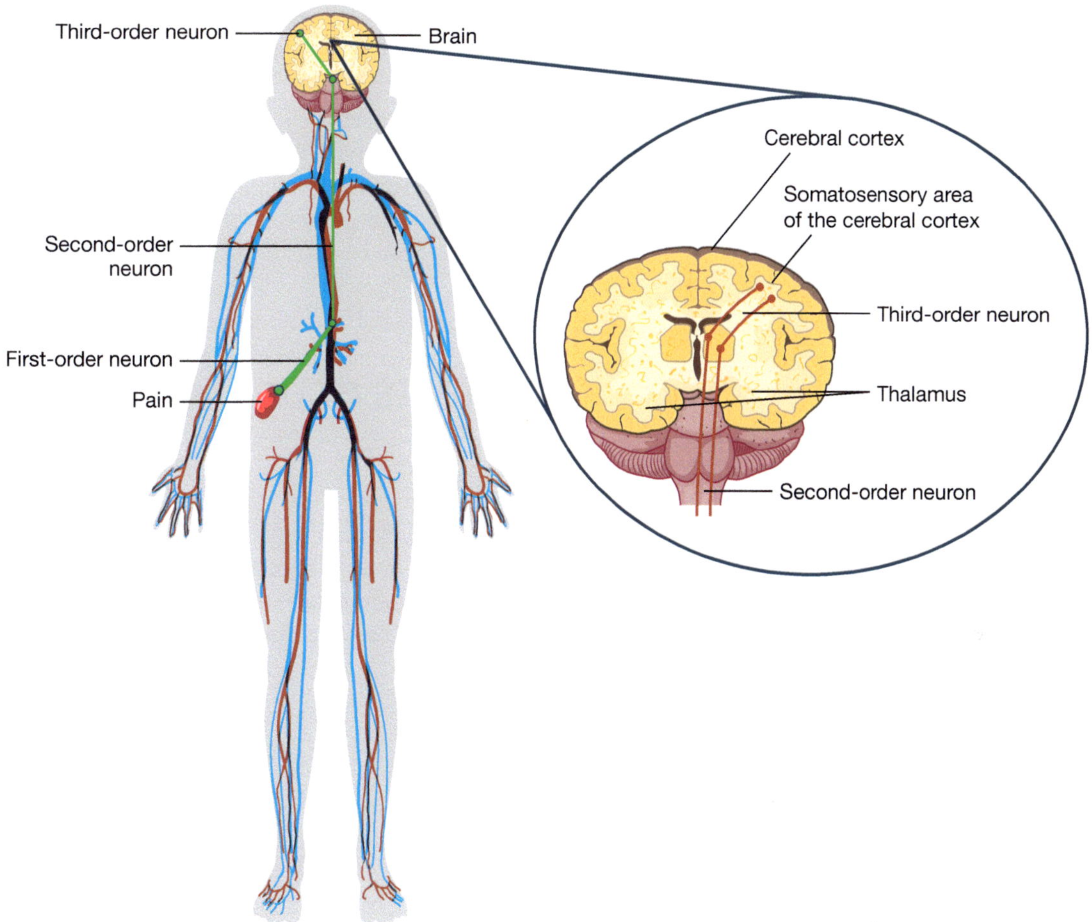

FIGURE 8.2 The ascending pain pathway.

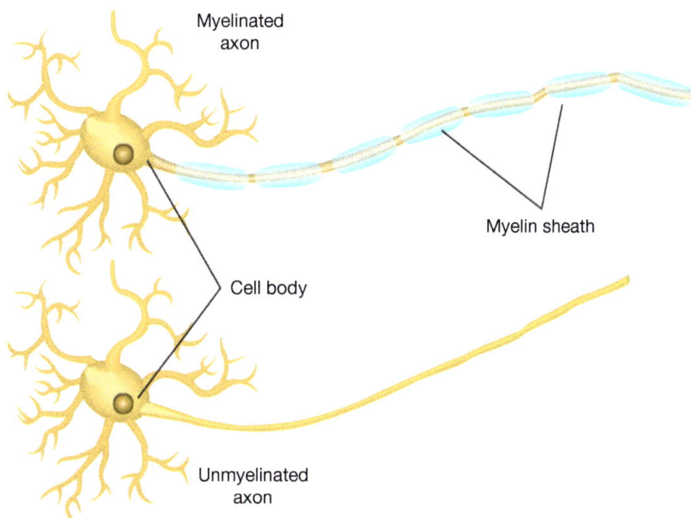

FIGURE 8.3 Basic structure of myelinated and unmyelinated nerve fibres.

TABLE 8.2 Size and speed of first-order sensory fibres

Sensory fibre	Diameter (μm)	Myelinated	Speed of conduction (m/s)
A-beta (Aβ) fibres	6–12	Yes	35–75
A-delta (Aδ) fibres	1–5	Yes	5–35
C fibres	0.2–1.5	No	0.5–2

Source: Peate (2021).

Gate control theory

A number of theories exist to explain how pain is experienced, but the one continuing to hold widespread support is the gate control theory (Fig. 8.4) (Melzack & Wall, 1965).

In essence, the theory is that the pain impulse has to pass through a theoretical gate to enable the brain to receive, perceive and interpret the impulse as painful. Broadly, the theory works on the basis that stimulation of A-delta fibres and C fibres pushes the gate open, and the stimulation of A-beta fibres pushes the gate closed, but also the presence (or absence) of other factors like fear or distraction may open or close the gate (McCaffery & Beebe,1989).

Effects of pain on vital signs

Pain involves more than anatomical and physiological processes, and its effects extend beyond physical reactions. However, it can still significantly impact children's vital signs. Common deviations in vital signs can be:

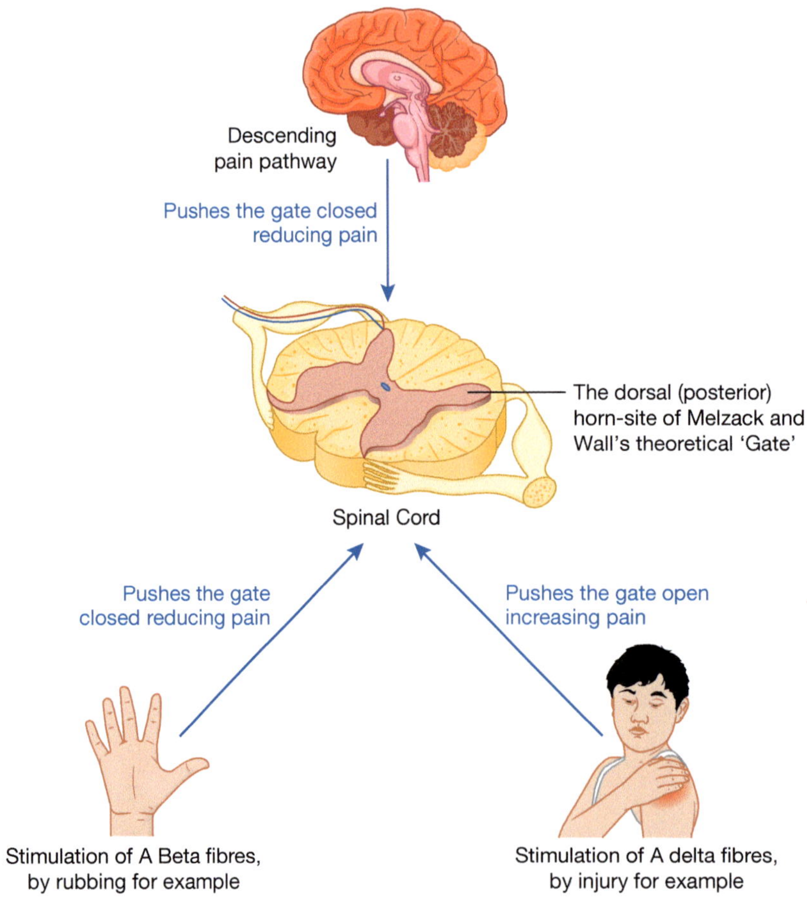

FIGURE 8.4 The gate control theory of pain.

- increased heart rate (tachycardia)
- increased rate of breathing (tachypnoea)
- high blood pressure (hypertension)
(Twycross *et al.*, 2009)

Children's pain has additional complexities, particularly concerning anatomical structures, some of which are not fully developed, along with developing emotional and cognitive states.

Nociceptive pain

Pain is often classified as somatic or visceral. Somatic pain arises from the skin, tissues, bones or joints and is usually sharp and well localised (Mears & Mears, 2023). Visceral pain originates from internal organs and is poorly localised due to fewer nociceptors and limited cortical representation. Because visceral and somatic pathways overlap, visceral pain may be felt in surrounding tissues or distant sites (Webb & Steeds, 2022).

Neuropathic pain

Neuropathic pain, caused by nervous system dysfunction, is less well understood than nociceptive pain and often harder to assess and manage (Twycross *et al.*, 2014). Pain from peripheral nerve damage is termed 'neuropathic', while central nerve damage produces 'central pain' (Webb & Steeds, 2022). Normally, non-painful stimuli, such as light touch, can be perceived as intensely painful (McCaffery & Pasero, 1999).

Nociplastic pain

This is a relatively new term.

IASP (2023) describes this pain as arising from altered nociception, without clear tissue damage or somatosensory system lesions. It is associated with conditions such as fibromyalgia and irritable bowel syndrome (Fitzcharles *et al.*, 2021).

Transient, acute and chronic pain

There are many types of pain documented; acute and chronic are two of the types most commonly referred to. More recently, transient pain has been a term used to describe a short episode of pain, temporary discomfort and self-limiting (Wheeldon, 2021).

Acute pain

Melzack and Wall (1996) describe acute pain as pain accompanied by tissue damage and anxiety, with eventual recovery. Modern definitions emphasise that acute pain arises suddenly, is often sharp or intense, serves as a warning of injury or illness and typically lasts from minutes to under 6 months, resolving once the underlying cause is treated (IASP, 2021a).

Chronic pain

In contrast, chronic pain persists beyond healing, is no longer a symptom of injury or disease and serves no useful function (Melzack & Wall, 1996). While its definition is less precise than acute pain, it is generally considered chronic if it lasts longer than 3 months (IASP, 2021b).

In contrast, chronic pain persists beyond healing, is no longer a symptom of injury or disease and serves no useful function (Melzack & Wall, 1996). While its definition is less precise than acute pain, it is generally considered chronic if it lasts longer than 3 months (IASP, 2021b).

Common approaches to assessing pain in infants, children and young people

Pain assessment is a vital component of pain management and should be conducted as standard practice. There are several common approaches to pain assessment. The nurse needs to understand the context of the pain experience for infants and CYP, and be able to identify and select appropriate validated pain assessment tools for use. Since the mid-1990s, there have been significant advances in how pain is assessed and managed amongst this age group. Developments in research and education have enriched understanding, helping to challenge misconceptions about pain and associated myths.

Pain assessment is essential for effective management and should be standard practice. Nurses must understand the pain experience in infants and CYP, and select appropriate validated assessment tools. Since the mid-1990s, research and education have advanced pain assessment and management in this age group, challenging misconceptions and myths about pain.

The pain experience for children

Pain is difficult to measure objectively because it is a biopsychosocial experience, shaped by age, development, communication skills, prior experience, gender, culture and family influences. Children may experience pain from accidents, injuries, surgery or routine procedures, and may also suffer chronic or recurrent pain from conditions such as sickle cell disease or juvenile idiopathic arthritis (Edwards & Coyne, 2019). Children's experiences of pain evolve with development, influencing how they interpret and cope with it over time.

Procedural pain is particularly significant and often the most distressing aspect of medical care (Howard *et al.*, 2010). Most hospitalised children undergo at least one painful procedure within 24 hours of admission, including venepuncture, cannulation, catheterisation or lumbar puncture (Stevens *et al.*, 2012). Early exposure to needle-related pain is linked to longer-term consequences, with 20–50% of adolescents developing persistent fears or phobias (McLenon & Rogers, 2019).

> Healthcare professionals (HCPs) must recognise and respect the individual experience of pain in children and their families, avoiding labelling, stereotyping or stigmatisation.

Factors affecting children and young people's perceptions of pain

- previous experiences, good or bad
- inability to communicate effectively
- peer pressure
- gender
- culture
- coping mechanisms
- anxiety
- lack of control
- support from parents/family
- developmental considerations
- fatigue
- professional attitudes/environment culture
- type and amount of information given
- understanding of the meaning of pain
- fear

Cognitive development and the perception of pain

Understanding children's perception of pain is improving, but each child and family experiences and expresses pain differently. A biopsychosocial approach, informed by the child's cognitive development, supports more accurate assessment. Whenever possible, children should self-report pain, recognising the added complexity when parents, carers or HCPs advocate on their behalf.

Infancy (0–12 months)

Neonates and infants respond to pain through physiological and behavioural changes, including bradycardia, apnoea, high-pitched crying, body stiffening and facial grimacing. Repeated untreated pain can affect growth, brain development, cognition and infection risk (Campbell-Yeo *et al.*, 2022; Cruz *et al.*, 2016). Pain in neonates should therefore be anticipated and managed proactively.

Early childhood (1–5 years)

For pre-school children, both physical pain and the context of events are important, as memory and imagination influence their play. They cannot fully explain illness and may perceive it as punishment, so immediate, simple explanations are needed (Edwards & Coyne, 2019). Separation from loved ones may cause more distress than the pain itself (Carter & Simons, 2014). Minimising psychological distress is therefore as important as relieving physical pain, and familiar comfort objects, like a favourite toy or themed plaster, can provide significant reassurance.

Middle childhood (6–12 years)

As children progress through school, cognitive development becomes more logical and less egocentric, though language skills may not reflect true cognitive ability (Edwards & Coyne, 2019). Psychological stress from pain or illness can cause developmental regression. Imagination can amplify fear, leading to misconceptions and concerns about mutilation, modesty, privacy and separation from school or peers (Carter & Simons, 2014; Edwards & Coyne, 2019).

Adolescence (13–18 years)

Adolescents can think abstractly, understand pain and communicate their feelings, but assumptions based on age should be avoided, as emotional immaturity and limited coping skills may persist. Anxiety, depression, self-esteem and emotional state influence pain perception (Forgeron & Stinson, 2014). Pain without a clear medical cause may be under-assessed (Igler *et al.*, 2017), so adolescents require compassion and understanding despite their growing independence.

Children with cognitive impairments

Children with cognitive impairments, including learning disabilities, present challenges for pain assessment due to altered processing and communication abilities, often compounded by complex medical conditions requiring painful procedures. Those with profound impairments rely on parents, carers and HCPs for effective assessment and management, making accurate evaluation crucial. Evidence suggests these children may receive inadequate pain relief (Best *et al.*, 2019). A tailored approach combining self-report (when possible), proxy report and validated observational tools, alongside physiological monitoring, is recommended (Albani *et al.*, 2022). Neurodiverse children may face additional challenges, including communication differences, social difficulties, resistance to routine changes and varied sensory responses. Regular, careful assessments in collaboration with parents or carers, who understand the child's typical behaviours and needs, are essential (Palese *et al.*, 2021).

Cultural aspects of pain

Pain meanings and behaviours are shaped by parents, peers, family, community and social experiences. HCPs must demonstrate cultural awareness when assessing children's pain, as both the child's and family's reporting is influenced by cultural background (Givler & Maani-Fogleman, 2023). HCPs' own cultural perspectives can also affect their interpretation, potentially leading to inaccurate assessments, so awareness is essential to prevent bias and inequality (Rogger *et al.*, 2023).

Cultural factors can influence how pain is expressed, for example:

- Some cultures value enduring pain with courage, sometimes linking it to spiritual growth.
- Pain may be seen as a sign of healing rather than a negative symptom.
- Stoicism is common in certain communities, with minimal outward expression despite severe discomfort.
- Religious beliefs may frame pain as a test of faith, spiritual cleansing, or a consequence of past actions.

(Givler & Maani-Fogleman, 2023)

When HCPs do not understand patients' and families' cultural beliefs, it can damage trust and hinder effective, family-centred pain assessment. Awareness of cultural and spiritual contexts enables HCPs to assess pain with greater empathy, reducing misunderstandings and strengthening the therapeutic relationship.

Language barriers

A major challenge arises when the child or family speak a different language, as translations can alter meaning and lead to inaccurate pain assessments. Using family members as translators may cause miscommunication. Nurses should distinguish between advocacy and translation roles and use professional interpreters to ensure accurate, sensitive communication.

Gender identity and pain

HCPs should be aware of potential gender bias in pain assessment, as females are often more likely to have their pain dismissed. Labaka *et al.* (2023) highlight a lack of gender equity skills among nurses and call for education to address bias and discrimination. Pain assessment for transgender and gender-diverse (TGD) children requires an individualised approach. Although research is limited, Engstrom *et al.* (2025) found that while pain assessments in the emergency department did not differ by gender identity or sexual orientation, cisgender children were more likely to receive opioids than TGD peers.

> Pain assessment scales should be culturally appropriate and gender-neutral, such as the Faces Pain Scale, Numeric Rating Scale or Visual Analogue Scale. HCPs should also consider that some children and families may not interpret scales horizontally or left to right, which can affect results.

Assessing pain in children and their families is complex and requires a holistic, non-judgemental approach. Psychosocial factors and the risk of stigmatisation should be considered before applying specific assessment techniques.

Methods of pain assessment

Accurate pain assessment is crucial in helping HCPs to identify the type and intensity of pain experienced and guide decisions about the best approach for pain relief (see Table 8.3). Bruce (2022) notes that a wide variety of pain assessment tools are available and necessary to address the needs of infants, CYP at different ages and development stages. It is recommended that pain be routinely assessed and recorded using an appropriate, validated pain assessment tool developed and supported by research (Association of Paediatric Anaesthetists of Great Britain and Ireland [APAGBI] 2012, Department of Health, 2004a, Royal College of Nursing, 2009). Where possible, children's self-report of their pain is the preferred approach. Often, it is pertinent for a carer to report and assess pain on a child's behalf (Zhang *et al.*, 2023).

A more comprehensive and detailed algorithm appears within the guidelines with evidence for the validated tools cited in the aforementioned sources.

TABLE 8.3 Validated, age-appropriate pain assessment tool suggestions

Age range	Tools available
Infants and neonates *Behavioural and physiological tools used*	COMFORT **C**rying, **R**equires O_2 for saturation above 95, **I**ncreased vital signs, **E**xpression and **S**leeplessness (CRIES) **P**remature **I**nfant **P**ain **P**rofile (PIPP) **N**eonatal **I**nfant **P**ain **S**cale (NIPS) **N**eonatal **P**ain, **A**gitation and **S**edation **S**cale (N-Pass)
Toddlers and young children *Behavioural tools used and some self-report tools are possible to use*	**F**aces, **L**egs, **A**ctivity, **C**ry, **C**onsolability (FLACC) and FLACC – Revised **C**hildren's **H**ospital of **E**astern **O**ntario **P**ain **S**cale (CHEOPS) COMFORT Visual analogue scales such as: Wong-Baker FACES scale Faces Pain Scale Revised The Oucher Poker Chip
Older children and young people *Self-report tools used*	Numeric or verbal rating scales (such as faces, numbers and poker chips) Colour analogue scale Word descriptor scale Pain diaries
Children with cognitive impairment and/or neurodiversity *Behavioural tools or self-report tools are possible to use alongside proxy assessments and physiological parameters*	Faces, Legs, Activity, Cry, Consolability (FLACC) Paediatric pain profile (PPP) Non-communicating children's pain checklist revised (NCCPC-R)

Sources: Bruce (2022)/John Wiley & Sons.

Behavioural cues

Plummer *et al.* (2024) highlight the importance of behavioural cues in pain assessment, though challenges arise when a child's behaviour does not match

TABLE 8.4 Pain and behavioural cues

Age of child	Common behaviours exhibited
Infants	Grimacing, high-pitched crying, changes in breathing pattern, difficulty in calming, quivering chin, difficulty sucking, hiccupping, avoiding eye contact, wanting to be still
Toddlers and young children	Increase in crying, irritability or restlessness, loss of interest in play, difficulty sleeping, reduction in eating or drinking, quiet or curled, need to be held, pulling at affected body part, saying something hurts, difficulty sleeping
School-age child	Difficulty sleeping, moaning/crying, holding or protecting area of discomfort, loss of interest in play, decrease in activity level, complaining of pain, reduction in eating or drinking
Adolescent	Increasingly quiet, loss of interest in friends and family, decrease in activity level, increase in anger or irritability, changes in eating habits
Children with cognitive impairment and/ or neurodiversity	Physiological changes, altered breathing, skin colour, sweating, verbal expressions such as aggressive behaviour, with or without altered body posture or movement, resistance to environmental change or changes in daily routines, plus responses to sensory stimuli.

Source: Adapted from Turner-Cobb (2014) and Albani *et al.* (2022).

self- or proxy-reported pain scores. These cues should be monitored and interpreted with input from the family, recognising that behavioural scales cannot always differentiate pain from distress or anxiety. Tamvaki *et al.* (2024) suggest biomarkers may help assess pain in critically ill children who cannot self-report or display behavioural cues (Table 8.4).

The common behaviours indicated in Table 8.4 may not be limited to a particular age, ethnicity, gender or culture.

Involving parents and family members in pain assessment

Parents contribute a valuable insight into pain assessment through intuition and knowledge of their child (Carter & Simons, 2014). Children's pain often elicits strong emotional reactions in parents, such as stress or worry, and parents' past pain experiences can shape their perceptions (Ndengeyingoma *et al.*, 2023). While parents value objective assessment, their own pain tolerance or sensitivity may influence how they interpret their child's discomfort, and children may mirror these behaviours.

Sibling influence is an under-researched factor, with notions of pain tolerance or competition affecting how children express pain, which can further complicate parental interpretation (Ndengeyingoma *et al.*, 2023). Zhang *et al.* (2023) highlight that parents may struggle to assess their child's pain and recommend providing family support and pain-related education to guide parental practices.

Pain assessment, which incorporates an individual, non-judgemental and respectful approach, demonstrates best practice.

Pain management

Pain management is a multidisciplinary responsibility which helps reduce treatment side effects and complications (Williams & Rose, 2015). Acute pain management teams for children, established in the 1990s on an evidence-based foundation (Royal College of Anaesthetists, 1990), may include clinical pain nurses, play therapists, pharmacists, psychologists and physiotherapists, led by an anaesthetist (Royal College of Anaesthetists, 2025).

The importance of the family in the management of pain cannot be underestimated. Parents and carers may know which analgesia works best for their child. Children who have impaired neurological conditions that impact communication may be solely reliant on their parents to manage their pain (Chen *et al.*, 2025).

Parental mood, such as depression or anxiety, can influence the perception of their child's pain, potentially leading to under- or over-medication, especially with opioids (Chen *et al.*, 2025).

Parents and carers are vital in pain management, particularly non-pharmacological strategies like providing distraction and comfort (Vasey *et al.*, 2019).

Optimal pain management requires a patient-centred, individualised, multidisciplinary approach using both pharmacological and non-pharmacological strategies (WHO, 2020). Accurate assessment is the first step to identifying appropriate treatment, addressing the biological, psychological and social aspects of the child. The overarching aims in managing pain in children are (APAGBI, 2012):

- early identification
- prevention
- administration of appropriate analgesia
- reduction of stress response
- multimodal approach
- prevention of adverse reactions
- consideration of emotional aspects
- continued control post-discharge.

Interventions

Psychological

- relaxation
- hypnosis
- biofeedback
- CBT
- acceptance and commitment therapy
- music therapy
- distraction

Physical

- TENS
- massage
- desensitisation
- acupuncture
- rehabilitation

Pharmacological

- non-opioid
- opioid
- adjuvants
- PCA/NCA
- local/regional anaesthesia

The WHO (1987) 3-step management of pain

The World Health Organization developed the 3-step pain ladder in 1986, and although its design is simple, it is still used widely as a guide for the pharmacological treatment of pain.

STEP1 – Mild pain – non-opioid +/– adjuvant
STEP 2 – Mild to moderate pain – 'weak' opioid +/– adjuvant
STEP 3 – Moderate to severe pain – 'strong opioid +/– non-opioid +/– adjuvant

Pharmacological management

The WHO pain ladder is guided by three principles: 'by the clock, by the mouth, by the ladder', meaning medications should be given orally, titrated from step one and administered at regular intervals rather than as needed (Anekar *et al.*, 2023). Its limitation is its one-dimensional approach, as it does not address emotional, physical or psychological causes of pain (Cuomo *et al.*, 2019).

Analgesia in children often relies on clinical experience due to limited evidence, resulting in frequent use of off-label or unlicensed medications (Garcia-Lopez *et al.*, 2020). Understanding pharmacokinetics (how the drug reaches the site of action) and pharmacodynamics (the drug's effect on the body) is crucial (Khan, 2020). Analgesics act either centrally, on opioid receptors in the spinal cord and brain or peripherally, by inhibiting prostaglandin production (Reaney & Trower, 2010).

Non-opioid analgesia

Mild pain is commonly treated with paracetamol or non-steroidal anti-inflammatory drugs (NSAIDs), such as ibuprofen, in children under 16 (Paediatric Joint Formulary

Committee, 2025). Combined with opioids, these form a multimodal approach for moderate to severe pain, defined by the ASA (2012) as using two or more drugs with different mechanisms of action. This approach should be individualised, with dosing optimised for efficacy.

Combining a non-opioid with an opioid results in a greater pain relief effect than is experienced when either drug is administered alone. It is important for optimum effect that the correct dosages be used (Joint Formulary Committee, 2025).

Opioid analgesia

Opioids, used alongside non-opioid analgesics, treat moderate to severe pain, with the route of administration chosen based on pain severity, duration and the child's condition. According to the WHO pain ladder, weak opioids (e.g., codeine phosphate for children over 12, dihydrocodeine) are used at step 2, and strong opioids (e.g., morphine, diamorphine and tramadol) at step 3 (Paediatric Joint Formulary Committee, 2025).

Routes of opioid administration

Opioid administration in children

Opioids can be administered via multiple routes depending on the drug, the child's needs and the desired effect. Guidance for administration must always be followed. Common routes include: enteral (oral, nasogastric tube [NGT], percutaneous endoscopic gastrostomy [PEG] and percutaneous endoscopic jejunostomy [PEJ]), intramuscular (IM), intravenous (IV), subcutaneous (SC), inhalation, transdermal, epidural/caudal, intrathecal (IT) and transmucosal (sublingual, buccal, intranasal and rectal).

> Concurrent use of opioids with benzodiazepines or similar drugs increases the risk of sedation, respiratory depression, coma and death (MHRA, 2020). Prolonged use (>3 months) carries a risk of dependence.

- **Oral:** Preferred route when possible; comfortable and as effective as IV morphine (Rieder & Jong, 2021).
- **IV bolus:** For children unable to take enteral opioids or with severe pain; short-acting, so continuous infusion may be needed (Gai *et al.*, 2020). Morphine is the preferred drug.
- **Subcutaneous:** Common for continuous morphine infusion, particularly in palliative care (Garcia-Lopez *et al.*, 2023).
- **Continuous morphine infusion (CMI):** Used for prolonged or intermittent pain when bolus doses are inappropriate, or the child cannot use patient-controlled analgesia (PCA).
- **Patient-controlled analgesia (PCA):** Suitable for children, typically over 6 years, who can understand and manage self-administration via a programmable pump (Hayes *et al.*, 2016).

Patient-controlled analgesia administration

Patient-controlled analgesia (PCA) is an intravenous analgesia method, commonly using morphine, allowing the child to control administration via a hand-held button on a programmable pump (Reaney & Trower, 2010). Doses are weight-based, and successful use requires thorough preparation and education of the child, family and nursing staff (Gai *et al.*, 2020).

PCA can be delivered in three ways, used alone or in combination:

- **Patient-administered bolus:** Set doses with a lockout to prevent overdose.
- **Nurse-controlled analgesia (NCA):** Administered by a nurse when the child cannot use PCA due to cognitive or physical limitations or end-of-life care (Franson, 2010).
- **Continuous opioid infusion:** Provides constant pain relief, typically with morphine; bolus doses can be prescribed for breakthrough pain (Macintyre *et al.*, 2010).

Local guidelines and protocols, including assessment schedules (e.g., Table 8.5), should always be followed, as practices may vary between organisations.

> Recent studies have shown that overestimation of oxygen saturations is higher in CYP with dark-toned skin (Hooli *et al.*, 2024).

TABLE 8.5 Patient observations during PCA administration and for 4 hours following discontinuation (other vital signs such as temperature and blood pressure may also be monitored as part of vital signs assessment)

Observation	Frequency	Rationale
Heart rate	Hourly	Opioids can cause bradycardia
Respiratory rate	Hourly	Opioids can cause respiratory depression
Sedation score	Hourly	Opioids can cause sedation
Pain score	Hourly	To assess effectiveness of analgesia
Nausea and vomiting	Hourly	Opioids can cause nausea and vomiting, particularly in the initial stages
Pruritus	At least 4-hourly	Opioids can cause itching and urticaria
Urinary retention	Regular output monitoring	Opioids can induce urinary retention
Oxygen saturations	Continuous	Opioids can cause respiratory depression

Regional analgesia

- Central blocks
- Peripheral blocks

Central blocks

Neuraxial analgesia involves administering drugs into the epidural or intrathecal space to block pain transmission, often as a single-dose caudal injection combined with a local anaesthetic to prolong the effect (APAGBI, 2012).

Children undergoing major surgery benefit from epidural or caudal analgesia (Thomas *et al.*, 2023). Those with chronic pain, such as Complex Regional Pain Syndrome, may receive epidural catheters, lumbar sympathetic blocks or peripheral nerve blocks (Mosquera-Moscoso *et al.*, 2024). Caudal or single bolus epidurals are used intraoperatively, while continuous epidural infusions manage postoperative pain.

RCoA Guidelines (2020) recommend using the lowest effective concentration of local anaesthetic to balance pain relief and motor function. Hospital protocols specify limited epidural solutions, with dosing tailored to age and weight, particularly in infants and neonates. Opioids like fentanyl can be added, but are avoided in infants under 5 kg due to risk of apnoea (APAGBI, 2012) (Table 8.6).

Please note these are suggested observations and requirements vary between organisations; readers are advised to follow local and institutional guidelines.

Peripheral blocks

Peripheral nerve blocks are increasingly used in children due to advances in point-of-care ultrasound (Frawley *et al.*, 2022). Most are performed under general anaesthetic, though older children may sometimes receive blocks awake (Roberts *et al.*, 2022). The block site depends on the surgical indication, e.g., brachial plexus for hand/forearm surgery or lumbar plexus for lower limb surgery (Merella & Mossetti, 2020).

Local anaesthetics, typically bupivacaine or levobupivacaine, can be given as a single perioperative dose or via continuous perineural catheter, for acute or chronic pain management. Regional anaesthesia reduces opioid requirements, lowers respiratory complications and promotes faster gut recovery. Epinephrine is the only approved adjunct in children, prolonging the block by delaying systemic absorption (Roberts *et al.*, 2022).

Post-block monitoring should include assessment for nausea, vomiting, persistent motor blockade, infection and catheter issues such as leakage or occlusion (Dadure & Capdevila, 2012).

Adjuvant drugs

These are medications that can be used in addition to basic and opioid analgesia and used especially in the treatment of neuropathic and visceral pain (Friedrichsdorf and Goubert, 2020). Children with chronic pain can be

TABLE 8.6 Suggested observations for children on a continuous epidural with levobupivacaine with or without fentanyl

Observation	Frequency	Rationale
Pain score (validated and appropriate)	Hourly	To monitor effectiveness of the analgesia
Sedation score	Hourly	Fentanyl can cause sedation
Heart rate	Hourly	Levobupivacaine can cause a decrease in heart rate
Respiratory rate	Hourly	To monitor for high motor block
Oxygen saturation	Continuous	To detect respiratory problems
Blood pressure	Hourly	Levobupivacaine can decrease blood pressure
Bromage score	4-hourly	Levobupivacaine can affect motor nerves
Sensory block	4-hourly	Monitor the spread of the block
Catheter site	6-hourly	To observe for leakage/redness
Pressure areas	At least 4-hourly	Local anaesthetic blocks can lead to loss of sensation
Agitation	Regularly	Levobupivacaine can cause agitation
Pruritus	Regularly	Fentanyl can cause itching
Nausea and vomiting	Hourly	Fentanyl is an emetic. Hypotension can lead to nausea
Temperature	4-hourly	Indication of catheter infection

prescribed anti-neuropathic drugs such as tricyclic antidepressants and anti-epileptic drugs, and these should be initiated by a consultation of a specialist (Paediatric Joint Formulary Committee, 2025).

Non-pharmacological management of pain

Opioids are the preferred treatment for moderate to severe pain, but may cause hypotension, delirium and respiratory depression (Maffeo *et al.*, 2024). Anxiety and stress can worsen pain perception, so personalised approaches combining pharmacological and non-pharmacological strategies are recommended.

Psychological interventions, such as Cognitive Behavioural Therapy (CBT), effectively reduce pain, especially in chronic pain (Checa-Peñalver *et al.*, 2024). Non-pharmacological methods, including massage, heat/cold, touch and vibration, stimulate unmyelinated C fibres to 'close the pain gate', preventing pain signals from reaching the brain (Gür & Apay, 2020). These low-cost interventions can reduce analgesic doses, improve medical compliance and mitigate short- and long-term pain effects (Wu *et al.*, 2022; Sönmez Düzkaya *et al.*, 2024).

Distraction techniques, such as music, virtual reality or video therapy, trigger beta-endorphin release and activate brain regions involved in pain modulation, blocking pain transmission (Ramdhanie *et al.*, 2024). Devices using vibration and cold stimulate enkephalin production and are effective for procedures like venepuncture or vaccinations in children (Bergomi *et al.*, 2018).

Infants (0–12 months)

Neonates and infants, especially in intensive care, experience multiple painful procedures such as cannula insertion and IM injections (Weng *et al.*, 2024). Effective non-pharmacological interventions include non-nutritive sucking, kangaroo care, breastfeeding and oral sucrose. Oral sucrose and skin-to-skin care are particularly beneficial for preterm and low-birth-weight infants, while direct breastfeeding is most effective for full-term infants (Hoarau *et al.*, 2021). Breast milk, especially colostrum, contains beta-endorphins, providing natural analgesia (Wu *et al.*, 2022).

Infants also respond positively to oral stimulation and physical comfort, which helps minimise procedural pain (Krauss *et al.*, 2016). Additional supportive interventions include mobiles, music and familiar objects to provide comfort and distraction.

Early childhood (1–5 years)

Preschool children benefit from physical comfort and distraction, especially from parents or primary caregivers. Both interactive and passive distractions help manage procedural pain. Procedures like cannulation can provoke high anxiety and reduce cooperation, particularly in children aged 12–18 months who struggle with self-regulation (Gennis *et al.*, 2024). Effective interventions include reassurance, praise, reading books, blowing bubbles, telling simple stories and offering simple choices.

Middle childhood (6–12 years)

Needle pain is a common fear in middle childhood, and can lead to needle phobias and avoidance behaviours (Guillari *et al.*, 2024). Interventions such as Kaleidoscopes and virtual reality can significantly reduce procedural anxiety and pain (Gotkas & Anvi, 2023). Children in this age group also benefit from hand-held games, relaxation techniques, role-play with medical equipment and being given appropriate information to make choices about their care.

Adolescents (13–18 years)

Adolescents are developing autonomy and decision-making skills, though they may still involve parents or caregivers in care (Hadiprodjo *et al.*, 2022). Needle pain remains a common fear (Guillari *et al.*, 2024). Effective non-pharmacological strategies include listening to favourite music, reading, playing computer games and using muscle relaxation and controlled breathing techniques to manage pain.

Case study: Amina

Amina is 1 day post-appendectomy, receiving pain relief via a morphine PCA and regular oral analgesia. Her mother, Leila, her primary caregiver, is concerned that Amina remains in pain despite PCA use. The family has a multicultural background, and Amina is typically reserved in expressing discomfort.

Leila will need to leave soon to collect Amina's younger brother, Sami, from nursery and take him to his father's home. Amina's parents are separated, sharing childcare amid work commitments and limited communication.

The clinical team must assess and manage Amina's pain effectively while considering cultural background, emotional needs, language preferences and the family's logistical challenges.

Discussion Questions

1. What pain assessment tools would be appropriate to assess Amina's pain, taking into account age and communication style?
2. What other factors should be considered when managing Amina's pain?
3. What non-pharmacological methods could be used to help Amina feel more comfortable during her hospital stay?

Case study: Joseph

Joseph, a 15-year-old autistic boy, presents to the ED after a playground fall, landing on his outstretched arm. He cried out immediately and is visibly distressed, shielding his face and covering his ears due to bright lights and noise. He communicates verbally but may become non-verbal when overwhelmed.

His mother, Kyla, explains that calm, clear communication and warning before touch help Joseph cope, and that previous hospital experiences have caused significant anxiety. The family is culturally diverse, English-speaking, with extended family potentially joining later.

Initial assessment indicates a displaced fracture of the left forearm. The care team must plan pain management while minimising distress and accommodating Joseph's sensory sensitivities, communication needs and anxiety.

Discussion Questions

1. What pain assessment tools are appropriate for Joseph?
2. What factors related to diversity and neurodiversity should be considered?
3. What strategies could be used to manage Joseph's pain effectively and reduce his distress in the ED?

Conclusion

While anatomical and physiological processes influence pain perception, a child's experience is also shaped by age, developmental stage, gender, cultural background and previous experiences within the family. Pain assessment should involve both the child and their family whenever possible. Because of these complexities, no single approach fits all; effective pain management requires a tailored, biopsychosocial and multimodal strategy, posing ongoing challenges for children's nurses.

References

Albani, E., Konstantinos, P., Saridi, M., *et al.* (2022). Pain assessment in children with cognitive disabilities: critical review and clinical implications. *International Journal of Caring Sciences* 15(3), 1784.

American Society of Anesthesiologists (ASA) (2012). Practice guidelines for acute pain management in the perioperative setting. an updated report by the American Society of Anesthesiologists Task Force on Acute Pain Management. *Anaesthesiology* 116(2), 248–273.

Anekar, A.A., Hendrix, J.M., & Cascella, M. (2023). *WHO Analgesic Ladder.* StatPearls Publishing, Treasure Island FL.

Association of Paediatric Anaesthetists of Great Britain and Ireland (APAGBI) (2012). Good practice in postoperative and procedural pain management, 2. In: *Pediatric Anesthesia*, Vol. 22, Suppl. 1, pp. 1–79. Wiley; https://onlinelibrary.wiley.com/doi/pdf/10.1111/j.1460-9592.2012.03838.x

Bergomi, P., Scudeller, L., Pintaldi, S., & Dal Molin, A. (2018). Efficacy of non-pharmacological methods of pain management in children undergoing venipuncture in a pediatric outpatient clinic: a randomized controlled trial of audiovisual distraction and external cold and vibration. *Journal of Pediatric Nursing* 42, e66–e72 https://doi.org/10.1016/j.pedn.2018.04.011.

Best, K.M., Asaro, L.A., Curley, M., & Randomized Evaluation of Sedation Titration for Respiratory Failure (RESTORE) Study Investigators (2019). Sedation management for critically Ill children with preexisting cognitive impairment. *The Journal of Pediatrics* 206, 204–211.e1 https://doi.org/10.1016/j.jpeds.2018.10.042.

Briggs, E. (2010). Understanding the experience and physiology of pain. *Nursing Standard* 25(3), 35–39.

Bruce, E.A. (2022). Pain management. In: Bruce, E.A. (ed). *The Great Ormond Street Hospital Manual of Children and Young People's Nursing Practices*, 2nd edn. Wiley-Blackwell EPUB. Chap. 24.

Campbell-Yeo, M., Erikson, M., & Benoit, B. (2022). Assessment and management of pain in preterm infants: a practice update. *Children* 2022(9), 244 https://doi.org/10.3390/children9020244.

Carter, B., & Simons, J. (2014). *Stories of Children's Pain: Linking Evidence to Practice.* Sage, London.

Checa-Peñalver, A., Lírio-Romero, C., Luiz Ferreira, E.A., *et al.* (2024). Effectiveness of non-pharmacological interventions in the management of pediatric chronic pain: a systematic review. *Children (Basel)* 11(12), 1420. https://doi.org/10.3390/children11121420.

Chen, T., Siu, J.M., Hubbard, B., *et al.* (2025). Effect of parental anxiety and catastrophizing on post-tonsillectomy opioid consumption in children. *International Journal of Pediatric Otorhinolaryngology* 194, 112374 https://doi.org/10.1016/j.ijporl.2025.112374.

Colbert, B., Ankney, J., & Lee, K. (2020). *Anatomy and Physiology for Health,Professionals*, 4th edn. Pearson, London.

Cruz, M.D., Fernandes, A.M., & Oliveira, C.R. (2016). Epidemiology of painful procedures performed in neonates: a systematic review of observational studies. *European Journal of Pain* 20, 489–498.

Cuomo, A., Bimonte, S., Forte, C.A., *et al.* (2019). Multimodal approaches and tailored therapies for pain management: the trolley analgesic model Multimodal approaches and tailored therapies for pain management: the trolley analgesic model. *Journal of Pain Research* 12, 711–714.

Dadure, C., & Capdevila, X. (2012). Peripheral catheter techniques. *Paediatric Anaesthesia* 22(1), 93–101.

Department of Health (DH) (2004). *Ill child Standard, National Service Framework for Children, Young People and Maternity Services.* Department of Health, London.

Eccleston, C., Fisher, E., Howard, R.F., *et al.* (2021). Delivering transformative action in paediatric pain: a Lancet Child & Adolescent Health Commission. *The Lancet Child & Adolescent Health* 5(1), 47–87.

Edwards, S and Coyne, I. (2019) A Survival Guide to Children's Nursing Revised and Updated Edition EPUB

Engstrom, K., Bellolio, F., Moore Jeffery, M., *et al.* (2025). Disparities in pain management among transgender patients presenting to the emergency department for abdominal pain. *Academic Emergency Medicine* 32, 130–136 https://doi.org/10.1111/acem.15027.

Fateh, Z., Sedighi, D., Biglari, M., & Khalili, A. (2024). Investigating the assessment tools for pain severity during venipuncture in preschool-age children: a systematic review. *Journal of Pediatrics Review* 12(2), 143–152 https://doi.org/10.32598/jpr.12.2.1166.1.

Fitzcharles, M.A., Cohen, S.P., Clauw, D.J., *et al.* (2021). Nociplastic pain: towards an understanding of prevalent pain conditions. *Lancet* 397(10289), 2098–2110.

Forgeron, P.A., & Stinson, J. (2014). Fundamentals of chronic pain in children and young people. Part 1. *Nursing Children and Young People* 26(6), 29–34.

Franck, L., Greenberg, C., & Stevens, B. (2000). Pain assessment in infants and children. *Pediatric Clinics of North America* 47(3), 487–512.

Franson, H. (2010). Postoperative patient-controlled analgesia in the pediatric population: a literature review. *American Association of Nurse Anesthetists Journal* 78(5), 374–378.

Frawley, G., Marchesini, V., Loh, B., *et al.* (2022). Pediatric lower limb peripheral nerve blocks: Indications, effectiveness, and the incidence of adverse events. *Pediatric Anesthesia* 32(8), 946–953 https://doi.org/10.1111/pan.14468.

Friedrichsdorf, S.J., & Goubert, L. (2020). Pediatric pain treatment and prevention for hospitalized children. *PAIN Reports* 5(1), e804 https://doi.org/10.1097/PR9.0000000000000804

Gai, N., Naser, B., Hanley, J., *et al.* (2020). A practical guide to acute pain management in children. *Journal of Anesthesia* 34(3), 421–433 https://doi.org/10.1007/s00540-020-02767-x.

García-López, I., Cuervas-Mons Vendrell, M., Martín Romero, I., *et al.* (2020). Off-label and unlicensed drugs in pediatric palliative care: a prospective observational study. *Journal of Pain and Symptom Management* 60(5), 923–932 https://doi.org/10.1016/j.jpainsymman.2020.06.014.

García-López, I., González, L.C., Martín-Romero, I., *et al.* (2023). Pediatric palliative care at home: a prospective study on subcutaneous drug administration. *Journal of Pain and Symptom Management* 66(3), e319–e326 https://doi.org/10.1016/j.jpainsymman.2023.05.011.

Gennis, H.G., Flora, D.B., McMurtry, C.M., *et al.* (2024). It takes two: the relative contributions of parent versus child-led regulatory behaviours on toddler vaccination pain. *European Journal of Pain* 28(3), 476–490 https://doi.org/10.1002/ejp.2197.

Givler, A., and Maani-Fogelman, P. A. (2023). The importance of cultural competence in pain and palliative care. National Library of Medicine; StatPearls Publishing. https://www.ncbi.nlm.nih.gov/books/NBK493154/

Godfrey, H. (2005). Understanding pain, part 1: physiology of pain. *British Journal of Nursing* 14(16), 846–852.

Goktas, N., & Avci, D. (2023). The effect of visual and/or auditory distraction techniques on children's pain, anxiety and medical fear in invasive procedures: a randomized controlled trial. *Journal of Pediatric Nursing* 73, e27–e35 https://doi.org/10.1016/j.pedn.2023.07.005.

Grass, J.A. (2005). Patient-controlled analgesia. *Anesthesia and Analgesia* 101(5 Suppl), S44–S61.

Guillari, A., Giordano, V., Catone, M., *et al.* (2024). Non-pharmacological interventions to reduce procedural needle pain in children (6–12 years): a systematic review. *Journal of Pediatric Nursing* 78, e102–e116 https://doi.org/10.1016/j.pedn.2024.06.025.

Gür, E.Y., & Apay, S.E. (2020). The effect of cognitive behavioral techniques using virtual reality on birth pain: a randomized controlled trial. *Midwifery 91*, 102856 https://doi.org/10.1016/j.midw.2020.102856.

Hadiprodjo, N.A., Dean, B.J., & Parson, J.A. (2022). In: Hadiprodjo, N.A., Dean, B.J., & Parson, J.A. (eds). *Integrating therapeutic play into nursing and allied health practice: a developmentally sensitive approach to communicating with children.* Springer.

Hayes, J., Dowling, J.J., Peliowski, A., *et al.* (2016). Patient-controlled analgesia plus background opioid infusion for post-operative pain in children: a systematic review and meta-analysis of randomized trials. *Anesthesia and Analgesia* 123(4), 991–1003 https://doi.org/10.1213/ANE.0000000000001244.

Hoarau, K., Payet, M.L., Zamidio, L., *et al.* (2021). "Holding-cuddling" and sucrose for pain relief during venepuncture in newborn infants: a randomized, controlled trial (CÂSA). *Frontiers in Pediatrics* 8, 607900 https://doi.org/10.3389/fped.2020.607900.

Hooli, S., Colbourn, T., Shah, M.I., *et al.* (2024). Pulse oximetry accuracy in children with dark skin tones: relevance to acute lower respiratory infection care in low- and middle-income countries. *The American Journal of Tropical Medicine and Hygiene* 111(4), 736–739 https://doi.org/10.4269/ajtmh.23-0656.

Howard, R.E., Lloyd-Thomas, A., Thomas, M., *et al.* (2010). Nurse-controlled analgesia (NCA) following major surgery in 10,000 patients in a children's hospital. *Paediatric Anaesthesia* 20(2), 126–134.

Igler, E.C., Defenderfer, E.K., Lang, A.C. *et al.* (2017). Gender differences in the experience of pain dismissal in adolescence. *Journal of Child Health Care* 21(4), 381–391.

International Association for the Study of Pain (2020) IASP announces revised definition of pain. Retrieved 11/04/2025 from: https://www.iasp-pain.org/publications/iasp-news/iasp-announces-revised-definition-of-pain/ (accessed April 2025).

International Association for the Study of Pain (2021a). Acute pain. Retrieved 11/04/2025 from: https://www.iasp-pain.org/resources/topics/acute-pain/#:~:text=Acute%20pain%20happens%20suddenly%2C%20starts%20out%20sharp%20or,a%20few%20minutes%20to%20less%20than%20six%20months (accessed April 2025).

International Association for the Study of Pain (2021b) Definitions of Chronic Pain Syndromes Retrieved 25/05/2025 from: Definitions of Chronic Pain Syndromes – International Association for the Study of Pain (IASP) (last accessed May 2025).

International Association for the Study of Pain (2023) Pain terms and definitions. Retrieved 11/04/2025 from: https://www.iasp-pain.org/resources/terminology/ (accessed April 2025).

Joint Formulary Committee (2025). The British National Formulary. https://bnf.nice.org.uk/. (accessed June 2025).

Khan, E. (2020). Pharmacokinetics and pharmacodynamics. In: Hood, P. & Khan, E. (eds). *Understanding Pharmacology in Nursing Practice*. Cham: Springer https://doi-org.hallam.idm.oclc.org/10.1007/978-3-030-32004-1_2.

Krauss, B.S., Calligaris, L., Green, S.M., & Barbi, E. (2016). Current concepts in management of pain in children in the emergency department. *Lancet* 387(10013), 83–92.

Labaka, A., Zamakola, A., Arrue, M., & Arrieta, H. (2023). Evaluating gender awareness, gender-related health knowledge and pain legitimisation among nursing students: A quasi-experimental study. *Nurse Education in Practice* 72. https://doi.org/10.1016/j.nepr.2023.103790.

Macintyre, P.E., Schug, S.A., Scott, D.A., *et al.* (2010). *Acute Pain Management: Scientific Evidence*, 3rd edn. ANZCA & FPM, Melbourne.

Maffeo, M., Bianchi, A., Fogli, B., *et al.* (2024). Use of non pharmacological therapies for pain management in children: a survey of pediatric healthcare provides. *Infermieristica Journal* 3(4), 287–294. doi:10.36253/if-2904.

Marieb, E. (2015). *Essentials of Human Anatomy and Physiology*, 11th edn. Pearson, London.

Marieb, E., & Keller, S. (2018). *Essentials of Human Anatomy and Physiology*, 12th edn. Pearson.

McCaffery, M., & Beebe, A. (1989). *Pain: Clinical Manual for Nursing Practice*. Mosby, St. Louis.

McCaffery, M., & Pasero, C. (1999). *Pain: Clinical Manual*, 2nd edn. Mosby, St. Louis.

McLenon, J., & Rogers, M.A. (2019). The fear of needles: a systematic review and meta-analysis. *Journal of Advanced Nursing* 75(1), 30–42 https://doi.org/10.1111/jan.13818.

Mears, L., & Mears, J. (2023). The pathophysiology, assessment, and management of acute pain. *British Journal of Nursing 32*(2).

Medicines and Healthcare products Regulatory Agency (2020). Drug Safety Update volume 13, issue 8: March 2020: 5

Melzack, R., & Wall, P. (1965). Pain mechanisms: a new theory. *Science* 150(3699), 971–979.

Melzack, R., & Wall, P. (1996). *The Challenge of Pain*, 2nd edn. Penguin, London.

Merella, F., & Mossetti, V. (2020). Ultrasound-guided upper and lower extremity nerve blocks in children. *BJA Education* 20(2), 42–50 https://doi.org/10.1016/j.bjae.2019.11.003.

Mosquera-Moscoso, J., Eldrige, J., Encalada, S., *et al.* (2024). Interventional pain management of CRPS in the pediatric population: a literature review. *Interventional Pain Medicine (Online)* 3 https://doi.org/10.1016/j.inpm.2024.100532.

Ndengeyingoma, A., Lebel, V., & Alvarez, S.B. (2023). Children and pain: assessment and management according to parents' perspective. *Research in Nursing & Health* 46, 93–100 https://doi.org/10.1002/nur.22271.

Paediatric Joint Formulary Committee (2025). *British National Formulary for Children*. Retrieved 2/4/25 from https://bnfc.nice.org.uk/treatment-summaries/analgesics/#related-treatment-summaries.

Palese, A., Conforto, L., Meloni, F., *et al.* (2021). Assessing pain in children with autism spectrum disorders: findings from a preliminary validation survey. *Scandinavian Journal of Caring Sciences* 35, 457–467.

Pancekauskaitė, G., & Jankauskaitė, L. (2018). Paediatric pain medicine: pain differences, recognition and coping acute procedural pain in paediatric emergency room. *Medicina* 54(6), 94 https://doi.org/10.3390/medicina54060094.

Peate, I. (2021). *Fundamentals of Applied Pathophysiology: An Essentials Guide for Nursing and Healthcare Students*, 4th edn. Wiley Blackwell.

Plummer, K., McCarthy, M., Newall, F., & Manias, E. (2024). Their bodies just give it away. *Cancer Nursing* 47(2), 151–162 https://doi.org/10.1097/NCC.0000000000001199.

Ramdhanie, G.G., Nurrohmah, A., Mulya, A.P., *et al.* (2024). A scoping review of audiovisual distraction techniques among children in reducing invasive procedure pain a scoping review of audiovisual distraction techniques among children in reducing invasive procedure pain. *Journal of Multidisciplinary Healthcare* 17, 4363–4372.

Reaney, R., & Trower, C. (2010). In: Trigg, E. & Mohammed, T. (eds). *Practices in Children's Nursing. Guidelines for Hospital and Community*, 3rd edn. Edinburgh: Churchill Livingstone Elsevier.

Rieder, M.J., & Jong, G. (2021). The use of oral opioids to control children's pain in the post-codeine era. *Paediatrics & Child Health* 26(2), 120–127 https://doi.org/10.1093/pch/pxaa133.

Roberts, S., Bali, S., & Misselbrook, K. (2022). Peripheral and local anaesthetic techniques for paediatric surgery. *Anaesthesia and Intensive Care Medicine* 23(5), 276–284 https://doi.org/10.1016/j.mpaic.2022.02.017.

Rogger, R., Bello, C., Romero, C.S., *et al.* (2023). Cultural framing and the impact on acute pain and pain services. *Current Pain and Headache Reports* 27, 429–436. https://doi.org/10.1007/s11916-023-01125-2.

Royal College of Anaesthetists (2025). Chapter 11: Guidelines for the provision of anaesthesia services for inpatient pain management. https://rcoa.ac.uk/node/21456 (accessed 18 June 2025).

Royal College of Anaesthetists (RCoA) (1990). *Commission on the Provision of Surgical Services: Report of a Working Party on Pain after Surgery*. RCoA, London.

Royal College of Anaesthetists (RCoA) (2020). Best practice in the management of epidural analgesia in the hospital setting. https://fpm.ac.uk/sites/fpm/files/documents/2020-09/Epidural-AUG-2020-FINAL.pdf. (accessed 13 June 2025).

Royal College of Nursing (RCN) (2009). The recognition and assessment of acute pain in children. Update of full guideline. RCN, London.

Sönmez Düzkaya, D., Karakul, A., Akoy, İ., & Andi, S. (2024). Effects of ShotBlocker® and the Helfer skin tap technique on pain and fear experienced during intramuscular injection among children aged 6–12 years in pediatric emergency units: a randomized controlled trial. *International Emergency Nursing 76* https://doi.org/10.1016/j.ienj.2024.101502.

Stevens, B.J., Harrison, D., Rashotte, J., *et al.* (2012). Pain assessment and intensity in hospitalized children in Canada. *Journal of Pain* 13(9), 857–865.

Tamvaki, E., Giannakopoulou, M., Bozas, E., & Zachpoulu, D. (2024). Use of biomarkers to objectively evaluate pain in critically ill children: a scoping review. *Critical Care Nurse* 44(1), 55–66.

Thomas, A., Bhasulamani, S.P., James, D., *et al.* (2023). A cross-sectional observation study to evaluate the efficacy and complications of epidural analgesia in paediatric population. *Journal of Anaesthesiology, Clinical Pharmacology* 39(2), 189–194 https://doi.org/10.4103/joacp.joacp_218_21.

Tortora, G., & Derrickson, B. (2021). *Principles of Anatomy and Physiology*, 16th edn. Wiley-Blackwell, Hoboken, NJ.

Turner-Cobb, J. (2014). *Child Health Psychology: A Biopsychosocial Perspective*. Sage, London.

Twycross, A., Dowden, S., & Bruce, E. (eds) (2009). *Managing Pain in Children: A Clinical Guide*. Wiley.

Twycross, A., Dowden, S., & Stinson, J. (eds) (2014). *Managing Pain in Children: A Clinical Guide for Nurses and Healthcare Professionals*, 2nd edn. Wiley, Oxford.

Vasey, J., Smith, J., Kirshbaum, M.N., & Chirema, K. (2019). Tokenism or true partnership: parental involvement in a child's acute pain care. *Journal of Clinical Nursing* 28(9–10), 1491–1505 https://doi.org/10.1111/jocn.14747.

Webb, C.M., & Steeds, C.E. (2022). The anatomy and physiology of pain. *Clinics in Integrated Care* 14, Article 100115.

Weng, Y., Zhang, J., & Chen, Z. (2024). Effect of non-pharmacological interventions on pain in preterm infants in the neonatal intensive care unit: a network meta-analysis of randomized controlled trials. *BMC Pediatrics* 24(1), 9 https://doi.org/10.1186/s12887-023-04488-y.

Wheeldon, A. (2021). Pain and Pain management in. In: Peate, I. (ed). *Fundamentals of Applied Pathophysiology: An Essential Guide for Nursing and Healthcare Students*, 4th edn. Wiley Blackwell.

Williams, G., & Rose, M. (2015). Managing acute pain in children and young people. In: Faculty of Pain Medicine of the Royal College of Anaesthetists (ed). *Core Standards for Pain Management Services in the UK*. London: RCoA.

World Health Organization (WHO) (2020). *Guidelines on the management of chronic pain in children*. WHO, Geneva.

Wu, Y., Zhao, Y., Wu, L., *et al.* (2022). Non-pharmacological management for vaccine-related pain in children in the healthcare setting: a scoping review non-pharmacological management for vaccine-related pain in children in the healthcare setting: a scoping review. *Journal of Pain Research* 15, 2773–2782.

Zhang, S.M., Chan, Y., Lai, L., *et al.* (2023). Parental postoperative pain management perceptions, attitudes, and practices in pediatric limb fractures. *Pain Management Nursing* 24, 506–512 https://doi.org/10.1016/j.pmn.2023.07.006.

CHAPTER 9

Disorders of the nervous system

Elizabeth Gormley-Fleming

AIM

The aim of this chapter is to provide the reader with an overview of the nervous system and an understanding of pathophysiological changes associated with disorders of this system.

LEARNING OUTCOMES

On completion of this chapter, the reader will be able to:

- Outline the organisation, structure and function of the nervous system.
- Understand the pathophysiology of common childhood neurological disorders.
- Consider the priorities of a neurological nursing assessment.
- Examine some key red flags in the assessment of neurological conditions.
- Discuss the management and nursing care of young patients with neurological disorders.

KEYWORDS

- central and peripheral nervous system (PNS)
- autonomic and somatic nervous system
- brain and spinal cord
- meninges
- cerebrospinal fluid (CSF)
- intracranial pressure (ICP)
- seizure
- haemorrhage
- tumour

Test your prior knowledge

1. List the two anatomical areas of the central nervous system (CNS).
2. Describe the functions of the central CNS.
3. Name the four main anatomical areas of the brain.
4. Describe the four main functions of cerebrospinal fluid (CSF).
5. Review the role of neurotransmitters in the CNS.
6. Outline the structure of the peripheral nervous system (PNS).
7. Compare the structure and function of the autonomic and sympathetic nervous systems.
8. Draw a diagram of a motor neurone cell.
9. Review foetal and childhood development of the nervous system.

Introduction

Along with the endocrine system, the nervous system interacts with all body systems to maintain homeostasis. It is a complex system coordinating and controlling voluntary and involuntary action. It orientates us to the internal and external environment through sensory mechanisms. The nervous system assimilates experiences and information through memory, intelligence, learning and dreaming. It provides us with instinctual information and reflexes, at birth and beyond.

Structure of the nervous system

While the nervous system functions as a whole, it is useful to subdivide its anatomical structure and physiological components (Table 9.1, Fig. 9.1) to assist in understanding its complexity.

Central and peripheral nervous systems

The nervous system may be divided into the central nervous system (CNS) and the peripheral nervous system (PNS).

Physiologically, the nervous system is subdivided and organised as shown in Fig. 9.1.

Cellular structure of the nervous system

Highly specialised neurones and neuroglia form the cellular foundation of the nervous system. Neurones transmit information, while neuroglial cells provide essential supportive functions.

TABLE 9.1 Anatomical structure of the nervous system

Central nervous system (CNS)	Peripheral nervous system (PNS)
• Brain • Spinal cord	• Cranial nerves • Spinal nerves • Sensory (afferent) neurones • Motor (efferent) neurones • Somatic nervous system (voluntary) • Autonomic nervous system (involuntary) • Sympathetic • Parasympathetic

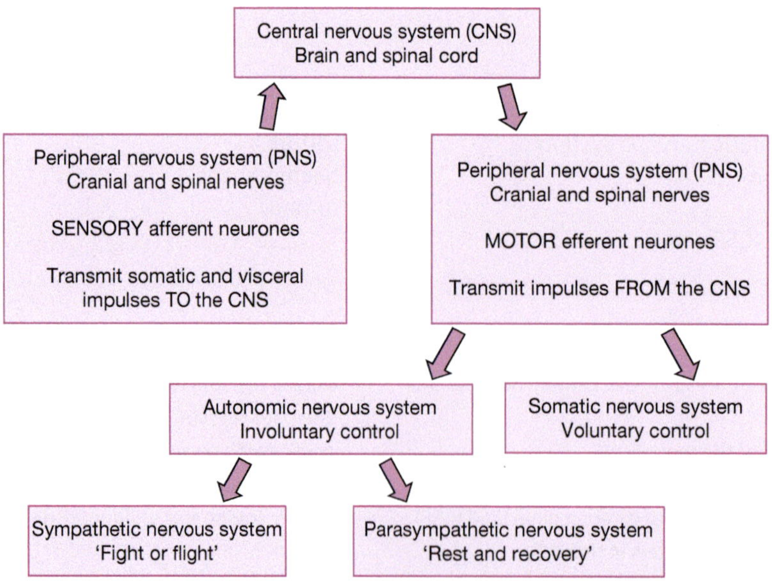

FIGURE 9.1 Organisation of the nervous system.

Transmission of nerve impulses

The nervous system uses three types of nerve impulse transmission. Simple linear transmission conducts electrical action potentials along neurones through sodium and potassium exchange, causing cycles of polarisation and depolarisation. Saltatory conduction occurs in myelinated neurones, where action potentials 'jump' between nodes of Ranvier, allowing much faster transmission. The third type involves chemical neurotransmitters at synapses. Key examples include acetylcholine in the CNS and neuromuscular junctions, dopamine and norepinephrine (noradrenaline) in the CNS and autonomic nervous system and other common transmitters such as serotonin and GABA.

Disorders of the nervous system

Introduction

This section outlines common neurological disorders in childhood. These conditions arise from dysfunction of the brain or nervous system and can lead to physical, behavioural and cognitive symptoms. Given the complexity of the nervous system, such disorders are categorised by their cause, including neurological and cerebral dysfunction, head and spinal trauma, motor disorders, neurological tumours, infections and seizures.

Causes of neurological dysfunction

Prenatal causes

These conditions arise in the womb. The nervous system begins developing in the third week of embryonic life, forming the neural tube through neurulation. Between the fourth and eleventh weeks, distinct brain regions develop. The PNS forms from the neural crest at around 4 weeks, alongside the spinal, cranial and autonomic systems. Growth continues so that by birth, all major nervous system structures are present. Exposure to harmful factors during pregnancy can disrupt this development and lead to intellectual, behavioural and developmental difficulties.

- **Neurotoxins** can cross the placenta and harm the foetal nervous system, leading to later neurological problems. Alcohol use in pregnancy is linked to foetal alcohol syndrome; tobacco use has been associated with challenging behaviours and developmental impairment; and exposure to lead or mercury can affect intelligence, memory, learning and overall development.
- **Nutritional deficiencies** in the final trimester can reduce the number of brain cells. Spina bifida is associated with inadequate maternal folic acid intake before conception or in early pregnancy.
- **Infections** can pass from mother to foetus via the placenta, causing developmental problems. Chorioamnionitis can lead to cerebral palsy. The Zika virus causes microcephaly, with reduced head size and incomplete brain development. Other infections affecting prenatal development include toxoplasmosis, rubella, cytomegalovirus, HIV, herpes simplex, hepatitis B and syphilis.
- **Birth complications**, such as hypoxic brain injury, may occur if the umbilical cord blood supply is reduced or interrupted during labour, depriving the foetus of oxygen and nutrients and resulting in potential brain damage.

Congenital causes

Genetic abnormalities can cause a wide range of neurological disorders. Most genetic disorders are inherited rather than arising from new mutations. They result from the combination of maternal and paternal chromosomes that form the foetal DNA. Human cells contain 22 pairs of autosomes and one pair of sex chromosomes, totalling 46 chromosomes. This DNA carries the code that determines our characteristics, and complex interactions between multiple factors can lead to neurological and other disorders.

- **Genetic mutations** can disrupt development and lead to neurological damage. Phenylketonuria (PKU) is an example in which a child inherits a faulty gene from both parents.
- **Chromosomal disorders** have widespread effects because each chromosome contains around 20 000 genes. Down syndrome results from an extra copy of chromosome 21, while Turner syndrome is caused by the loss of one sex chromosome. Microdeletions or microduplications of gene segments can lead to conditions such as Cri-du-chat, 5p– and Prader–Willi syndromes.
- **Metabolic disorders** can also cause neurological harm and require early detection. In PKU, babies cannot metabolise phenylalanine found in food; elevated levels damage brain cells and impair intellectual development. Many countries now routinely screen newborns for PKU.

Acquired causes

These develop after birth and may be caused by trauma, infection, exposure to toxins, autoimmune disorders, epilepsy and neurological tumours.

Cerebral dysfunction

Cerebral dysfunction may be focal or global, affecting brain function and processing. Focal dysfunction arises from structural abnormalities such as tumours, local haemorrhage or congenital and acquired malformations. Global cerebral dysfunction involves the entire brain and can result from metabolic, hypoxic, toxic, infective, haemorrhagic or traumatic causes.

Pathophysiology of raised intracranial pressure (ICP)

The brain contains four interconnected ventricles filled with cerebrospinal fluid (CSF), which circulates through the ventricles and the subarachnoid space around the brain and spinal cord.

Raised ICP is a major consequence of cerebral dysfunction. It can result from any increase in intracranial volume, including tumour growth, oedema, inflammation (e.g., meningitis), developmental abnormalities, excess CSF (hydrocephalus) or bleeding.

CSF has four key functions: providing mechanical protection against impact with the skull; supporting the brain's weight to prevent lower-region ischaemia; maintaining chemical stability by buffering pH and ionic changes; and circulating oxygen, nutrients and metabolic waste products such as carbon dioxide.

Changes in ICP directly affect cerebral blood flow. When ICP rises, blood flow falls, reducing the delivery of oxygen and glucose and rapidly causing cerebral hypoxia. Reduced blood flow also impairs CO_2 removal, leading to acidosis and a drop in pH.

As autoregulation and chemoregulation fail, cerebral vessels dilate in an attempt to increase blood and oxygen supply. However, within the rigid skull, this increase in blood volume has no space to expand into, causing fluid to leak from cerebral vessels. The resulting oedema further raises ICP and worsens blood-flow compromise. Because brain tissue can tolerate only about 3 minutes without oxygen, this rapidly leads to cell death.

As ICP continues to rise, CSF drainage from the ventricles is obstructed, increasing pressure further. Persistent elevation compresses and damages brain tissue. Ultimately, raised ICP can cause herniation of brain structures through the foramen magnum – known as coning, which compresses the brainstem and is invariably fatal.

Early signs

- Decreasing level of consciousness
- Headache worsening with coughing or straining
- Sluggish pupillary response to bright light
- Visual disturbances, including blurred vision from papilledema
- Seizures or convulsions
- Abnormal breathing patterns
- Impaired motor or sensory responses
- Speech and swallowing difficulties
- Altered mood or challenging behaviour

Late signs (if ICP continues to rise)

- Decerebrate or decorticate posturing
- Bulging anterior fontanelle (infants)
- Head enlargement if cranial sutures are not fused (infants)
- Vomiting
- High temperature without infection
- Cushing's reflex (vasopressor response), presenting as Cushing's triad:
  - Raised systolic blood pressure with widened pulse pressure
  - Bradycardia
  - Irregular, slow or shallow respirations

Management depends on the underlying cause, with the primary goal of reducing ICP.

This can be achieved by:

- Reducing cerebral volume, e.g., treating tumours or inflammation
- Draining excess CSF
- Decreasing cerebral blood volume
- Lowering the brain's metabolic demand for oxygen and nutrients, using prescribed sedation, anti-emetics and pharmacological seizure control

Hydrocephalus

Hydrocephalus causes global cerebral dysfunction due to excess CSF in the brain and spinal cord. It may be congenital or acquired.

- Congenital hydrocephalus is present at birth and can result from conditions such as spina bifida, tumours, inflammation or maternal infections during pregnancy (e.g., mumps or rubella).
- Acquired hydrocephalus develops after birth, usually following injury, illness or the growth of a brain tumour.

In both types, increased CSF raises ICP. Persistent pressure compresses and damages brain tissue, producing clinical signs caused by the rising CSF volume and ICP, resulting in:

- head enlargement in babies and children with congenital hydrocephalus
- bulging anterior fontanelle (babies only)
- dilated scalp veins and separation of skull sutures (later sign)
- downward eye gaze (also known as the 'setting-sun' sign)
- convulsions
- other signs of raised ICP.

Hydrocephalus is a life-threatening emergency requiring prompt treatment. Early diagnosis is crucial in older children, whose fused skull bones leave little room for swelling, rapidly leading to raised ICP.

Treatment typically involves a ventriculoperitoneal (VP) shunt, a thin tube implanted in the brain ventricles. Excess CSF drains through the shunt to another part of the body, usually the peritoneal cavity, where it is absorbed into the bloodstream. The shunt contains a valve to regulate CSF flow and prevent over-drainage (Yates *et al.*, 2025).

Altered respiration, fluctuating or elevated blood pressure with widened pulse pressure and bradycardia indicate a raised ICP with potential brainstem involvement. This is a medical emergency requiring immediate intervention to prevent brainstem herniation and death (Advanced Life Support Group, 2023).

Cerebral trauma

Fractured skull

Skull fractures can be linear, depressed or open. Linear fractures show no signs of skull depression and are treated conservatively. Depressed skull fractures with a depression of more than 1 cm and open skull fractures may need surgical intervention and repair of the damaged structure. Evidence of a meningeal tear, CSF leakage, cranial nerve damage, seizure activity or a risk of infection makes this more likely.

Table 9.2 illustrates specific signs and symptoms that may be present in a child with a fractured skull.

Urgent assessment using the ABCDE approach and a full neurological evaluation is essential. This includes the Paediatric Early Warning System (PEWS), Alert, Voice, Pain, Unresponsive (AVPU) and an age-appropriate Glasgow Coma Scale (GCS) to determine the child's level of consciousness and awareness (Table 9.3).

TABLE 9.2 Vital signs and symptoms of a fractured skull

Symptoms can include:

- Bruising around the eyes ('panda' or 'raccoon eyes') from a basal skull fracture; meningeal rupture allows blood to pool in the peri-orbital area via cranial sinuses
- Bruising over the mastoid bone ('Battle's sign'), indicating posterior cranial fossa fracture; often appears 24 hours post-injury
- Blood in the ear canal
- Cerebrospinal fluid (CSF) leakage from the nose or ears, typically due to a basal skull fracture
- Palpable dent or spongy area, suggesting a depressed skull fracture (Tsang & Whitfield, 2024)

Other possible signs depending on injury location:

- Evidence of raised intracranial pressure (ICP)
- Visual disturbances from optic nerve compression or elevated ICP
- Facial muscle weakness, altered facial sensation or loss of smell due to cranial nerve injury
- Speech impairment
- Hearing loss from inner ear haemorrhage or ruptured eardrum
- Dizziness, vertigo and balance problems
- Impaired motor or sensory function and responses

Important consideration:

- Always consider a cervical spine injury in any head injury

Source: Tsang and Whitfield (2024) and NICE (2023).

Mechanism of injury: if the child has fallen from a height of greater than 1 m or greater height, alert but irritable and/or altered behaviour should be flagged as an immediate risk.

Emergency nursing care involves supporting airway and breathing, including assisting with intubation and ventilation if the respiratory centre is compromised. Immobilise the cervical spine if a fracture is suspected. Continuously monitor vital signs for signs of rising ICP, using the GCS and PEWS charts, and perform a full neurological assessment, including level of consciousness, cranial nerves, motor and sensory function and cerebellar function. Assess for other injuries or open wounds, including skull fractures, but only treat or suture if it will not delay further investigations or transfer.

Pain should be assessed using an age-appropriate tool, with analgesia administered and its effectiveness evaluated. Prescribed anti-emetics should be given to prevent vomiting, which can further raise ICP. Family-centred care is essential, with clear communication and liaison with the child, family and carers. Provide information on known injuries, investigations, treatments and expected outcomes. Prepare the child and family for safe transfer to definitive care, either within the hospital, such as intensive care, or to an external neurological unit in a tertiary centre (NICE, 2023).

TABLE 9.3 Investigations to assess the level of consciousness

1. The AVPU response scale can be used quickly to assess the level of consciousness. A score lower than V is a cause for concern and requires urgent medical referral
    - A patient awake
    - V patient responds to verbal stimulation
    - P patient responds to painful stimulation
    - U patient is completely unresponsive.
2. The Glasgow Coma Scale (GCS) is used to provide a practical method for the assessment of conscious level in response to defined stimuli. The GCS can be used without modification for children over 5 years old. Under 5 years old, it will be difficult for children to 'obey commands' or give a verbal response that indicates that they are 'orientated'. Thus, the Paediatric Glasgow Coma Scale (PGCS) may be more appropriate (Amended PGCS stimuli are shown herewith in brackets.)

GCS stimuli include:

- Eye opening
    - 4. Eyes opening spontaneously
    - 3. Eye opening to speech
    - 2. Eye opening to pressure
    - 1. No eye opening or response
- Verbal response
    - 5. Orientated (smiles, oriented to sounds, follows objects, interacts)
    - 4. Confused (cries but consolable, inappropriate interactions)
    - 3. Words (inconsistently inconsolable, moaning)
    - 2. Sounds (inconsolable, agitated)
    - 1. No verbal response
- Motor response
    - 6. Obeys commands (infant moves spontaneously or purposefully)
    - 5. Localises (infant withdraws from touch)
    - 4. Normal flexion (infant withdraws from pressure)
    - 3. Abnormal flexion to pain (decorticate response)
    - 2. Extension to pain (decerebrate response)
    - 1. No motor response

Each response has a value and these should be considered individually and as a combined score. A combined score of less than eight represents a significant risk of mortality. The GCS should be recorded regularly on a GCS chart. This will allow the nurse to observe trends that can indicate improvement or deterioration of the patient's condition.

Source: Adapted from Glasgow Coma Scale (2018).

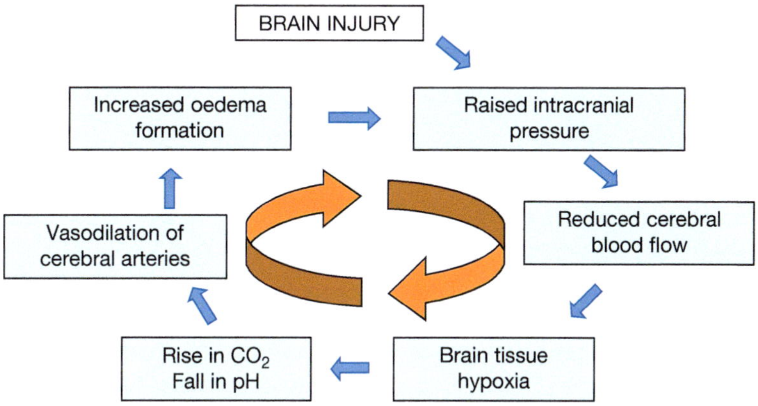

FIGURE 9.2 Focal and diffuse brain injury types.

Head injury

This occurs when trauma to the head results in damage to the brain. There are three main types of traumatic brain injury (TBI).

- Closed head injuries – where no damage is visible. Common in car accidents where the moving head suddenly stops or the child experiences a blow to the head.
- Open penetrating wounds – such as occur in conjunction with a fractured skull. Brain is exposed, may have been damaged by an object or a blow to the head.
- Crushing injuries – the head is crushed, brain damage occurs. Younger children are more at risk due to the pliability of their skulls.

Brain injuries may be classified as focal or diffuse (see Fig. 9.2). Focal injuries are localised to one area, whereas diffuse injuries occur throughout the brain and CNS.

The most common cause of severe head injury in infants under 12 months is non-accidental injury, often referred to as abusive head trauma or, in the media, 'shaken baby syndrome'. Safeguarding must always be considered whenever a child presents with a head injury (NICE, 2023).

Focal head injuries include contusions, lacerations and haemorrhage

Contusions occur when the brain strikes the hard inner skull, most commonly affecting the frontal and temporal lobes. The trauma can cause microscopic blood vessel leakage and, occasionally, meningeal tears, resulting in haemorrhage.

Lacerations are tears in brain tissue, often caused by a skull fracture or the entry of a foreign object, such as a bullet. They rupture larger blood vessels, leading to bleeding, haematoma formation, cerebral oedema and raised ICP.

Haemorrhage occurs when blood vessels are damaged, causing bleeding into the brain. Arterial blood is supplied via the internal carotid and vertebral arteries, while venous blood drains through the jugular veins and superior vena cava. The brain is highly sensitive to interruptions in blood flow, which rapidly deprives neural tissue of oxygen and glucose.

Haemorrhages are classified according to the space in which they occur (Fig. 9.3).

- Intracerebral haemorrhage occurs deep within the brain tissue.
- Subdural haemorrhage develops in the subdural space between the dura mater and arachnoid mater. It is commonly associated with abusive head trauma

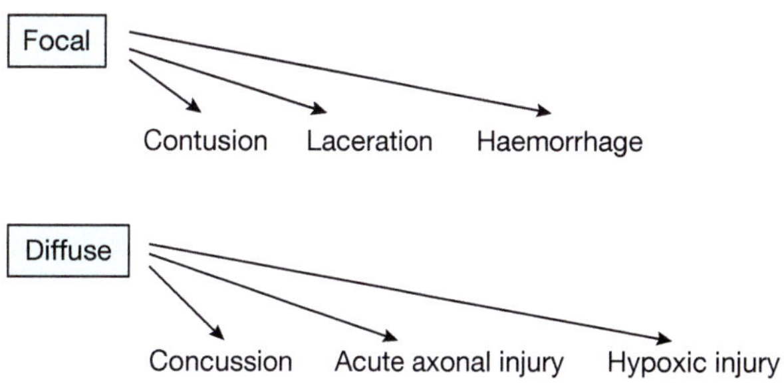

FIGURE 9.3 Anterior view of frontal section through the skull showing the cranial meninges.
Source: Tortora and Nielsen (2009)/John Wiley & Sons.

and is a major cause of serious head injury, although other symptoms must be considered for a full diagnosis (Zahl *et al.*, 2023).

- Subarachnoid haemorrhage occurs in the subarachnoid space between the arachnoid mater and pia mater. It may result from a tear in the pia mater, allowing blood to enter this space, or from the rupture of aneurysms or arteriovenous malformations, often located in the circle of Willis. The circle of Willis connects the cerebral arteries, enabling rapid redistribution of blood to dependent areas of the brain.

Diffuse head injuries include concussion, acute axonal injury and hypoxic injury.

Concussion is usually a mild, diffuse injury and the most common type of brain trauma. It may cause temporary loss of consciousness (minutes to hours), confusion, amnesia, visual disturbances, vestibular imbalance, headaches and nausea or vomiting.

Acute axonal injury typically results from high-speed acceleration or deceleration, causing diffuse haemorrhages throughout the brain and often leading to deep unconsciousness.

Hypoxic injury occurs due to oxygen deprivation, such as during cardiac arrest or near drowning. It may occur without direct head trauma but can worsen the effects of an existing brain injury.

Sudden loss of the Moro reflex, tonic neck reflex and withdrawal reflexes in young infants indicates a neurological emergency.

Spinal trauma

Spinal cord injury

The spinal cord extends from the medulla oblongata to the second lumbar vertebra and has three main functions: transmitting efferent motor signals to muscles, transmitting afferent sensory information to the brain (both via the white matter) and coordinating autonomic and somatic reflexes through the central grey matter.

The main causes of spinal cord injury are car accidents, falls and sports-related trauma. Benign or cancerous spinal tumours can also compress the cord and nerves, producing similar dysfunction.

Types of spinal injury vary in severity. Contusions and concussions may temporarily disrupt motor and sensory function, while compression must be relieved promptly to prevent ischaemia and permanent damage. Crush or penetrating injuries to the lower spine can cause cauda equina syndrome, a rare medical emergency resulting from compression of the nerve roots at the base of the spinal cord.

The following symptoms could be a sign of cauda equina syndrome, which needs urgent medical treatment to prevent permanent damage to the spinal cord.

S: Saddle anaesthesia – loss of feeling around the buttocks and genital area
P: Pain – severe nerve pain in the back or legs
I: Incontinence – bladder and bowel incontinence/retention/constipation
N: Numbness – weakness and loss of sensation in the legs
E: Emergency treatment needed (National Health Service England, 2025a, 2025b).

Full spinal cord transection results in complete paralysis and loss of sensation below the level of injury.

Spinal shock occurs immediately after injury, causing loss of reflexes, flaccid paralysis, loss of sensation and loss of bowel and bladder control below the lesion. Disruption of sympathetic nerve pathways also leads to hypotension, poor venous return, sweating and peripheral vasodilation. Impaired thermoregulation causes the child's body temperature to match the environment. Spinal shock typically lasts days to weeks; the return of reflexes, hyperreflexia and spasticity signals its resolution.

Motor dysfunction

Cerebral palsy

Cerebral palsy is a non-progressive disorder of movement, muscle tone and posture caused by injury or abnormal development of the immature brain during foetal development or the first year of life. Brain damage leads to corresponding motor dysfunction and may also cause epileptic seizures, learning difficulties, incontinence, dysarthria, scoliosis and visual or hearing impairments.

Causal factors include impaired embryonic implantation, genetic abnormalities, maternal infections, trauma, radiation, toxins, diabetes, toxaemia and nutritional deficiencies. Perinatal neurological injury is most commonly due to anoxia, trauma or infection, with low birth weight and birth asphyxia as notable risk factors. CNS trauma during birth and vascular issues such as infarction or haemorrhage may also contribute.

Cerebral palsy is classified by the affected brain region and resulting motor effects:

- **Spastic (pyramidal)** – 80% of cases; caused by corticospinal pathway damage, leading to hypertonia, stiff/weak muscles, abnormal tendon reflexes and primitive reflexes (NICE, 2024a).
- **Dyskinetic** – caused by basal ganglia or thalamic injury; muscle tone fluctuates between hypertonia and hypotonia, causing uncontrolled, jerky movements and impaired fine motor coordination.
- **Ataxic** – caused by cerebellar injury; presents with balance, gait and coordination problems, clumsy movements and involuntary tremors.
- **Mixed** – features of more than one type.

Management depends on age, type, severity and associated disorders. A multidisciplinary, patient-centred approach involving medical, social and educational support is recommended, respecting the wishes of the child and family (NICE, 2024a).

Developmental delays, such as not sitting by 8 months, not walking by 18 months or showing asymmetrical hand preference before 1 year, along with abnormal muscle tone (hypotonia, spasticity or dystonia), late head control, delayed rolling or crawling, abnormal fidgety movements or feeding difficulties, should be thoroughly investigated, as they may indicate cerebral palsy.

Spina bifida

Spina bifida is a neural tube defect resulting from incomplete closure of the posterior vertebral laminae during foetal development, causing incomplete fusion of the spine and surrounding membranes. While there is no single cause, folic acid deficiency in early pregnancy increases the risk. The incidence is lower in developed countries (0.4 per 1000) compared to developing countries (1.9 per 1000), with Ireland having the highest live birth rate in Europe (1:1000) (McKeating & Turner, 2017). The most common forms are meningocele and myelomeningocele.

Spina bifida meningocele

A meningocele occurs when the meninges herniate through a vertebral defect without involving the spinal cord or nerve roots. The cyst contains CSF but often causes no neurological deficit. It can appear anywhere along the spine, depending on the vertebral defect, sometimes presenting as a small lump on the baby's back at birth. Surgical correction is possible.

When a vertebral defect is present without herniation, it is called spina bifida occulta, the mildest form of posterior neural tube defect. It usually causes no neurological problems, and most individuals are unaware they have it.

Spina bifida myelomeningocele

A **myelomeningocele** occurs when the meninges, CSF, spinal cord and nerves herniate through the posterior vertebral arch. Most are in the lumbar or sacro-lumbar regions, the last part of the neural tube to close. A thin, often transparent membrane covers the defect, which may be intact or leak CSF, requiring urgent surgical repair at birth to prevent infection and further nerve damage. Most cases are detected prenatally via blood tests or ultrasound, and delivery is usually by Caesarean section to reduce trauma.

Myelomeningocele is one of the most common developmental nervous system abnormalities. It damages the spinal cord, causing loss of motor, sensory, reflex and autonomic function below the defect. Symptoms may include muscle weakness, paralysis, sensory loss and bowel or urinary incontinence. Severity depends on the defect's location and the presence of hydrocephalus.

Neurological tumours

Neurological tumours can occur anywhere in the nervous system, but are most common in the brain, spinal cord and sympathetic nervous system. Their cause is unknown.

Central nervous system tumours

Neurological tumours of the brain and spinal cord, part of the CNS, are the second most common childhood cancers, accounting for over a quarter (26%) of cases (Cancer Research UK, 2023a).

Brain tumours may be benign or malignant. Benign tumours remain in situ and do not spread, but can still

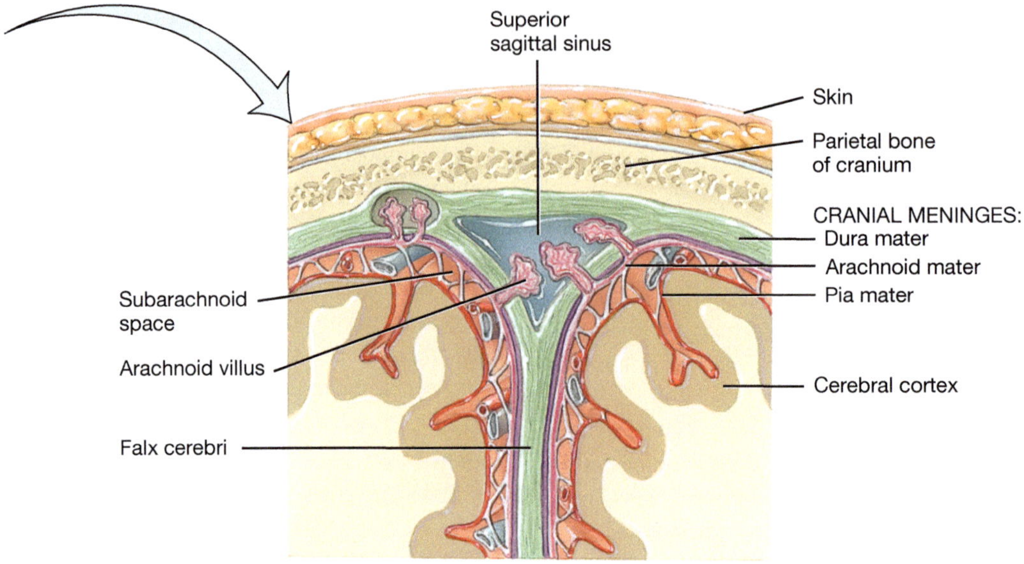

FIGURE 9.4 Raised intracranial pressure (ICP).

cause pressure and neurological damage similar to malignant tumours.

Intracranial tumours compress cerebral tissue as they grow, affecting the ventricular system, obstructing CSF flow and raising ICP. If untreated, elevated ICP can cause permanent brain damage or death (Fig. 9.4).

Malignant tumours are cancerous, invade surrounding tissue and carry a high risk, making early diagnosis essential. In children, the most common types are glial and embryonal, named according to the originating cell type.

Glial tumours or gliomas

Astrocytomas arise from supportive neuroglial cells in the nervous system, specifically astrocytes, which help form the blood–brain barrier by wrapping around neuronal synapses and capillaries, regulating endothelial permeability. Astrocytomas are the largest subgroup of childhood malignant brain tumours (WHO, 2021) and are classified as astrocytoma IDH mutant with three grades: grade 2 – diffuse, grade 3 – anaplastic and grade 4.

Treatment options include surgery, chemotherapy, radiotherapy and proton beam therapy (Cancer Research, 2022a, 2022b).

Embryonal tumours

These are the second most common malignant paediatric brain tumours (Cancer Research UK, 2023a), arising from immature nerve cells. Previously called primitive neuroectodermal tumours (PNETs), they are now classified as CNS embryonal tumours. They can occur anywhere in the CNS, though most are found in the posterior fossa (cerebellum) or supratentorial compartment (Ronsley *et al.*, 2024). The tumour types in this group include:

- medulloblastoma
- CNS neuroblastoma
- CNS ganglioneuroblastoma
- Embryonal tumour with multilayer rosettes

The most common and fast-growing CNS embryonal tumour is the medulloblastoma (Cancer Research UK, 2023b). It typically arises in the cerebellum and can spread to other brain regions or the spinal cord. Treatment and surgical removal can be challenging, depending on tumour location and growth rate.

Initial investigations include a detailed medical history, full examination and imaging with CT or MRI (see Table 9.4 for vital signs and symptoms of paediatric brain tumours). Treatment may involve surgery for diagnostic biopsy, tumour resection and reduction of ICP. Tumours located in the brainstem, thalamus or deep grey matter are usually inoperable. Adjunct therapies include chemotherapy, radiotherapy and dexamethasone to reduce cerebral oedema (Bailey *et al.*, 2025).

Postoperative nursing care involves initial support in the paediatric intensive care unit (PICU), followed by monitoring during recovery for neurological, endocrine and wound complications. Rehabilitation, parental education and a multidisciplinary approach are essential to support the child and family (NICE, 2017, 2025c).

TABLE 9.4 Vital signs and symptoms of paediatric brain tumours

Can be difficult to ascertain in young children who are unable to verbalise. Symptoms can mimic common childhood ailments and can include: • seizures • limb weakness • difficulty walking • speech impairments • swallowing difficulties • strange sensations • learning impairments • challenging behaviours • vision/hearing impairments	Signs and symptoms can be predicted by the location of the tumours. • ataxia – posterior fossa • visual disturbances – optic nerve of posterior fossa • seizures – temporal lobe • behavioural changes – frontal lobe • hormone imbalance – pituitary gland

TABLE 9.5 Staging of neuroblastoma

Stage 1 (INRGSS L1)	Tumour is localised and can be completely removed by surgery
Stage 2a (INRGSS L2)	Tumour is localised and cannot be completely removed by surgery
Stage 2b	Tumour is localised but has spread to lymph nodes
Stage 3 (INRGSS L2)	Tumour crosses the midline, may or may not have lymph node involvement and cannot be surgically removed
Stage 4 (INRGSS M)	Tumour has spread to distant lymph nodes, bone marrow, liver, bones and possibly other organs. Likely to need intensive treatment
Stage 4s (INRGSS MS)	Tumour is localised (Stage 1, 2a or 2b) with spread to the liver, skin and/or bone marrow in a child under 1 year of age.

Source: Royal Marsden 2025 / NHS / www.cancerresearchuk.org/about-cancer/childrens-cancer/neuroblastoma/risk-groups-staging / last accessed Oct. 15, 2025.

Sympathetic nervous system tumours

These can be malignant or benign, akin to tumours found in the brain and CNS. Neuroblastoma is a common malignant tumour, and neurofibromatosis type 1 (NF1) is classed as a benign tumour.

Neuroblastoma

Nearly all the malignant tumours of the sympathetic nervous system are neuroblastoma, accounting for 8–10% of all childhood cancers and contributing to 15% approximately of childhood cancer-related deaths. Neuroblastoma is a cancer of the neural crest cells in the sympathetic nervous system, and it is the most frequently occurring cancer in children under the age of one. Globally, the incidence of neuroblastoma has been found to be lower in much of South East Asia and the United States, the prevalence of neuroblastoma is lower in black children (8.5% per million) than in white children (11.5% per million) (Nong *et al.*, 2025).

Forty-six percent of neuroblastomas develop in the adrenal gland, 26% in other abdominal sites and 13% in thoracic sites (Cancer Research UK, 2025a). Hence, initial symptoms can vary depending on the site of the primary tumour. The most common sign is an abdominal mass, which can cause pain, lack of appetite, weight loss and constipation. A tumour in the neck or chest can cause difficulties swallowing and breathing if it becomes enlarged. Difficulty walking and passing urine may be signs of a tumour pressing on the peripheral spinal nerves. Bone metastasis can cause joint and bone pain and bone marrow abnormalities such as anaemia, bleeding, pallor and blood cell production.

The staging system commonly used (Table 9.5) will determine the most appropriate treatment. The International Neuroblastoma Risk Group Staging System (INRGSS) may also be utilised to determine the stage of the tumour.

Neuroblastoma investigations include X-ray, ultrasound, CT, MRI, bone marrow aspirate and trephine and metaiodobenzylguanidine (MIBG) bone scan to determine tumour location and spread. Neuroblastoma cells excrete vanillylmandelic acid (VMA) and homovanillic acid (HVA), detectable in urine, with 90% of affected children showing elevated VMA levels (Royal Marsden, 2025).

Treatment depends on tumour location and stage. Localised tumours are managed with surgery alone, while high-risk or aggressive neuroblastoma requires multi-agent chemotherapy, primary tumour resection and autologous stem cell transplant. Radiotherapy may be used following surgery or high-dose chemotherapy. The 5-year survival rate ranges from 50% to 90% (NICE, CKS, 2025a).

Neurofibromatosis type 1 (NF1)

NF1 is the most common benign nervous system tumour disorder, caused by a spontaneous mutation or autosomal dominant inheritance of the NF1 gene on chromosome 17q11.2 (Kehrer-Sawatzki & Cooper, 2022). It affects

1 in 3000 live births in the United Kingdom, with around 25 000 people diagnosed. Children with NF1 have an increased risk of malignant tumours: 5% develop brain tumours, 10% a malignant peripheral nerve sheath tumour and 15% an optic pathway glioma (Peduto *et al.*, 2023).

Clinical features include café-au-lait spots and freckles in the armpits, groin or under the breast, which may be less visible in darker skin. Neurofibromas, benign tumours on nerve sheaths, vary in size and number. Cognitive and behavioural effects are common: 60% of children have mild learning difficulties, and 50% have attention-deficit/hyperactivity disorder (ADHD). Physical complications include scoliosis, macrocephaly, epilepsy, renal disorders, depression, anxiety and vision problems from optic pathway gliomas (NHS, 2025).

Management focuses on regular monitoring and a multidisciplinary approach. Assessments should include skin checks for new or changing neurofibromas, blood pressure, vision, bone health and monitoring school progress to identify learning or developmental issues.

Intercranial infection

The most commonly seen infection includes meningitis, which is an infection of the meninges lining the brain and cranium. Encephalitis is an infection of the brain that causes acute and rapid swelling.

Meningitis

The meninges are three protective layers surrounding the brain, continuous with the spinal cord meninges (Fig. 9.3). They are the dura mater, arachnoid mater and pia mater, with CSF circulating in the subarachnoid space between the arachnoid mater and pia mater.

Meningitis is an acute inflammation of the pia mater and arachnoid mater and spinal cord, most commonly caused by bacterial or viral infection, with fungal meningitis being rare. Bacterial meningitis is life-threatening. Diagnosis in infants and young children is challenging, which is significant as the peak incidence occurs in children under 5 years. A second peak occurs in 15–19-year-olds, a pattern unique to meningitis among infectious diseases (Oxford Vaccine Group, 2025).

> Bacterial meningitis is a life-threatening condition and, if suspected, immediate treatment is required.

The main bacterial causes of meningitis are meningococcal infection (*Neisseria meningitidis*, gram-negative) and pneumococcal infection (*Streptococcus pneumoniae*, gram-positive). Group B streptococcus (GBS) is the leading cause of infection in neonates. Bacterial meningitis can lead to brain damage, hearing loss or learning disability in 10–20% of survivors (NICE, 2024b).

Viral meningitis is caused by viruses such as mumps, enteroviruses and Epstein–Barr virus. It is less life-threatening and does not require antibiotics. Nursing care focuses on symptom relief, such as managing headache, vomiting and photophobia, as most children recover within 7–14 days.

Assessment and diagnosis: Risk stratification for suspected sepsis should be applied. Definitive diagnosis relies on a lumbar puncture (LP) to detect bacteria in CSF, performed once the child is stabilised. Blood cultures identify the causative organism, and a throat swab may be taken specifically for meningococcal culture.

Treatment

- **Bacterial meningitis:** IV antibiotics are usually started empirically before confirmation; if viral infection is confirmed, antibiotics are stopped. In meningococcal cases, prophylactic antibiotics are given to close contacts.
- **Viral meningitis:** Supportive care only.

Critically ill children require PICU care for airway, breathing and circulation (ABC) support. Conscious children need close monitoring of neurological and cardiovascular functions, including vigilance for deteriorating consciousness, increased ICP or shock. GCS and PEWS scoring aid ongoing assessment (see Table 9.6). Nursing management also includes maintaining fluid balance, a quiet environment, reduced stimulation and effective communication and support for parents.

> An unwell child who develops a purpuric, non-blanching petechial rash may have overwhelming meningococcal disease and sepsis. This constitutes a medical emergency (NICE, 2024c).

Meningococcal disease

Meningococcal disease encompasses meningococcal meningitis and meningococcal septicaemia, which may occur individually or together, causing a life-threatening

TABLE 9.6 Vital signs and symptoms of meningitis and meningococcal disease

Meningitis	Meningococcal disease/septicaemia
Early symptoms are non-specific and may include: • fever • vomiting • irritability • drowsiness In infants under 18 months • a tense or bulging anterior fontanelle is a sign of raised ICP • a distinctive high-pitched or moaning cry may be present In older children • headache • neck stiffness • photophobia At any age • seizures • positive Kernig's sign (inability to extend the knee when the leg is flexed at the hip when lying down) • positive Brudzinski's sign (severe neck stiffness causes a patient's hips and knees to flex when the neck is flexed) • confusion • sleepy and difficult to wake	Early symptoms are non-specific, but the child becomes rapidly unwell. • A rash will be present in more than 50% of cases. This can be: – sparse or profuse – tiny petechial spots to large non-blanching purpuric lesions – pale or mottled skin. • fever • cold hands and feet • shivering • high respiratory rate • cardiovascular instability • neurological instability: – raised ICP – altered GCS • GI symptoms, including abdominal pain, vomiting and diarrhoea • myalgia (muscle pain) in the legs • joint pain • weakness • restlessness • confusion • sleepy and difficult to wake

systemic infection. It carries a high mortality rate: approximately 1 in 20 cases result in death, and 1 in 5 survivors experience permanent effects such as limb amputation, skin scarring, hearing loss or brain damage. Disease incidence peaks in children under 5 years and young people aged 15–19 years. Early diagnosis and aggressive treatment are essential for improving outcomes.

Neisseria meningitidis is capable of causing large epidemics. Of the 13 identified serogroups, six (A, B, C, W, X and Y) can trigger epidemics (WHO, 2025), with B, C, W and Y being most common in the United Kingdom (Oxford Vaccine Group, 2025).

Since the introduction of the MenC vaccine in 1999, there has been a significant fall in the number of cases of type C meningococcal disease. Hence, childhood vaccinations should be promoted to maintain healthy lives.

Nursing management of meningococcal disease and bacterial meningitis focuses on stabilising the child and monitoring for early complications. Key actions may include:

- ABC assessment, recording on a PEWS chart and following the NICE (2024b) algorithm for early management. Initiate resuscitation if needed. Monitor cardiovascular function, including blood pressure, ECG, capillary refill and core temperature. Restore circulatory volume with fluids and, if necessary, inotropes.
- Neurological assessment using GCS to detect early signs of raised ICP (Table 9.3).
- **Laboratory support:** Assist with rapid collection of blood samples (FBC, U&Es, blood cultures, clotting screen, blood glucose and meningococcal serology). Prepare the child for an LP and ensure prompt CSF analysis, taking a blood glucose sample close to the LP for comparison.
- **Medication administration:** Give antibiotics, analgesia and anti-emetics as prescribed, monitoring efficacy. Antibiotics should ideally be administered

within 1 hour of hospital arrival, with diagnostic tests performed beforehand where possible.
- **Parental support:** Provide psychological support, facilitate clear communication and keep parents informed about progress and procedures to reduce anxiety.

A capillary refill time of 3 seconds or more should be considered abnormal in children (APLG, 2023).

Encephalitis

Encephalitis is acute brain inflammation; when combined with meningitis, it is called meningoencephalitis. Young children are at higher risk due to an immature immune system.

Infective encephalitis is usually viral (e.g., rabies, polio and measles) but can also be bacterial (e.g., syphilis, toxoplasmosis, Lyme disease and malaria). Chronic encephalitis may develop slowly from conditions such as HIV, and autoimmune encephalitis can be initially difficult to diagnose, causing abnormal movements and seizures.

Symptoms in young children are often non-specific, resembling meningitis. Diagnosis involves CT/MRI, LP and electroencephalogram (EEG). Treatment depends on the cause and may include antibiotics, antivirals or steroids. Most children require PICU admission, close monitoring and intensive care.

Long-term neurological consequences can include memory problems, behavioural changes, speech impairments and epilepsy.

Seizure disorders

Pathophysiology of a seizure

Seizures are transient events caused by abnormal, excessive or synchronous brain activity. A seizure does not necessarily indicate epilepsy. They are broadly classified as focal (localised to one hemisphere) or generalised (involving both hemispheres). Abnormal electrical discharges in sensory, motor or autonomic regions can produce various seizure types, with levels of consciousness described as aware, impaired or unknown.

The International League Against Epilepsy (ILAE, 2017) has introduced a new operational classification to provide clinicians with greater flexibility in naming seizure types.

Epilepsy

Epilepsy is the term used to describe a group of neurological conditions of the brain characterised by an enduring predisposition to generate epileptic seizures. The ILAE (Fisher *et al.*, 2017) task force proposed that epilepsy is considered a disease of the brain, defined by any of the following conditions:

- At least two unprovoked (or reflex) seizures occurring >24 hours apart.
- One unprovoked (or reflex) seizure and a probability of further seizures similar to the general recurrence risk (at least 60%) after two unprovoked seizures, occurring over the next 10 years.
- Diagnosis of an epilepsy syndrome.

Epilepsy is considered resolved for individuals who had an age-dependent epilepsy syndrome but are now past the applicable age. This also includes those who have remained seizure-free for the last 10 years, with no anti-seizure medicines for the last 5 years. International consensus via a task force has sought to classify seizures into groupings (Fig. 9.5) for the purpose of communication in clinical care, teaching and research.

Diagnostic tests for seizures include CT and MRI to detect scarring, tumours or brain damage that may cause epilepsy. An EEG records current brain electrical activity and can help localise seizure onset, but it cannot detect past or future seizures and should not be used alone for diagnosis. An ambulatory EEG may be required for extended monitoring. A 12-lead ECG helps identify arrhythmias or cardiac conditions that can cause altered

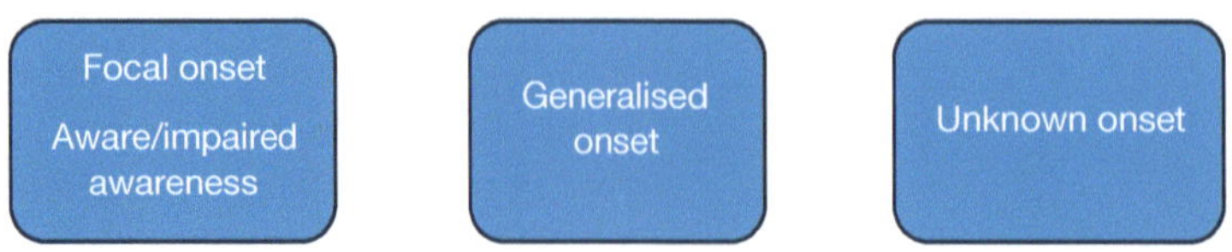

FIGURE 9.5 Basic operational classification of seizure type.
Source: Adapted from ILAE (2017).

consciousness. Baseline blood tests are necessary at new-onset seizure diagnosis and before starting anti-seizure medication.

Immediate first aid for seizures: Ensure the child's safety without restraining or moving them unless in danger. Cushion the head and do not put anything in the mouth. Time the seizure and stay until full recovery. Do not attempt to wake the child or give fluids during the seizure. Once it ends, place the child in the recovery position. Remain calm and reassuring, and check for an epilepsy identity card, jewellery or individual healthcare plan (Epilepsy Action, 2025).

Emergency help should be called if:

- the seizure lasts for more than 5 minutes
- one tonic–clonic seizure follows another one without the child regaining consciousness
- it is the child's first seizure
- an injury has occurred during the seizure (Epilepsy Action, 2025).

Management of status epilepticus

Immediate treatment is essential to prevent prolonged seizures. In the community, call an emergency ambulance. In the hospital, seek urgent assistance, secure the airway, provide oxygen, assess cardiac and respiratory function and check blood glucose. Establish intravenous access and follow the age-appropriate status epilepticus algorithm (NICE, 2025b).

Initial treatment usually includes anti-convulsant medication, oxygen and, if necessary, anaesthesia for intubation and ventilation. Provide support for the family throughout.

Ongoing management focuses on controlling seizures to prevent recurrence. Monotherapy is preferred if possible (NICE, 2025b). Some anti-seizure medications require regular blood tests to monitor liver function; this should be explained to both children and parents.

Children taking anti-epileptic medication should be advised to take extra precautions in summer as some anti-epileptic medication may make them more photosensitive, increasing their risk of sunburn and long-term skin damage.

Children experiencing seizures are more at risk of accidents and seizures may put them at an academic and social disadvantage. Risk assessment of activities of daily living should be considered as epilepsy is associated with an increased risk of premature death, including a risk of sudden unexpected death in epilepsy (SUDEP). Children and young people will need to be supported to understand this and agree on ways of mitigating risks.

Stevens–Johnson syndrome (SJS) is a rare but serious side effect of some anti-epileptic medications, such as lamotrigine and sodium valproate. It may begin with flu-like symptoms followed by a rapidly spreading rash on the upper body, face, arms and legs. The rash is usually not itchy. Blisters can develop on the lips, oral cavity, urethra and conjunctiva. Urgent medical attention is required if SJS is suspected.

Case study 9.1

Alice is a 16-and-a-half-year-old female who has been newly diagnosed with focal seizures. She had one seizure when she was 14 years old and then a second when she was 16 years old. Her first seizure was reported as being generalised, loss of consciousness and no incontinence. She sustained a head injury as she fell to the pavement. She was taken to the emergency department and discharged with no further follow-up. Her second seizure were seizures of short duration; there was no loss of consciousness, but there was limb involvement, right arm twitching and in a clenched position and twitching of her face and eye. She has occasional 'vague' episodes also. She was referred to a neurologist by her GP. From an MRI scan, it is evident that there is a gliosis on the left side of her brain. Alice is commenced on Lamotrigine. She is keen to start driving as soon as she turns 17 years old. She loves sports and likes to relax by taking a bath after a day of studying. She has a part-time job as a swimming teacher's assistant. She has a boyfriend and likes to have an occasional drink. Alice is planning to go to University. She very much wants to be treated as not different from her friends.

What advice would you give to Alice if you were the Clinical Nurse Specialist for Epilepsy?

Febrile convulsion

Febrile convulsions are seizures associated with a high temperature **without CNS infection** and are distinct from epilepsy. Their pathophysiology is not fully understood, but a **genetic predisposition** is suggested. They occur in children **6 months to 5 years**, affecting about **1 in 50** by age 5. Most children **outgrow** this condition.

Febrile convulsions usually occur when a child's temperature rises above 39 °C, most commonly due to viral infections, ear, throat, gastrointestinal infections or post-immunisation reactions. They resemble tonic–clonic seizures, with loss of consciousness, jerking limb movements and sometimes loss of continence. These seizures are brief (<5 minutes) in simple cases and do not cause lasting brain damage.

First aid and emergency guidance are the same as for epileptic seizures (Epilepsy Action, 2025). Hospital admission is generally unnecessary after a first febrile seizure unless it lasts >15 minutes, recurs within 24 hours or shows focal features, indicating a complex febrile seizure. The postictal period of drowsiness, irritability or confusion usually lasts up to 60 minutes, with full recovery thereafter.

Even short, simple febrile seizures require assessment of the cause and the risk of serious illness to exclude CNS infections such as meningitis, meningococcal disease or encephalitis (CKS, 2024). Complex febrile seizures – lasting >15 minutes or involving features such as one-sided weakness – carry a higher risk of developing epilepsy.

Antipyretics (paracetamol or ibuprofen) may reduce fever but do not prevent recurrence (CKS, 2023). Dehydration should also be avoided. Immunisation-related febrile seizures rarely recur, so parents should continue routine vaccinations (CKS, 2024).

Children with recurrent febrile seizures may have a treatment plan for benzodiazepine rescue medication.

Conclusion

Although most of the nervous system is formed at birth, rapid development continues throughout childhood. The brain grows, cognitive abilities develop and neural pathways are stabilised. Myelination of neurones allows for refined motor control. Trauma or disease can disrupt this developmental trajectory, but the plasticity of the nervous system enables compensation by creating new neural pathways to re-learn or re-pattern damaged areas.

References

Advanced Life Support Group (2023). *Advanced Paediatric Life Support: A Practical Approach to Emergencies*, 7th edn. Wiley Publishing West Essex.

Bailey, S., Jacobs, S., Kourti, M., *et al.* (2025). Medulloblastoma therapy: Consensus treatment recommendations from SIOP-Europe and the European Reference Network. *EJC Paediatric Oncology* 5, 100205.

Cancer Research UK (2022a). Decisions about treatment for children's brain tumours. Available at: https://www.cancerresearchuk.org/about-cancer/childrens-cancer/brain-tumours/treatment/decisions-about-treatment (accessed 1 August 2025).

Cancer Research UK (2022b). Children's cancers-brain tumours. Available at: https://www.cancerresearchuk.org/about-cancer/childrens-cancer/brain-tumours/about (accessed 1 August 2025).

Cancer Research UK (2023a). Children's cancer. Available at: https://www.cancerresearchuk.org/about-cancer/childrens-cancer (accessed 1 August 2025).

Cancer Research UK (2023b). Medulloblastoma. Available at: https://www.cancerresearchuk.org/about-cancer/childrens-cancer/brain-tumours/types/medulloblastoma (accessed 1 August 2025).

Cancer Research UK (2025a). Neuroblastoma. Available at: https://www.cancerresearchuk.org/about-cancer/childrens-cancer/neuroblastoma (accessed 1 August 2025).

Clinical Knowledge Summaries (CKS) (2023). Feverish children – risk assessment and management. Available at: https://cks.nice.org.uk/topics/feverish-children-risk-assessment-management/ (accessed 31 July 2025).

Clinical Knowledge Summaries (CKS) (2024). Febrile seizures. Available at: https://cks.nice.org.uk/topics/febrile-seizure/ (accessed 31 July 2025).

Epilepsy Action (2025). First Aid for seizures. Available at: https://www.epilepsy.org.uk/info/firstaid (accessed 1 August 2025).

Fisher, R.S., Cross, J.H., & French, J.A. (2017). Operational classification of seizure types by the International League Against Epilepsy: Position Paper of the ILAE Commission for Classification and Terminology. *Epilepsia* 58(4), 522–530.

Glasgow Coma Scale (2018). The Glasgow structured approach to assessment of the Glasgow Coma Scale. Available at: http://www.glasgowcomascale.org (accessed 31 July 2025).

International League Against Epilepsy (ILAE) (2017). Operational classification of seizure types. Available at: www.ilae.org/guidelines/definition-and-classification/operational-classification-2017 (accessed 31 July 2025).

Kehrer-Sawatzki, H., & Cooper, D.N. (2022). Challenges in the diagnosis of neurofibromatosis type 1 (NF1) in young children facilitated by means of revised diagnostic criteria including genetic testing for pathogenic *NF1* gene variants. *Human Genetics* **141**, 177–191.

McKeating, A., & Turner, M.J. (2017). The prevention of neural tube defects in Ireland. *Irish Medical Journal* 110(6) Editorial.

National Health Service England (NHSE) (2025a). Neurofibromatosis type 1 (NF1) https://www.nhs.uk/conditions/neurofibromatosis-type-1/ (accessed 31 July 2025).

National Health Service England (NHSE) (2025b). Spinal Surgery: National Suspected Cauda Equina Syndrome (CES) Pathway. Getting it Right First Time. https://gettingitrightfirsttime.co.uk/wp-content/uploads/2025/03/National-Suspected-Cauda-Equina-Pathway-February-2025.pdf (accessed 31 July 2025).

National Institute for Health and Care Excellence (NICE) (updated 2017). Improving outcomes for people with brain and other central nervous system tumours. Cancer service guideline [CSG10]. Available at: https://www.nice.org.uk/guidance/csg10 (accessed 1 August 2025).

National Institute for Health and Care Excellence (NICE) (2023). Head injury: assessment and early management NG232 Available at: https://www.nice.org.uk/guidance/ng232 (accessed 1 August 2025).

National Institute for Health and Care Excellence (NICE) (2024a). Cerebral palsy in under 25s: assessment and management. NG62. Available at: https://www.nice.org.uk/guidance/ng62/resources/cerebral-palsy-in-under-25s-assessment-and-management-pdf-1837570402501 (accessed 2 August 2025).

National Institute for Health and Care Excellence (NICE) (2024b). Meningitis (bacterial) and meningococcal disease: recognition, diagnosis and management Available at: https://cks.nice.org.uk/topics/meningitis-bacterial-meningitis-meningococcal-disease/ (accessed 31 July 2025).

National Institute for Health and Care Excellence (NICE) (2024c). Sepsis: recognition, diagnosis and early management. Available at: https://cks.nice.org.uk/topics/sepsis/ (accessed 31 July 2025).

National Institute for Health and Care Excellence (NICE) (2025b). Epilepsies in children, young people and adults. NG217. Available at https://www.nice.org.uk/guidance/ng217 (accessed 1 August 2025).

National Institute for Health and Care Excellence (NICE) (2025c). Childhood cancers-recognition and referral. Available at: https://cks.nice.org.uk/topics/childhood-cancers-recognition-referral/ (accessed 31 July 2025).

National Institute for Health and Care Excellence (NICE) Clinical Knowledge Summary (2025a) Childhood cancers – recognition and referral NICE https://cks.nice.org.uk/topics/childhood-cancers-recognition-referral/ (accessed 1 August 2025).

Nong, J, Cheng, S., Changhua, C. et al. (2025) Global, regional, and national epidemiology of childhood neuroblastoma (1990–2021): a statistical analysis of incidence, mortality, and DALYs. Vol. 79. eClinical Medicine, The Lancet.

Oxford Vaccine Group (2025). Meningococcal disease. Available at: https://vaccineknowledge.ox.ac.uk/meningococcal-disease (accessed 1 August 2025).

Peduto, C., Zanobio, M., Nigro, V., *et al.* (2023). Neurofibromatosis Type 1: Pediatric aspects and review of genotype–phenotype correlations. *Cancers 15*, 1217.

Ronsley, R., Cole, B., Ketterl, T., *et al.* (2024). Pediatric central nervous system embryonal tumors: presentation, diagnosis, therapeutic strategies, and survivorship – a review. *Pediatric Neurology* 161, 237–246.

Royal Marsden NHS Foundation Trust (2025). Neuroblastoma. Available at: https://www.royalmarsden.nhs.uk/your-care/cancer-types/paediatric-cancers/neuroblastoma (accessed 31 July 2025).

Tortora, G.J., & Neilsen, M.T. (2009). *Principles of Human Anatomy*, 11th edn. Wiley, Chichester.

Tsang, K. Whitfield, P (2024) Skull fractures-Symptoms, diagnosis and treatment. British Medical Journal. Best practice. Available at: https://bestpractice.bmj.com/topics/en-gb/398 (accessed 1 August 2025).

World Health Organisation (WHO) (2021). WHO Classification of Tumours. Available at: https://tumourclassification.iarc.who.int/welcome/ (Accessed 1 August 2025).

World Health Organization (WHO) (2025). WHO guidelines on meningitis diagnosis, treatment and care. Available at: https://www.who.int/publications/i/item/9789240108042 (accessed 1 August 2025).

Yates, C.F., Colditz, M.J., Maclachlan, L., *et al.* (2025). Paediatric ventriculoperitoneal shunt obstruction and cerebrospinal fluid protein. *Journal of Clinical Neuroscience* 137, 111341.

Zahl, S.M., Andersson, J., Wester, K., & Wikström, J. (2023). Neuroradiological findings in children with subdural hematoma and suspected abusive head trauma. *Annals of the Child Neurology Society* 1, 44–52.

CHAPTER 10

Blood disorders

Sarah Brazel-Terris

AIM

The aim of this chapter is to provide the readers with the material to develop their understanding of the applied pathophysiology of a variety of blood disorders.

LEARNING OUTCOMES

On completion of this chapter, the reader will be able to:

- Recognise a range of blood disorders.
- Discuss the normal physiology and consider the abnormal physiology occurring in common blood disorders.
- List common signs and symptoms associated with blood disorders.
- Outline the care of children and young people who have blood disorders.

KEYWORDS

- blood
- blood disorders
- lifelong effects
- red blood cell
- white blood cells
- platelets
- haematology
- bone marrow aspirate

Test your prior knowledge

1. What are the three main classes of blood cells?
2. What are the functions of the three main classes of blood cells?
3. How many types of white blood cells are there, can you name them?
4. What are the main functions of blood?
5. What is the process of haematopoiesis?

Introduction

Blood, often called the 'river of life', circulates through the body to nourish tissues, transport oxygen and defend against disease. It is composed of red blood cells (RBCs), white blood cells (WBCs), platelets and plasma, each with a unique role in maintaining health. This chapter explores the components of blood and their functions, and how disruptions can lead to blood disorders. Understanding these conditions helps recognise symptoms, guide treatment and appreciate the complexity of blood function. A basic knowledge of haematopoiesis and the haematological system is essential, as understanding 'normal' is key to recognising the effects of the 'abnormal'.

Recap of the functions of blood

Blood is a specialised body fluid pumped by the heart, with three main roles: transportation, regulation and protection against infection. It consists of RBCs, WBCs, platelets and plasma (see Fig. 10.1).

- RBCs transport oxygen from the lungs to tissues and carry waste products, such as carbon dioxide, back to the lungs.
- WBCs protect the body against infection and disease.
- Platelets aid in blood clotting, preventing blood loss and opportunistic infection.
- Plasma, the liquid portion, supports transportation and regulation, allowing the cellular components to circulate efficiently.

Each blood component can be assessed using a full blood count (FBC). Laboratory analysis allows each component to be measured and compared with age- and sex-specific normal ranges (see Table 10.1).

Haemopoiesis is the process by which blood cells are produced. After birth, it occurs primarily in the bone marrow, gradually becoming limited to certain bones, such as the pelvis.

Bone marrow is a soft, fatty myeloid tissue within bones, composed of fat and blood-forming cells. All blood cells originate from multipotent (pluripotent) stem cells (Jones, 2020). These divide into haemocytoblasts, which further differentiate into myeloid or lymphoid stem cells (see Fig. 10.2).

- Myeloid stem cells give rise to:
  - Erythrocytes (RBCs) from proerythroblasts
  - Eosinophils, neutrophils and basophils from myeloblasts
  - Monocytes/macrophages from monoblasts
  - Platelets (thrombocytes) from megakaryoblasts
- Lymphoid stem cells develop into lymphoblasts, which mature into lymphocytes and plasma cells.

When interpreting blood results, it is important to use accurate, universally recognised terminology. Table 10.2 lists commonly used clinical terms and their definitions.

Special considerations

Duffy-null associated neutropenia, commonly known as benign ethnic neutropenia (BEN), is a condition in which individuals, particularly of African, Middle Eastern and West Indian descent, have a lower-than-average neutrophil count. 'Duffy-null' refers to the absence of the Duffy antigen. The condition is linked to a variation in the Duffy Antigen Receptor for Chemokines (DARC), present in around 80% of people of African descent versus less than 1% of Asian or Caucasian descent (Merz *et al.*, 2023).

Importantly, this lower neutrophil count does not increase infection risk. Misinterpretation of results can lead to unnecessary invasive investigations, while assuming BEN in other populations may delay the diagnosis of serious conditions.

Many advocate renaming BEN to 'Duffy-null Associated Neutrophil Count' to avoid historical inequities (Merz *et al.*, 2023). Both terms are used in this textbook to reflect current usage and raise awareness of systemic inequalities in healthcare.

Classification of blood disorders

Blood disorders affect the various components of blood, RBCs, WBCs, platelets and plasma. Understanding these conditions is essential for high-quality patient care, early recognition of symptoms and timely interventions. Blood disorders can broadly be classified into the following categories:

Red blood cell disorders: Conditions affecting the oxygen-carrying capacity of blood, such as myriad anaemias and sickle cell disease (SCD).

White blood cell disorders: Conditions resulting in over-, under- or abnormal production of white cells, such as leukaemia and immune deficiencies.

Platelet disorders: Conditions impacting platelet count or function, such as medication-induced thrombocytopenia and thrombotic thrombocytopenic purpura (TTP).

Plasma and clotting disorders: Conditions affecting proteins and clotting factors in plasma, such as haemophilia and Von Willebrand Disease (VWD).

Red blood cell disorders

There are approximately 4–5.5 million RBCs per cubic millimetre of blood (Marieb & Hoehn, 2022). Abnormalities in the shape, function or production of RBCs can adversely

Blood is a connective tissue that consists of blood plasma (liquid) plus formed elements (red blood cells, white blood cells and platelets).

Functions of Blood

1. Transports oxygen, carbon dioxide, nutrients, hormones, heat and wastes.
2. Regulates pH, body temperature and water content of cells.
3. Protects against blood loss through clotting and against disease through phagocytic white blood cells and proteins such as antibodies, interferons and complement.

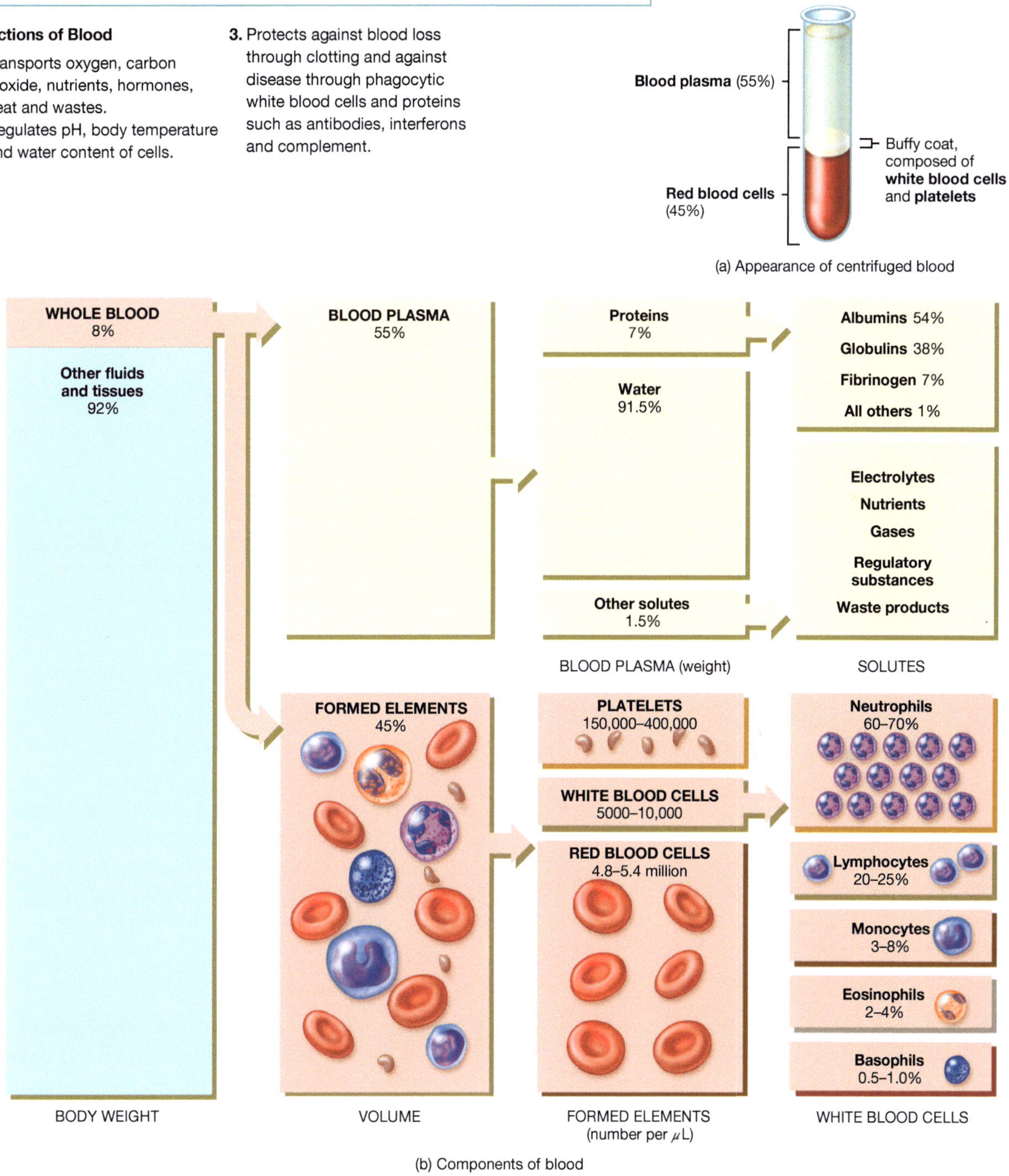

FIGURE 10.1 Components of blood Image.
Source: Tortora and Derrickson (2017) / with permission of John Wiley & Sons.

TABLE 10.1 Normal values

Age	Hb (g/L)	RBC ($\times 10^{12}$/L)	HCT (L/L)	Platelets ($\times 10^9$/L)	WBC ($\times 10^9$/L)	Neutrophils ($\times 10^9$/L)
Birth	149–237	3.7–6.5	0.47–0.75	150–400 at all ages	10.0–26.0	2.7–14.4
2 weeks	134–198	3.9–5.9	0.41–0.65		6.0–21.0	1.8–5.4
4 weeks	94–130	3.1–4.3	0.28–0.42		6.0–18.0	1.2–7.5
2–6 months	114–141	3.9–5.5	0.31–0.41		6.0–17.5	1.0–8.5
6 months to 1 year	115–135	4.1–5.3	0.33–0.41		6.0–17.5	1.5–8.5
1–6 years	115–135	3.9–5.3	0.34–0.40		5.0–17.0	1.5–8.5
6–12 years	115–155	4.0–5.2	0.35–0.45		4.5–14.5	1.5–8.0
12–18 years (female)	120–150	4.1–5.1	0.36–0.46		4.5–13.0	1.8–8.0
12–18 years (male)	130–160	4.5–5.3	0.37–0.49		4.5–13.0	1.8–8.0

Note: The reference ranges presented are compiled from recent textbooks and national guidelines. Blood results should not be interpreted in isolation; clinicians must consider the child or young person's clinical status, symptoms and history. These ranges refer to sex assigned at birth and not gender identity, and should be used alongside relevant clinical guidelines.

affect the body. RBC disorders encompass any condition impacting these cells, including haemoglobin defects or underproduction of RBCs.

Anaemia

The most common RBC disorders are anaemias, derived from the Greek 'anaimia' meaning 'lack of blood'. Today, anaemia refers to a deficiency of RBCs or haemoglobin rather than blood volume.

Anaemias are often classified by RBC size:

1. Microcytic anaemia (small RBCs), e.g., iron-deficiency anaemia (IDA)
2. Macrocytic anaemia (large RBCs), e.g., Vitamin B12 deficiency
3. Normocytic anaemia (normal-sized RBCs), e.g., aplastic anaemia, sickle cell anaemia

RBC size is measured via mean corpuscular volume (MCV) in femtoliters (fL) as part of an FBC:

- Newborns: 95–121 fL
- 6 months–2 years: 70–86 fL
- After 2 years: 70–100 fL

There is no significant variation between males and females.

Microcytic anaemia

Microcytic anaemia is characterised by smaller-than-normal RBCs, reflected as a low MCV on blood tests. The most common cause is iron deficiency, as iron is essential for haemoglobin production. Low iron levels reduce haemoglobin synthesis, resulting in smaller RBCs.

Macrocytic anaemia

Macrocytic anaemia, also called megaloblastic anaemia, is caused by folate and/or vitamin B12 deficiency. These nutrients are essential for DNA maturation, so their deficiency leads to the production of unusually large RBCs that are wider and thicker and have a higher total volume.

Normocytic anaemia

Normocytic anaemia features normal-sized RBCs but an insufficient number. It can result from chronic disease or acute blood loss and is less common than other anaemias. While thalassaemia is usually microcytic, co-existing

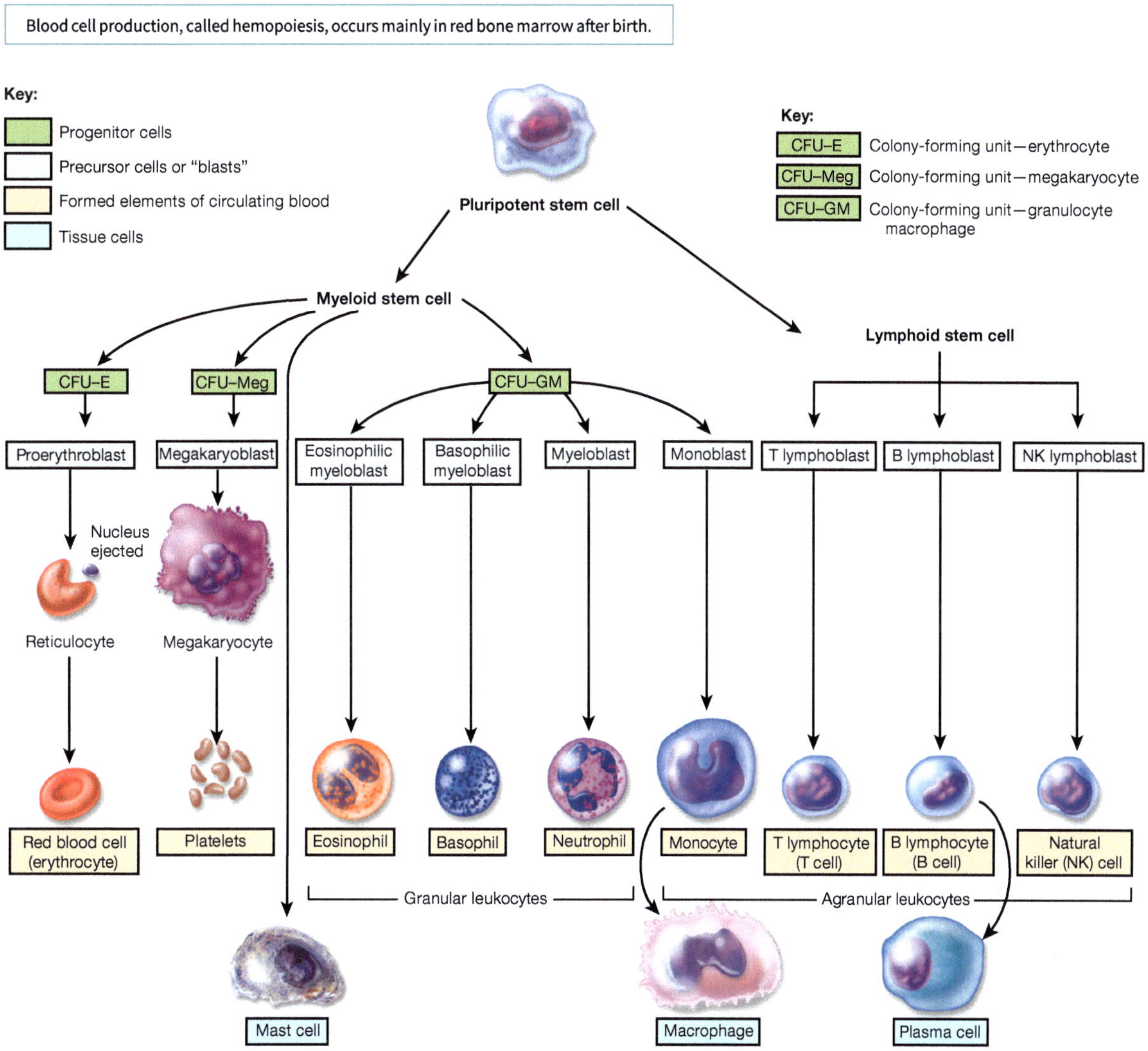

FIGURE 10.2 The development of blood cells.
Source: Tortora and Derrickson (2017) / with permission of John Wiley & Sons.

TABLE 10.2 Terms used in association with blood results

Terminology	Definition
Anaemia	Lower than normal red blood cells
Thrombocytopenia	Lower than normal platelet count
Leukopenia	Lower than normal white cell count
Neutropenia	Lower than normal neutrophil count
Lymphopenia	Lower than normal lymphocyte count
Cytopenia	Lower than normal red blood cells, white blood cells of any kind or low platelets
Pancytopenia	Lower than normal red blood cells, white blood cells of any kind and low platelets

conditions may alter RBC size. Around 5% of the global population carries genes for haemoglobin disorders, mainly SCD and thalassaemia (WHO, 2025).

Anaemia is often a symptom of an underlying condition rather than a primary diagnosis, a topic explored later in this chapter.

Special consideration

Iron-deficiency anaemia (IDA) is the most common haematological disorder in children (Moscheo *et al.*, 2022). It is primarily nutritional, often caused by insufficient iron-rich foods due to developmental food aversions or socio-economic factors limiting diet quality. IDA can also result from gastrointestinal issues, causing malabsorption or iron loss through haemorrhage.

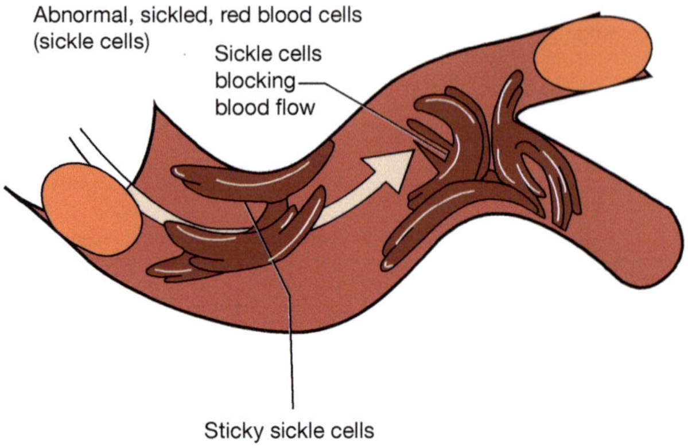

FIGURE 10.4 Sickle cell in microcirculation.
Source: Peate (2017) / with permission of John Wiley & Sons.

Sickle cell disease

Pathophysiology

SCD refers to a group of inherited disorders affecting RBCs, caused by a mutation in the HBB gene that alters haemoglobin structure. It is inherited in an autosomal recessive pattern, requiring two copies of the gene for the condition to manifest. (See Fig. 10.3 for comparison of a sickle cell and a normal RBC.)

SCD is caused by defective haemoglobin, the oxygen-carrying protein in RBCs. Normally, RBCs are flexible and move easily through vessels, but in SCD, deoxygenated RBCs adopt a rigid, sickle shape (see Fig. 10.4). These sickled cells are sticky, prone to blockages and have weakened membranes, leading to premature destruction and anaemia. The bone marrow compensates by producing more RBCs, often immature, which can further complicate circulation. SCD is most common in individuals of African or Caribbean descent. Carriers (sickle trait) gain malaria resistance, an example of heterozygote advantage.

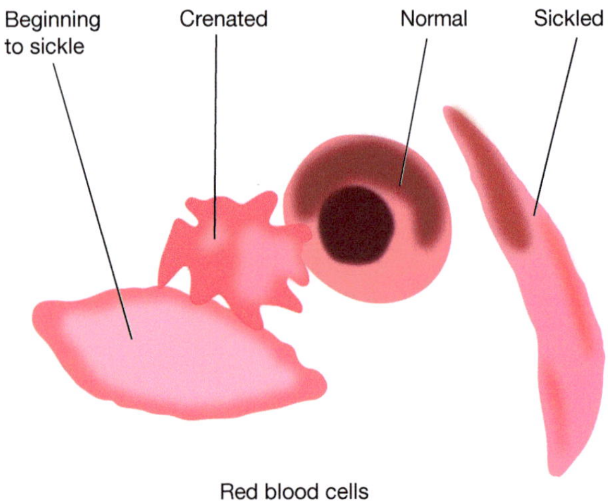

FIGURE 10.3 Sickle cell and red blood cell (RBC).

In the United Kingdom, pregnancy screening for SCD is offered, and testing is included in the newborn blood spot programme.

Clinical manifestations

The main symptoms of SCD are:

- **Pain:** Secondary to 'Sickle Cell Crises', which can be severe and last for days or weeks.
- **Sickle cell crisis:** This is caused by an occlusion of blood vessels, leading to ischaemic pain and organ damage. This commonly affects the chest, back, extremities and abdomen. Sickle cell crisis can lead to fatal complications, such as a stroke or pulmonary hypertension.
- **Chronic anaemia:** Results from premature RBC destruction caused by recurrent sickling. The resulting hypoxia stimulates the bone marrow to produce more RBCs, which, over time, can lead to expansion of RBC-producing marrow, including in the skull.

- **Increased risk of infection:** Sickle-shaped RBCs can cause occlusions, leading to splenic ischaemia and damage. This impairs the spleen's ability to filter microorganisms and reduces the number of memory B cells, increasing susceptibility to infection.
- **Organ damage:** Over time, recurrent ischaemic episodes in SCD can cause damage to organs, including the kidneys, heart, lungs, liver and spleen.

Treatment and management

SCD treatment primarily focuses on preventing and managing complications, as curative options are limited. A stem cell (bone marrow) transplant can potentially cure severe cases but requires a well-matched donor to minimise risk. Advances in gene therapy (GT) aim to correct the underlying genetic defect; in 2024, the first GT was licensed in the United Kingdom for SCD and transfusion-dependent beta-thalassaemia (NICE, 2024a).

Pharmacological and non-pharmacological management

- **Hydroxyurea:** Increases foetal haemoglobin (HbF) production, reducing sickling and frequency of pain crises.
- **Pain management:** Opioids (such as morphine) and non-steroidal anti-inflammatories (such as Diclofenac) for management of vasoocclusive pain crises.
- **Folic acid supplementation:** To support healthy RBC production.
- **L-glutamine therapy:** Reduces oxidative stress and sickling episodes.
- **Blood transfusions:** Treatment aims to increase the volume of healthy RBCs, enhance oxygen-carrying capacity and reduce complications such as sickle cell crises.
- **Antibiotics (such as penicillin prophylaxis):** To prevent common infections due to the risk of the person being immunocompromised.
- **Immunisations:** All infants should follow national immunisation schedules. Individuals with SCD should also receive lifelong booster vaccines, including annual influenza, to reduce infection risk.
- **Hydration:** Adequate fluid intake to help prevent dehydration-induced crisis.
- **Environmental factors:** Avoiding cold or extreme environments to reduce vasoconstriction.

Nursing considerations

- Assess and manage pain using age-appropriate validated scales.
- Administer prescribed analgesics promptly, monitoring for opioid side effects.
- Encourage hydration and provide IV fluids as needed.
- Monitor oxygen saturation and give supplemental oxygen if hypoxic.
- Conduct regular neurovascular assessments to detect early ischaemic damage.
- Educate patients and families on medication adherence, hydration and avoiding triggers such as cold, high altitude or dehydration.
- Address mental health concerns related to chronic pain and disease burden.

Special considerations

Chronic illness impacts both patients and caregivers. Adolescents with SCD may experience stress from parental restrictions, affecting independence (Coco *et al.*, 2023). Caregivers and family members are also at risk of poorer mental health, with research suggesting routine mental health screening for SCD caregivers is recommended (Bruzzese *et al.*, 2023). Understanding the lived experience of chronic illness is vital for high-quality care.

Thalassaemia

Pathophysiology

Thalassaemia is an inherited blood disorder caused by reduced or absent synthesis of globin chains in haemoglobin. It is autosomal recessive, requiring two copies of the gene for disease expression. Haemoglobin normally has two alpha (α) and two beta (β) chains; mutations lead to an imbalance, resulting in alpha-thalassaemia (α chain deficiency) or beta-thalassaemia (β chain deficiency).

Patients may have transfusion-dependent thalassaemia (TDT) or non-transfusion-dependent thalassaemia (nTDT). Severity varies with the specific mutation and number of affected gene copies, from asymptomatic carriers to life-threatening disease, influencing management strategies.

Thalassaemia predominantly affects people of Mediterranean, South Asian, Southeast Asian and Middle Eastern descent, but can occur in all populations worldwide.

Clinical manifestations

- **Chronic anaemia:** Premature RBC destruction leads to anaemia, causing breathlessness, pallor and lethargy. Hypoxia stimulates the bone marrow to produce more RBCs, potentially causing marrow expansion in bones such as the skull.
- **Hepatosplenomegaly:** The liver and spleen enlarge as they filter abnormal RBCs and compensate for inadequate bone marrow production by acting as alternate sites for RBC formation.
- **Slowed growth and delayed puberty:** Chronic anaemia can impair growth rates and pubertal development if not managed effectively.

Treatment and management

Thalassaemia treatment primarily focuses on preventing and managing complications, as curative options are limited. A stem cell transplant may offer a cure in severe cases with a well-matched donor, while GT is an emerging option; in 2024, the first GT was licensed in the United Kingdom for transfusion-dependent beta-thalassaemia and SCD (NICE, 2024b).

- **Blood transfusions:** Used to manage anaemia, ensuring effective oxygen transport and normal body function.
- **Iron overload management:** In TDT, iron overload occurs earlier and must be managed proactively. Chelation therapy is typically started after 10–12 units of packed RBCs to prevent organ damage or failure from excess iron (Shah *et al.*, 2022).

Nursing considerations

- Deliver care promptly to prevent complications.
- Educate patients and families on medication and treatment adherence.
- Ensure awareness of anaemia symptoms and when to seek hospital care.
- Address mental health concerns, including depression and anxiety related to disease and treatment.
- Promote infection prevention, including vaccinations, as patients are susceptible to infections.

Early signs include fatigue, breathlessness and changes in skin colour (blue-tinged in lighter skin or darker in darker skin), which can be confused with anaemia, making transfusions potentially worsen iron overload.

In the United Kingdom, chelation therapy is used to treat iron overload, binding iron for excretion via urine or stool. Untreated, iron overload can cause irreversible and fatal organ damage.

Iron overload

Repeated blood transfusions may lead to iron overload, where excess iron accumulates in organs such as the liver and heart, damaging lipids, proteins and DNA, resulting in inflammation, fibrosis and cell death. Diagnosis is made by measuring ferritin levels and using MRI to assess iron burden (Shah *et al.*, 2022).

White blood cell +disorders

WBCs are crucial for immune defence, protecting the body against infection and disease. In children, WBC counts naturally fluctuate, rising during bacterial infections and sometimes falling during viral illnesses, as part of a normal immune response.

Persistently abnormal counts or dysfunctional cells may indicate a WBC disorder, ranging from benign, transient conditions to serious diseases such as immunodeficiencies, bone marrow failure syndromes and leukaemias. Early recognition and timely investigation are vital in paediatric care.

Leukaemia (acute lymphoblastic and acute myeloid)

Leukaemia refers to a group of disorders originating in the bone marrow, causing overproduction of immature or abnormal WBCs that enter circulation. Types of leukaemia are classified by the affected white cell subset. For example, acute lymphoblastic leukaemia (ALL) affects lymphocytes, while acute myeloid leukaemia (AML) affects myeloid cells, which normally develop into various WBCs, RBCs and platelets (see Fig. 10.5).

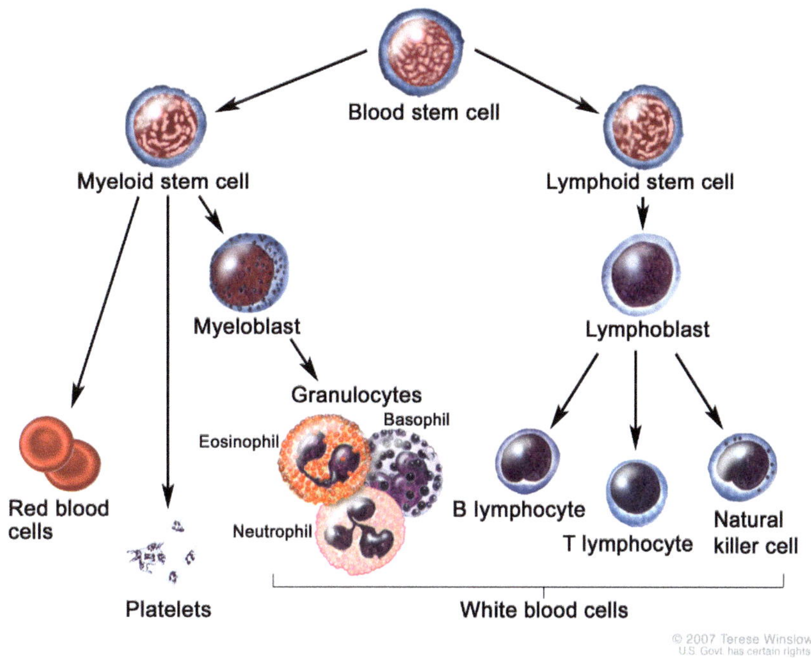

FIGURE 10.5 Image of stem cell and the myeloid/lymphoid lineage.
Source: USA.gov/white blood cell/https://www.cancer.gov/publications/dictionaries/cancer-terms/def/white-blood-cell/Public Domain/last accessed on October 15,2025.

Identifying the specific subset is essential for treatment planning and nursing care. Understanding normal WBC production is key to grasping how leukaemia impacts children and young people.

Leukaemia is the most common type of cancer diagnosed in children, with ALL being the most commonly occurring of those cancers (National Health Service England, 2024). ALL has the best outcome of all leukaemic variants found in children and young people, with over 85% of patients being cured on standard protocol (Moorman *et al.*, 2022).

In its most simplistic form, ALL is a fast-developing blood cancer, stemming from the bone marrow. The bone marrow will make too many B or T lymphocytes, which subsequently are not fully developed, so they do not work normally. They are often referred to as blast cells. They grow and divide quickly, taking up space within the bone marrow and stopping the development of functional WBCs. Additionally, they can spill out of the bone marrow, into places such as lymph nodes, liver, spleen, brain and spinal cord, blood and, in males, testicles. Being 'acute', this type of leukaemia develops quickly and intensively.

However, in AML, whilst it is also a rapidly developing subtype of leukaemia, it affects cells in the myeloid lineages. The bone marrow produces immature myeloid cells at an accelerated rate, causing them to grow and divide uncontrollably. These abnormal cells accumulate in the bone marrow, impeding healthy blood cell production, and may eventually enter the bloodstream. These cells can also be found in the lymph nodes, liver and spleen.

Ultimately, in both ALL and AML, the bone marrow produces an excessive number of abnormal WBCs. These immature cells multiply rapidly and crowd the bone marrow, leaving insufficient space for the production of healthy blood cells. As a result, levels of functional WBCs, RBCs and platelets are reduced. Although WBCs are essential for fighting infections, the abnormal cells produced in leukaemia do not function properly. This makes the individual more vulnerable to infections and less able to recover from them. The reduced number of RBCs (anaemia) impairs oxygen transport throughout the body, leading to symptoms such as fatigue and shortness of breath. A low platelet count increases the risk of bleeding and bruising, as platelets are critical for blood clotting. This may present as frequent nosebleeds, easy bruising or prolonged bleeding from minor cuts.

In some cases, the abnormal white cells can also accumulate in other organs, such as the liver, spleen or lymph nodes. This can cause abdominal discomfort, swelling or a feeling of fullness. In certain types of leukaemia, these cells may even spread to the brain or central nervous system, potentially leading to neurological symptoms such as gait abnormalities, facial palsy, headaches or significant changes in behaviour. It is important to consider that this is where the disease can infiltrate and indicate relapse during or after treatment can be isolated to these areas. As an example, if a young male is being treated for leukaemia of any kind and develops testicular swelling or pain, this must be assessed for isolated testicular disease relapse.

Diagnosis of leukaemia can be made in different ways, depending on where the disease is located. If the leukaemia has already left the bone marrow, leukaemic blast cells will be detectable on a blood film test. A blood film, also known as a blood smear or peripheral blood smear, is a microscopic examination of a thin layer of blood spread on a slide. This process allows healthcare professionals to analyse the individual characteristics of blood and, therefore, see any frank leukaemic cells. Additionally, if there is suspicion of disease but nothing evident on the blood film, a sample can be analysed for flow cytometry (commonly known as a 'flow' sample). This technique will analyse cells within the sample to identify their properties and types. It will be able to determine if the WBCs are fully matured, or diagnostic for leukaemia. If the leukaemia is caught earlier than this stage of disease, it will be detected in a bone marrow aspiration.

Leukaemia is the most common childhood cancer, with ALL being the most frequent type (NHS England, 2024). ALL generally has the best prognosis, with over 85% of children cured using standard protocols (Moorman *et al.*, 2022).

ALL is a fast-developing cancer originating in the bone marrow. It produces excessive immature B or T lymphocytes (blast cells) that do not function properly. These cells crowd the bone marrow, reducing the production of healthy WBCs, RBCs and platelets, and can spread to lymph nodes, liver, spleen, brain, spinal cord, blood and, in males, testicles.

AML also develops rapidly, affecting myeloid cells. Immature myeloid cells multiply uncontrollably, accumulating in the bone marrow and sometimes spreading to the bloodstream, lymph nodes, liver and spleen.

In both ALL and AML, the overproduction of abnormal cells leads to:

- Reduced immunity, increasing infection risk
- Anaemia, causing fatigue and shortness of breath
- Low platelet count, increasing bleeding and bruising

Abnormal cells can also infiltrate organs, causing hepatosplenomegaly, lymph node swelling, abdominal discomfort or CNS involvement with neurological symptoms. Isolated relapse may occur in sites like the testicles, requiring careful assessment.

Diagnosis depends on disease location:

- Blood film (peripheral smear) can reveal leukaemic blast cells
- Flow cytometry can confirm immature or abnormal WBCs
- Bone marrow aspiration detects leukaemia at an earlier stage

This diagnostic approach ensures accurate identification and guides treatment planning.

Clinical manifestations

- Lethargy: Often due to anaemia from disrupted RBC production; circulating RBCs are usually normal in size but reduced in number (normocytic anaemia).
- Nosebleeds and bruising: Result from thrombocytopenia caused by impaired platelet production.
- Frequent fever and infections: Caused by the release of immature, non-functional WBCs, reducing immunity.
- Swollen lymph nodes: Accumulation of blast cells in lymph nodes, palpable on examination.
- Hepatosplenomegaly: Accumulation of blast cells in the liver and spleen, causing organ enlargement detectable on palpation.

Management and treatment

Survival depends on disease stage, genetic features of leukaemic cells and treatment tolerance. Untreated leukaemia can be fatal within weeks or months, usually due to infection, haemorrhage or organ failure.

Treatment typically involves a combination of steroids and chemotherapy, tailored by the specialist team. Plans often follow clinical trials to optimise cure rates while minimising side effects. Factors influencing treatment choice include:

- Age at diagnosis
- WBC count at diagnosis
- Type of leukaemia
- Location of leukaemia cells (e.g., CSF or brain)
- Previous cancer history
- Underlying conditions increasing leukaemia risk (e.g., Trisomy 21)

The most frequently used medications within (related to guidelines) are:

- **Steroids:** Used in high doses to reduce inflammation, suppress the immune system and induce death in leukaemia cells by influencing gene expression.
- **Chemotherapy:** Targets rapidly dividing cells, including cancer cells, by damaging DNA/RNA, disrupting cell division and triggering apoptosis. It also affects normal rapidly dividing cells such as those in the mucosa, skin and hair follicles.
- **Monoclonal antibodies ('mabs'):** Lab-produced molecules designed to mimic the immune system, targeting specific antigens on cancer cells.
- **CAR-T-cell therapy (Chimeric Antigen Receptor T-cell therapy):** Uses the patient's own T cells to recognise and destroy cancer cells. Currently used mainly for B-cell ALL; trials are ongoing for T-cell ALL.
- **Radiotherapy:** Not standard for leukaemia, but used prior to stem cell transplant to destroy remaining cancer cells, suppress immunity and make space for new stem cells.

Nursing considerations

- **Assessment:** Ensure timely assessments and treatments without delay.
- **Psychosocial support:** Provide family-centred care, recognising the emotional impact of a cancer diagnosis on patients and their families.
- **Education:** Help patients and families understand the treatment plan and identify red flags requiring urgent support.
- **Interpretation of blood results:** Blood results guide many treatment steps; nurses must be able to interpret and act on them appropriately.
- **Infection prevention and control:** These patients are highly vulnerable to life-threatening infections and may require isolation and strict infection control measures.

Risks of prolonged steroid use

Steroids are powerful medications used in treating various blood disorders. Prolonged use can lead to serious side effects, including:

- Increased appetite
- Mood changes
- Kidney damage
- Hypertension
- Steroid-induced diabetes
- Osteoporosis
- Adrenal insufficiency

Adrenal insufficiency occurs when prolonged steroid use suppresses natural cortisol production by the adrenal glands. When reducing or stopping steroids, such as prednisolone, one must consider the risk of secondary adrenal insufficiency. Management includes oral hydrocortisone replacement and monitoring cortisol levels, usually via an early morning blood test.

During physiological stress (illness, trauma and fever), cortisol requirements rise. Untreated adrenal insufficiency can cause adrenal crisis, which is life-threatening and requires immediate intramuscular hydrocortisone and hospitalisation (British Society for Paediatric Endocrinology and Diabetes, 2025).

Severe combined immunodeficiency

Severe combined immunodeficiency (SCID) is a rare but life-threatening primary immunodeficiency disorder in which infants are born with little to no functioning immune system. SCID most commonly affects both T cells and B cells (and sometimes NK cells), causing them to be either absent or not fully functioning. These cells are essential for fighting off viruses, bacteria and fungi. Without them, even common infections can become severe or fatal. The type of SCID an infant is diagnosed with will be dependent on the genetic testing to identify the specific mutation causing the disorder.

Historically, this would be identified when an infant had an overwhelming infection, leading to sepsis and intensive care admissions. Most commonly, this would happen when the infant would stop breastfeeding or earlier if they were not breastfed, as the breastmilk provided some protection from infections. However, in the United Kingdom, an evaluation of newborn screening for SCID was launched in September 2021. This means infants are diagnosed far earlier, before encountering overwhelming infections.

Clinical manifestation

Since the newborn screening was started for SCID, symptoms of this condition are far less commonly seen in patients, as they can be medically managed until progressing onto curative bone marrow transplant (BMT). However, as some patients will not undergo newborn screening or may have been born outside of the United Kingdom, symptom awareness is still crucial.

- Multiple and severe infections: Due to the inability of the WBCs to function properly to protect the infant from infection
- Poor weight gain
- Chronic loose stools

Treatment and management

The only known cures for SCID are a Haematopoietic Stem Cell Transplant (BMT) or, in some cases, GT.

- **Bone marrow transplant (BMT):** Replaces faulty immune cells with healthy donor cells. Early diagnosis through newborn screening allows infants to undergo BMT infection-free, reducing transplant-related mortality.
- **Gene therapy:** Available for adenosine deaminase-deficient (ADA) SCID, where a faulty ADA gene is corrected in stem cells to restore lymphocyte function.
- **Supportive care:** Before curative treatment, infants require protective isolation, prophylactic antibiotics and antifungals, IV immunoglobulin (IVIG) infusions for temporary immunity, and avoidance of live vaccines. Post-BMT, vaccinations can resume per national guidelines.

Nursing considerations

Providing nursing care for infants with SCID requires a strong focus on psychosocial support, education, infection control and close monitoring. Psychosocial support is vital, as the diagnosis can be confusing and distressing for families, particularly if they have never encountered SCID before. Nurses play a key role in offering compassionate, family-centred care and, because SCID is genetic, supporting families to consider implications for future pregnancies, including possible genetic counselling.

Education is essential to ensure parents understand the treatment plan, including curative options such as BMT or GT, and the supportive measures needed beforehand. Teaching families to recognise red flags – such as fever, feeding difficulties, lethargy or respiratory symptoms – helps them seek help promptly.

Strict infection prevention and control measures are crucial, as infants with SCID are highly vulnerable to life-threatening infections. Effective hand hygiene, isolation precautions and limiting exposure to others are central to maintaining safety.

Close monitoring is also required throughout care, as deterioration can occur rapidly. Regular assessment supports early recognition of complications and timely intervention, promoting safer outcomes for the infant and family.

Neutropenic sepsis

Neutropenic sepsis is a life-threatening emergency in immunocompromised patients. Whether neutropenia is primary (as in SCID) or acquired (for example, following chemotherapy or BMT), the approach to treatment is the same.

Rapid recognition and intervention are essential, with the 'golden hour' being critical. From the first sign of fever, patients must immediately undergo the following:

- Take blood cultures from all central venous access devices; if a double-lumen line is present, both lumens must be sampled.
- Perform FBC and C-reactive protein (CRP) testing.
- Start intravenous antibiotics promptly. For most patients, this will be a single broad-spectrum agent such as piperacillin/tazobactam. Those with known resistance may require alternative agents. Post-BMT patients need dual therapy: a broad-spectrum antibiotic (e.g., piperacillin/tazobactam) plus an aminoglycoside such as gentamicin or amikacin.

Febrile Neutropenia Clinical Guideline, National Institute for Health and Care Excellence (2020).

Platelet disorders

Haemostasis, the mechanism that prevents excessive bleeding, depends on the precise coordination of platelets and coagulation factors. Disruption to this balance can cause bleeding or thrombosis. Platelet and coagulation disorders include a broad range of inherited conditions, such as haemophilia, and acquired disorders linked to autoimmune disease, infection, medications, liver disease or malignancy. Disorders affecting platelets can be broadly categorised into three groups:

1. Thrombocythemia – an abnormally high platelet count.
2. Thrombocytopenia – an abnormally low platelet count.
3. Platelet dysfunction disorders – a normal platelet count, but impaired platelet function.

Immune thrombocytopenic purpura (ITP)

Pathophysiology

Immune thrombocytopenia (ITP), previously called idiopathic thrombocytopenic purpura, is an autoimmune disorder in which the immune system mistakenly destroys platelets, leading to thrombocytopenia. This process is primarily mediated by IgG antibodies that bind to platelet surface antigens, causing their removal by macrophages in the spleen and liver. Antibodies may also impair platelet production in the bone marrow, further reducing platelet counts. ITP can be primary (occurring alone) or secondary to infections, autoimmune diseases or medications.

In children, ITP often follows a viral illness, with around 55% of cases appearing within a month of infection, though many cases have no identifiable cause. Some children are asymptomatic, with the condition discovered incidentally on blood tests. Common presentations include bruising, petechiae, mucosal bleeding (such as nosebleeds), purpura or heavy menstrual bleeding in adolescents.

Clinical manifestations

- **Easy bruising and petechiae:** Due to the significantly impaired function or low number of platelets
- Bleeding gums
- Blood in stool or urine
- For menstruating females – prolonged and heavy periods, also known as menorrhagia
- **Spontaneous intracranial bleeding:** This is a very serious and significant brain bleed and requires emergency management.

Treatment and management

Most children with ITP do not require treatment unless they are actively bleeding or experiencing sporadic bleeding episodes. Treatment options include:

- **Tranexamic acid:** Helps blood clotting but does not increase platelet count. It is effective for gum bleeding, nosebleeds or menstrual bleeding. It should be avoided if blood is present in the urine to prevent urethral obstruction.
- **Steroids:** Short-term steroid therapy can reduce platelet destruction and temporarily raise platelet counts. Counts typically return to baseline once the dose is reduced.
- **Intravenous immunoglobulin (IVIG):** Works similarly to steroids by blocking the destruction of antibody-coated platelets.
- **Splenectomy:** Reserved for severe, unresolving cases with life-threatening bleeding. Removal of the spleen decreases platelet destruction but renders the child immunocompromised for life.

Platelet transfusions are generally not beneficial in ITP, except in life-threatening bleeding, as transfused platelets are also rapidly destroyed (Goel *et al.*, 2019).

Approximately 80% of children with ITP experience a return to normal platelet counts within 6 months, and often much sooner, sometimes within 6 weeks (Bennett *et al.*, 2018). If low platelet counts persist beyond 6 months, the condition is classified as chronic ITP.

In most younger children, even if recovery extends beyond a year, full resolution is still likely over time, often within a few years. For adolescents, however, if platelet levels remain low after 12 months, they may have a form of ITP more akin to the adult chronic type, where platelet counts may not fully recover, and long-term management may be necessary.

Nursing considerations

- **Management:** Close monitoring for blood loss and fast interventions can be life-saving for children and young people with ITP.
- **Education:** For patients and their families on the condition and management options.

Plasma disorders

Plasma disorders in children are a key group of paediatric haematological conditions, involving deficiencies or abnormalities in the clotting proteins found in plasma. These disorders impair the body's ability to form stable blood clots, increasing the risk of prolonged or spontaneous bleeding. Unlike platelet disorders, which affect the initial clot formation, plasma disorders primarily disrupt the secondary haemostasis, where soluble clotting factors work together to stabilise the clot. Table 10.3 details the individual clotting factors and their roles in this process.

TABLE 10.3 Clotting factors

Factor	Alternative names
I	Fibrinogen
II	Prothrombin
III	Tissue factor (thromboplastin)
IV	Calcium ions
V	Proaccelerin Labile factor Accelerator globulin
VII	Serum prothrombin conversion accelerator Stable factor Proconvertin
VIII	Antihaemophilic factor Antihaemophilic factor A Antihaemophilic globulin
IX	Christmas factor Plasma thromboplastin component Antihaemophilic factor B
X	Stuart factor Power factor Thrombokinase
XI	Plasma thromboplastin antecedent Antihaemophilic factor C
XII	Hageman factor Glass factor Contact factor
XIII	Fibrin-stabilising factor Fibrinase

In children, the most prevalent are Haemophilia A, Haemophilia B and VWD. These disorders can lead to spontaneous or prolonged bleeding episodes, significantly impacting quality of life if not properly managed.

Haemophilia A and B

Pathophysiology

Haemophilia is an inherited bleeding disorder caused by a deficiency or dysfunction of specific clotting factors, impairing the formation of a stable fibrin clot and leading to prolonged or spontaneous bleeding. Haemophilia A results from a deficiency of factor VIII, while Haemophilia B (Christmas disease) is due to a deficiency of factor IX. Both are X-linked recessive conditions, primarily affecting males, as females have a second X chromosome that often compensates for the affected one. However, females can still be affected. Severity is classified according to the percentage of clotting factor activity (Thachil *et al.*, 2023):

- Severe: < 1% activity
- Moderate: 1–5% activity
- Mild: 5–40% activity

In severe cases, spontaneous bleeding into joints and muscles is common, leading to complications like haemarthrosis and potential joint damage.

Clinical manifestations

- **Spontaneous or prolonged bleeding:** Caused by the blood's inability to clot normally, leading to extended bleeding episodes.
- **Internal or external bleeding:** External bleeding can result in anaemia or hypovolaemic shock, while internal bleeding – particularly into joints – can cause long-term damage or, if uncontrolled, be life-threatening.
- **Easy bruising:** Impaired clotting leads to significant and frequent bruising, even after minor trauma.

Medication and treatment

Treatment for haemophilia can be narrowed down into the following subsections:

In severe haemophilia cases

- **Factor replacement therapy:** This involves regular infusions or injections of clotting factor VIII (for haemophilia A) or factor IX (for haemophilia B) to prevent bleeding episodes. These infusions can be self-administered at home, often multiple times a week. This is considered a prophylactic (or preventative) treatment.

- **Emicizumab (Hemlibra):** This medication is a monoclonal antibody that mimics the function of factor VIII, preventing bleeding by activating other clotting factors. It's administered as a subcutaneous injection.

In less severe Haemophilia cases and on-demand treatment

- **Factor replacement therapy:** In less severe cases (and in addition to the aforementioned, in severe cases), injections of clotting factor VIII (for haemophilia A) or factor IX (for haemophilia B) to prevent bleeding that has already started or prior to dental work or surgery.
- **Antifibrinolytics (such as tranexamic acid):** These medications help stabilise blood clots by preventing their premature breakdown, making them effective for controlling bleeding episodes and for use around surgical or dental procedures.

Some patients develop antibodies, or 'inhibitors', against infused clotting factors, making treatment less effective. This usually occurs within the first 50 days of therapy, most often in the first 20 days. Children with severe haemophilia are more likely to develop inhibitors early, while those with mild or moderate disease may develop them later.

The main treatment for inhibitors is immune tolerance induction (ITI), which involves frequent, sustained exposure to the clotting factor (VIII or IX) to train the immune system to recognise it as harmless.

Nursing considerations

- **Psychosocial support:** This diagnosis may be very stressful for patients and their families, even if it is commonly occurring in their family. A nursing role in this aspect is to consider how to provide effective and thorough family-centred care.
- **Education:** Ensuring the patient and their family understand the treatment regimen and any red flags to seek support.
- **Medication compliance:** Encouraging patients and their families to adhere to treatment plans.

Von Willebrand Disease (VWD)

VWD is caused by quantitative or qualitative defects in Von Willebrand Factor (VWF), a protein essential for platelet adhesion and as a carrier for factor VIII. VWD is classified into:

Type 1: Partial quantitative deficiency of VWF.
Type 2: Qualitative defects in VWF function, with subtypes 2A, 2B, 2M and 2N.
Type 3: Virtually complete deficiency of VWF, leading to severe bleeding tendencies. This is considered the most severe subtype of VWD.

VWD is almost always inherited. Types 1 and 2 VWD are inherited in an autosomal dominant pattern, where only one parent needs to pass on a faulty VWF gene. With each pregnancy, there is a 50% chance the child will inherit the condition.

Type 3 VWD, the rarest and most severe form, is inherited in an autosomal recessive manner. This means a child must inherit a faulty gene from both parents to develop the condition. Even within the same family, symptoms can vary significantly, and a child's symptoms may differ from those of their parents. In some cases, individuals may carry a faulty VWF gene without showing any symptoms. However, they can still pass the gene on to their children.

For most people with VWD, the condition causes few problems and rarely disrupts daily life, except during surgery, childbirth or serious injury. However, all forms of VWD can lead to bleeding complications, and in rare, severe cases, internal bleeding into muscles and joints may occur, like haemophilia.

Clinical manifestations

VWD may not cause noticeable symptoms unless triggered by an injury. In many cases, it is only diagnosed after experiencing unusual or excessive bleeding following surgery or dental work.

Possible symptoms of Von Willebrand Disease

- **Bruising easily:** As the blood is unable to clot and prevent further bleeding, patients with VWD can bruise easily and significantly.
- **Nose bleeds:** Even slight trauma in the highly vascular area within the nostrils can result in significant and prolonged bleeding. This can also be in the absence of trauma.
- Bleeding for longer and more significantly than peers after what appears to be a small injury.

- Bleeding gums when tooth brushing
- Blood in stool and urine

Due to the lack of symptoms in most people, VWD is not diagnosed quickly. In most cases, until a child or young person undergoes surgery or has a significant family history, a diagnosis will not be made.

Treatment and management

In Types 1 and 2 of VWD, the children or young people (CYP) would only need treatment if they were to bleed. In Type 3, prophylactic treatment to prevent bleeding would also be encouraged:

- **Avoidance of infection:** By maintaining a healthy lifestyle and good dental hygiene, patients with VWD can avoid unnecessary procedures.
- **Avoidance of NSAIDs:** Medications such as ibuprofen can reduce the blood's ability to clot, but reducing platelet counts. This, in combination with an underlying condition such as VWD, would result in a higher risk of prolonged bleeding.
- **Antifibrinolytics (such as tranexamic acid):** These medications help stabilise blood clots by preventing their premature breakdown, making them effective for controlling bleeding episodes and for use around surgical or dental procedures.
- **Factor replacement therapy:** Necessary for Type 3 as a prophylactic measure; however, can be given in Type 1 and Type 2 in the event of uncontrolled bleeding.
- **Desmopressin (DDAVP):** Effective for many types of VWD; it stimulates the release of VWF and factor VIII.

Nursing considerations

- **Psychosocial support:** This diagnosis may be very stressful for patients and their families, even if it is commonly occurring in their family. A nursing role in this aspect is to consider how to provide effective and through family centred care.
- **Education:** Ensuring the patient and their family understand the treatment regimen and any red flags to seek support.
- **Medication compliance:** Encouraging patients and their families to adhere to treatment plans.

A thorough understanding of the pathophysiology, prevalence, and management of Haemophilia A, Haemophilia B and VWD is essential for effective nursing care. Early diagnosis, personalised treatment plans and detailed patient and family education can greatly improve outcomes for children with these plasma disorders.

Case study 10.1

Arun, a previously healthy 3-month-old infant, was brought to the children's emergency department with a 10-day history of high fever (up to 39.5 °C), increasing irritability and poor oral intake. Arun's weight has recently dropped off their usual centile, with the weight on admission as 7.2 kg. Arun's parents also reported reduced activity, pale skin and a recent episode of vomiting. No recent travel.

Observations	
Temperature	39.3 °C
Heart rate	172 beats per minute (tachycardic)
Respiratory rate	52 breaths per minute
Oxygen saturation (SpO_2)	97% self-ventilating in room air
Blood pressure	74/45 mmHg (low-normal)
Capillary refill time	3–4 seconds

On examination, Arun is found to have pale mucosa, and his parents state his skin tone is different to his usual. He is noted to have hepatosplenomegaly, palpable 4 cm below the coastal margin. Blood tests are as follows:

Blood test	Result	Normal ranges
Haemoglobin (Hb)	78 g/L	10.5–13.5 g/dL
White cell count (WBC)	2.1×10^9/L	6–17.5 × 10^9/L
Platelets	48×10^9/L	150–400 × 10^9/L
Ferritin	42 000 ng/L	25–300 ng/L
Triglycerides	4.8 mmol/L	< 1.5 mmol/L
Fibrinogen	0.9 g/L	1.5–4.0 g/L
AST	210 U/L	< 48 U/L
ALT	190 U/L	< 55 U/L
Lactate dehydrogenase (LDH)	850 U/L	100–250 U/L

Arun is admitted to the children's ward for further investigations into his symptoms and blood results.

The following day, Arun undergoes a bone marrow aspirate, which shows the presence of haemophagocytosis, where cells are engulfing other blood cells.

Haemophagocytic lymphohistiocytosis (HLH) in infants can progress rapidly and be life-threatening. Prompt recognition and initiation of immunosuppressive therapy is critical. Arun's severe cytopenias, markedly elevated ferritin and haemophagocytosis on bone marrow are classical features of primary HLH.

Conclusion

This chapter has reviewed a selection of blood disorders, highlighting the crucial role nurses play in recognising, managing and supporting patients with these conditions. Blood disorders often present subtly but can rapidly lead to serious complications if not identified early. From anaemias and clotting disorders to immune-mediated conditions such as HLH or ITP, nurses are central to early detection, patient and family education, monitoring for complications and providing both physical and emotional care.

Proficiency in interpreting haematological values, recognising signs of bleeding or clotting and understanding laboratory findings is essential. Nurses act as advocates within multidisciplinary teams, ensuring timely interventions, safe administration of blood products or medications and adherence to clinical protocols. Through vigilance, continued education, clinical experience and compassionate care, nurses enhance patient safety, outcomes and overall holistic care for individuals living with blood disorders, underpinning excellence in haematological nursing practice.

References

Bennett, C.M., Neunert, C., Grace, R.F., *et al.* (2018). Predictors of remission in children with newly diagnosed immune thrombocytopenia: data from the Intercontinental Cooperative ITP Study Group Registry II participants. *Pediatric Blood & Cancer* 65(1), e26736. https://doi.org/10.1002/pbc.26736.

British Society for Paediatric Endocrinology and Dissbetes (BSPED) (2025). *BSPED Adrenal Insufficiency Consensus Guidelines.* https://www.bsped.org.uk/clinical-resources/bsped-adrenal-insufficiency-consensus-guidelines/ (accessed 01 May 2025).

Bruzzese, J., Usseglio, J., Iannacci-Manasia, L., *et al.* (2023). Mental and emotional health of caregivers of youth with sickle cell disease: a systematic review. *Journal of Health Care for the Poor and Underserved* 34(3), 1070–1104 https://muse.jhu.edu/article/903064.

Coco, M., Henderson, W.A., Park, C.L., & Starkweather, A.R. (2023). Growing beyond sickle cell disease: a metasynthesis of children, adolescents, and young adult experiences living with sickle cell disease. *Research in Nursing & Health* 46(3), 299–312 https://doi.org/10.1002/nur.22310.

Goel, R., Chopra, S., Tobian, A.A.R., *et al.* (2019). Platelet transfusion practices in immune thrombocytopenia related hospitalizations. *Transfusion* 59(1), 169–176 https://doi.org/10.1111/trf.15069.

Jones, N. (2020). The circulatory system. In: Peate, I. & Evans, S. (eds). *Fundamentals of Anatomy and Physiology For Nursing and Healthcare Students*, 3rd edn. Chichester: Wiley-Blackwell.

Marieb, E.N., & Hoehn, K. (2022). *Human Anatomy and Physiology*, 12th edn. Pearson Benjamin Cummings.

Merz, L.E., Story, C.M., Osei, M.A., *et al.* (2023). Absolute neutrophil count by Duffy status among healthy Black and African American adults. *Blood Advances* 14(3), 317–320 https://doi.org/10.1182/bloodadvances.2022007679.

Moorman, A.V., Antony, G., Wade, R., *et al.* (2022). Time to cure for childhood and young adult acute lymphoblastic leukaemia is independent of early risk factors: Long -term follow-up of the UKALL2003 trial. *Journal of Clinical Oncology* 40(36), 4228–4239.

Moscheo, C., Licciardello, M., Samperi, P., *et al.* (2022). New insights into iron deficiency anemia in children: a practical review. *Metabolites* 12, 289 https://doi.org/10.3390/metabo12040289.

National Health Service England (2024). Cancer Registration Statistics, England, 2022. https://digital.nhs.uk/data-and-information/publications/statistical/cancer-registration-statistics/england-2022# (accessed 01 May 2025).

National Institute for Health and Care Excellence (2020). Neutropenic sepsis: prevention and management in people with cancer. https://www.nice.org.uk/guidance/CG151 (accessed 16 May 2025).

National Institute for Health and Care Excellence (2024a). *Sickle Cell Disease.* Available at: https://cks.nice.org.uk/topics/sickle-cell-disease/ (accessed 12 May 2025).

National Institute for Health and Care Excellence (2024b). World's first gene editing therapy for blood disorder to be available to hundreds of patients in England. https://www.nice.org.uk/news/articles/worlds-first-gene-editing-therapy-for-blood-disorder-to-be-available-to-hundreds-of-patients-in-england. (accessed 20 April 2025).

Peate, I. (2017). *Fundamentals of Applied Pathophysiology: An Essential Guide for Nursing and Healthcare Students.* John Wiley & Sons.

Shah, F.T., Porter, J.B., Sadasivam, N., *et al.* (2022). Guidelines for the monitoring and management of iron overload in patients with haemoglobinopathies and rare anaemias. *British Journal of Haematology* 196, 336–350 https://doi.org/10.1111/bjh.17839.

Thachil, J., Connors, J.M., Mahlangu, J., & Sholzberg, M. (2023). Reclassifying hemophilia to include the definition of outcomes and phenotype as new targets. *Journal of Thrombosis and Haemostasis* 21(7), 1737–1740 https://doi.org/10.1016/j.jtha.2023.03.016.

Tortora, G.J., & Derrickson, B.H. (2017). *Principles of Anatomy and Physiology*, 15th edn. Pearson Benjamin Cummings.

World Health Organization (2025). *Sickle Cell Disease.* Available at: https://www.afro.who.int/health-topics/sickle-cell-disease (accessed 29 April 2025).

CHAPTER 11

Disorders of the cardiac system

Sheila Roberts

AIM

The aim of this chapter is for readers to develop their understanding of the anatomy and physiology of the cardiac system in order to appreciate various disorders of this system; to do this effectively, the reader also has to understand pathophysiological mechanisms.

LEARNING OUTCOMES

On completion of this chapter, the reader will be able to:

- Discuss the normal and consider the abnormal anatomy and physiology of the heart.
- Understand why some heart defects are considered cyanotic and some acyanotic.
- Discuss the signs and symptoms of heart failure across the age ranges.
- Identify which heart conditions are congenital and which are acquired.

KEYWORDS

- heart
- circulation
- congenital
- acquired
- disorders
- heart failure

Test your prior knowledge

1. Draw and label the heart.
2. Draw the flow of blood through the heart.
3. Consider the adaptations required by the foetal circulation.
4. What is the difference between the pulmonary circulation and the systemic circulation?
5. What is the difference between a congenital and an acquired disease?

Introduction

The cardiovascular system is responsible for providing the body with a continuous supply of oxygen and nutrients while also transporting the waste materials, such as carbon dioxide, that need to be expelled from the body. The cardiovascular system includes:

- the heart, which pumps deoxygenated blood to the lungs, where gas exchange takes place and oxygenated blood gets transported to the rest of the body;
- the veins, which are the blood vessels that transport the blood from the body back towards the heart;
- the arteries, which are the blood vessels that transport the blood away from the heart;
- the capillaries, which are very small blood vessels connecting the arteries to the veins.

This chapter will provide a brief overview of the anatomy of the heart. It will then consider a range of anomalies that can affect the heart and the impact that these may have on the infant, child or young person.

Anatomy of the heart

The heart is comprised of four chambers: the left atrium and left ventricle and the right atrium and right ventricle. Deoxygenated blood enters the heart from the superior and inferior vena cava directly into the right atrium. Contraction of the muscle of the right atrium causes an increase in pressure within the right atrium, allowing the one-way valve, the right atrioventricular valve (the tricuspid valve), situated between the right atrium and right ventricle, to open and allow the blood to pass through to the right ventricle.

As the atrium empties of blood and the ventricle fills, the atrium relaxes, and the muscles of the right ventricle begin to contract, increasing the pressure within the right ventricle. The atrioventricular valve closes, and the blood is then forced through the pulmonary valve into the right and left pulmonary arteries. As the right ventricle empties of blood, the pulmonary valve closes to prevent backflow of blood from the pulmonary .arteries into the right ventricle.

The deoxygenated blood is transported via the right and left pulmonary arteries to the lungs, where gaseous exchange takes place. Carbon dioxide is expelled and replaced with oxygen.

The oxygenated blood returns to the heart via the pulmonary veins directly into the left atrium. The left atrium fills with blood, the muscles of the left atrium contract and the resulting increase in pressure forces the blood through the left atrioventricular valve (the mitral or bicuspid valve) into the left ventricle.

Contraction of the left ventricle pumps the oxygenated blood through the aortic valve into the aorta for transportation around the body. Again, the aortic valve closes to prevent backflow. Refer to Fig. 11.1 for a diagrammatic representation of the blood flow through the heart. For a more complete understanding of the anatomy and physiology of the heart, refer to Roberts (2025).

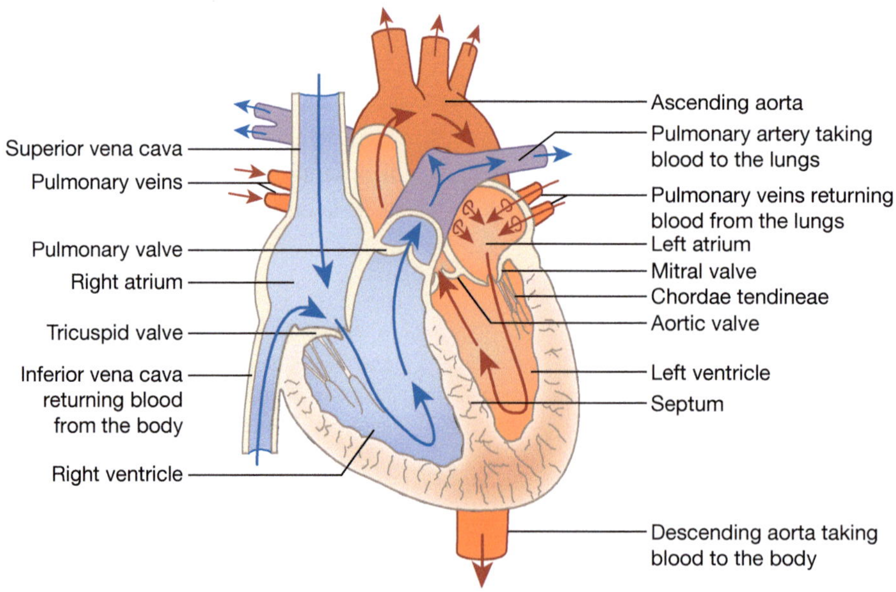

FIGURE 11.1 The blood flow through the heart.
Source: Reproduced with permission of Roberts (2025)/John Wiley & Sons.

Congenital disorders of the heart

A congenital heart defect (CHD) is an anatomical malformation of the heart and/or great vessels, which occurs during foetal development (Rao & Rao, 2022). A CHD is the most common of all defects that affects the newborn baby and is apparent in 0.8–1.2% of live births worldwide (Wu *et al.*, 2020). There are regional variations, with developing countries having a significantly higher incidence of CHDs than developed countries. The overall incidence of CHDs increases in spontaneous miscarriage, stillborn and premature babies. The reasons for CHD are generally unknown, although there are situations where there is a known increased risk (Table 11.1).

TABLE 11.1 **Possible causes for CHD**

Risk factor	Possible congenital heart defect
Mother with type 1 or type 2 diabetes	Transposition of the great arteries
Alcohol intake during pregnancy	Atrial septal defect Ventricular septal defect
Genetic conditions, e.g., babies with Down syndrome	Septal defect
Noonan syndrome	Pulmonary valve stenosis
Turner syndrome	Coarctation of the aorta
Exposure to the rubella virus	Patent ductus arteriosus/ pulmonary artery stenosis
Medication, e.g., benzodiazepines (anti-convulsion medication) and ibuprofen (analgesic medication)	Atrial or ventricular septal defects
Mothers with phenylketonuria who do not adhere to a low-protein diet	Coarctation of the aorta and tetralogy of Fallot
Mother's exposure to organic solvents	Various

Source: Adapted from NHS Choices (2021).

The incidence of CHD is often scrutinised, and sociodemographic factors feature as a possible cause. Maternal age, race, ethnicity and poverty are factors which may lead to a higher incidence of CHD and poorer outcomes for the infant. Maternal education is also a consideration in the incidence of CHD. This may be for a variety of reasons: lower maternal education is associated with a poor diet and nutrition, reduced uptake of supplements such as folic acid and vitamins and can impact prenatal care (Tran *et al.*, 2023). Awareness of the sociodemographic factors that may impact the foetus in an attempt to ensure healthcare equality for all is important.

Cardiac or heart failure

Cardiac failure (CF) occurs when the heart is unable to pump enough blood and therefore oxygen to meet the needs of the metabolising cells. Heart failure is a syndrome characterised by either or both pulmonary and systemic venous congestion, generally leading to inadequate peripheral oxygen delivery. It is caused by cardiac dysfunction. CHDs are the most common reason for CF in infants; at what age this occurs depends on the severity of the defect. In the older child, CF may result from a range of problems (Table 11.2).

CF can be categorised simply as caused by abnormal structures within the heart versus a normal heart, or more accurately, according to the haemodynamic changes that occur:

- **Preload increase or volume overload:** Commonly caused by large left-to-right shunts, such as ventricular septal defect (VSD) and patent ductus arteriosus (PDA). Very rare before 6–8 weeks of age, as pulmonary vascular resistance does not fall low enough to cause the large shunt before this age, but then causes congestive CF (CCF) in the first 6 months of life.
- **Excessive afterload or pressure overload:** Commonly caused by obstructive abnormalities, such as coarctation of the aorta or valve stenosis. The left ventricle is unable to generate sufficient pressure to overcome the fixed downstream obstruction, and it cannot, therefore, maintain cardiac output (Panesar & Burch, 2016).
- **Impaired contractility:** The contractility is the ability of the myocardium (heart muscle) to contract. Impaired contractility is caused by any factor that affects the myocardium and its ability to contract, such as cardiomyopathy or myocarditis.

TABLE 11.2 Possible causes of CF not associated with congenital heart defects

Approximate age of child	Aetiology leading to heart failure
Toddlers	Viral myocarditis
1–4 years	Myocarditis associated with Kawasaki disease
School-age children	Acute rheumatic carditis
Older children	Rheumatic valvular disease
Any age during childhood/ adolescence	Cardiomyopathy
Newborns	Metabolic abnormalities, e.g., severe hypoxia, hypocalcaemia
Early infancy	Supraventricular tachycardia
Any age	Hyperthyroidism
Any age	Severe anaemia
School-age children	Acute systemic hypertension with glomerulonephritis

Source: Park & Salmat (2021)/with permission of Elsevier.

- **Rhythm disturbances:** Arrhythmias can induce heart failure as a result of an inadequate heart rate. Tachycardia leads to inadequate filling of the heart chambers and, therefore, decreased cardiac output. Bradycardia leads to an increase in ventricular filling volume, leading to ventricular dilatation.
- **Distensibility disorders:** Distensibility refers to the ability of the chambers and vessels of the heart to increase in volume without a significant increase in pressure. When the heart is unable to do this, cardiac output is affected.
- **Ischaemia:** Relatively rare in children, it appears as a consequence of congenital coronary abnormalities or as a complication following surgical procedures for congenital heart disease (CHD). Kawasaki disease is the primary cause of acquired coronary disease in children (Jui *et al.*, 2021).

Signs and symptoms

The severity of the symptoms will always depend on the severity of the heart condition. Symptoms also vary according to whether the left or the right side of the heart is primarily affected. Signs and symptoms across the age spectrum include:

Infant

- Poor weight gain, although the infant may be of average length – this is because the baby with CF has an increased metabolic rate and therefore needs additional calories; however, they tire easily and are unable to meet this calorific demand.
- Poor feeding due to fatigue.
- Diaphoresis (excessive sweating), especially when feeding, due to a catecholamine (epinephrine and norepinephrine) surge that occurs when babies are challenged with feeding while in respiratory distress.
- Tachypnoea – left-sided heart failure causes congestion of the pulmonary veins and respiratory symptoms, such as breathlessness and grunting.
- Hepatomegaly (enlargement of the liver) is caused by congestion from right-sided heart failure.

Child

- Respiratory distress, tachypnoea and hepatomegaly persist.
- Increased shortness of breath during activities.
- Orthopnoea (shortness of breath when lying flat) may be evident in older children, caused by increased distribution of blood to the pulmonary circulation.
- Tire easily.
- Oedema of the eyelids or feet, along with jugular venous distension caused by congestion of the right side of the heart.
- Weight gain may be present due to oedema.
- Dizziness due to a lack of blood supply and therefore oxygen to the brain.
- Abdominal pain, nausea and vomiting, especially after eating, due to mesenteric ischaemia; this is caused by poor blood supply to the mesentery.

General

- Tachycardia as the body attempts to pump more blood around the body.
- Gallop rhythm refers to an abnormal rhythm of the heart on auscultation. It includes three or even four sounds, thus resembling the sounds of a gallop. The normal heart rhythm contains two audible heart sounds, the 'lub-dub' rhythm caused by the closing of the heart valves.

- Hypotension due to poor cardiac output.
- Cool peripheries with a weak, thready pulse due to decreased circulation combined with tachycardia.
- Decreased urinary output due to low circulatory output.
- Cardiomegaly seen on chest X-ray is nearly always present.

Management

The management of CF in children involves treating the underlying cause, such as correcting anaemia, surgically correcting CHDs where possible or treating infections. Management also involves control of heart failure through the use of medication (Table 11.3), along with general supportive measures, such as rest and help with feeding. This may include high-calorie feeds through a nasogastric tube and elimination of salt in the older child's diet. Too much salt in the body causes water to be retained, which in turn increases fluid retention, further increasing oedema and breathing difficulties.

Babies and CYP with heart failure may require oxygen therapy. All healthcare professionals must remember that oxygen needs to be prescribed by a suitably qualified practitioner, and oxygen use must be documented for each patient.

Oxygen concentrations will vary from patient to patient depending on their individual condition. Inappropriate concentrations can have serious implications ranging from lung damage, convulsions and retinal damage, particularly in neonates.

In patients who have long-term severe lung disease, additional oxygen may slow their breathing sufficiently for carbon dioxide to build up to dangerous levels.

Healthcare professionals need to be aware of the dangers of administering too much oxygen. Saturation monitors and arterial blood gases will provide a measure of blood oxygen levels, although it should be noted that while internal oxygen levels may under normal circumstances be 100% (see Fig. 11.3), oxygen saturation monitor readings taken peripherally on a child receiving additional oxygen should not be 100%, as this may indicate that the child is receiving too much oxygen.

TABLE 11.3 Drugs that may be used in the treatment of heart failure

Drug	How it works	Possible side effects
Angiotensin-converting enzyme (ACE) inhibitors, e.g., captopril	Prevents conversion of angiotensin I to angiotensin II. Dilate the blood vessels, making it easier for the heart to pump blood to the body	Hyperkalaemia in children with impaired renal function Hypotension Persistent dry cough
Beta-blockers, e.g., atenolol	Decreases the activity of the heart by blocking the action of hormones such as epinephrine	May precipitate asthma Bradycardia Sleep disturbance in some instances
Diuretics, usually loop diuretics, e.g., furosemide	Inhibits the body's ability to reabsorb sodium at the ascending loop (loop of Henle) in the nephron, which leads to an excretion of water in the urine	Hypokalaemia Dehydration
Aldosterone antagonists, e.g., spironolactone	Inhibits sodium resorption in the collecting duct of the nephron in the kidneys. This interferes with sodium/potassium exchange, reducing urinary potassium excretion and weakly increasing water excretion	Hyperkalaemia Hyponatraemia Dehydration
Positive inotropic drugs, e.g., digoxin	Increases the force of contraction of the myocardium	Dizziness Irregular heartbeat
Anticoagulation, e.g., heparin	Interruption of the process involved in the formation of blood clots	Bleeding, which may cause, e.g., haematuria or nosebleeds

Source: Adapted from Joint Formulary Committee, (2025).

Classification of congenital heart defects

CHDs can be categorised into cyanotic and acyanotic defects. A baby or child with a cyanotic defect will present with a blue discolouration to their lips and extremities, whereas a baby or child with an acyanotic heart defect will retain their normal colouring. However, a child with an acyanotic defect may become cyanosed, and a child with a cyanotic defect may not show signs of cyanosis, and therefore, a more accurate classification involves blood flow (Fig. 11.2).

1. Increased pulmonary blood flow
2. Decreased pulmonary blood flow
3. Obstruction to blood flow out of the heart
4. Mixed blood flow.

Cyanosis occurs when there is an inadequate amount of oxygenated blood circulating in the body. The percentage of oxygen saturation varies through the heart chambers, with the left side reaching 100% oxygen saturation as the blood returns from the lungs. Oxygen saturation on the right side of the heart is 75% as the deoxygenated blood returns from the body. The left side of the heart has higher pressure than the right side, as the left ventricle is responsible for pumping blood throughout the body, whereas the right ventricle is only pumping blood to the lungs. Where there are defects, blood will flow from areas of higher pressure to lower pressure (Figs 11.3 and 11.4).

Special consideration

Cyanosis is routinely assessed through visual assessment of skin colour, with terms such as 'pink' or 'blue' being used to describe skin colour. In infants, children and young people with darker skin tones, this terminology is both controversial and inaccurate. A child with a darker skin tone may present with grey/white skin, which may be observed on the palms of the hands, soles of the feet, lips, tongue or inside the eyelids. Assessment of cyanosis should also include pulse oximetry, which, although better than visual assessment, may also be inaccurate in dark skin tones, specifically in neonates (Fair *et al.*, 2024).

Cardiac investigations

Diagnosing a CHD involves:

- History taking
- Gestational and perinatal history
- Postnatal and present history
- Family history
- Physical examination
- General appearance, e.g., respiratory state, colour including cyanosis, nutritional state
- Pulse including peripheral pulses and auscultation of the heart
- Blood pressure including four limb measurements
- Electrocardiogram

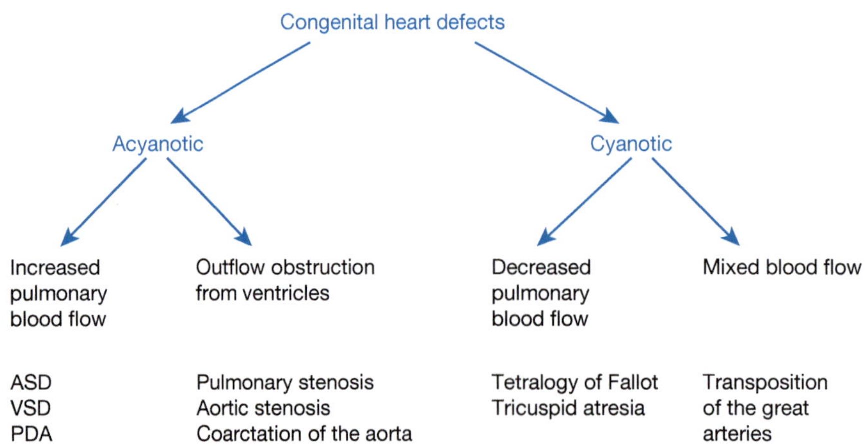

FIGURE 11.2 Classification of CHD.

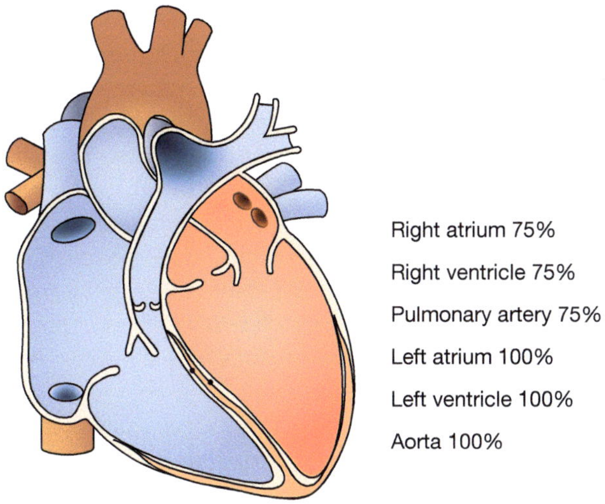

FIGURE 11.3 Oxygen saturation levels within the heart.

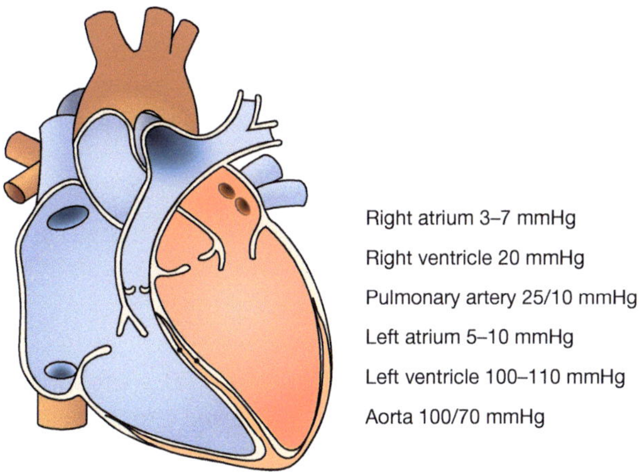

FIGURE 11.4 Pressure in mmHg within the heart.

- Chest X-ray to consider heart size
- Echocardiogram
- Magnetic resonance imaging (MRI) and cardiac computed tomography (CT) may occasionally be required
- Cardiac catheterisation.

Investigation

Cardiac catheterisation is an invasive procedure that is used:

- to inject a contrast medium to show up veins in and around the heart
- to open or widen narrow or blocked blood vessels or valves with the use of a balloon on the end of the catheter with or without stents, e.g., in PDA or pulmonary atresia
- to close holes or blood vessels, e.g., atrial septal defects (ASDs)
- to determine pressures within the heart
- to assess cardiomyopathy or myocarditis.

Depending on the age of the child, a general anaesthetic or sedation in the older child is required. A needle is inserted into the femoral vein with a guide wire; the catheter is then threaded through the vein to the heart. X-rays are used to show the position of the catheter.

Children need to recover from the anaesthetic/sedation by resting, tolerating fluids and diet and passing urine before being discharged home. There is a very small risk of bleeding from the injection site, and some discomfort may be experienced. Cardiac catheterisation is not without risk; complications can range from mild bruising around the injection site to death or cerebral infarction.

Acyanotic congenital heart defects

Increased pulmonary blood flow

Atrial septal defect

The interatrial septum is the wall of tissue that separates the right atrium from the left atrium. It develops in stages during the first and second months of foetal development. During development, a small section of the wall is left open, covered by a small flap; this is the foramen ovale, which is a vital part of foetal circulation as it allows blood to bypass the lungs. During foetal circulation, blood entering the heart bypasses the right ventricle, passing directly through the foramen ovale into the left atrium, through the left atrioventricular valve to the left ventricle and is then pumped back to the body via the aorta. The foetus receives oxygen from the mother through the placenta. The flap of the foramen ovale closes at birth as the pressures within the heart adjust to normal circulation.

An ASD occurs when the interatrial septum fails to develop correctly, leaving a hole in the atrial wall. Blood is forced back from the higher-pressure left atrium to the lower-pressure right atrium (Fig. 11.5).

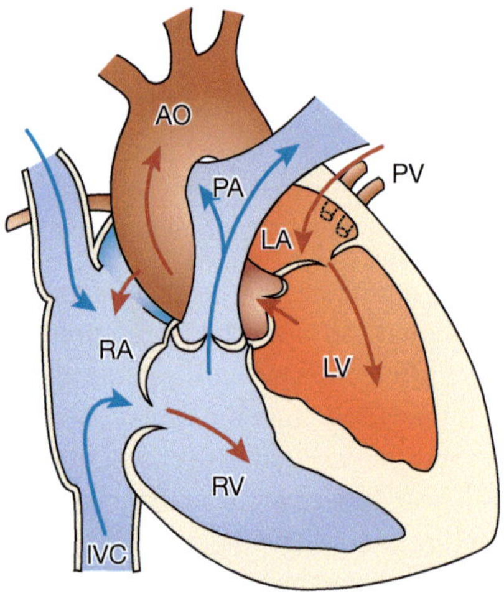

FIGURE 11.5 Diagram of ASD showing oxygenated blood flowing from the left atrium to the right atrium.

Types of ASD

- **Secundum ASD:** This is the most common type of ASD, accounting for 70% of all ASDs. It is in the centre of the atrial wall and is caused because the foramen ovale fails to close after birth, i.e., patent foramen ovale (PFO).
- **Primum ASD:** This accounts for about 25% of ASDs and arises from the lower end of the atrial septum.
- **Sinus venosus ASD:** This defect accounts for only 5% of ASDs and arises from the upper end of the atrial septum.

Pathophysiology

The slightly higher pressure within the left atrium causes oxygenated blood to flow from the left atrium through the septal defect to the right atrium, a left-to-right shunt, causing an increase in oxygenated blood through the right side of the heart. This additional flow is generally well tolerated, although it can cause the right side of the heart to stretch and enlarge.

Signs and symptoms

Small defects are mainly asymptomatic; a murmur may be heard on auscultation of the chest, and the defect may be detected during a routine health check.

Larger defects may cause symptoms of a left-to-right shunt with extra strain on the right-hand side of the heart. Babies may become breathless, especially during feeding and, therefore, struggle to gain weight. Older children may have poor exercise tolerance. Frequent chest infections may be an additional indication. Left untreated, CF or pulmonary hypertension may develop in later life.

Treatment

Eighty percent of small, secundum defects close spontaneously in the early years and may not require any treatment. A defect larger than 8 mm is unlikely to close spontaneously, nor is spontaneous closure likely to occur after the age of 4 years (Park & Salamat, 2021).

Larger defects may be closed through a cardiac catheterisation procedure using a septal occluder to cover the defect. A small catheter is inserted into a vein in the groin and fed through the vein to the heart. If this is not possible, open-heart surgery and cardiopulmonary bypass will be required.

Ventricular septal defect (VSD)

A VSD is a congenital defect (hole) of the interventricular septum, which is the wall separating the right and left ventricles (Fig. 11.6). At 4–8 weeks' gestation, the previously single ventricular chamber of the heart is remodelled, and development of the septum occurs to form a four-chambered heart (Chamley *et al.*, 2005), two ventricles and two atria. An error at this stage will result in a VSD.

Types of VSD

- Membranous VSD, which accounts for 80% of all VSDs.
- Muscular VSD.

Pathophysiology

Higher pressure in the left ventricle causes a left-to-right shunt of blood into the right ventricle and into the pulmonary artery. Increased blood volume in the right ventricle is pumped into the pulmonary artery and to the lungs. The increased blood flow to the lungs will, over a period of time,

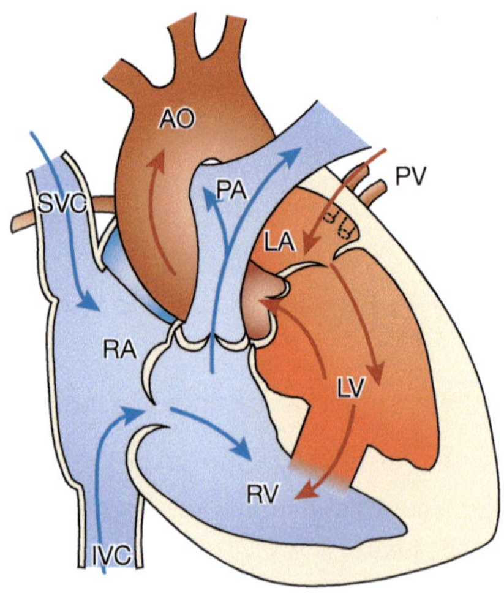

FIGURE 11.6 Diagram of VSD showing oxygenated blood flowing from the left ventricle to the right ventricle.

increase pulmonary vascular resistance. The increased pressure within the right ventricle and the increased pulmonary vascular resistance will cause the muscle of the right ventricle to hypertrophy. The right atrium may also enlarge as it attempts to overcome the resistance within the right ventricle.

Signs and symptoms

Infants and children with small VSDs may be asymptomatic. Larger defects will cause problems with growth and development as infants struggle to feed adequately. They may suffer from repeated chest infections, have a decreased exercise tolerance and develop CF. The degree and position of a murmur will depend on the severity of the defect, and a chest X-ray may show cardiomegaly (enlargement of the heart).

Treatment

Small VSDs may spontaneously close in 30–40% of cases (Park & Salamat, 2021). Surgical treatment is most likely to be required. Complete repair using sutures or a patch is common; this requires open heart surgery and cardiopulmonary bypass. Depending on size and location, it may be possible to close the VSD through a cardiac catheterisation procedure. Medical treatment for heart failure may be required prior to surgery. Surgery may be delayed in asymptomatic children until the age of 4 or 5 years. Those who respond well to medical treatment may have surgery delayed until approximately 18 months of age, whereas those with large defects and those who do not respond well to medical treatment should be operated on sooner.

Patent ductus arteriosus

Normal foetal circulation involves a small vessel, the DA, which connects the pulmonary artery to the aorta (Fig. 11.7). The foetal circulation bypasses the lungs due to oxygenation taking place at the placenta; blood is therefore diverted from the pulmonary artery directly into the aorta to return to the body. A PDA is the failure of the vessel to close at or shortly after birth; it accounts for 5–10% of all CHDs, excluding premature infants (Table 11.4).

Pathophysiology

Higher pressure within the aorta shunts the blood from the aorta into the pulmonary artery, resulting in the blood being returned to the lungs and then back to the left side of the heart. This increases the volume of blood in the left side of the heart, thus increasing the workload of the left side of the heart and pulmonary vascular congestion.

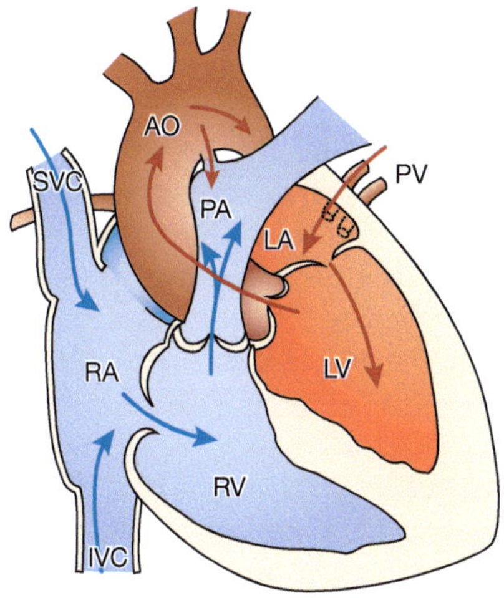

FIGURE 11.7 Diagram of PDA showing oxygenated blood returning to the heart from the aorta.

TABLE 11.4 Patent ductus arteriosus (PDA) in the premature infant

- PDA appears in 45% of infants weighing less than 1.7 kg at birth and in about 80% of infants weighing less than 1.2 kg (Park & Salamat, 2021).
- Additional problems are evident in infants with respiratory distress syndrome caused by the lack of surfactant in the lungs of premature infants. The pulmonary vascular resistance of the premature infant is reduced through improved oxygenation, but the ductus arteriosus remains open because its response to oxygen remains immature. This results in the shunt of blood from the aorta to the pulmonary artery and the resulting increased blood volume through the immature lungs and left side of the heart. Weaning an infant off ventilation becomes increasingly difficult.
- Episodes of bradycardia or apnoea may be evident in infants not requiring ventilation. A murmur and bounding peripheral pulses may be present.
- Pharmacological treatment for closure of a PDA may be achieved with intravenous ibuprofen or indomethacin.

Signs and symptoms

If the defect is small, infants may be asymptomatic; larger defects can increase the occurrence of chest infections, leading to heart failure and faltering growth. A murmur may be heard, and an echocardiogram may show cardiomegaly.

Treatment

A PDA found incidentally through an echocardiogram and causing no symptoms does not require closure. Closure via cardiac catheterisation is recommended when the PDA causes heart failure or concerns about the infant's growth and development. Surgical closure is indicated in some cases.

Outflow obstruction from ventricles

Outflow obstruction from the ventricles means that the blood leaving the heart from the ventricles, left or right, is met with an anatomical defect, a stenosis or narrowing. This causes an obstruction, which in turn causes an increase in pressure below the stenosis, usually in the ventricles, and a decrease in pressure beyond the stenosis in one of the great arteries. The stenosis is usually found near the valves.

Pulmonary stenosis

Blood leaves the right ventricle through the pulmonary artery, the entrance to which is guarded by the pulmonary valve. The valve consists of three semilunar cusps, and their function is to prevent backflow of blood into the right ventricle. Pulmonary stenosis (Fig. 11.8) is the narrowing of the pulmonary artery and accounts for 5–8% of all CHDs (Park & Salamat, 2021). Location of pulmonary stenosis may be:

- valvular – at the pulmonary valve (most common manifestation)
- subvalvular – narrowing below the valve
- supravalvular – narrowing of the pulmonary artery above the valve.

Pulmonary atresia is the most extreme form of pulmonary stenosis. There is no blood flow through the pulmonary artery, and survival is only possible if there is also an interatrial defect, such as an ASD, present.

Pathophysiology

Resistance to blood flow into the pulmonary artery causes increased pressure within and hypertrophy of the right ventricle. As the right ventricle fails, the pressure within the right atrium will increase, which may cause the foramen ovale to reopen. As the pressure will be higher in the right atrium, deoxygenated blood will be shunted across the foramen ovale and into the left atrium to the left ventricle through the aorta to the body – systemic cyanosis will be present. Severe pulmonary stenosis will lead to heart failure.

Signs and symptoms

Depending on the degree of obstruction, an infant or child may be asymptomatic, have mild cyanosis or have signs and symptoms of heart failure. A heart murmur will be present, and an echocardiogram will show a thickened pulmonary valve. The severity of the obstruction does not usually increase in mild cases, but may progress with age in moderate to severe cases.

Treatment

Balloon valvuloplasty is the treatment of choice where possible. A catheter, with a small collapsed balloon at the end, is inserted into the femoral vein and passed into the heart and the pulmonary artery. The balloon is then positioned in the narrowed valve, is inflated, stretching the valve open, before being deflated and removed. Surgery may be required if this procedure is unsuccessful or not indicated, for example, due to the position of the stenosis.

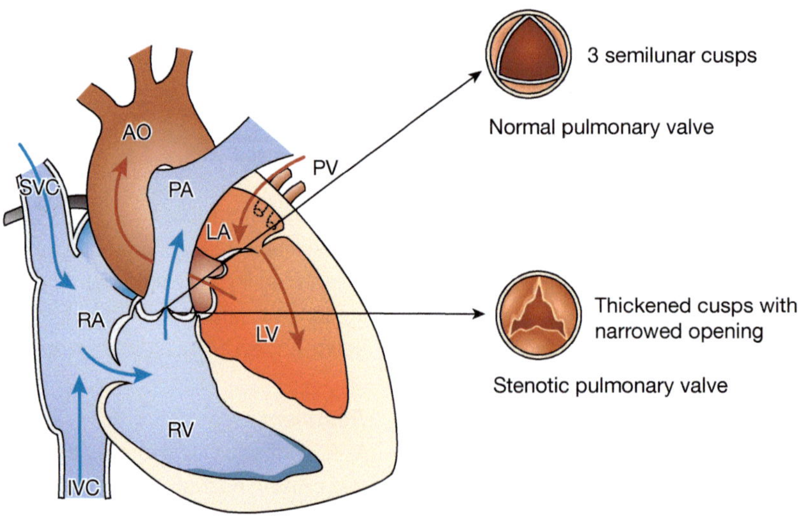

FIGURE 11.8 Diagram of pulmonary stenosis with right ventricular hypertrophy.

Aortic stenosis

The aorta is the body's largest artery. It begins in the left ventricle of the heart, ascends for a short distance before arching backwards and descending through the thoracic cavity, and on into the abdominal cavity. Blood is pumped from the muscular left ventricle through the aortic valve into the aorta and to the body. The aortic valve, formed of three semilunar cusps, guards the entrance of the aorta and prevents backflow of blood into the left ventricle. Aortic stenosis (Fig. 11.9) causes outflow obstruction from the left ventricle and accounts for 10% of all CHDs (Park & Salamat, 2021). Aortic stenosis location may be:

- valvular – at the aortic valve is the most common manifestation and is generally caused by malformation of the cusps, resulting in a bicuspid rather than a tricuspid valve, or from the fusion of the cusps. Many cases of bicuspid aortic valve go unnoticed in childhood (Park & Salamat, 2021);
- subvalvular – narrowing of the aorta below the valve;
- supravalvular – narrowing of the aorta above the valve.

Aortic atresia is the most extreme form of aortic stenosis. There is no blood flow through the aorta, and survival is only possible if the DA remains open. Aortic atresia usually occurs in combination with other heart defects, typically hypoplastic left heart syndrome.

Pathophysiology

Resistance to blood flow into the aorta causes increased pressure within the left ventricle. The extra workload causes hypertrophy (thickening) of the left ventricle. As the left ventricle fails, the pressure within the left atrium will increase, which in turn causes increased pressure within the pulmonary veins and leads to pulmonary oedema/congestion.

Signs and symptoms

Children with mild to moderate degrees of aortic stenosis may be asymptomatic, although they may be exercise-intolerant, presenting with signs of chest pain and dizziness. Blood pressure is generally normal, as is an electrocardiogram (ECG). Diagnosis is confirmed with an echocardiogram. In the case of aortic stenosis, the severity may worsen with time as a result of calcification (Park & Salamat, 2021).

Neonates with severe aortic stenosis will show signs of reduced cardiac output, weak pulses, hypotension, tachycardia and poor feeding.

Treatment

The critically ill neonate will need medical treatment for heart failure, such as inotropic drugs and diuretics, along with prostaglandin to keep the DA open. Balloon valvuloplasty (see pulmonary atresia) of the aortic valve is the first line of treatment to stretch the aortic valve and increase blood flow. Surgical repair or replacement of the valve may be indicated if valvuloplasty is unsuccessful or as the condition worsens.

Medicine management

A newborn infant with a congenital heart defect (CHD) that is reliant on the DA remaining open to provide some blood circulation, e.g., in the case of aortic atresia, is given prostaglandin E1 or prostaglandin E2, which are strong vasodilators.

Naturally occurring prostaglandin E2 is produced by both the placenta and the DA itself, and is the most potent of the E prostaglandins. It is what keeps the DA open in the unborn child. Prostaglandin E1 also has a role in keeping the DA open. Immediately after birth, the levels of prostaglandin significantly reduce, allowing the DA to close.

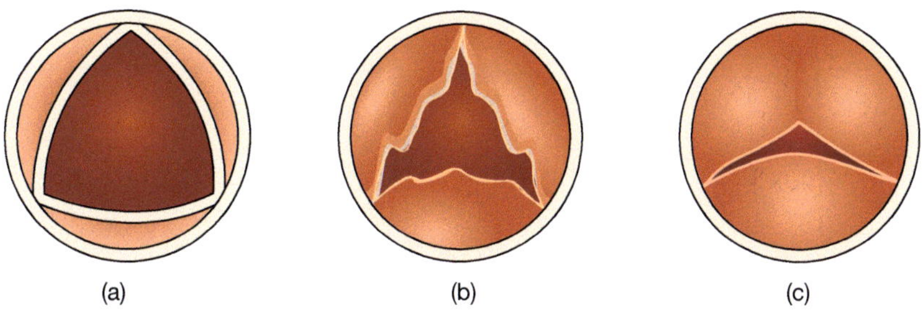

FIGURE 11.9 Diagram showing (a) normal tricuspid aorta valve; (b) stenotic tricuspid aorta valve; (c) abnormal bicuspid aorta valve.

Prostaglandin is given intravenously, and the dose is calculated according to the body weight of the infant.

During the infusion, the baby requires careful monitoring of heart rate, blood pressure, respiratory rate and core body temperature as the side effects of prostaglandin include apnoea, severe bradycardia, hypotension and fever. In the event of such occurrences, the infusion may be stopped temporarily and restarted at a lower dose, or the baby may require ventilator support in order for the prostaglandin to continue (Joint Formulary Committee, 2025).

Coarctation of the aorta

As the aorta arches backwards and begins its descent, there is a narrowing of the vessel. This is known as coarctation of the aorta (Fig. 11.10) and accounts for 8–10% of all CHDs (Park & Salamat, 2021). The most common manifestation is distal to the left subclavian artery, and this may be before or after the DA.

Pathophysiology

As the narrowing of the aorta causes an obstruction to the blood flow, there is increased pressure proximal (before) to the defect and decreased pressure distal (after) to it. The increased pressure affects the head and upper extremities, where the blood is supplied from the carotid and subclavian arteries, respectively, and also the heart, as the blood is unable to move normally through the aorta. Decreased pressure affects the remainder of the body.

Signs and symptoms

Infants and children fall into one of two categories: symptomatic and asymptomatic.

Asymptomatic children and young people may occasionally complain of headaches, epistaxis, leg pains and cramps with exercise or decreased exercise ability (Raza *et al.*, 2023). The pulse in the legs is weak or absent, and the blood pressure is lower in the lower limbs than in the upper limbs. ECG and chest X-ray are generally normal; however, an echocardiogram will reveal the altered blood flow.

Symptomatic infants often have additional heart defects, such as transposition of the great arteries (TGA), VSD or PDA, and they present with signs of heart failure with poor feeding, dyspnoea and oliguria. Heart murmurs are not usually present, but a loud gallop is present along with weak and thread pulses. Chest X-ray shows signs of cardiomegaly, and an echocardiogram confirms the site and size of the coarctation and any other defects.

Treatment

For the older infant and child, balloon angioplasty may be performed to widen the narrowing of the aorta. A catheter, with a deflated balloon, is passed through the femoral artery to the aorta; on reaching the narrowing, the balloon is inflated to make the narrowing wider. An expandable stent may also be put in position at this stage, although this is generally used in children of at least 8 years of age.

Surgical correction of resection of the narrowed segment with an end-to-end anastomosis is the surgical treatment of choice.

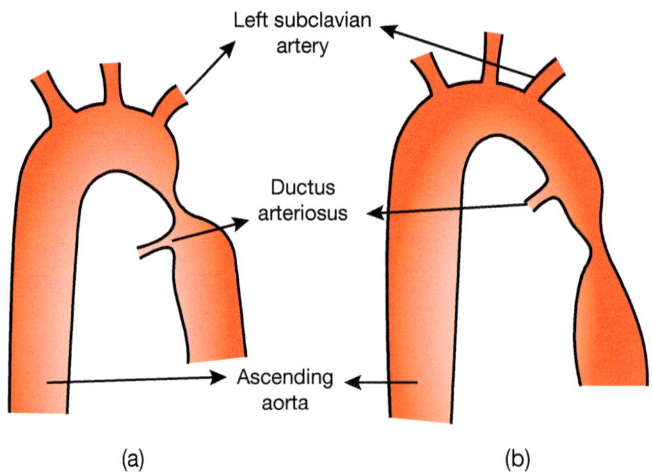

FIGURE 11.10 Diagram showing (a) preductal coarctation of the aorta; (b) post-ductal coarctation of the aorta.

Cyanotic congenital heart defects

Decreased pulmonary blood flow

Tetralogy of Fallot

Tetralogy of Fallot (TOF) accounts for about 10% of all CHDs and occurs equally in boys and girls. It is associated with several genetic conditions, including trisomy 21 (Down syndrome) and DiGeorge syndrome, in which airway difficulties are commonly found (Heriwardito & Aristya, 2022). TOF (Fig. 11.11) consists of four defects:

1. ventricular septal defect – this is generally large
2. pulmonary stenosis – usually affecting the valve
3. overriding aorta – the aorta is positioned above the VSD
4. right ventricular hypertrophy.

Pathophysiology

Narrowing of the pulmonary valve, causing outflow obstruction from the right ventricle, causes the right ventricle to work harder, and hence it becomes hypertrophied. The large VSD equalises the pressures in the two ventricles, although a shunt may still be evident depending on the pulmonary vascular resistance versus the systemic resistance; this will depend on the degree of pulmonary stenosis. A right-to-left shunt will be evident if the resistance is greater in the pulmonary arteries, forcing unoxygenated blood into the overriding aorta and giving the child a cyanotic presentation.

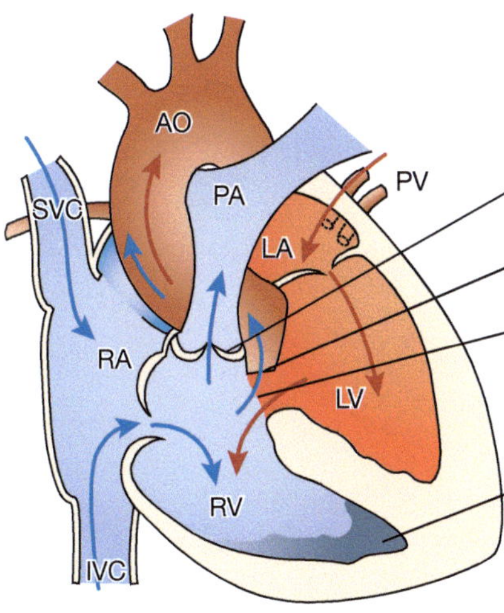

FIGURE 11.11 Diagram of tetralogy of Fallot.

Signs and symptoms

Children with an acyanotic TOF that is a left-to-right shunt, demonstrating that the pulmonary resistance is not too high, are often asymptomatic.

Symptomatic infants may be acutely cyanosed at birth or develop worsening cyanosis over a period of time as the pulmonary resistance increases. The children may suffer from dyspnoea, clubbing and acute episodes of cyanosis and hypoxia (known as hypercyanotic spells). These occur when the body's oxygen requirement cannot be met, for example, during feeding or crying. The right-to-left shunt stimulates the respiratory centre to increase breathing, which in turn increases the venous return and further increases the right-to-left shunt. A heart murmur will be present, and a chest X-ray will demonstrate a boot-shaped heart, caused by the right ventricular hypertrophy, although an echocardiogram will be the definitive diagnosis.

Treatment

Hypercyanotic spells, during which the infant becomes acutely cyanosed with deeper and faster breathing, occur most frequently in the morning with crying, feeding or when passing a stool. Treatment includes calming the baby and holding the baby in the knee-chest position, which increases systemic vascular resistance and therefore decreases the right-to-left shunting and aims to break the cycle. A severe hypercyanotic spell can lead to limpness, convulsions, risk of emboli or death (Park & Salamat, 2021). If the hypercyanotic spell continues, medical treatment to suppress the respirations, for example, morphine, may be administered, along with treatment of the acidosis with sodium bicarbonate.

Treatment of TOF includes medication to control hypercyanotic spells until surgery is indicated; dilation of the pulmonary artery may be performed as an interim step prior to full surgical correction.

Clubbing of the fingers and toes is characterised by a thickening and flattening of the tips of the digits. Clubbing is associated with cyanotic CHDs and bacterial endocarditis. It is thought to occur because of chronic tissue hypoxaemia and polycythaemia – an overproduction of red blood cells due to low oxygen levels.

Healthcare professionals need to be aware that the presence of clubbing is known to significantly compromise the registration of SaO_2 on the extremities, with the result that readings are underestimated. Alternative sites, such as the earlobe, should be considered. However, blood gases remain the gold standard for measuring blood oxygen levels.

Tricuspid atresia

The atrioventricular valves begin to develop between weeks 5 and 8 of gestation. Initially, bicuspid, the right atrioventricular valve develops a third cusp in the third month (Chamley *et al.*, 2005). Failure of this tricuspid valve to develop results in tricuspid atresia (Fig. 11.12); blood is unable to flow from the right atrium to the right ventricle. However, blood will flow through the PFO to the left atrium, through the left atrioventricular valve to the left ventricle and then through a VSD to the right ventricle and into the pulmonary artery for oxygenation in the lungs.

Pathophysiology

At birth, it is imperative that the foramen ovale remains open, and a VSD is required for circulation and therefore survival. The right ventricle and pulmonary artery are hypoplastic (underdeveloped), and there is often an associated TGA. All blood entering the heart is shunted across from the right atrium to the left atrium, causing dilation and hypertrophy of the right atrium. The left atrium and ventricle are enlarged as all blood, systemic and pulmonary, is shunted through the left side of the heart.

Signs and symptoms

Cyanosis is present at birth with associated tachycardia, dyspnoea and difficulty in feeding. Older children may have clubbing as a result of chronic hypoxia. A murmur is heard on auscultation, chest X-ray may show a boot-shaped heart, while an echocardiogram provides the diagnostic test.

Treatment

Intravenous prostaglandin is required to keep the DA open, and a balloon septostomy may be performed to enlarge the shunt between the right and left atria. Staged surgery occurs over the first 1–2 years to correct abnormalities associated with tricuspid atresia.

Mixed blood flow

Transposition of the great arteries

TGA accounts for 5% of all CHDs. In normal circulation, the pulmonary artery leaves the right ventricle and goes to the lungs, where blood is oxygenated. The aorta leaves the left ventricle, and blood is delivered to the rest of the body. In TGA, the pulmonary artery leaves the left ventricle, and the aorta leaves the right ventricle. With no other defects, this provides two independent circulatory systems and is not compatible with life (Fig. 11.13).

Pathophysiology

For survival, additional defects such as ASD, VSD and PDA are required. A VSD is present in about 40% of cases, while in 40% of cases, there is only a small ASD or PDA (Park & Salamat, 2021). Hypoxia quickly progresses in neonates with minimal mixing of blood, and early death can occur.

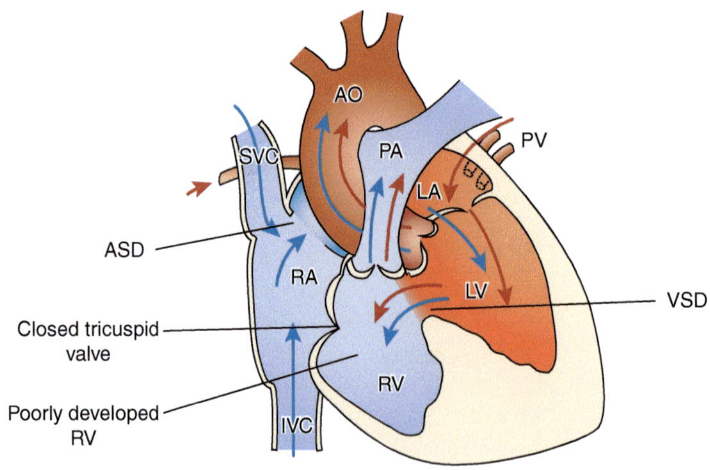

FIGURE 11.12 Diagram of tricuspid atresia.

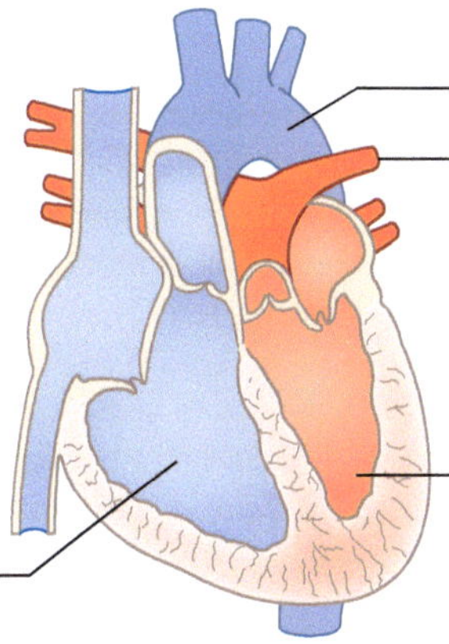

FIGURE 11.13 Transposition of the great arteries. The aorta takes blood from the right ventricle, and the pulmonary artery takes blood from the left ventricle.
Source: Reproduced with permission of Peate & Gormley-Fleming (2015)/John Wiley & Sons.

Signs and symptoms

Cyanosis is evident as blood returning from the body is recirculated to the body without oxygenation. Signs of heart failure may be seen as the heart attempts to overcome the defects, especially when a VSD is present. There is no murmur if there is no VSD; however, a murmur will be present if there is an associated VSD. Chest X-ray shows cardiomegaly, and an echocardiogram will demonstrate the extent of the problems.

Treatment

Prostaglandin infusion is required to keep the DA open, and in the absence of a VSD, a balloon atrial septostomy is performed to increase the flow of oxygen-rich blood to the body. Signs of heart failure need to be treated with the appropriate medication. Surgery to swap the great vessels back to the correct position occurs within a few weeks of birth.

Children and young people with CHD are at an increased risk of morbidity, with psychiatric disorders being the most common. Separation anxieties, intensive care stressors, disruption of 'normal' routine from school and peers and concerns of body image in adolescence can lead to increased anxiety and stress. Adolescents face vulnerability when they are attempting to find their independence; they face uncertain futures in terms of health, which in turn affects education and future career pathways. Additionally, adolescents face the stress of transitioning from children to adult healthcare services. Depressive symptoms and loneliness among adolescents with CHD are closely linked and have been associated with poorer quality of life (Kovacs *et al.*, 2022).

Case study 11.1

Ben is a newborn, delivered by normal vaginal delivery at 38 weeks' gestation after his mother, Sally, went into labour spontaneously. Sally had a traumatic pregnancy as her first ultrasound scan at 12 weeks' gestation identified concerns about the condition of her unborn baby's heart. Following more scans in the second trimester, Sally was informed that Ben had hypoplastic left heart syndrome. Ben was delivered in a specialist unit and admitted to the cardiac unit for stabilisation. Hypoplastic left heart syndrome is a congenital defect of the heart characterised by underdevelopment of the left ventricle with associated stenosis or atresia of the aortic valve and also the mitral valves. The ascending aorta is also hypoplastic, as there is restricted foetal blood flow through the aorta. Ben's in utero blood returning from the lungs entered the left atrium and was then diverted across the foramen ovale, into the right atrium, to the right ventricle, into the pulmonary artery and through the DA to enter the aorta, and on to the rest of the body.

Vital signs

The following vital signs were noted and recorded immediately after birth (Fig. 11.14):

Vital sign	Observation	Normal
Temperature	36.1 °C	36.5–37.5 °C
Pulse	160 beats per minute	100–170 beats per minute
Respirations	56 breaths per minute	40–60 breaths per minute
Blood pressure	52/31 mmHg	65/41 mmHg
Oxygen saturations	93%	98–100%
Colour	Mild cyanosis	Pink
PEWS score	0	

- Reflect and consider why immediately after birth, Ben's vital signs of pulse, respiration and blood pressure fall within normal parameters.
- Without treatment, what is the likely outcome for Ben?

Within 12 hours, Ben is looking critically ill. The following vital signs were noted and recorded:

Vital sign	Observation	Normal
Temperature	37.1 °C	36.5–37.5 °C
Pulse	190 bpm	100–170 bpm
Respirations	75 breaths per minute	40–60 breaths per minute
Blood pressure	50/30 mmHg	65/41 mmHg
Oxygen saturations	86%	98–100%
Colour	Cyanosed	Pink
PEWS score	4	

Other signs include:

Poor peripheral pulses
Gallop rhythm
Hepatomegaly
Pulmonary crackles

- Reflect and consider what changes are occurring within Ben's heart, causing him to deteriorate so rapidly.
- What investigations may be required?
- What immediate treatment will be required?

Investigations

- Full physical examination plus chest X-ray, which shows a mildly enlarged heart and pulmonary venous congestion
- Echocardiogram
- Electrocardiogram

Electrocardiogram

An ECG is used to check the heart's rhythm and electrical activity. Leads are attached to the patient and a trace is recorded on the monitor. The normal P, QRS and T waves are representative of the electrical activity within the heart during one full cardiac cycle. In a normal sinus rhythm, the P wave represents atrial contraction, the QRS complex represents the depolarisation of the ventricles causing them to contract and the T wave is the repolarisation or relaxation of the ventricles.

The child and family need to be fully informed and prepared for the procedure. An ECG may be recorded with 3, 6 or 12 leads. The electrodes are placed on the child (see Fig. 11.15):

Chest

- V1 – 4th intercostal space to right of sternum
- V2 – 4th intercostal space to left of sternum
- V3 – midway between V2 and V4
- V4 – 5th intercostal space at mid-clavicular line
- V5 – 5th left intercostal space, midway between V4 and V6
- V6 – 5th left intercostal space

Limbs

- One on each arm at wrist level
- One on each leg, just above the ankle

Treatment

Initial treatment for hypoplastic left heart syndrome is stabilisation of the infant, including ventilation and inotropes to correct heart failure. Prostaglandin infusion is required to keep the DA open and ensure adequate systemic circulation. A balloon atrial septostomy may be performed to ensure the patency of the left and right atria.

It is not possible to correct hypoplastic left heart syndrome, but surgery can be carried out to allow the heart to function more adequately. Surgery is done in stages and is either the Norwood procedure or the hybrid approach. Heart transplantation is an alternative option.

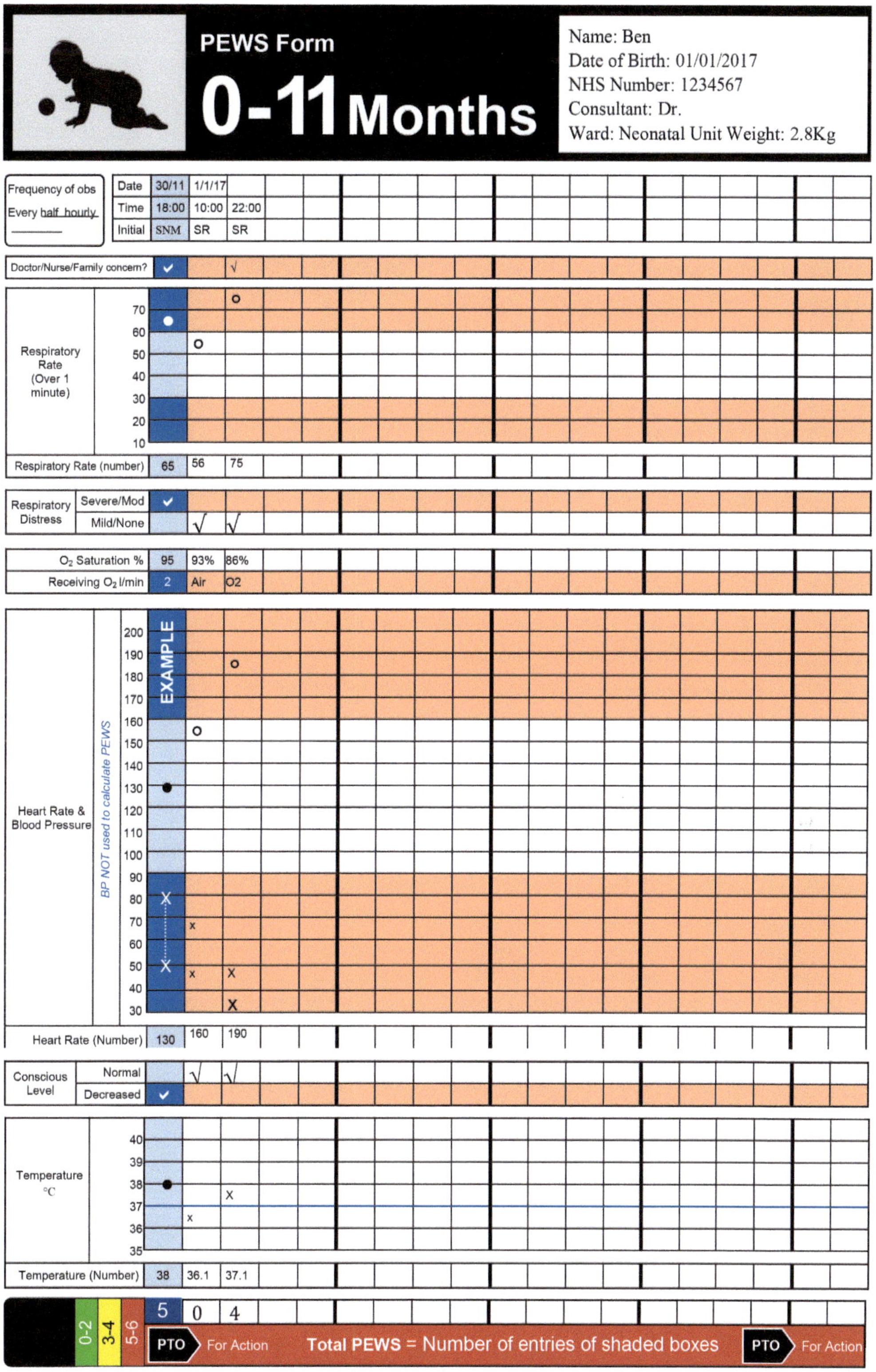

FIGURE 11.14 PEWS chart.

Source: NHS (2024).

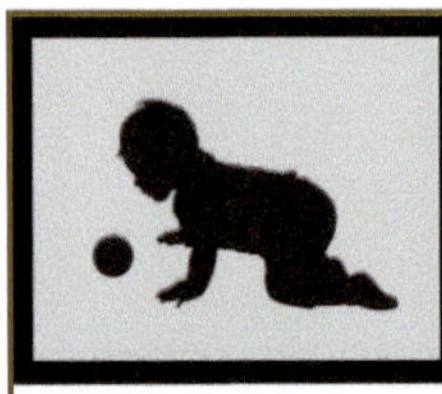

PEWS Form

0-11 Months

Name
Date of Birth
NHS Number
Consultant
Ward Weight

PEWS Escalation Aid

S **Situation:**
I am (name), a nurse on ward (X)
I am calling about (child X)
I am calling because I am concerned that…
(e.g. BP is low/high, pulse is XXX
temperature is XX, Early Warning Score is XX)

B **Background:**
Child (X) was admitted on (XX date) with
(e.g. respiratory infection)
They have had (X operation/procedure/investigation)
Child (X)'s condition has changed in the last (XX mins)
Their last set of obs were (XXX)
The child's normal condition is…
(e.g. alert/drowsy/confused, pain free)

A **Assessment:**
I think the problem is (XXX)
and I have…
(e.g. given O2 /analgesia, stopped the infusion)
OR
I am not sure what the problem is but child (X) is deteriorating
OR
I don't know what's wrong but I am really worried

R **Recommendation:**
I need you to…
Come to see the child in the next (XX mins)
AND
Is there anything I need to do in the meantime?
(e.g. stop the fluid/repeat the obs)

Download SBAR prompt cards and pads at
www.institute.nhs.uk/SBAR

Remember: If you feel you need more help at any time, call for help – regardless of PEW Score

Score	Action
0 1	Continue monitoring
2	Nurse in charge MUST review
3	Nurse in charge & Doctor MUST review
4	Nurse in charge & Doctor MUST review & inform Consultant
5 6	Nurse in charge & Consultant MUST review

Record Call When PEWS 3 Or More				Record Time of Review, Who by & Plan		
Date	Time	PEWS	Print Name (nurse)	Time	Plan	Print Name
01/01/12	09:00	5	SN Morton	09:15	ED consultant called Anaesthetic review	Sister JACKS

NHS Institute for Innovation and Improvement

Download documents to use or edit at
www.institute.nhs.uk/PEWScharts

FIGURE 11.14 *(Continued)*

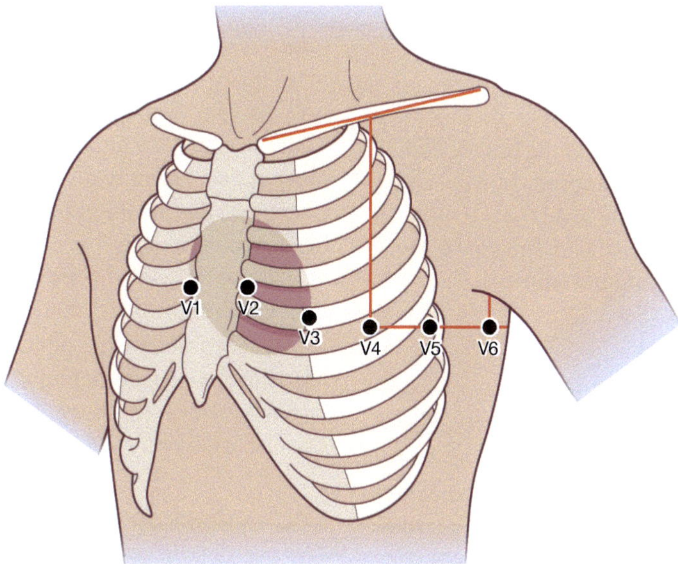

FIGURE 11.15 Position of chest ECG leads.
Source: Nair and Peate (2017)/with permission of John Wiley & Sons.

Special Considerations for Children with a CHD

CHD can lead to an increased risk of neurodevelopmental concerns in children and young people, including learning difficulties and behavioural problems. This increased risk may be as a result of the greater incidence of CHD with other factors, e.g., Down syndrome, but also as a result of potential episodes of hypoxia, surgical interventions and the stress of ongoing medical interventions. Silva *et al.* (2024) suggest that children with 'simple' heart defects have more favourable outcomes than those with complex conditions requiring a greater level of medical intervention. Infants and toddlers with CHD are at a greater risk of impaired motor development, specifically in the first 18 months of life (Huisenga *et al.*, 2022). Ongoing developmental assessment and support are essential in ensuring these CYP are able to reach their full potential.

It is important for children and young people with a CHD to consider exercise. Despite the benefits, the paediatric cardiologist must be consulted prior to starting to exercise, as there may be restrictions in some incidences, e.g., children and young people with a pacemaker. Moderate exercise, where the heart beats faster, but the individual is still able to speak, is beneficial for a range of reasons: promotes sleep, reduces anxiety and depression, promotes a sense of belonging with peers and is known to improve overall quality of life.

Acquired heart disease

Acquired heart disease in children refers to conditions that occur after birth or which affect an otherwise normal heart. They occur for a variety of reasons, such as infection, autoimmune responses or environmental factors.

Kawasaki disease

Pathophysiology

Kawasaki disease predominantly affects infants and young children, although it can occasionally affect older children and adolescents. It is an acute, self-limited disease causing vasculitis of small- and medium-sized vessels. Initially affecting the small capillaries, it progresses to affect the medium-sized vessels, including the coronary arteries. Left untreated, approximately 1 in 4 children will develop dilation of the coronary arteries and formation of coronary artery aneurysms, making Kawasaki disease the most common cause of acquired heart disease in children. The precise cause of Kawasaki disease is unknown, although one or multiple infectious triggers is/are most likely, combined with potential abnormalities of the immune system. Other arteries, such as the iliac, femoral, axillary and renal, may also be affected but with less frequency.

Signs and symptoms

- Fever > 39 °C, for at least 5 days, not responding to antipyretic medication or antibiotics
- Bilateral conjunctivitis
- Red cracked lips
- Strawberry tongue – the coating of the tongue comes off, leaving the large papillae exposed
- Oedematous hands and feet
- Erythema of palms and soles leading to peeling of skin on the fingers and toes in the later stages.

Cardiac involvement

Tachycardia, gallop rhythm, cardiomegaly and other signs of CF may be present. When coronary artery aneurysms appear (rarely before 10 days of onset of illness (Park & Salamat, 2021)), they vary in size; the larger aneurysms can thrombose or clot, causing myocardial infarction. Aneurysms that heal do so with stenosis, causing myocardial ischaemia months or even years later. Symptoms of myocardial infarction in children include abdominal pain, pallor, restlessness and shock. Younger children rarely complain of chest pain. Additionally, children may develop myocarditis, valvular regurgitation or pericardial effusion, all of which lead to poor cardiac function.

Treatment

The aim of the treatment is to reduce inflammation within the coronary arteries and to prevent thrombosis by inhibiting platelet accumulation (Park & Salamat, 2021).

- Intravenous immunoglobulin reduces the incidence of coronary artery aneurysms from about 20% to less than 5% (Nadig *et al.*, 2023).
- Aspirin is used for its antiplatelet effect.
- Corticosteroids.

Medicine management

Aspirin (acetylsalicylic acid) is unlicensed for children under the age of 16 years. An unlicensed drug is a medication that does not have a marketing authorisation provided by the Medicines and Healthcare products Regulatory Agency (MHRA). The MHRA is responsible for ensuring medicines are safe. Prescribing unlicensed medicines to children increases the prescriber's potential liability; the prescription must therefore be justified, and the child (if age appropriate) and the child's carer must be informed (Joint Formulary Committee, 2025).

Infective endocarditis

Infective endocarditis is an infection of the valves and inner lining of the heart, which can lead to valve damage and varying degrees of morbidity or even mortality. Children who have undergone surgery for major CHDs are most at risk (Vicent *et al.*, 2022), and children with a prosthetic heart valve are at particularly high risk. It can also occur spontaneously.

Various organisms are responsible for causing infective endocarditis, including *Streptococcus*, most commonly seen following dental procedures. *Enterococci* found following genitourinary or gastrointestinal surgery, and *Staphylococcus* found in post-operative endocarditis can also cause infective endocarditis.

Pathophysiology

The microorganisms grow on a section of the endocardium, where there is or has been an abnormal flow or pressure of blood. The change in the endocardium makes it susceptible to the growth of invading organisms, which form a vegetation. These lesions may invade surrounding heart tissue, such as the valves or myocardium, or they may break off and cause an embolism somewhere within the body.

Signs and symptoms

Signs and symptoms include a low-grade prolonged pyrexia along with other non-specific symptoms such as malaise, headaches and weight loss. A heart murmur is likely to be heard, and splenomegaly is common. Petechiae may be seen on the skin or mucous membranes, and signs that result from embolus formation elsewhere in the body may be present.

Routine blood tests, including full blood count (FBC) and C-reactive protein (CRP), are required. Positive blood cultures, raised erythrocyte sedimentation rate (ESR) and anaemia, along with ECG changes and an echocardiogram, will all aid diagnosis.

Treatment

High doses of intravenous antibiotics are required for a prolonged period of time; these should be modified as blood culture results become available. Early treatment of infective endocarditis generally has a successful outcome, but when treatment is delayed, emboli are present, or heart valve involvement has occurred, prognosis may be less favourable. Death occurs as a result of heart failure or myocardial infarction.

Rheumatic fever

Rheumatic fever is caused by group A haemolytic streptococcal infection of the pharynx. The child, commonly 6–15 years of age, will present with a recent history (1–5 weeks) of a streptococcal throat infection. Rheumatic fever causes the body to attack its own tissues, causing widespread inflammation, affecting joints, skin and the brain, with the most serious complication being cardiac valve damage.

Signs and symptoms

Signs and symptoms are described as major or minor (Table 11.5) and are accompanied by a history of streptococcal throat infection or elevated streptococcal antibody titre. Streptococcal antibody titre is a blood test that measures the amount of antibodies within a person's blood; an elevated level is diagnostic of a recent streptococcal infection. Diagnosis requires the presence of two major or one major and two minor manifestations, plus the evidence of a recent streptococcal infection (Chowdhury *et al.*, 2025).

TABLE 11.5 Manifestations of rheumatic fever

Major manifestations	Minor manifestations
Arthritis, swelling, pain, redness and heat, involving one or several of the large joints	Fever, low grade, but may spike in the early evening
Carditis resulting in tachycardia, a heart murmur, pericarditis, cardiomegaly and signs of heart failure	Arthralgia or joint pain
Erythema marginatum is a type of erythema (redness of the skin or mucous membranes) involving pink rings on the trunk and inner surfaces of the limbs. The rash disappears in the cold and reappears in the warm.	Blood results reflect inflammatory responses, raised erythrocyte sedimentation rate (ESR) and C-reactive protein (CRP)
Subcutaneous nodules are small non-tender swellings, which may be found singularly or in crops over bony prominences, such as feet, hands, elbows or scalp.	An ECG would demonstrate a prolonged PR interval, indicating some degree of heart block
Sydenham chorea is a disorder characterised by rapid, uncoordinated jerking movements primarily affecting the extremities and it reflects the involvement of the central nervous system	

Treatment

Following diagnosis, benzathine penicillin is the antibiotic of choice. Anti-inflammatory medication is required for the treatment of arthritis and carditis. Bed rest is indicated in all cases, ranging from a week or two for mild symptoms to a couple of months for severe symptoms. Prophylactic antibiotics are recommended for all children who have had rheumatic fever, the duration of which depends on the severity of the condition, but may be lifelong.

Medicine management

Penicillin refers to a group of antibiotics that includes benzylpenicillin (penicillin G) and phenoxymethylpenicillin (penicillin V). They are bactericidal and act by interfering with bacterial cell wall synthesis. Penicillins diffuse into the body tissues and are excreted in the urine (Joint Formulary Committee, 2025).

Penicillin is commonly associated with an *allergic reaction*, and a patient's history or family history of allergy to penicillin must be checked. Common signs and symptoms of penicillin allergy include urticaria, diarrhoea and fever. Severe reactions include anaphylaxis, a life-threatening condition that affects multiple body systems.

Patients who are allergic to one penicillin will be allergic to them all because the hypersensitivity is related to the basic penicillin structure.

Cardiomyopathy

Cardiomyopathy is a chronic and progressive disease in which the myocardium is abnormally enlarged and thickened. Cardiomyopathy generally begins in the ventricles and progresses to affect the atria. The muscle cells become damaged, the heart weakens and is unable to pump blood efficiently and heart failure develops. In approximately 50% of cases, the cause of cardiomyopathy is unknown, although some known causes include:

- myocarditis, the most known cause of dilated cardiomyopathy
- familial, the common inheritance mode is autosomal dominant (Ullah, 2023)

- infections, predominantly viral, but may be bacterial and fungal
- arrhythmias, e.g., supraventricular tachycardia or bradycardia
- endocrine disorders, e.g., hyper-/hypothyroidism or congenital adrenal hyperplasia
- storage disease, e.g., glycogen storage disease
- nutritional deficiencies, e.g., protein, thiamine or vitamin E/D
- ischaemia, e.g., hypoxia, birth asphyxia or drowning
- toxins, e.g., radiation, penicillin sensitivity, iron or copper
- systemic disorders, e.g., systemic lupus, juvenile idiopathic arthritis

Cardiomyopathy in children is divided into three categories according to the type of abnormal structure and the dysfunction present:

- dilated cardiomyopathy,
- hypertrophic cardiomyopathy,
- restrictive cardiomyopathy.

Dilated cardiomyopathy

Dilated cardiomyopathy is rare but the most common type of cardiomyopathy in children.

Pathophysiology

A weakening of the systolic contraction, that is, the contraction of the ventricles and specifically the left ventricle, is associated with dilation of all four heart chambers. Thrombus formation is common in the apical portion of the ventricles or in the atrial appendages, which may lead to pulmonary and systemic embolisation (Park & Salamat, 2021). Dilated cardiomyopathy may progress to heart failure and is associated with an increased risk of arrhythmia, and may lead to end-stage heart failure within 1–5 years (Ullah, 2023).

Signs and symptoms

The signs and symptoms include tiredness and general signs of heart failure; see the previous section on heart failure. An echocardiogram will be diagnostic, although cardiac catheterisation may give a more complete aetiology.

Treatment

Treatment is associated with heart failure, along with treating the underlying cause if known. Children may progress to needing a heart transplant.

Hypertrophic cardiomyopathy

Hypertrophic cardiomyopathy is the second most common form of the heart disease affecting the heart muscle. It is genetically transmitted in many cases. Hypertrophic cardiomyopathy is the most common cause of sudden cardiac death in adolescents (Park & Salamat, 2021).

Pathophysiology

An abnormal growth of muscle fibres leads to thickening (hypertrophy) of the heart walls, typically the left ventricle and specifically the septum is most often affected, this is known as asymmetric septal hypertrophy. However, the distribution, location and degree of hypertrophy may vary. Symmetric ventricular hypertrophy refers to evenly distributed hypertrophy throughout the ventricles, and apical hypertrophy refers to thickening at the apex of the heart. The thickened muscle walls cause the heart to be stiff and small, leading to difficulties with blood flow. Progressive hypertrophy leads to obstruction of blood flow.

Signs and symptoms

Dyspnoea, tiredness, palpitations and chest pain are often the presenting signs and symptoms. Heart murmurs are heard, ECG abnormalities are common and echocardiograms will demonstrate varying degrees of hypertrophy. Sudden death may occur during exercise, and atrial fibrillation may cause a stroke.

Treatment

Treatment includes reducing the left ventricular outflow obstruction and increasing the ventricular compliance. Beta-blockers reduce the degree of obstruction, decrease the incidence of angina pain and have anti-arrhythmic actions (Park & Salamat, 2021).

Restrictive cardiomyopathy

Restrictive cardiomyopathy is extremely rare in children, and it is generally idiopathic with a poor outlook.

Pathophysiology

The ventricles are normal in size and pumping (systolic) function, but have abnormal diastolic filling due to the stiff ventricular walls and an inability to expand. As a result, the atria are dilated, and as the disease progresses, blood flow is restricted.

Signs and symptoms

Exercise intolerance, tiredness, dyspnoea and chest pain may be present. Heart murmurs are audible on auscultation, and hepatomegaly may be present. An echocardiogram will demonstrate dilation of the atria.

Treatment

Treatment is to alleviate symptoms with the use of drugs. A pacemaker may be indicated for permanent heart block, and a heart transplant may be considered before pulmonary hypertension develops.

Cardiac arrhythmias

Normal heart rates vary with age; the younger the child, the faster the heart rate. Cardiac arrhythmias occur in children:

- with or without a CHD
- following surgical repair of a heart defect
- with cardiomyopathy
- who have a cardiac tumour
- secondary to metabolic or electrolyte imbalance.

Regular sinus rhythm refers to a normal heart rhythm at an age-related normal rate.

Sinus tachycardia refers to a normal heart rhythm at an age-related elevated rate.

Sinus bradycardia refers to a normal heart rhythm at an age-related low rate.

Cardiac arrhythmias generally arise in the right atrium due to abnormalities in impulse generation; some are self-limiting, while others cause poor cardiac output, with associated symptoms. Treatment of arrhythmias depends on the cause, e.g., correcting electrolyte imbalance will correct the arrhythmia; others may require medication or even pacemaker placement.

Case study 11.2

Mei is 12 years old; she has recently become interested in hockey. However, when she plays, she is aware of her heart beating very fast, but she has put this down to being unfit. During a match, Mei experiences the same feelings of a very fast heart rate; she also feels dizzy and faints. The school calls an ambulance, and she is taken to the local children's emergency department. Her parents arrive shortly afterwards.

Vital signs

The following vital signs were recorded:

Vital sign	Observation	Normal range
Temperature	36.8 °C	36.3–37.5 °C
Pulse	116 bpm	70–120 bpm
Respirations	22 breaths per minute	20–30 breaths per minute
Blood pressure	112/62 mmHg	100–130 mmHg

An FBC was performed: no abnormalities found

An ECG shows a normal sinus rhythm

Reflect on this brief history and consider the following:

1. With all current investigations within normal limits being normal, what additional tests may be required?
2. Mei and her parents are understandably feeling anxious. What steps will the healthcare professional take to provide reassurance?

Mei is fitted with a Holter monitor, which will provide a 24-hour ECG. During this time, she is advised to sleep, play and exercise as normal. Results of the 24-hour ECG demonstrated one episode of:

- Pulse: 240 bpm
- ECG: an earlier than normal deflection of the QRS complex

Wolff-Parkinson-White syndrome

Wolff-Parkinson-White (WPW) syndrome is a congenital abnormality that involves the presence of abnormal electrical conductive circuits between the atria and ventricles (Chhabra *et al.*, 2023). The accessory pathways are congenital, and in children with WPW syndrome, the electrical signals in the heart do not travel along the normal route because of the extra (accessory) pathway, known as the bundle of Kent. The accessory pathway directly connects the atrium to the ventricle, and therefore, this pathway allows atrial activity to bypass the normal bundle of His and Purkinje system, allowing the ventricle to become excited before it would normally do so, resulting in an abnormal ECG. This also gives rise to the alternative name for the WPW syndrome or 'pre-excitation syndrome'. Type 'A' pre-excitation pathway refers to the left atrium and left ventricle, and type

'B' pre-excitation pathway exists between the right atrium and the right ventricle.

WPW syndrome can occur on its own, but it is associated with additional congenital cardiac defects, such as Ebstein anomaly or TGA.

Signs and symptoms

- There are two arrhythmias associated with WPW syndrome:
  - supraventricular tachycardia (SVT);
  - atrial fibrillation (AF) – although rare in children, when it does occur, the accessory pathway will send fast, irregular signals from the atria to the ventricle, causing ventricular fibrillation, which is potentially life-threatening.
- Chest pain
- Palpitations
- Dyspnoea
- Tachycardia
- Dizziness
- Syncope

Treatment

Treatment consists of stopping the acute episode of supraventricular tachycardia and preventing further episodes.

Acute episodes of SVT:

- Vagal manoeuvres are techniques designed to stimulate the nerve that slows down the electrical signals in your heart. Techniques include:
  - Valsalva manoeuvre – this is a moderately forceful attempt at exhalation against a closed airway, usually done by closing the mouth, pinching the nose shut and pressing out as if blowing up a balloon.
  - Carotid sinus massage – the neck is massaged in the region of the carotid sinus in an attempt to stimulate the vagus nerve.
  - Splashing cold water/ice water on the face may have a similar effect to the Valsalva manoeuvre.
  - Medication – adenosine is the drug of choice for terminating supraventricular tachycardia, including those associated with WPW syndrome (Joint Formulary Committee, 2025).
  - Cardioversion may be required if neither of the aforementioned works.

Preventing further episodes

- Medication – an anti-arrhythmic drug such as amiodarone slows down the electrical impulses in the heart.
- Catheter ablation – a catheter is guided from the femoral vein to the heart. The catheter records the electrical activity of the heart in order to pinpoint the exact location of the problem. High-frequency radio waves are used to destroy the tissue that causes the arrhythmia. It is effective in around 95% of cases.

A diagnosis of a heart defect either during pregnancy or after the baby has been born, or the diagnosis of heart disease in a child or young person, is devastating for the family. Fear of the unknown, concerns as to whether the child will survive, and questions relating to long-term health will affect the family. Healthcare professionals caring for a child with congenital or acquired heart disease need to be mindful of the need for holistic care. Up-to-date evidence-based care needs to be applied to the assessment, planning and care of the child to ensure the best possible outcome.

Consideration must be given to the child's need for rest, sleep and nutrition, along with the more procedural aspects of care, such as monitoring the child's condition and response to treatment. Family-centred care is fundamental when caring for a baby, child or young person and should be considered at all times.

Conclusion

Although CHDs are the most common of congenital problems to affect babies, it is important to remember that each individual condition is rare. This chapter has considered a range of diseases and defects that affect the heart. There are other congenital and acquired conditions which the reader needs to be aware of. Understanding the anatomy and physiology of the heart is essential to the understanding of heart disease.

References

Chamley, C., Carson, P., Randall, D., & Sandwell, M. (2005). *Developmental anatomy and physiology of children.* Churchill Livingstone, London.

Chhabra, L., Goyal, A., & Benham, M.D. (2023). Wolff-Parkinson-White Syndrome. In: *StatPearls* [Internet]. Treasure Island (FL): StatPearls Publishing.

Chowdhury, S., Koziatek, C.A., Tristram, D., & Rajnik, M. (2025). Acute rheumatic fever. In: *StatPearls [Internet].* Treasure Island (FL): StatPearls Publishing.

Fair, F., Furness, A., Higginbottom, G., *et al.* (2024). Systematic review of Apgar scores & cyanosis in Black, Asian, and ethnic minority infants. *Pediatric Research* https://doi.org/10.1038/s41390-024-03543-3 97, 939–952.

Heriwardito, A., & Aristya, L. (2022). Tetralogy of fallot. *Journal of Anesthesia and Critical Care: Open access* 14(6), 215–218.

Huisenga, D., Gemert, S., Van Bergen, A., *et al.* (2022). Motor development in infants with complex congenital heart disease: a longitudinal study. *Developmental Medicine and Child Neurology* 65(1), 117–125.

Joint Formulary Committee. (ed) (2025). *British National Formulary for Children 2024–2025.* BMJ Group and Pharmaceutical Press, London.

Jui, E., Singampalli, K.L., Shani, K., *et al.* (2021). The immune and inflammatory basis of acquired pediatric cardiac disease. *Frontiers in Cardiovascular Medicine* 8, 701224.

Kovacs, A., Brouillette, J., Ibeziako, P., *et al.* (2022). Psychological outcomes and interventions for individuals with congenital heart disease: a scientific statement from the American Heart Association. *Circulation: Cardiovascular Quality and Outcomes* 15.

Nadig, P.L., Joshi, V., Pilania, R.K., *et al.* (2023). Intravenous immunoglobulin in Kawasaki disease—evolution and pathogenic mechanisms. *Diagnostics* 13, 2338.

Nair, M., & Peate, I. (2017). *Fundamentals of Anatomy and Physiology: For Nursing and Healthcare Students*, 2nd edn. Wiley, Oxford.

NHS Choices (2021). Congenital heart disease. Available at: https://www.nhs.uk/conditions/congenital-heart-disease/ (accessed 21 April 2025).

Panesar, D., & Burch, M. (2016). Understanding and treating heart failure in children. *Paediatrics and Child Health.*

Park, M., & Salamat, M. (2021). *Park's The Pediatric Cardiology Handbook*, 6th edn. Elsevier, Missouri.

Rao, P., & Rao, P. (2022). Introductory Chapter: Introduction to recent advances in the diagnosis and management of congenital heart defects. In: Rao, P. (ed). *Congenital Heart Defects – Recent Advances.* London: IntechOpen.

Raza, S., Aggarwal, S., Jenkins, P., *et al.* (2023). Coarctation of the aorta: diagnosis and management. *Diagnostics (Basel)* 13(13).

Roberts, S. (2025). The cardiac system. In: Peate, I. & Gormley-Fleming, E. (eds). *Fundamentals of Children's Anatomy and Physiology.* Oxford: Wiley.

Silva, C., Rodrigues, L., Oliveira, P., *et al.* (2024). Impact of Congenital Heart Disease on the Cognitive and Psychological Development of Children at Different stages of Childhood. *International Journal of Health Science* 4(97), 1–7.

Tran, M., Miner, A., Merkel, C., *et al.* (2023). Sociodemographic profile associated with congenital heart disease among infants <1 year old. *Journal of Pediatric Nursing* 73.

Vicent, L., Luna, R., & Martínez-Sellés, M. (2022). Pediatric infective endocarditis: a literature review. *Journal of Clinical Medicine* 11(11).

Wu, W., He, J., & Shao, X. (2020). Incidence and mortality trend of congenital heart disease at the global, regional, and national level, 1990-2017. *Medicine (Baltimore)* 99(23), e20593.

CHAPTER 12

Disorders of the respiratory system

Elizabeth Mills

AIM

To understand the pathophysiology of the respiratory system during an acute illness phase, and the care and management required by children and young people and their families.

LEARNING OUTCOMES

On completion of this chapter, the reader will be able to:

- Explain the process of respiratory assessment.
- List common signs and symptoms of respiratory illness.
- Describe the altered physiology that occurs in common childhood respiratory disorders.
- Explain the nursing care and management that children and young people and families require during an acute respiratory illness.

KEYWORDS

- airway
- internal and external respiration
- ventilation
- oxygen
- carbon dioxide
- transportation of gases
- hypoxia
- apnoea
- dyspnoea
- inspiration
- expiration
- upper and lower respiratory tract
- chemoreceptors
- respiratory disorders

Test your prior knowledge

1. State the normal respiratory rate range for the following age ranges? Newborn, 1 year, 5 years, 12 years.
2. List four components of a respiratory assessment.
3. List three causes of upper airway obstruction.
4. List three causes of lower airway obstruction.
5. Name two respiratory illnesses which are preventable by vaccination.

Introduction

Respiratory illness is very common in infants and children and is the most frequent reason for children to attend the General Practitioner (GP) or be admitted to hospital. Different types of respiratory illness and conditions range from mild and self-limiting to severe and life-threatening, and if the child has other medical issues, such as a long-term, complex condition, then an acute respiratory illness can have a very serious effect on the child's health (Advanced Life Support Group [ALSG], 2023).

Infants and young children have an increased susceptibility to respiratory illnesses and subsequent respiratory distress and progressive failure, potentially leading to respiratory arrest. This is due to a number of important factors (ALSG, 2023):

- Immaturity of the immune system makes babies and young children vulnerable to infections.
- Upper and lower airways are narrow and small, making them easily blocked with mucus and restricted by swelling and oedema; this is particularly important in infants aged 0–6 months, who tend to be obligatory nose breathers and unable to breathe through their mouth.
- Infants have a particularly soft, compliant chest wall, which is easily sucked in during respiratory distress and increases the work of breathing, causing the classic sign of recession. Along with this, infants have a round-shaped rib cage and horizontally positioned ribs, which have a limited effect in assisting with increasing chest expansion.
- A smaller number of alveoli, as the lungs are not fully mature until approximately 8 years of age, by which time the lungs will contain around 500 million alveoli, and a large surface area for gaseous exchange.

Respiratory assessment

Respiratory assessment is a fundamental skill of the nurse caring for the sick child. Assessing differing elements of respiratory function will give you an overall indication of the child's respiratory status.

A full respiratory assessment will include the following observations:

- Respiratory rate – an increased respiratory rate usually indicates an increased demand for oxygen within the body. Therefore, it is important to know the 'normal' expected respiratory rate of different age groups, as respiratory rates vary widely from birth to 16 years of age. Best practice states that a respiratory rate should be measured for a full minute to identify breathing irregularities in rhythm and rate (Royal College of Nursing [RCN], 2017). During this time, it is useful to be able to observe other aspects of the respiratory assessment, for example, chest movement.

> Apnoea is a brief period of time with no breathing activity, which lasts for approx. 10–20 seconds.

Infants are particularly prone to apnoea as they become exhausted from respiratory distress and the increased work of breathing. Seek senior help immediately if you think an infant or child is experiencing apnoea, as this is a sign that respiratory arrest may be imminent.

- Observe chest movement – observe the chest movement during the respiratory cycle; if possible, you should undress the child to visualise the chest wall. Check for equal movement on both sides of the chest; unequal lung expansion could indicate an area of collapse or consolidation within the lung fields, or a pneumothorax. Look for other indications of respiratory distress and observe for any recession and use of other accessory muscles. Recession occurs when a child has increased work of breathing due to the compliant (soft) chest wall. In babies and young children, recession can occur at lower levels of respiratory distress, and in-drawing of the chest wall will increase as respiratory distress increases. Recession can be seen in different areas of the chest wall:
  - *Intercostal recession* – in-drawing between the rib spaces
  - *Subcostal recession* – in-drawing underneath the rib cage
  - *Suprasternal recession* – in-drawing above the rib cage
  - *Sternal recession* – in-drawing of the sternum, which is the large flat bone on the front of the rib cage. This indicates significant respiratory distress in any age group.
- As children increase in age, the chest wall and rib cage become more calcified and rigid, and less likely

to be sucked in during increased respiratory effort. Therefore, an older child with recession is a sign of more severe respiratory distress.

- Accessory muscle use – in addition to recession, children may show other signs of increased respiratory effort that you need to consider:
  - *Head bobbing* – infants tend to head bob in an attempt to increase respiratory effort as their respiratory distress increases.
  - *Diaphragmatic breathing* – infants use the diaphragm as a major muscle in the respiratory cycle. The diaphragm and abdominal muscles will be working extra hard at times of respiratory distress and, therefore, a 'see-saw' breathing pattern may be observed with increasing respiratory distress (paroxysmal breathing).
  - *Tracheal tug* – the soft tissue around the trachea will be in-drawn in respiratory distress and is a sign in all age groups that the respiratory distress is increasing.
  - *Nasal flaring* – a sign of increased respiratory distress, which is seen particularly in infants. This is because, below 6 months of age, infants are primarily nose breathers and do not know how to mouth breathe.

Respiratory noises

Listen for audible noises made during the respiratory cycle (inspiration and expiration).

Types of noises you may hear are:

- *Stridor* – this is a 'harsh' respiratory noise made on inspiration and usually indicates a partial upper airway obstruction. It is typically heard in conditions such as croup or foreign body obstruction.
- *Wheeze* – this is a softer 'musical' sound, usually heard on expiration and is produced in the lower respiratory tract. This is often due to air being trapped in the alveoli and small airways. It is the typical noise heard in asthma.
- *Grunting* – a sound produced by infants in severe respiratory distress. It is a noise produced when the epiglottis is used to partially close the trachea on expiration to stop the alveolar collapsing and ease the work of breathing. It is an indication of severe respiratory distress, and help should be sought immediately.

Measuring oxygen saturations

Using an oxygen saturation monitor with an infrared probe enables a measurement of the amount of oxygen dissolved in the blood to be made. Normal oxygen saturation levels should be 95% and above. In some groups of children, however, a lower measurement is acceptable, for example, children with chronic lung problems or children with certain cardiac conditions – please refer to local guidelines and policies.

Skin colour

Pale skin colour can be an indication of inadequate oxygen delivery to the cells and/or inadequate circulatory perfusion to the skin. However, it is always best to seek clarification from parents or carers on the child's normal skin colour, as some children are usually pale. This can also be difficult to detect in the child with a darker skin tone, and you will need to carefully observe the mucous membranes (inside the mouth and eyelids, for example) (Don't Forget the Bubble, 2025).

> Cyanosis is a type of discolouration that appears in mucous membrane and skin when children are severely hypoxic. This is a severe warning sign, and help should be sought immediately.

Heart rate

Children in respiratory distress will have a raised heart rate too due to the circulatory system compensating for a lack of oxygen. However, check that the heart rate is increased in a comparable amount to the increased respiratory rate. A significantly increased heart rate may be an indicator of other underlying issues, for example, a cardiac condition which may be causing the respiratory distress or another diagnosis.

> Bradycardia is a severe warning sign and could indicate that cardiorespiratory arrest is imminent; therefore, immediate senior help is required.

Mental status

The effect of hypoxia on the brain is to alter the mental status; this could mean that a child becomes floppy or irritable and then more drowsy as the hypoxia progresses. Using a neurological assessment tool is useful, for example, AVPU or the Glasgow Coma Scale, to objectively measure mental status.

Case study 12.1

Rosie is a 4-week-old baby who is being admitted to a medical ward with respiratory distress and poor feeding. She is waiting to be reviewed by the medical staff, when Rosie's mum comes to find you and says that Rosie has gone a 'funny colour'.

When you assess Rosie:

Respiratory rate – 65 bpm
Severe intercostal and subcostal recession, and diaphragmatic breathing. Nasal flaring
Oxygen saturations – 90% in air
Heart rate – 185 bpm; capillary refill time – 2 seconds; BP – 80/55
Skin colour – pale
Mental status – responds to mum's voice (AVPU)
Investigations – nasopharyngeal aspirate (NPA) taken in the emergency department, result is RSV +ve

Oxygen therapy

Due to the low levels of oxygen in Rosie's blood, delivering oxygen is the first priority. In this emergency situation, use a non-rebreathe oxygen mask with the oxygen flow metre turned to 15 L. The non-rebreathe mask has a reservoir bag which will fill with oxygen and deliver a high concentration of oxygen.

However, once Rosie becomes more stable, it may be more appropriate to use an oxygen mask, which will deliver a lower concentration of oxygen, or nasal prongs. If Rosie continues to require a high level of oxygen to maintain her oxygen blood levels, then she would need to be nursed in an area that can deliver high-flow nasal cannula oxygen therapy or non-invasive continuous positive airway pressure (CPAP) or that can potentially intubate and ventilate Rosie should her condition require this (e.g., high-dependency area, children's critical care or intensive care) (NICE, 2021).

Clearance of nasal and oral secretions

While observing the effect of the oxygen, Rosie appears to have white, bubbly secretions coming from her nostrils and in her mouth. Because of the small size of an infant's nostrils and airways, these can easily become blocked with secretions produced during a respiratory illness such as bronchiolitis. This can be a problem for infants, particularly as they like to nose breathe, which is difficult once the nostrils become blocked. Often, these secretions can be wiped away with a tissue. Some babies benefit from saline nose drops to keep the mucus loose and easily cleared from the nostrils.

In a clinical ward, it may be appropriate to use gentle suctioning to clear secretions in the nostrils and mouth. This is a clinical skill which should only be performed when the need for it has been assessed, such as in respiratory distress or feeding difficulties, and it should not be performed routinely on infants with bronchiolitis (NICE, 2021). Refer to local guidelines and policies when performing suction, and only undertake this skill when you have been assessed as competent or under direct supervision with a qualified healthcare professional.

Infection control precautions

Bronchiolitis is highly infectious, and infection control measures must be undertaken with regard to local policies and guidelines. In particular, good hand hygiene and grouping (cohorting) of infectious patients in restricted areas. Parents managing infants at home with bronchiolitis should be advised on hand hygiene and washing of toys and equipment.

Bronchiolitis

Bronchiolitis is a common lower respiratory tract illness affecting children under the age of 2 years. It is most commonly seen in those under 1 year, and peak incidence is at age 3–6 months. It is estimated that a third of all children in the United Kingdom will have had bronchiolitis in their first year of life, and approximately 3% of children with bronchiolitis will need hospitalisation for supportive care (UK Health Security Agency, 2024a).

What is bronchiolitis?

The disease is caused by a viral infection; approximately 80% of cases are caused by respiratory syncytial virus (RSV), but bronchiolitis can also be caused by other viruses, such as adenovirus and rhinovirus.

The infection causes inflammatory obstruction of the lower airways and alveoli due to necrosis of the cell lining. Ciliary damage impedes secretion clearance of the lower lung fields, combined with increased mucus production. Air becomes trapped below the obstruction of secretions, and it becomes more difficult for the infant to exhale. Hence, a wheezy noise develops, and respiratory distress follows. In severe cases, a consolidation or collapse occurs in the affected area of lung, and gaseous exchange may be impaired (UK Health Security Agency, 2025a).

Bronchiolitis normally presents as a cough with increased effort in breathing; it often affects the infant's ability to feed. It can be confused with the 'common cold' as there are common features. However, the presence of lower respiratory tract infection, such as wheeze or crackles, can be heard on auscultation. The symptoms are usually mild, but in some cases, they will be severe, particularly if the infant has associated risk factors, such as chronic lung disease, congenital heart disease, premature birth, neuromuscular disorder or an immunodeficiency disorder (NICE, 2021; UK Health Security Agency, 2025a).

Very young infants, for example, those under 6 weeks of age, may have apnoea (periods of no respiratory effort, which may or may not be self-resolving). Symptoms usually peak at 3–5 days of the disease trajectory, and the cough normally resolves within 3 weeks. Some children can be left with a residual wheeze.

Treatment

Treatment for bronchiolitis is mainly supportive. It may include giving oxygen therapy for low oxygen saturation (usually 90% and below), which may be via nasal cannula or in a head box. Ideally, oxygen should be humidified and warmed if it is given for any prolonged length of time. The amount of oxygen given should be titrated to the level of oxygen saturations of the infant to avoid over-delivery of oxygen, which has been shown to have harmful effects if given in excess over a prolonged period of time (ALSG, 2023).

Support with hydration and feeding may be required for infants with severe infection. This may include intravenous fluids to correct dehydration and/or nasogastric feeding. Due to respiratory distress, infants can have difficulty feeding adequately; this needs to be assessed on an individual basis. Secretion clearance from the nostrils, either with suction or saline nose drops, can often facilitate more effective feeding.

No medication is recommended to treat bronchiolitis, although the use of paracetamol and ibuprofen may be used if the child is old enough to treat discomfort (NICE, 2021). The use of antibiotics is not recommended for bronchiolitis; however, it may be required if the child develops a post-viral bacterial infection. Risk factors for severe illness include infants under the age of 2 months, prematurity, congenital heart disease and chronic lung disease.

Parental/carer support is required, as this can be a frightening experience for parents and may be the first illness for their infant. Parents/carers at home with a child with bronchiolitis should be given advice about what to expect and when they need to call for advice or help (NICE, 2021).

Upper airway disorders

Babies and young children are vulnerable to upper airway problems because of the small size of their anatomy, as discussed previously.

Croup

Croup is a common condition, also known as acute viral laryngotracheobronchitis, often caused by the parainfluenza virus. The peak incidence for croup is 2 years of age; however, it can occur from 6 months up to 5 years of age.

Children with croup have the distinctive 'croup' sound on inspiration; this is called a stridor. This is due to swelling and oedema of the upper airway, causing a partial airway obstruction. They may also have a barking cough, a mild fever and a hoarse voice.

Inhalation of warm, moist air is often recommended; however, there is little evidence of benefit. Oral or nebulised steroids may be given to reduce the severity and length of the illness (NICE, 2022).

Epiglottitis

Epiglottitis is swelling of the epiglottis and surrounding tissues due to infection. It is treated as a potentially life-threatening emergency, as total obstruction of the larynx can occur. Urgent hospital admission is required for a child with suspected epiglottitis (Watts & Kay, 2023).

This condition has become much rarer in children since the introduction of the HIB vaccination, as it is primarily caused by the *Haemophilus influenzae* bacteria. The most common age occurrence is 2–6 years (Watts & Kay, 2023).

Children presenting with epiglottitis typically present with the 4 Ds: dyspnoea, dysphagia, drooling and dysphonia (muffled 'hot potato' voice) and look very unwell, due to the overwhelming infection and pyrexia. It is very important not to upset the child whom you may suspect has epiglottitis. Do not insist that they lie flat, as they often find their own most effective position for breathing, which will often be leaning forward, and they may prefer to sit on a parent's lap. Causing the child unnecessary distress, for example, attempting cannulation, may invoke a complete obstruction of the upper airway and require emergency airway management.

Antibiotic therapy will be required once the airway has been secured, and this will usually be with intubation. After antibiotic therapy has been established, recovery is normally rapid.

Aspiration of a foreign body

This is an uncommon occurrence in children; however, because infants and children are inquisitive and put objects in their mouths or are learning to eat different types of food, aspiration of a foreign body is a possibility.

Children often have a sudden onset of respiratory distress and a history of choking. Children with suspected aspiration of a foreign body will need a laryngobronchoscopy to remove the object from the airway.

Children who present with an acute choking episode need to be treated with the choking algorithm (ALSG, 2023) (Fig. 12.1).

Pneumonia

Pneumonia is globally recognised as the leading cause of death from infection in the under-fives, accounting for approximately 14% of all deaths of children under 5 years old worldwide (World Health Organization, 2022).

Pneumonia is an infection affecting the lower respiratory tract and can be caused by viral, bacterial or fungal pathogens (World Health Organization, 2022). Infants, children and young people are affected by different organisms. Infection can occur via the bloodstream or through

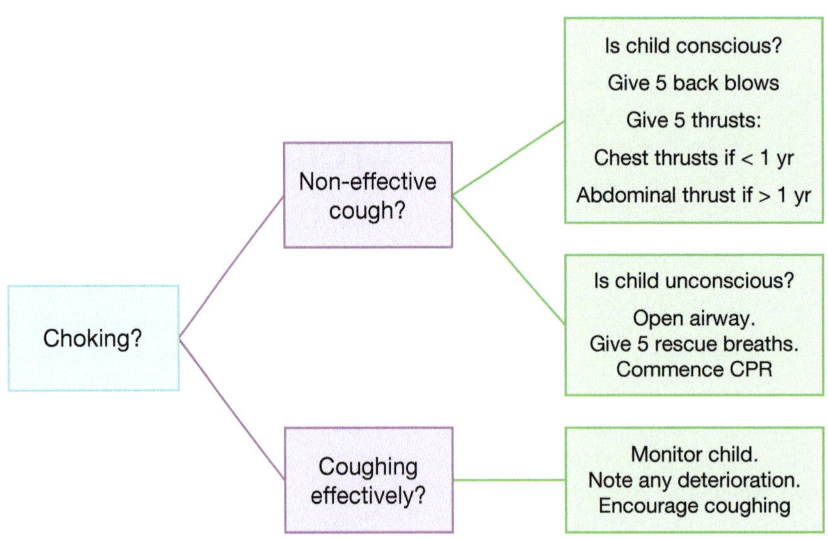

FIGURE 12.1 Choking algorithm.
Source: ALSG (2023)/John Wiley & Sons.

inhalation via the airway epithelium. It is characterised by inflammation of the lung parenchyma leading to consolidation of alveoli. There are different classifications of pneumonia, which can relate to the anatomical distribution of the disease, the infective pathogen responsible for the disease or whether the disease is community-acquired or hospital-acquired (nosocomial).

According to Kesley and Rylatt (2021), pneumonia can be classified by the site of its anatomical distribution:

- Lobar pneumonia involves a large portion of an entire lobe of a lung and is predominantly caused by *Streptococcus pneumoniae.*
- Bronchopneumonia begins in the terminal bronchioles, which become congested with exudate and form patches of consolidation involving several lobes of the lungs; it usually follows another respiratory illness, such as whooping cough or bronchiolitis.
- Interstitial pneumonia involves the walls surrounding the alveoli and bronchioles and is usually caused by viral or mycoplasma infections. The inflammatory process is confined within the alveolar walls and the peribronchiolar and interlobular tissues.

Altered physiology

Bacterial pneumonia

Infectious organisms spread to the lower respiratory tract via the bloodstream or upper airways, prompting an immune response in the lungs. This leads to leaky lung capillaries, causing plasma proteins, red blood cells (RBCs) and inflammatory mediators to enter the alveoli, reducing the functional area for gaseous exchange. Consequently, breathing rate increases to address oxygen demand and rising carbon dioxide levels. Increased mucus production and continued fluid accumulation in the alveoli further impair lung function. As the disease advances, the alveoli fill with fluid and debris from the intense white blood cell (WBC) activity, eventually solidifying into areas of consolidation where gas exchange becomes severely limited.

Viral pneumonia infects the walls of the alveoli and the parenchyma of the lung. The ciliated epithelial cells become damaged as the virus replicates in the alveolar epithelial cells, leading to rupturing of the walls of the alveoli and the bronchioles.

Diagnosis

Distinguishing between viral and bacterial infections can be difficult, and it can also be hard to obtain a definitive diagnosis of bacterial infection in babies and young children. Recommendations suggest that in children where there is persistent or repetitive fever greater than 38.5 °C together with chest wall recession and a raised respiratory rate, a diagnosis of bacterial pneumonia should be considered (Ebeledike & Ahmad, 2023). A chest X-ray is only indicated when a child fails to respond to treatment or if complications are suspected.

Signs and symptoms

Signs and symptoms are often non-specific and vary according to the age of the child and the causative pathogens. Respiratory assessment is the most important diagnostic tool.

- Neonates and infants may present with cough, lethargy, poor feeding, fever or labile temperature.
- Pre-school children may present with cough, fever, chest pain, abdominal pain and vomiting.
- Older children may present with fever, cough, chest pain and dyspnoea.
- Children with community-acquired pneumonia may present with fever, tachypnoea, breathlessness or difficulty in breathing, cough, wheeze or chest pain. They may also present with abdominal pain and/or vomiting and may have a headache.

Investigations

Chest X-ray is only necessary if there is failure to respond to treatment or if complications are suspected.

Full blood count, C-reactive protein and blood cultures should be performed, and a blood gas to assess respiratory function may be indicated if there is acute respiratory distress.

Nasopharyngeal aspirate for viral immunofluorescence and/or sputum specimen for microscopy, culture and sensitivity may also be considered.

Assessment and treatment

The priority for managing a child with pneumonia is prompt identification and treatment of respiratory distress. Full respiratory assessment should be undertaken, including pulse oximetry, and supplementary oxygen should be administered if the oxygen saturation reading is below 92% (ALSG, 2023).

Children demonstrating signs of severe respiratory distress and decreasing levels of consciousness may require tracheal intubation and artificial ventilation to maintain adequate oxygenation.

Assessment of the nutritional status of the child is important in preventing dehydration (see Red Flag box). Symptoms of respiratory distress, such as tachypnoea and recession, can impede the ability to swallow, and children should be assessed for dehydration. Dependent upon the severity of the respiratory distress, it may be necessary to commence intravenous fluids or enteral feeding via a nasogastric tube. Presence of a nasogastric tube, however, can exacerbate respiratory distress if it occludes too much of the airway.

Antimicrobial therapy is usually started with a diagnosis of bacterial pneumonia, and the type of drug and route of administration will depend upon the age of the child, the severity of the illness and the causative pathogen (if known).

Children who do not require oxygen and are drinking adequately can be managed at home with a course of oral antibiotics (WHO, 2024).

Complications

If the pneumonia fails to respond to treatment, there is a risk of developing empyema. Empyema is a serious respiratory condition which is caused by the pleural fluid within the pleural space becoming infected. Left untreated, the pus thickens and causes sections of the pleura to stick together, forming pockets of pus. The thickening deposits can extend to the outer layer of the lung, which prevents adequate lung expansion. Empyema is treated with insertion of a small chest drain connected to an underwater seal to allow the infected fluid to drain.

Dehydration

Dehydration can be a common adjunct to respiratory infection as a result of difficulties in coordinating breathing and swallowing mechanisms. In addition, paroxysmal coughing can result in episodes of vomiting. Infants and children should be assessed for signs of dehydration and managed accordingly. Parents of children who are diagnosed with a respiratory infection but who are not admitted to hospital should be informed about what symptoms to look out for and advised when to contact a healthcare professional should symptoms persist.

Signs of clinical dehydration, as identified by the NICE (2020), appear in Table 12.1.

TABLE 12.1 Signs of clinical dehydration

Altered responsiveness, for example, irritable or lethargic	Decreased urine output
Normal skin colour	Sunken eyes
Warm extremities	Tachycardia
Dry mucous membranes	Tachypnoea
Normal peripheral pulses	Normal capillary refill time
Reduced skin turgor	Normal blood pressure

Whooping cough (pertussis)

Pertussis is a highly contagious acute respiratory infection, which is predominantly caused by the bacterium *Bordetella pertussis*. Incidence of the disease is relatively low as a result of the 5-in-1 vaccine given as part of the routine vaccination schedule to infants at 8 weeks, 12 weeks and 16 weeks of age (see Table 12.2: 'Vaccinations'). The introduction of pertussis vaccination in pregnancy from October 2012 has seen a reduction in the deaths of babies from pertussis, with maternal vaccine effectiveness against death of infants from pertussis estimated at around 97% effective (UK Health Protection Agency, 2024b). Young unimmunised infants, particularly premature babies, babies under 3 months of age and babies born to unimmunised mothers, are identified as the most vulnerable group, with the highest rates of complications and deaths (UK Health Protection Agency, 2024b). However, since 2023, there has been a continued increase in the number of pertussis cases across all age groups, with 4793 confirmed cases reported between January and April 2024 (UK Health Protection Agency, 2024c).

Presenting symptoms in the catarrhal stage include mild fever, runny nose and occasional cough lasting 7–10 days. The paroxysmal stage can last for up to 10 weeks, and during this stage, the cough gradually develops into a paroxysmal cough causing a characteristic inspiratory 'whoop', vomiting and exhaustion. The convalescent stage involves a general recovery with a gradual resolution of the cough over a 2–3-week period. Diagnosis can often be delayed in older children who present with a persistent cough rather than a characteristic 'whooping' cough. The infection can be more serious in infants, as paroxysms of coughing can result in episodes of apnoea.

TABLE 12.2 Vaccination schedule

When to give	Diseases protected against
8 weeks of age	6-in-1 vaccine: diphtheria, tetanus, pertussis (whooping cough), polio, Hib (*Haemophilus influenzae* type b) and Hepatitis B Meningococcal group B (MenB) Rotavirus
12 weeks of age	6-in-1 vaccine: diphtheria, tetanus, pertussis (whooping cough), polio, Hib (*Haemophilus influenzae* type b) and Hepatitis B Meningococcal group B (MenB) Rotavirus
16 weeks of age	6-in-1 vaccine: diphtheria, tetanus, pertussis (whooping cough), polio, Hib (*Haemophilus influenzae* type b) and Hepatitis B Pneumococcal
One year old (on or after the child's first birthday)	Pneumococcal Measles, mumps, rubella and varicella Meningococcal group B (MenB)
18 months	6-in-1 vaccine: diphtheria, tetanus, pertussis (whooping cough), polio, Hib (*Haemophilus influenzae* type b) and Hepatitis B
3 years 4 months of age	4-in-1 pre-school booster: Diphtheria, tetanus, pertussis and polio
Boys and girls aged 12 to 13 years	Cancers and genital warts caused by specific human papillomavirus (HPV) types
14 years old (school year 9)	Tetanus, diphtheria and polio Meningococcal groups A, C, W and Y

Source: UK Health Security Agency (2025)/GOV.UK/Public Domain.

Vigorous, persistent coughing can cause nosebleeds and subconjunctival haemorrhage.

Pertussis is spread person to person by droplet infection, and the incubation period is 7–10 days. A case is infectious from day seven of exposure up to 21 days after the onset of paroxysmal cough, if not receiving antibiotic treatment, and symptoms can persist for 3 months. Where antibiotic treatment is commenced, the infectious period reduces to 48 hours post the commencement of the appropriate antibiotic (UK Health Protection Agency, 2024c). It is worth noting that a single episode of pertussis offers lifetime immunity.

Management

Pertussis is treated by administration of an antimicrobial therapy to reduce the period of infectivity. Antimicrobial therapy, however, does not shorten the course of the illness or manage other associated symptoms. Close contacts and other household members also require treatment with antimicrobial therapy (UK Health Protection Agency, 2024c). Infants and children can become very anxious during episodes of coughing and require supportive care in managing their fear and distress. Fluid intake and nutrition need to be carefully monitored, as paroxysmal coughing often causes vomiting of mucus.

Complications

Complications of whooping cough include lobar pneumonia, atelectasis and bronchiectasis. In addition, prolonged episodes of coughing can result in nosebleed, subconjunctival haemorrhage and inguinal hernia.

Notifiable diseases

Pertussis is a notifiable disease in accordance with the Health Protection Legislation (England) Guidance 2010 (Department of Health, 2010). Suspected cases should be notified by telephone to the local health protection team as soon as is practicable and written notification sent within 3 days, with confirmation of the identified pathogen within 7 days (UK Health Protection Agency, 2024c).

Vaccinations

The vaccines identified in Table 12.2 form part of the routine vaccination schedule that is freely available through the NHS to all babies and children in the United Kingdom. Significant protection against respiratory infections is provided within this schedule, and the importance of having babies and children vaccinated should be discussed with parents.

The following is an optional vaccination offered in addition to the routine vaccinations to 'at-risk' groups of babies or children (UK Health Security Agency, 2025).

BCG (Bacillus Calmette-Guérin) tuberculosis vaccine:

Protects against: Tuberculosis (TB)
Given to: Babies and children who have a high chance of coming into contact with TB
Given at: Birth to 16 years of age

In the United Kingdom, the BCG vaccine is not routinely administered as part of the NHS vaccination schedule. It is specifically targeted at children and adults considered to be at elevated risk of TB. Universal vaccination at birth is advised for infants in the 11 high TB incidence areas identified within the United Kingdom (UK Health Security Agency, 2025). The UK Health Security Agency (2025) publication 'Immunisation against infectious disease' provides detailed information on UK vaccine policies and procedures.

Tuberculosis is a chronic, specific, inflammatory infectious disease caused by the slow-growing bacterium *Mycobacterium tuberculosis*. In the United Kingdom, pulmonary TB is the most common form, accounting for nearly 80% of all cases (UK Health Security Agency, 2025d). Although TB primarily affects the lungs, it can also affect other areas of the body. Children are most often infected by inhaling infectious droplet nuclei from infectious individuals within their immediate family or with whom they have regular contact. Children with TB are generally not infectious. Therefore, when a child is diagnosed with TB, public health notification is essential for contact tracing to identify the source case.

Inhaled bacilli implant in the distal airspaces of the lower part of the upper lobe or the upper part of the lower lobe of the lungs. In many cases, the infection is contained by the immune system and does not cause the disease; however, there is a residual area of infection present in the lung called the Ghon focus and enlargement of the mediastinal lymph nodes referred to as the primary complex. Infection may be spread via the bloodstream, distributing the infection to other parts of the body where it may lodge. The organism may remain inactive indefinitely or may reactivate at a later stage to cause pulmonary or extrapulmonary TB dependent upon the site of the infection.

Extra-pulmonary TB can manifest in various ways, including cervical lymph node enlargement, spinal TB, TB meningitis, TB arthritis, and, less commonly in children, abdominal and genitourinary TB (Smyth, 2013). The clinical presentation varies depending on the strength of the immune response, ranging from localised containment and dormancy to widespread, disseminated infection.

The majority of infants and children infected with *Mycobacterium tuberculosis* do not progress to active TB and remain asymptomatic. When symptoms do occur, they typically develop gradually and may include cough and other respiratory symptoms, weight loss, failure to thrive, anorexia, dyspnoea and fever. Diagnostic approaches depend on whether the infection is detected through *passive case finding* (examination of children presenting with signs and symptoms) or *active case finding* (contact tracing or routine immigration screening). Diagnosis relies on chest X-rays, tuberculin testing, sputum testing and gastric aspiration.

Early diagnosis is crucial for identifying the source case who transmitted the disease to the child and for initiating long-term anti-tuberculosis drug therapy. Treatment and preventative therapy are managed by a specialist clinician and may involve a 3- to 6-month course of anti-tuberculosis drugs. Adherence to the treatment regimen is essential for effective disease management and to minimise the risk of drug resistance. This can be challenging, as children may become symptom-free after only a few weeks, making long-term preventative medication use problematic without proper guidance. Children with active disease typically require multiple medications over an extended period.

Parents need to be alerted to the following signs and seek immediate hospital treatment should any be present:

- Worsening effort of breathing (e.g., grunting, nasal flaring and/or marked chest recession)
- fluid intake is 50–75% of normal or no wet nappy for 12 hours
- apnoea or cyanosis
- exhaustion (e.g., not responding normally to social cues, wakes only with prolonged stimulation)

(NICE, 2024)

The incidence of TB in England has increased; in 2024, 5480 cases were reported, representing a 13% rise (UK Health Security Agency, 2025d). While the majority (81.5%) of these cases occurred in people born outside the United Kingdom, there is a growing number of cases in the UK-born population. Factors contributing to TB transmission in the United Kingdom include social deprivation, residence in large urban areas, homelessness, drug and alcohol dependency and involvement with the criminal justice system (UK Health Security Agency, 2025d).

Case study 12.2

Olivia Hinchcliffe is a 13-year-old girl who has visited her GP on several occasions over the past month with a history of persistent cough, wheeze and shortness of breath. She has been treated for a viral respiratory tract infection. During physical education (PE), she became distressed and found it difficult to breathe. The school rang the emergency services for an ambulance. Olivia has no further medical history, and the school has contacted her mum to let them know what has happened.

Vital signs
Physical and blood
The following vital signs were noted and recorded:

Pulse	120
Respiratory rate	30
SaO_2	92%
Blood pressure	110/70
Temperature	36.8 °C

A full blood count was performed.

Test	Result	Guideline normal values
White blood cells (WBCs)	6×10^9/L	$4–11 \times 10^9$/L
Neutrophils	4.4×10^9/L	$2.0–7.5 \times 10^9$/L
Lymphocytes	2.8×10^9/L	$1.3–4.0 \times 10^9$/L
Red blood cells (RBCs)	5.1×10^9/L	$4.5–6.5 \times 10^9$/L
Haemoglobin (Hb)	14 g/dL	11.5–16.5 g/dL
Platelets	320×10^9/L	$150–440 \times 10^9$/L

Reflect on the care of Olivia and consider the following:

1. What could be the most likely diagnosis?
2. What further information do you require from Olivia and her mum in order to ensure that safe and effective family-centred care is provided for her?
3. List any further investigations that Olivia might require.
4. What treatment options are available for Olivia?

Investigations

Chest X-ray

An X-ray is a diagnostic test that uses small amounts of radiation to generate a picture of organs, tissues and bones of the body. When an X-ray of the chest is taken, it can help identify abnormalities or disease of the airways, heart, lungs, blood vessels and bones. Chest X-rays can also be used to identify the presence of fluid in the lungs or fluid and air around the lungs. A chest X-ray can be requested for a variety of reasons, including to assess injury after an accident or to monitor the progression of a disease (cystic fibrosis).

A chest X-ray is a quick, easy and effective test that has been used for decades in the assessment and treatment of patients.

Prolonged increased effort of breathing

Increased effort of breathing is tiring, and the body cannot maintain this for long periods of time. Identifying this early can reduce the risk of respiratory arrest. Early indicators that the body is starting to get into difficulty can be easily identified. These include:

- Altered neurological state: vacant look, restless, irritable, sitting very still
- Increased effort of breathing: nasal flaring, shoulder bobbing, clavicle or tracheal tug, intercostal and subcostal recession (using the small muscles within the rib cage to assist with breathing)
- Tripoding: using arms to alter position to enable more chest expansion to try and assist/ease the effort of breathing
- Respiratory arrest: breathing stops and does not spontaneously restart.

Asthma

Due to its nature, there is no clear definition of asthma, which makes it difficult to provide recommendations for a diagnosis of asthma that is evidence-based (British Thoracic Society/Scottish Intercollegiate Guideline Network [BTS/SIGN], 2024). The recognised symptoms of asthma can include wheeze, breathlessness, chest tightness, cough and variable airway obstructions. However, the symptoms of asthma are individual to each

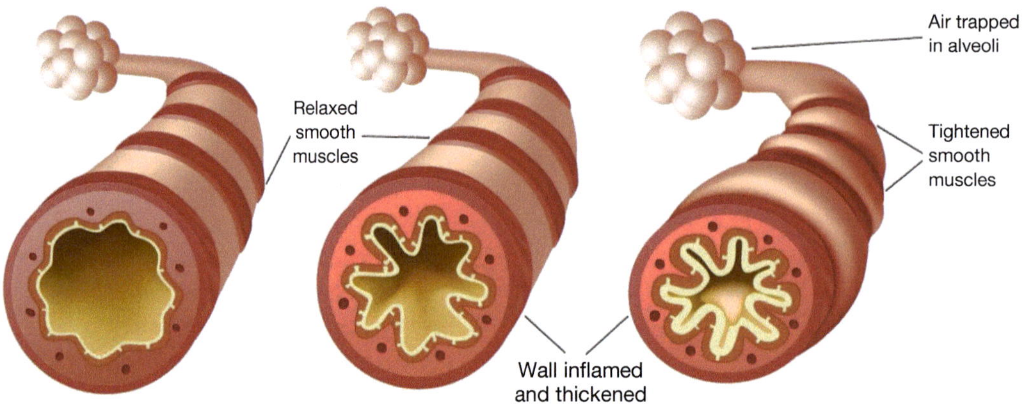

FIGURE 12.2 Difference between a normal airway and an asthmatic airway.

patient, which can increase the difficulty of diagnosis. The presenting symptoms are usually reversible with drug therapy or can be spontaneously reversed without it.

In the airways of an asthmatic, there is increased inflammation and hyper-responsiveness to identified stimuli or triggers (Fig. 12.2); these can include exercise, stress and allergens (pollen, dust and pet dander). The airways present with a bronchospasm, which is the narrowing of the bronchial walls due to an uncontrolled smooth muscle contraction because of hyper-responsiveness to an identified stimulus. At the same time, inflammation within the airways occurs, causing the airways to become hyper-responsive and narrow easily in reaction to the stimulus. There is further narrowing of the airways through invasion by the inflammatory cells, as the body responds to protect itself. Inflammatory cells contain chemical mediators, including histamine, prostaglandins and leukotrienes, which cause vasodilation and increased capillary permeability. This results in mucus production and oedema occurring within the airways (Kelsey & Rylatt, 2021).

Altered pathophysiology

Within a normal airway structure, the bronchial wall and basement membrane are thin, with a thin viscous layer of fluid covering the epithelial surface. The smooth muscle is relaxed, leaving the airway wide open for good airflow. In an asthmatic airway structure, however, the bronchial walls and basement membrane are inflamed and thickened, with inflammatory exudate covering the lumen of airways. The smooth muscle is constricted and in spasm, leading to bronchospasm and airway obstruction. This reduces the size of the airway, leading to poor airflow and a wheeze being produced.

Medication

Salbutamol (blue inhaler): Can cause fine muscle tremors throughout the body; this includes the heart muscle, leading to tachycardia and palpitations.

Beclomethasone (brown inhaler): Can cause a dry mouth and oral thrush. To reduce the incidence of this happening, encourage the child to brush their teeth after using their inhaler.

Inhaler technique: Ensuring correct inhaler technique is the cornerstone of effective asthma management and treatment. All patients (and parents) need to have regular checks that they are using the inhaler correctly.

Oral steroids: Long-term use of oral steroids can lead to poor bone health and cataract development (Bhatt *et al.*, 2013).

Assessment

When undertaking a nursing assessment of a child with a suspected or known asthma attack, there are some specific questions that need to be answered to assist in their treatment. These include the following:

- What symptoms does the child have?
- Do they have a cough? If so, is it persistent, nocturnal, productive or episodic?
- Do they have a wheeze? If so, is it inspiratory/expiratory or nocturnal, and is it caused by anything specific, like exercise, emotions or feeding, for example?

- Are they breathless? If so, is it persistent or variable (e.g., can they complete a sentence without becoming breathless if they are talking to you; if an infant, what is their cry like)?
- How long have they had the symptoms, and when did the symptoms begin?
- How long do the symptoms last?
- Does the child look distressed, or are they in distress?
- Is there any family history of asthma, eczema or hay fever in the family?

Care and treatment

When planning the nursing treatment for a child with asthma, the ultimate goal is to restore a normal breathing pattern, as asthma is a reversible condition. The use of continuous monitoring of vital signs until the child is stabilised is paramount to monitor the effectiveness of the inhaled medication. The maintenance of oxygen saturation levels above 92% is essential to ensure adequate oxygenation, but also to assist in the effort of breathing (ALSG, 2023). This is done through the safe administration of prescribed oxygen via a non-rebreather mask. The administration of prescribed bronchodilators and oral steroids is the most effective way to control asthma. When administering medication, it is important to follow the Nursing & Midwifery Council (NMC) (2018) Code, professional standards of practice and behaviour for nurses, midwives and nursing associates. During care delivery, it is important that comfort and reassurance are given to both the child and parent, as dyspnoea (shortness of breath) is very frightening to both the child and parent. Giving reassurance to a parent will help reduce their own anxiety, which in turn will help the child relax and breathe more easily.

Once the child's asthma is under control, the next step is to develop or review the child's asthma plan; this is best done by an asthma specialist nurse who will work with the child and their family to discuss their educational needs, support and care pathway (BTS/SIGN, 2024). As part of this ongoing support and treatment, if it is felt to be appropriate, the introduction of regular peak expiratory flow rate (PEFR) measurement will be considered and implemented.

Investigations

Peak flow readings

These are objective lung function measurements of the peak expiratory flow (PEF). This is the maximum flow of air achieved during expiration, delivered with the maximum force. The PEF is recorded in litres per minute (L/min). It is done using a simple and portable device that can be used in the home and in the hospital, and which is suitable for children over the age of 6 years.

The negative side is that they are not as sensitive as spirometry readings, which require more sophisticated equipment that is usually non-portable and requires specialist training to undertake the procedure and interpret the readings.

Peak flow zones

Peak flow zones are based on the traffic light concept: red means danger, yellow means caution and green means safe. Based on the patient's personal best, the three peak flow zones include:

Green: 80–100% of your personal best PEFR; asthma is under control.

Yellow: 50–79% of your personal best PEFR; asthma is getting worse; may need to use quick-relief medications.

Red: below 50% of your personal best PEFR; medical alert, take quick-relief medication; GET medical help *immediately*.

Management of acute/severe or life-threatening asthma (see Table 12.3)

Asthma treatment protocols are subject to regular review. Clear guidelines have been produced in relation to (BTS/SIGN, 2024):

- the management of acute asthma in children in the emergency department
- the management of acute asthma in children in hospital
- the management of acute asthma in infants aged and children under 5

Difficult asthma

Asthma that is not under control may be a result of several different reasons, which need to be considered. These reasons include the individual not receiving the right level of support or not accessing care when they

TABLE 12.3 Features of acute/severe and life-threatening asthma

Main symptoms of asthma	Features of acute/severe asthma	Features of life-threatening asthma
Cough that may become productive	Peak flow less than 50% of predicted or best	Peak flow less than 33% of predicted or best
Dyspnoea and chest tightness	Dyspnoea - unable to complete a sentence in one breath	Oxygen saturation less than 92%
Wheeze	Tachypnoea	Silent chest
Peak flow less than predicted or best	Tachycardia	Weak and feeble respiratory effort
		Cyanosis
		Bradycardia or hypotension
		Confusion, exhaustion or coma

Source: Adapted from BTS/SIGN (2024).

need it. This could be a result of a lack of information or understanding about asthma, or a lack of services available to the individual. Concordance with medication can be an issue. This is where the rule of thirds applies: one-third of children will take medication as directed, one-third will partially follow instructions, and one-third do not take medication at all (Tate, 2010 and Klok *et al.*, 2013). People may not understand what their medicines are for and how to take them, or they may not be taking their medicines as prescribed. Some people do not have access to effective healthcare or medicines because of language, cultural or social barriers, whereas others are unable, unwilling or unaware of the need to avoid persistent exposure to triggers such as cigarette smoke or exposure to workplace substances. People may have other underlying health conditions that have not been identified and which may make their asthma symptoms worse, or they may be misdiagnosed with asthma and thus asthma medicines will not help their symptoms.

The National Respiratory Audit Programme (NRAP, 2024) found deficiencies in both the routine care of people with asthma and the treatment of attacks (Royal College of Physicians, 2024). In many instances, neither doctors nor patients recognised the signs of deteriorating asthma; they also did not react quickly enough when these were seen.

When reviewing a child's respiratory health, all factors of the child's life need to be taken into consideration, including environment, housing, socioeconomic status and habits. In recent years, there has been a landmark case where poor air quality and pollution have been identified as contributing factors to the death of a child with asthma (Royal College of Paediatric and Child Health, 2021). In 2020, poor housing conditions, specifically mould, was identified as a contributing factor to the death of a 2-year-old child within the coroner's report (Kearsley, 2022). These factors need to be recognised, and questions should be asked about housing and environment when taking a history from the child and their parents/carers. Asking older children and young people about habits, including smoking and vaping need to be included in routine admission questions (Royal College of Physicians, 2024). Where smoking or vaping is identified, support can be offered to help with stopping, which will have a positive impact on future long-term lung health (Royal College of Physicians, 2024).

Conclusion

Respiratory illnesses in children are common as a result of developmental differences in the respiratory systems of infants and young children. Effective respiratory assessment enables early detection and appropriate care and management of the sick child. It is important to consider all aspects of life that can impact the respiratory health of a child. These areas include immunisation status, housing, the environment, both inside and outside the house and socially accepted behaviours, including smoking and vaping, especially in young people. Undertaking a good respiratory assessment that includes questions about all of these areas will enable a clear picture of the disease trajectory and compounding factors that need to be taken into consideration when caring for a child who has presented with a respiratory illness.

References

Advanced Life Support Group (2023). *Advanced Paediatric Life Support: A Practical Approach to Emergencies*, 7th edn. Wiley, Oxford.

Bhatt, J., Vyas, H., & Forster, D. (2013). Management of asthma and allergy. In: Mighten, J. (ed). *Children's Respiratory Nursing.* Oxford: Wiley.

British Thoracic Society/Scottish Intercollegiate Guidelines Network (BTS/SIGN) (2024). Joint guidelines for the diagnosis, monitoring and chronic asthma management (BTS,NICE, SIGN) NICE Guideline [NG245] Available at Asthma | British Thoracic Society | Better lung health for all (accessed 3 July 2025).

Department of Health (2010). Health protection legislation guidance 2010. Public Health England, London.

Don't Forget the Bubble (2025). Skin Deep. Available at https://dftbskindeep.com/ (accessed 3 June 2025).

Ebeledike, C and Ahmad T (2023). Pediatric pneumonia. Available at https://www.ncbi.nlm.nih.gov/books/NBK536940/ (accessed 3 July 2025).

Kearsley J (2022). Regulation 28:report to prevent future deaths. Available at: https://www.judiciary.uk/wp-content/uploads/2022/11/Awaab-Ishak-Prevention-of-future-deaths-report-2022-0365_Published.pdf (accessed 17 April 2025).

Kesley, J., & Rylatt, L.A. (2021). Respiratory illness in children. In: In Glasper, A., Richardson, J., & Randall, D.A. (eds). *Textbook of Children's and Young People's Nursing*, 3rd edn. Oxford: Churchill Livingstone.

Klok, T., Kaptein, A.A., & Brand, P.L.P. (2013). Improving adherence in paediatric respiratory disease. *Breather* 9(4), 268–277. doi:10.1183/20734735.002513.

National Institute for Health and Care Excellence (NICE) (2020). Intravenous fluid therapy in children and young people in hospital. NICE guideline [NG29]. Available at: https://www.nice.org.uk/guidance/ng29/chapter/Recommendations#principles-and-protocols-for-intravenous-fluid-therapy (accessed 2 July 2025).

National Institute for Health and Care Excellence (NICE) (2021). Bronchiolitis in children: diagnosis and management. NICE guidelines [NG9]. Available at: https://www.nice.org.uk/guidance/ng9 (accessed 3 June 2025).

National Institute for Health and Care Excellence (NICE) (2022). Croup. Available at: https://cks.nice.org.uk/topics/croup/ (accessed 3 June 2025)

National Institute for Health and Care Excellence (NICE) (2024). Tuberculosis. NICE guideline [NG33] Available at Recommendations | Tuberculosis | Guidance | NICE (accessed on 3 July 2025).

Nursing & Midwifery Council (NMC) (2018). The Code. Professional standards of practice and behaviour for nurses, midwives and nursing associates. Available at *The Code* (accessed 3 July 2025).

Royal College of Nursing (RCN) (2017). *Standards for assessing, measuring and monitoring vital signs in infants, children and young people.* RCN Publications, London.

Royal College of Paediatric and child health (2021). 2021-0113-Response-from-Royal-College-of-Paediatrics-and-Child-Health Available at: https://www.judiciary.uk/wp-content/uploads/2021/04/2021-0113-Response-from-Royal-College-of-Paediatrics-and-Child-Health-Redacted.pdf (accessed 17 April 2025).

Royal College of Physicians (2024). Why asthma still kills. Available at: https://www.hqip.org.uk/resource/nrap-breathing-well/ (accessed April 2025).

Smyth, A.R. (2013). Management of lung infection in children. In: Mighten, J. (ed). *Children's Respiratory Nursing.* Chichester: Wiley.

Tate, P. (2010). *The Doctor's Communication Handbook*, 6th edn. Radcliffe Publishing, Oxford.

UK Health Protection Agency (2024c). Guidance on the management of cases of pertussis in England during the re-emergence of pertussis in 2024. Available at https://assets.publishing.service.gov.uk/media/66c4a642808b8c0aa08fa7e7/UKHSA-guidance-on-the-management-of-cases-of-pertussis-during-high-activity-august-2024.pdf (accessed 3 July 2025).

UK Health Security Agency (2024a). New RSV vaccine could prevent 5,000 infant hospitalisation, Press Release. Available at https://www.gov.uk/government/news/new-rsv-vaccine-could-prevent-5000-infant-hospitalisations.

UK Health Security Agency (2024b). Health Protection report volume 18, issue 1: News(1 and 26 February 2024) Update on pertussis activity in England. Available at *HPR volume 18 issue 1: news (1 and 26 February 2024) - GOV.UK* (viewed 3 July 2025).

UK Health Security Agency (2025). Immunisation schedule Available at: https://www.gov.uk/government/publications/routine-childhood-immunisation-schedule/routine-childhood-immunisations-from-1-july-2025-babies-born-from-1-july-2024 (accessed February 2025).

UK Health Security Agency (2025a). Respiratory syncytial virus (RSV): the Green Book, Chapter 27a. Available at https://www.gov.uk/government/publications/respiratory-syncytial-virus-the-green-book-chapter-27a.

UK Health Security Agency (2025d). Tuberculosis cases in England continued to increase in 2024. Available at Tuberculosis cases in England continued to increase in 2024 - GOV.UK (accessed 3 July 2025).

Watts E and Kay R (2023) Epiglottitis. Available at https://teachmepaediatrics.com/ent/throat/epiglottitis/ (accessed 3 June 2025).

World Health Organization (WHO) (2022). Pneumonia in children. Available at https://www.who.int/news-room/fact-sheets/detail/pneumonia (accessed on 3 June 2025).

World Health Organization (WHO) (2024). Guideline on management of pneumonia and diarrhoea in children up to 10 years of age. Available at https://www.who.int/publications/i/item/9789240103412 (accessed on 2 July 2025).

CHAPTER 13

Disorders of the endocrine system

Julia Petty

AIM

The aim of this chapter is to offer an overview of the anatomy and physiology of the endocrine system along with the altered pathophysiology.

LEARNING OUTCOMES

On completion of this chapter, the reader will be able to:

- List the organs and hormones of the endocrine system along with their key functions.
- Discuss normal and abnormal pathophysiological changes that may occur in the endocrine system.
- Outline the diagnosis and assessment of a range of endocrine disorders.
- Outline the care of children and/or young people with endocrine disorders.

KEYWORDS

- endocrine system
- endocrine glands
- hormones
- endocrine disorders
- hormone replacement
- lifelong effects

Test your prior knowledge

1. Outline the role and functions of the endocrine system, considering each endocrine gland and its associated hormone(s).
2. For each endocrine gland, identify disorders that can occur and the associated pathophysiology.
3. Outline how endocrine disorders are diagnosed, including key signs and symptoms.
4. Discuss the treatment and care of children and/or young people with a range of endocrine disorders.
5. Discuss how disorders of the endocrine system can impact health and well-being, both physical and emotional.

Introduction

The endocrine system regulates many vital bodily functions (Hinson *et al.*, 2022; Jameson & De Groot, 2022). This chapter outlines the major endocrine glands and hormones and examines the pathophysiology that arises from disease, injury or dysfunction. It also reviews key endocrine conditions along with their diagnosis, treatment and care.

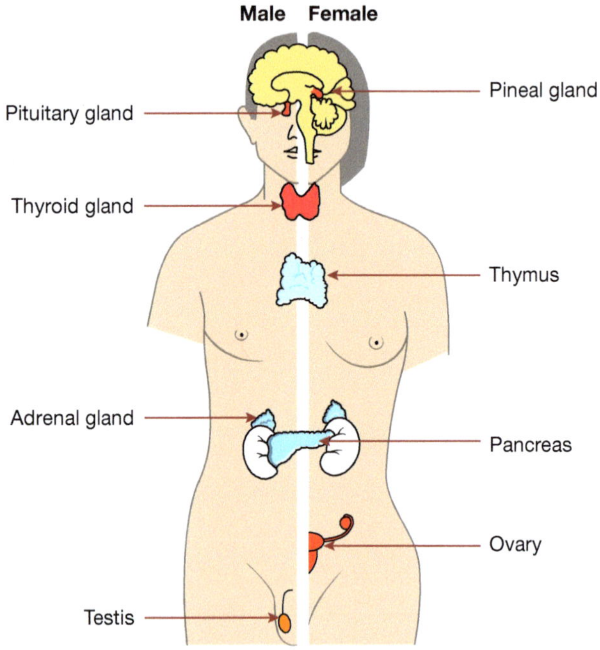

FIGURE 13.1 The endocrine system.
Source: Unknown/Wikimedia/ http://commons.wikimedia.org/wiki/File:Illu_endocrine_system.jpg/Public Domain/last accessed on October 15, 2025.

Endocrine anatomy and function

The endocrine and nervous systems transmit vital messages and regulate key bodily functions (Knight, 2021; Ashwell, 2022). While the nervous system relies on electrical impulses, the endocrine system consists of ductless, highly vascular glands that secrete hormones directly into the bloodstream. These hormones travel to distant target tissues or organs (Molina, 2023), where they exert specific effects. Endocrine activity is regulated by neural stimulation, blood-borne chemical receptors and hormones released by other glands (Waugh & Grant, 2022). Through the regulation of organ function, the endocrine system helps maintain homeostasis. Hormones underpin essential physiological processes, including growth and development, sexual maturation, glucose and mineral balance and the stress response (Petty, 2021). The anatomy of the endocrine system is shown in Fig. 13.1.

The integrity of this system is crucial for healthy body weight, growth and physical and emotional development. Consequently, damage or disease affecting endocrine glands can have significant effects on a child or young person.

A summary of the endocrine organs, their functions and associated disorders can be seen in Table 13.1.

Endocrine disorders

Referring to the systems in Table 13.1, this chapter discusses each associated disorder, outlining the pathophysiology, diagnosis and presenting signs along with a brief overview of care and management. For all conditions involving the endocrine system, referral to a paediatric endocrinology team and/or other health professionals, as appropriate, is necessary for ongoing follow-up and management.

Psychological and social factors may influence development differently in children with endocrine disorders and can significantly affect emotional well-being.

- **Body image and self-esteem:** Conditions such as growth hormone deficiency or early/late puberty can result in noticeable differences in height, weight or physical development. These may make children feel different from their peers, contributing to low self-esteem, anxiety or social withdrawal.
- **Social integration and peer relationships:** Chronic endocrine conditions often involve frequent medical appointments, dietary restrictions or physical limitations that disrupt school and social participation. As a result, some children may struggle to build and maintain peer relationships, increasing the risk of social isolation.

TABLE 13.1 Overview of the endocrine system, its associated functions and disorders

Endocrine organ	Function	Associated disorders
Hypothalamus	Acts as the central endocrine control centre, communicating with the pituitary gland and regulating functions such as growth, thermoregulation, hunger and thirst, sexual development and stress responses.	Hypothalamic disease can cause the disorders explained further.

Pituitary gland	Regulated by hypothalamic releasing and inhibiting hormones, the pituitary gland controls many endocrine functions. Hormones include: posterior pituitary, ADH and oxytocin; anterior pituitary, growth hormone (somatotropin), TSH, ACTH, FSH, LH, prolactin, melanocyte-stimulating hormone and beta-endorphin.	• Hypopituitarism
		• Pituitary dwarfism/poor somatic growth
		• Gigantism
		• Diabetes insipidus
		• Pituitary tumours, such as:
		  • craniopharyngioma
		  • prolactinoma
		  • pituitary adenoma

Pineal gland	Produces the hormone melatonin, helping to regulate the human sleep–wake cycle, the circadian rhythm	• Pineal disease/dysfunction, e.g., disruption to the sleep–wake cycle (circadian rhythms)
Thyroid gland	Releases thyroxine, which regulates metabolism, stimulates oxygen and energy use, supports growth through protein synthesis and influences nervous system activity. Calcitonin helps lower blood calcium levels.	• Hypothyroidism • Hyperthyroidism (Graves')
Parathyroid gland	Releases parathyroid hormone, raises blood calcium level and decreases phosphate level by increasing the rate of calcium absorption from the intestine into the blood.	• Hypoparathyroidism • Hyperparathyroidism
Thymus gland	Releases thymosin and other related hormones, plays an integral role in the maturation of T cells, part of the immune system.	• Thymus disease/dysfunction, e.g., interference with normal immune response
Adrenal gland	Produces mineralocorticoids, which stimulate kidney sodium reabsorption, increasing blood sodium and water levels; corticosteroids, which promote gluconeogenesis, fat breakdown, metabolism, stress resistance and increased blood glucose; and gonadocorticoids, which influence masculinisation (virilisation) in both sexes. Adrenaline and noradrenaline from the adrenal medulla play key roles in the body's fight-or-flight stress response.	• Adrenal insufficiency: Addison's disease • Cushing disease • Congenital adrenal hyperplasia
Pancreas	Produces and releases insulin which results in target cells taking up free glucose so lowering blood levels. Conversely, glucagon is also released that targets the liver to break down glycogen into glucose which increases blood glucose levels.	• Diabetes mellitus • Hyperinsulinemia/nesidioblastosis
Testes and ovaries	Release sex hormones, testosterone or oestrogen, from either the testes or the ovaries.	• DSD or ambiguous genitalia • Gonadotropin deficiency – failure to initiate or complete puberty • Precocious puberty • Ovarian disease

For full details of endocrine system function and specific hormones as relevant to children, see Petty (2021).
ACTH, adrenocorticotropic hormone; ADH, anti-diuretic hormone; DSD, disorder of sex development; FSH, follicle-stimulating hormone; LH, luteinizing hormone; PG, pineal gland; TSH, thyroid-stimulating hormone.

Medical and lifestyle support are vital for healthy growth in children with endocrine disorders. Key approaches include:

- **Consistent medical management and monitoring:** Regular follow-up with a paediatric endocrinologist and adherence to prescribed treatments (such as hormone therapy, medication or dietary plans) help control the condition and promote normal growth and development.
- **Balanced nutrition and physical activity:** A nutritious, condition-appropriate diet and suitable physical activity support overall health, strengthen bones and muscles and contribute to healthy growth.

Growth and development

Growth and development vary across age groups, making age-specific care essential in managing paediatric endocrine disorders (Gibney *et al.*, 2022). Key points include:

- Age-appropriate communication with the child and family;
- Multidisciplinary care (e.g., endocrinologist, paediatrician, psychologist and dietitian);
- Regular growth and pubertal assessments;
- Awareness of the psychosocial impact of visible symptoms (e.g., short stature and early puberty).

In the neonatal period, congenital conditions such as hypothyroidism and adrenal hyperplasia require urgent screening, diagnosis and hormone replacement to prevent severe complications. Infancy involves rapid growth, with treatment supporting normal brain and physical development. Early childhood may reveal growth hormone deficiency or adrenal disorders, emphasising developmental monitoring and emotional support. In middle childhood, delayed or early puberty can affect peer comparison and self-esteem, requiring psychological support. Adolescents face hormonal changes, body image concerns and potential treatment non-compliance, making education, emotional support and transition planning essential.

Disorders of the hypothalamus and pituitary gland

Hypothalamic disease

This disorder arises from damage due to malnutrition (including anorexia and other eating disorders), genetic disorders, radiation, surgery, head trauma, lesions, tumours or other physical injury. Such damage can affect any hormones listed in Table 13.1 and the associated endocrine systems. Because many hypothalamic hormones regulate the pituitary gland, hypothalamic disease can disrupt pituitary function (Yu, 2014) and the organs it controls, including the adrenal glands, ovaries, testes and thyroid (Ashwell, 2022).

Hypothalamic damage may lead to disturbances in body temperature, growth, weight, fluid and sodium balance, lactation, emotions and sleep cycles. Conditions arising from hypothalamic disease include hypopituitarism, neurogenic diabetes insipidus (DI), hypothyroidism and altered pubertal development. The signs, symptoms and care for these conditions are discussed in the following sections.

Hypopituitarism

Due to the pituitary gland's wide-ranging functions (El Sayed *et al.*, 2019; Marquez, 2024), hypopituitarism is associated with numerous disorders. It refers to the pituitary gland's inability to produce sufficient hormones, either from inadequate pituitary function or insufficient hypothalamic-releasing hormones. Reduced pituitary hormone output lowers target gland hormone production due to a lack of trophic stimulation. Normally, low target hormone levels trigger increased pituitary hormone release, but in hypopituitarism, this response is absent, suboptimal or inappropriate, causing progressive secondary target gland failure (BMJ Best Practice, 2025a). The condition often involves multiple hormone deficiencies and can be chronic unless underlying disorders are successfully treated (Child Growth Foundation, 2025).

Children with hypopituitarism typically present with low target hormone levels alongside low or inappropriately normal trophic hormone levels (Iglesias, 2024). Pituitary function is assessed through target gland function rather than isolated pituitary hormone measurements. Symptoms vary with the type, severity and speed of hormone loss, as well as the resulting condition (Endocrine Society, 2024).

Specific conditions caused by hypopituitarism include growth disorders, DI and pituitary tumours.

Growth disorders

Growth disorders may arise from various constitutional and genetic causes, including achondroplasia, hypothyroidism, Cushing syndrome, Silver-Russell syndrome, nutritional short stature, intrauterine growth restriction and bone disorders (Murray & Clayton, 2022). In the context of this chapter, the focus is on short stature caused by pituitary hormone deficiency in hypopituitarism. This disorder is marked by very slow or delayed growth early in childhood, before bone cartilage ossification, due to insufficient pituitary growth hormone secretion (Boguszewski, 2021).

Symptoms usually appear from late infancy through the mid-teens, with the most obvious sign being slow growth. Children may show low blood glucose or obesity, but generally have average body proportions and intelligence (Human Growth Foundation, 2025). Long-term treatment with synthetic human growth hormone (HGH) injections can help these children achieve average height.

In contrast, acromegaly results from excessive growth hormone, rarely affecting children. When it occurs between ages 15 and 17, it can cause gigantism, leading to excessive growth and abnormal bone development.

Diabetes insipidus

Diabetes insipidus (DI) can be classified by cause: neurogenic (cranial) DI, due to reduced ADH production by the pituitary; nephrogenic DI, where the renal tubules are unresponsive to ADH; and idiopathic DI, where hypothalamic cells are damaged by an autoimmune response, halting ADH production (Levy *et al.*, 2019; Hui *et al.*, 2024).

ADH (also known as arginine vasopressin) regulates blood water levels. Osmoreceptors in the hypothalamus detect blood osmotic pressure and signal the pituitary to release ADH. ADH increases water reabsorption in the distal tubule and collecting ducts, concentrating urine and regulating thirst. Reduced ADH leads to excessively dilute urine and increased thirst, causing neurogenic DI (Christ-Crain *et al.*, 2019; Khardori, 2024). Prolonged DI may result in dehydration and can occur alone or with other pituitary hormone deficiencies. For presenting signs, see case study 13.1.

Treatment of neurogenic DI is synthetic ADH analogue desmopressin (DDAVP) (D'Alessandri-Silva *et al.*, 2019; Baldeweg *et al.*, 2018). Parents should be educated on fluid replacement in infants and young children unable to express thirst or access fluids. Gastrointestinal illnesses causing reduced intake or increased fluid loss require prompt attention to prevent life-threatening electrolyte and fluid imbalances (Christ-Crain *et al.*, 2019).

Medication alert

Hormone therapy for endocrine conditions – such as DI, hypothyroidism and diabetes mellitus – is often long-term or lifelong. Education of the child and family is essential, emphasising the importance of regular, timely administration, correct self-administration and integration into daily routines. They must understand the risks of missed doses or sudden cessation, particularly with hormones such as steroids, where abrupt withdrawal can be dangerous.

Investigations: Assessing endocrine function

Endocrine function and hormone levels can be assessed in several ways (Hadded *et al.*, 2019):

- **Measuring hormone effects:** Indirect assessment, such as using blood glucose to evaluate insulin availability.
- **Laboratory testing:** Hormone levels are often very low, requiring sensitive assays such as radioimmunoassays, immunoradiometric assays (IRMA) and ELISA (Barth, 2014; Jacobsen *et al.*, 2024). Blood tests may measure stimulating hormones (e.g., TSH) alongside target hormones (e.g., thyroxine).
- **Urine testing:** Hormone metabolites can be measured, typically using 24-hour collections.
- **Stimulation and suppression tests:** Dynamic tests assess gland function. Stimulation tests evaluate hypofunction by administering trophic hormones, while suppression tests confirm hyperfunction when glands fail to respond to normal negative feedback.
- **Imaging:** Supports diagnosis and follow-up. Isotopic imaging (e.g., thyroid scans) and non-isotopic methods (MRI, CT) visualise the hypothalamus, pituitary, adrenal and abdominal organs. Ultrasound provides clear imaging of the thyroid and adjacent structures.

Case study 13.1: pituitary insufficiency – diabetes insipidus

A 4-year-old boy is admitted to the children's emergency department with his mother, presenting with signs of dehydration. He has a history of excessive thirst, polyuria and poor growth, with both weight and height below the 10th centile and a drop of one centile over the past year. He is admitted for further investigation with a provisional diagnosis of DI.

The following vital signs were noted and recorded:

Vital sign	Observation	Normal
Temperature	37.9 °C	36.5–37.5 °C
Pulse	165 beats per minute	95–150
Respiration	50 breaths per minute	25–35
Blood pressure	75/40 mmHg	80–100 mmHg
CRT	4 seconds	<3 seconds
PEWS		
Behaviour	2: Irritable	
Cardiovascular	2: Prolonged capillary refill time and tachycardia	
Respiratory	1: > 10 above normal rate	
TOTAL SCORE	**5**	

The following parameters were also seen:

Test	Result	Guideline normal values
Urine output	6–7 mL/kg/hour	<4 mL/kg/hour
Urine: specific gravity	1.002	1.005–1.020
Urine osmolarity	300 mOsm/kg	500–800 mOsm/kg
Blood osmolarity	360 mOsm/kg	275–295 mOsm/kg
Blood sodium	147 mmol/L	135–145 mmol/L
Blood potassium	4 mmol/L	3.5–5 mmol/L
Blood creatinine	0.9 mg/dL	0.5–1.0 mg/dL
Blood urea	15 mg/dL	5–25 mg/dL

Reflect on this case and consider the following:

1. Why do the aforementioned signs and symptoms present in this condition?
2. What are the possible causes of this situation?
3. What are the goals and priorities of treatment?
4. What advice and education are required for the child and family in relation to the short- and long-term care?

Tumours of the pituitary gland

Pituitary tumours can cause pituitary dysfunction, usually benign, either through local effects or by altering hormone production (Jouinot *et al.*, 2022; Casar-Borota *et al.*, 2025). Common types include:

- **Craniopharyngioma:** A benign tumour near the pituitary, most often affecting children aged 5–10 years.
- **Pituitary adenoma:** A small benign tumour, usually < 1 cm, often producing excess ACTH, stimulating cortisol release (Russ *et al.*, 2023). Most paediatric Cushing syndrome cases, excluding steroid-induced, are caused by pituitary adenomas.
- **Prolactinoma:** Non-cancerous tumour producing excess prolactin.
- **Other hormone-secreting tumours:** GH-, TSH- or LH-/FSH-secreting tumours, named for the hormone they overproduce (Tidy, 2023a).

Mechanisms of symptoms

- Increased intracranial pressure causing headache, nausea, vomiting and balance difficulties.
- Pituitary dysfunction leading to hormone imbalances, e.g., DI or stunted growth.
- Optic nerve damage causing visual problems, often permanent and sometimes worsened post-surgery.

Investigations

- Endocrine hormone evaluation for imbalances (see Investigations: Assessing endocrine function);
- CT or MRI of the brain;
- Neurological examination (Children's Cancer and Leukaemia Group, 2021).

Clinical features

- **Craniopharyngioma:** Headache, nausea, vomiting, hormone imbalances and visual problems.

- **Pituitary adenoma/Cushing disease:** Growth failure, weight gain, facial plethora, round face, temporal fat pad, increased fine hair and diabetes.
- **Prolactinoma:** Reduced fertility, breast changes, headaches, delayed growth or puberty.

Management

- **Pituitary adenoma:** First-line is surgical adenomectomy; radiation if surgery fails (Sharma, 2023).
- **Prolactinoma:** Usually managed with dopamine agonist medication (Petersenn *et al.*, 2023).
- Tumours not fully resectable require radiation therapy.

Prognosis depends on tumour removal, neurological deficits and hormonal imbalances. Long-term issues with hormones, vision or neurology may persist and recurrence is possible (Molitch, 2017; Esposito *et al.*, 2019a).

Multi-system effects and symptoms of endocrine disorders

Healthcare professionals should recognise the multi-system manifestations of endocrine disorders in children and young people, given the widespread effects of hormones (Davies & Bryan, 2022). Unexplained or persistent signs may indicate an undiagnosed endocrine disorder. Examples include:

- **Neurological:** Headache, altered consciousness, abnormal muscle tone, strength or gait, movement difficulties and developmental delay (Jeesuk, 2014).
- **Skin:** Hypothyroidism – hair loss, cold and pale skin and myxedematous changes (hands and periorbital region). Cushing syndrome – centripetal obesity, moon facies, supraclavicular fat pads and abdominal striae. Addison's disease – hyperpigmentation, mainly on face, neck and hands; in darker-skinned children, lip colour changes are more reliable (Tong & Ooi, 2021; Ohanenye *et al.*, 2024).
- **Pulmonary:** Acute and chronic infections are common in diabetes mellitus; hypo- and hyperthyroidism may alter lung function and central respiratory drive.
- **Hypoparathyroidism:** Hypocalcaemia can cause laryngospasm, stridor and airway obstruction.

Endocrine disorders may also be more common in children with disabilities or those who have received childhood chemotherapy or radiotherapy (Gebauer *et al.*, 2019).

Medication alert

The methods of administering hormones

Hormones can be administered via various routes depending on the type of hormone, the child's age or preference. Examples include: oral (steroids and thyroxine), subcutaneous (insulin and growth hormone), intramuscular (testosterone), intranasal (vasopressin) and transdermal patches (female sex hormones). Dosages may be weight-based or adjusted according to monitoring, such as blood glucose levels for diabetes.

Regardless of the route, it is essential to monitor for side effects and educate the child or young person on what to watch for.

Disorders of the pineal gland

The pineal gland produces melatonin, regulating circadian rhythms, particularly the sleep–wake cycle, with secretion occurring in darkness during sleep. Benign pineal cysts are common and usually harmless in children (Arendt & Aulinas, 2022), while pineal dysfunction is rare. Circadian disruption may result from environmental factors (e.g., night-time light and jet lag), genetic factors, impaired melatonin production or pineal damage/tumours. Sleep problems can occur but are also common in 15–25% of children and adolescents (Esposito *et al.*, 2019b; Delahoyde *et al.*, 2024).

Studies indicate melatonin can provide short-term sleep benefits for children with insomnia, ADHD, autism, neurological or visual conditions, with minimal side effects. Evidence on long-term safety and efficacy, however, remains limited (Dack & Garstang, 2022; Paton *et al.*, 2024).

Disorders of the thyroid gland

The pituitary gland secretes thyroid-stimulating hormone (TSH), regulating thyroid hormone production via a feedback loop. The pituitary adjusts TSH based on circulating thyroid hormone levels. Hypothyroidism occurs when TSH is elevated, and thyroid hormone is low or low-normal, while hyperthyroidism occurs when TSH is low or suppressed and thyroid hormone is elevated.

Hypothyroidism

Congenital hypothyroidism (CH) is the absence of thyroid hormones at birth, which, if untreated, can cause irreversible neurological damage and poor growth (van Trotsenburg *et al.*, 2021; Bowden & Goldis, 2023). Some cases are due to hypothalamic or pituitary dysfunction, often alongside other pituitary hormone deficiencies such as growth hormone deficiency (Feldt-Rasmussen *et al.*, 2021).

Primary hypothyroidism may develop after birth and does not usually cause irreversible neurological damage. Causes include thyroid aplasia, hypoplasia, ectopic tissue or inherited defects in hormone metabolism (e.g., TSH unresponsiveness and thyroglobulin defects), while transient hypothyroidism can occur due to maternal medications (e.g., carbimazole) or maternal antibodies. Several genetic defects are also linked to CH (Cole, 2022; Stoupa *et al.*, 2025).

Infants are typically normal at birth due to maternal thyroid hormone, but later symptoms can include feeding difficulties, lethargy, constipation, macroglossia, hypotonia, prolonged jaundice, umbilical hernia, low temperature, myxoedema, genital and extremity oedema and cardiomegaly (Patil *et al.*, 2023). Older children may show short stature, hypertelorism, narrow palpebral fissures, eyelid oedema and goitre (Daniel, 2023).

Diagnosis is by blood tests measuring TSH and T4. Low T4 with high TSH confirms hypothyroidism (Knowles *et al.*, 2018; Nallagonda *et al.*, 2023). Presenting signs are detailed in case study 13.2.

Treatment involves prompt thyroxine replacement, ideally immediately after diagnostic blood sampling. Delaying treatment beyond 6 weeks increases the risk of

Case study 13.2: hypothyroidism

A two-and-a-half-week-old infant presents with low central temperature, cool, pale skin and bradycardia. At birth, she was floppy, slow to feed and difficult to rouse, and has since developed constipation and poor weight gain. Other signs include prolonged jaundice (more than 10 days), hoarse cry and a large abdomen. Recent blood spot screening, delayed due to a family move, indicates a high risk of CH, prompting urgent referral to a paediatric endocrine team. The infant and family are admitted for further investigations and diagnostic confirmation.

On admission to the endocrine ward, the following vital signs were noted and recorded:

Vital sign	Observation	Normal
Temperature	35 °C	36.5–37.5 °C
Pulse	85–90 beats per minute	100–190
Respiration	40–50 breaths per minute	30–40
Blood pressure	70/40 mmHg	70–90 mmHg (systolic)
O_2 saturation	94%	95%

Other test results were performed with the following results:

Test	Result	Guideline normal values
Thyroid-stimulating hormone (TSH)	35	<20 mU/L[a]
Thyroxine (T4)	5	9–25 mmol/L (free T4)
Calcium	1.6 mmol/L	1–1.3 mmol/L (ionised)

[a]UK NHS newborn bloodspot screening programme (2013, updated 2024).

Reflect on this case and consider the following:

1. Why does the infant present in this way?
2. What are the goals and priorities of treatment?
3. What are the potential short-term and long-term effects of this condition?
4. What advice and education are required for the child and the family?

cognitive delay. Newborns with elevated TSH are treated until at least 2 years of age to prevent permanent deficits. Serum T4 and TSH are monitored monthly until normal, then every 3 months until age 3 and regularly thereafter (Sinha, 2022). The goal is normalisation of thyroid function and elimination of all hypothyroid symptoms (van Trotsenburg *et al.*, 2021).

Hyperthyroidism

Hyperthyroidism refers to elevated thyroid hormone levels; thyrotoxicosis is a synonymous term. Common causes include Graves' disease, the most frequent, and autoimmune thyroiditis (Hoang *et al.*, 2022). While most prevalent in women aged 20–50 years, hyperthyroidism can also affect children and young people, often with a family history of thyroid or other autoimmune diseases, such as diabetes, rheumatoid arthritis or myasthenia gravis.

Symptoms include restlessness, irritability, emotional lability, poor sleep, tremor, weight loss, palpitations, sweating, diarrhoea, shortness of breath, skin changes (hair thinning, itching), menstrual irregularities, fatigue and muscle weakness (NICE, 2025). In Graves' disease, the thyroid often enlarges, forming a goitre, and some children may develop proptosis, eye discomfort, watering or double vision due to eye muscle involvement. For presenting vital signs in a 12-year-old with hyperthyroidism, see the Vital Signs box.

As with hypothyroidism, blood tests can diagnose hyperthyroidism or rule it out if symptoms suggest the condition. High blood T4 suppresses pituitary TSH release, so low TSH with high T4 confirms hyperthyroidism. If results are borderline, tests may be repeated after a few weeks, as other illnesses can temporarily affect hormone levels (Mathew *et al.*, 2023).

Treatment of hyperthyroidism aims to normalise T4 levels and manage symptoms, using medications, radioiodine or surgery (BMJ Best Practice, 2024a). Carbimazole reduces T4 production, while beta-blockers (e.g., propranolol and atenolol) temporarily relieve tremor, palpitations, sweating, agitation and anxiety. Surgery may remove part of the thyroid, but if too much is removed, thyroxine replacement is needed.

Treatment dosing can be challenging: excessive therapy may cause low T4, while insufficient treatment leaves T4 high. Regular blood tests monitor T4 levels. In some cases, a single high dose of carbimazole or radioiodine stops thyroid hormone production entirely, requiring daily thyroxine to maintain normal levels.

Long-term follow-up is essential (NICE, 2023). Even after successful treatment, thyroid function must be monitored as hyperthyroidism can recur, or hypothyroidism may develop, which is easily managed with thyroxine replacement.

Vital sign	Observation	Normal
Temperature	37.8 °C	36.5–37.5 °C
Pulse	140 beats per minute	60–100
Respiration	25 breaths per minute	15–20
Blood pressure	130/85 mmHg	100–120 mmHg (systolic)
PEWS	3	0–1
Other	Low thyroid-stimulating hormone (TSH) and high T4 (thyroxine), low calcium	

Long-term effects need to be prevented by early referral and treatment.

There are potential permanent and long-term effects of hormone deficiency on the developing brain and nervous system. To avoid damage in the long term, it is vital that identification, diagnosis and treatment are undertaken as early as possible. A key example is CH, which is screened for using the 5-day bloodspot test. If a high-risk sample is identified, urgent referral and further investigation are required in order to confirm diagnosis or not. If positive, the baby must be started on thyroxine therapy. This highlights the need for accurate and timely screening (Boelen & Heijboer, 2025).

Parathyroid disorders

As seen in Table 13.1, parathyroid hormone (PTH) is secreted by the four parathyroid glands, located in the neck behind the thyroid gland. It regulates serum calcium and phosphate levels and also plays a part in bone metabolism.

Hyperparathyroidism

Hyperparathyroidism occurs due to excessive secretion of PTH, leading to high serum calcium and low serum phosphate (Tidy, 2023b).

- **Primary hyperparathyroidism (PHPT):** Excess PTH from one or more parathyroid glands, most commonly due to a single adenoma; less commonly from hyperplasia or carcinoma.
- **Secondary hyperparathyroidism:** Rare, usually from kidney failure or vitamin D deficiency.

Diagnosis follows detection of hypercalcaemia. Symptoms result from calcium resorption from bone and may include osteopenia, bone pain, pathological fractures, muscle weakness, proximal myopathy, fatigue, renal calcium loss and renal calculi, the most common presentation.

Management in children and adolescents requires distinguishing familial hypocalciuric hypercalcaemia (usually no treatment) from other PHPT forms, which are best treated with subtotal or total parathyroidectomy (Bandeira *et al.*, 2022). Medical therapy is generally unsatisfactory, as no agents reliably block PTH release or hypercalcaemia long-term.

Hypoparathyroidism

Hypoparathyroidism occurs when PTH is insufficient or dysfunctional, leading to low blood calcium and high phosphate levels (National Organization for Rare Disorders) (NORD, 2024). The most common causes are accidental damage during surgery or radiation, with autoimmune destruction also possible. Low calcium can cause symptoms such as muscle cramps, pain and twitching. Treatment includes calcium and vitamin D supplementation, with regular blood monitoring to maintain appropriate levels (BMJ Best Practice, 2024b).

Disorders of the thymus gland

The thymus gland has both endocrine and immune functions, playing a key role in T lymphocyte development (West, 2023). Thymus disorders include thymoma (cancer), congenital athymia (absence of thymus) and DiGeorge syndrome or congenital thymic hypoplasia, a rare condition caused by deletion of part of chromosome 22 (Lackey & Muzio, 2025). Affected children are vulnerable to infections and may have heart defects, cleft palate, abnormal facial features and low calcium, leading to bone and muscle problems such as hypotonia, scoliosis, clumsiness, leg pain, arthritis and muscle weakness.

Disorders of the adrenal glands

The adrenal glands produce a range of hormones with various effects, so adrenal dysfunction can impact many different functions. The two conditions covered in this subsection are adrenal insufficiency, known as Addison's disease, and congenital adrenal hyperplasia (CAH).

Adrenal insufficiency: Addison's disease

Adrenal insufficiency is a reduction in adrenal hormone release, including glucocorticoids and/or mineralocorticoids. Primary insufficiency occurs when the adrenal glands cannot produce enough hormones, with Addison's disease being the autoimmune form. Secondary insufficiency results from inadequate pituitary or hypothalamic stimulation. The condition is rare in children.

Symptoms include fatigue, weakness, anorexia, nausea, vomiting, weight loss, cramps, dizziness and confusion (NICE, 2024a). Chronic insufficiency may cause exhaustion and skin hyperpigmentation, though this may be less obvious in children with darker skin; lip colouration should also be assessed (Tong & Ooi, 2021; Ohanenye *et al.*, 2024).

Families must be aware of the risk of adrenal crisis, an emergency triggered by sudden cortisol deficiency, which can disrupt stress responses, including glucose and metabolic regulation. Treatment involves lifelong hormone replacement (BSPED, 2022).

Congenital adrenal hyperplasia

Congenital adrenal hyperplasia (CAH) is a group of autosomal recessive disorders caused by enzyme deficiencies, most commonly 21-hydroxylase, which is needed for cortisol and aldosterone synthesis, while androgen production is unaffected (Orphanet, 2022). Clinical manifestations depend on the degree of cortisol and/or aldosterone deficiency. Reduced cortisol and aldosterone impair stress response and can lead to life-threatening salt loss, while androgen excess affects both sexes.

- **Females:** Severe 21-hydroxylase deficiency may cause ambiguous genitalia at birth (classic virilising CAH). Mild forms present later with precocious pubic hair, clitoromegaly and accelerated growth or skeletal maturation (simple virilising CAH).
- **Males:** Genitalia are usually normal, so severe cases present at 1–4 weeks with salt-wasting, including failure to thrive, vomiting, dehydration, hypotension, hyponatraemia, hyperkalaemia and shock (classic salt-wasting CAH). Milder deficiencies may present later with early pubic hair, phallic enlargement, accelerated growth and skeletal maturation (simple virilising CAH) (Yau *et al.*, 2016).

For an example of presenting vital signs in a 5-month-old with CAH, see the Vital Signs box.

Vital sign	Observation	Normal
Temperature	36.8 °C	36.5–37.5 °C
Pulse	180 beats per minute	110–160
Respiration	65 breaths per minute	30–40
Blood pressure	60/40 mmHg	70–90 mmHg
PEWS	4	0–1
CRT	4 seconds	<3 seconds
Other	Blood sodium low	

Children with CAH are cared for by a multidisciplinary team, including endocrinologists and genitourinary specialists. Initial management involves stabilisation with intravenous fluids to correct electrolytes, followed by lifelong cortisol and/or aldosterone replacement. Regular blood tests guide dosing and adjustments. As with Addison's disease, children are at risk of adrenal crisis during stress or illness, requiring close monitoring. Many children may develop short stature and benefit from growth hormone therapy (Sharma *et al.*, 2025).

Females may require surgery for virilised genitalia and additional hormone therapy if precocious puberty occurs. Fertility is usually normal in males; females may need assistance to conceive and may require caesarean delivery. As CAH is inherited, genetic counselling is recommended for families (Simpson & Rechitsky, 2019).

Endocrine reasons for childhood obesity

In the light of recent public health concerns about the increasing level of childhood obesity, the potential for endocrine causes needs consideration (Park & Ahima, 2023). Such causes may be as follows:

- Some classic endocrine disorders are associated with weight gain, such as hypothyroidism, growth hormone deficiency and Cushing syndrome.
- Obesity may arise after injury to, or congenital malformation of, the hypothalamus.
- Leptin, a hormone produced by adipose tissues, may be disrupted.

While obesity is not a disease, the long-term effects are well documented, and so endocrine reasons need to be ruled out.

Medication alert

Careful titration of hormones is essential.

For hormones such as steroids, insulin and other replacements, careful dose titration is essential. Hormones should never be stopped suddenly, especially cortisol, as the body's natural steroid production is absent or suppressed. Dosages should be adjusted as the child grows or as clinical circumstances change. Regular follow-up and therapy review with the endocrine or paediatric multidisciplinary team is a vital part of ongoing care.

Disorders of the pancreas

The pancreas is not strictly an endocrine gland, but because it produces and secretes the hormones insulin and glucagon, it is included in this chapter. The two conditions caused by abnormal insulin metabolism are: diabetes mellitus and congenital hyperinsulinemia.

Diabetes mellitus

Diabetes mellitus is a disease caused by a deficiency or diminished effectiveness of endogenous insulin. There are several types of diabetes in children and young people. Type 1 diabetes mellitus results from the body's failure to produce sufficient insulin (NICE, 2024b) as a result of an autoimmune response of the body, which damages the beta cells of the pancreas. Type 2 results from resistance to insulin (Lima, 2019) and arises due to lifestyle risk factors, such as obesity and poor diet. Gestational diabetes occurs in pregnant women who have high blood glucose levels during pregnancy. Maturity-onset diabetes of the young (MODY) involves beta-cell function and impaired insulin secretion, usually manifesting as mild hyperglycaemia at a young age (Hoffman *et al.*, 2023). MODY is caused by a mutation in a single gene; if a parent has this gene mutation, any child has a chance of inheriting the condition from them. Secondary diabetes accounts for a small incidence of diabetes mellitus and can be due to pancreatic disease and endocrine conditions, such as Cushing syndrome, acromegaly, thyrotoxicosis and glucagonoma, for example.

Diabetes mellitus is characterised by hyperglycaemia, deranged metabolism and chronic complications. The presentation includes key signs, such as polyuria, polydipsia, lethargy, weight loss, dehydration and ketonuria. Diabetes can be diagnosed on the basis of one abnormal plasma glucose (random $\geq$ 11.1 mmol/L or fasting $\geq$ 7 mmol/L) (NICE, 2015, updated 2023) in the presence of diabetic symptoms such as thirst, increased urination, recurrent infections, weight loss, drowsiness and, in the worst-case scenario, coma. DKA is caused by a critical relative or absolute deficit of insulin, resulting in intracellular starvation of insulin-dependent tissues (muscle, liver and adipose), stimulating the release of the counter-regulatory hormones glucagon, catecholamine, cortisol and growth hormone (Vakharia, 2022). Acidosis caused by high levels of blood ketones ensues. The severity of DKA is determined by the degree of acidosis. For an example of presenting vital signs in an 8-year-old child with moderate to severe diabetic ketoacidosis, see the following Vital Signs box.

Referral to a specialised paediatric diabetes team is required for ongoing management. The main goal of diabetes management is to restore blood glucose levels and carbohydrate metabolism to a normal state. To achieve this, children with type 1 diabetes and an absolute deficiency of insulin require insulin replacement therapy, given through injections or an insulin pump. Children with type 2 may be controlled initially by lifestyle modifications, such as increased physical activity and dietary changes with lower caloric intake; weight loss reduces the rate of progression to more serious diabetes (Syeda *et al.*, 2023). Insulin may be required if such modifications are not successful. Ketoacidosis is an emergency situation leading to cerebral oedema and coma if rapid insulin administration and/or resuscitation measures are not implemented. It is essential to follow recent, evidence-based guidelines in the care of diabetes as for any other clinical disorder; in this case, see those produced by BSPED (2021). The use of glucagon must be considered in the emergency care of severe hypoglycaemia, when blood glucose levels are poorly stabilised and fluctuate between high and low.

Vital sign	Observation	Normal
Temperature	36.8 °C	36.5–37.5 °C
Pulse	140 beats per minute	80–120
Respiration	40 breaths per minute	20–15
Blood pressure	85/45 mmHg	90–110 mmHg (systolic)
Blood gas	pH 7.15, bicarbonate 10 mmL/L (metabolic acidosis)	
PEWS	4	0–1
CRT	4 seconds	< 3 seconds
Other	Ketonaemia, glucosuria and ketonuria Glasgow Coma Score 12 Oxygen saturation 91%	

Hyperinsulinemia

Congenital hyperinsulinism (CHI), often termed nesidioblastosis (Shaikh *et al.*, 2023), is a rare pancreatic disorder causing unregulated insulin secretion, leading to hypoglycaemia. Symptoms often appear soon after birth and include jitteriness, hypotonia, lethargy and seizures. Urgent stabilisation with glucose is critical to prevent brain injury. Children with suspected CHI should be transferred to a specialist centre with the expertise to carry out blood glucose monitoring needed to deliver treatment. Management includes high-carbohydrate feeds and medications such as diazoxide or octreotide. If ineffective, surgery may remove part of the pancreas. Total removal is a last resort and carries risks such as diabetes or pancreatic insufficiency.

Disorders of the gonads

Two conditions will be discussed under this final system in the chapter: disorders of sex development (DSD) (formerly known as intersex conditions) and problems with the onset of puberty.

Disorders of sex development (DSD)

When a newborn's sex is not immediately clear, the term DSD is used, encompassing conditions such as CAH, ovotesticular DSD and mixed gonadal dysgenesis (MGD) (Ahmed *et al.*, 2021; Abdelhalim, 2023). Infants may appear male or female but present with genital abnormalities, such as severe hypospadias, undescended testes, clitoral hypertrophy, non-palpable gonads or a single vulval opening.

DSD requires urgent referral to a specialised multidisciplinary team, with sensitive communication to parents. Naming and registration of sex should be delayed. Investigation aims to determine sex of rearing, anticipate and treat early medical issues, explain the aetiology and develop a long-term management plan, usually confirmed via biochemical and genetic testing (Ahmed *et al.*, 2021).

Treatment may include sex assignment, corrective surgery and hormone replacement. Pubertal development may prompt gender identity considerations and hormone therapy for transition should be distinguished from therapy for endocrine disorders. A detailed discussion of DSD management is beyond this chapter's scope.

The emotional and psychological effects of endocrine disorders.

Lifelong endocrine conditions can significantly affect emotional and psychological development through childhood, puberty and adolescence. This is particularly relevant for young people with DSD, delayed or precocious puberty or gender dysphoria, who may receive hormones to induce characteristics of their identified sex or puberty-suppressing drugs. A sensitive, supportive and consistent approach to counselling and guidance for the child and family is essential (BSPED, 2017; Ahmed *et al.*, 2021).

Medication alert

Drugs may be required that suppress hormone action or counteract their effects.

In some cases, it is necessary to suppress or counteract a hormone. For example, anti-thyroid medications reduce thyroid hormone production in hyperthyroidism and gonadotropin-releasing hormone analogues block luteinising hormone release in precocious puberty. In DSD or gender dysphoria, sex hormone suppression may be required. Hormone action may also need to be countered in emergencies, such as administering glucagon to oppose insulin during hypoglycaemia.

Delayed or precocious puberty

Generally, puberty begins at any point between the ages of 8 and 13 years in girls, and 9 and 14 years in boys. However, there are wide variations in the age of onset that are still the norm (NICHD, 2021). That said, there are *some* cases when early puberty or delayed puberty, also known as precocious puberty, could be a sign of an underlying condition that may need to be treated (Kaplowitz, 2024).

Precocious puberty: It is not always clear what causes early puberty, and it may not have an obvious cause, particularly in girls. In boys, it is less common and so is more likely to be linked to an underlying problem. In any sex, it can be caused by damage to hypothalamic–pituitary function as a result of a tumour, infection, surgery or radiotherapy, ovarian dysfunction (BSPED, 2021), thyroid dysfunction or due to a genetic disorder, such as McCune–Albright syndrome (MAS).

Delayed puberty refers to the onset of puberty past the expected norms for age. In boys, there may be no sign of testicular development, and in girls, the absence of breast development and the onset of menstruation.

Conversely, delayed puberty tends to be common in boys, and there may be no known cause. Documented causes include: chronic illness, such as cystic fibrosis, diabetes, coeliac disease or kidney disease, malnutrition, eating disorders or a problem with endocrine control of the sex hormones because of damage to the ovaries, testes, thyroid gland and/or the pituitary gland. Certain DSDs can also lead to delayed puberty, such as androgen insensitivity syndrome or genetic conditions, such as Kallmann syndrome and Klinefelter syndrome.

Tests for precocious or delayed puberty include blood tests to check sex hormone levels and possibly scanning to exclude tumours. Treating any underlying cause is a key aim. Precocious puberty can be managed by using medication to reduce hormone levels and delay sexual development for a few years. GnRH agonists are used in central precocious puberty, as well as for other aetiologies, including MAS and testotoxicosis. These come in a number of depot preparations. They work by overstimulating the pituitary, causing desensitisation and thereby reducing the release of LH and FSH. They continue until the time for normal puberty arrives. Delayed puberty can be treated by using medication such as testosterone in boys or oestrogen in girls, to increase hormone levels and trigger the start of puberty (BMJ Best Practice, 2025b). Management with drugs, however, is only undertaken if it is thought that early or delayed puberty will cause emotional or physical problems.

Special considerations

Understanding endocrine disorders in children requires consideration of diverse demographic criteria and environmental influences. These factors significantly impact incidence, diagnosis, treatment and support, making inclusivity essential in paediatric endocrine care.

Recognising diversity in endocrine disorders: Ethnic differences influence the prevalence and clinical presentation of endocrine conditions in children, shaped by genetic, environmental and socioeconomic factors. This underlines the need for culturally sensitive healthcare approaches.

- **Type 1 diabetes (T1D):** T1D is more common in white populations, especially among children of northern European descent. It is less frequent in Asian and African American populations, though global incidence is rising (Gherbon, 2025). Presentation may vary by ethnicity – Hispanic and African American children often present with higher body mass index and increased rates of diabetic ketoacidosis at diagnosis compared to non-Hispanic white peers (Gandhi *et al.*, 2017).
- **Type 2 diabetes (T2D):** T2D disproportionately affects minority groups. In the United States, non-Hispanic Black, Hispanic, Native American and Asian/Pacific Islander youth have higher incidence rates. Non-Hispanic Black youth report 50.1 per 100 000 versus 5.5 per 100 000 in non-Hispanic whites (Pinhas-Hamiel & Zeitler, 2023). In the United Kingdom, children of Asian and mixed ethnic backgrounds show elevated T2D rates, with mixed-ethnicity children displaying poorer glycaemic control (Khanolkar *et al.*, 2016).
- **Congenital hypothyroidism (CH):** CH incidence is significantly higher among Asian and Black children compared to white populations (Knowles *et al.*, 2017).
- **Precocious puberty:** African American girls typically experience earlier sexual maturation, including earlier menarche, compared to white girls (Bleil *et al.*, 2017).

Gender identity: Endocrine care must address the unique needs of transgender and gender-diverse youth in parallel with medical and/or psychological support for gender incongruence (Dwyer & Greenspan, 2021; Hannema *et al.*, 2024).

- **Early identification and support:** Differentiating between gender nonconformity and dysphoria is essential. Multidisciplinary care involving endocrinologists, mental health professionals and social support is key.
- **Puberty blockers:** GnRH analogues are used at Tanner Stage 2 to pause puberty, allowing exploration of gender identity.
- **Cross-sex hormone therapy:** Typically initiated after age 16, with careful monitoring of bone health, growth and fertility.
- **Fertility preservation:** Discussions around egg/sperm preservation should be introduced early.
- **Diagnostic challenges:** In children with DSDs, assessing gender identity and timing of interventions is critical to avoid premature, irreversible decisions.

Environmental influences

Children's endocrine systems are especially sensitive to environmental factors.

- **Endocrine-disrupting chemicals (EDCs):** Bisphenol A (BPA), phthalates, pesticides and Polychlorinated Biphenyls (PCBs) can disrupt hormone signalling, contributing to early/delayed puberty, thyroid dysfunction, obesity and reproductive issues (Di Pietro *et al.*, 2023).
- **Nutrition and obesity:** Poor diet and excess weight are linked to insulin resistance, T2D and precocious puberty. Adipose tissue also produces oestrogen, impacting pubertal timing.
- **Stress and socioeconomic status:** Chronic stress and low socioeconomic conditions can affect HPA axis activity, influencing growth and adrenal function.
- **Micronutrient deficiencies:** Iodine and other nutrients are vital for thyroid health; deficiencies may cause hypothyroidism or goitre.
- **Climate and geography:** Sunlight exposure and altitude impact vitamin D synthesis, growth and puberty onset.

Conclusion

This chapter has provided insight into the normal and abnormal anatomy and physiology of the endocrine system, as well as providing a discussion on a number of pathological changes that may occur in this system in the child or young person. Emphasis has been placed on the provision of key information points to assist the reader to understand the complex physical, emotional and lifelong issues encountered by children, young people and their families who are living with an endocrine disorder.

References

Abdelhalim, A. (2023). Ambiguous genitalia and intersexuality, Medscape. Available at: http://emedicine.medscape.com/article/1015520-overview (accessed May 2025).

Ahmed, S.F., Achermann, J., Alderson, J., *et al.* (2021). Society for Endocrinology UK Guidance on the initial evaluation of a suspected difference or disorder of sex development (Revised 2021). *Clinical Endocrinology* 95(6), 818–840.

Arendt, J., & Aulinas, A. (2022). Physiology of the pineal gland and melatonin. [Updated 2022 Oct 30]. In: Feingold, K.R., Ahmed, S.F., Anawalt, B. *et al.* (eds). *Endotext [Internet].* South Dartmouth (MA): MDText.com, Inc.; 2000-. Available from: https://www.ncbi.nlm.nih.gov/books/NBK550972/.

Ashwell, E. (2022). The endocrine system and associated disorders. *British Journal of Nursing* 31(6), 316–320.https://www.britishjournalofnursing.com/content/clinical-pathophysiology/the-endocrine-system-and-associated-disorders

Baldeweg, S.E., Ball, S., Brooke, A., *et al.* (2018). Society for Endocrinology clinical guidance: inpatient management of cranial diabetes insipidus. *Endocrine Connections* 7(7), G8–G11 https://doi.org/10.1530/EC-18-0154.

Bandeira, F., de Moura, N.J., de Oliveira, L.B., & Bilezikian, J. (2022). Medical management of primary hyperparathyroidism. *Arch Endocrinology and Metabolism* 66. https://doi.org/10.20945/2359-3997000000558, 689–693.

Barth, J.H. (2014). How are hormones measured? A journey into endocrinology. *The Endocrinologist* 111, 2–32.

Bleil, M.E., Booth-LaForce, C., & Benner, A.D. (2017). Race disparities in pubertal timing: Implications for cardiovascular disease risk among African American women. *Population Research and Policy Review* 36(5), 717–738 https://doi.org/10.1007/s11113-017-9441-5.

BMJ Best Practice (2024a). Graves disease. BMJ publishing Group. https://bestpractice.bmj.com (accessed 14 February 2026).

BMJ Best Practice (2024b). Hypoparathyroidism. https://bestpractice.bmj.com/topics/en-gb/132 (accessed 14 February 2026).

BMJ Best Practice (2025a). Hypopituitarism https://bestpractice.bmj.com/topics/en-gb/521 (accessed May 2025).

BMJ Best Practice (2025b). Delayed puberty. https://bestpractice.bmj.com/topics/en-gb/1126 (accessed 14 February 2026).

Boelen, A., & Heijboer, A.C. (2025). Newborn screening and the screening laboratory: past, present and future. *European Thyroid Journal* 1.

Boguszewski MCS (2021). Growth hormone deficiency and replacement in children. *Reviews in Endocrine & Metabolic Disorders.* 22(1), 101–108 https://doi.org/10.1007/s11154-020-09604-2.

Bowden, S.A., & Goldis, M. (2023). Congenital hypothyroidism. [Updated 2023 Jun 5]. In: *StatPearls [Internet].* Treasure Island (FL): StatPearls Publishing; 2025 Available from: https://www.ncbi.nlm.nih.gov/books/NBK558913/.

British Society for Paediatric Endocrinology and Diabetes (BSPED) (2017). Clinical Standards for Management of an Infant or Adolescent presenting with suspected differences of sex development (DSD) https://www.bsped.org.uk/media/1577/clinical-standards-for-management-of-an-infant-or-adolescent-presenting-with-suspected-differences-of-sex-development-dsd-jan-19.pdf (accessed 14 February 2026).

British Society for Paediatric Endocrinology and Diabetes (BSPED) (2021). Recommended guideline for the management of children and young people under the age of 18 years with diabetic ketoacidosis. Available at: https://www.bsped.org.uk/media/v2ydcuv0/bsped-dka-guideline-v3.pdf (accessed June 2025).

British Society for Paediatric Endocrinology and Diabetes (BSPED) (2022). BSPED Adrenal Insufficiency Consensus Guidelines. https://www.bsped.org.uk/clinical-resources/bsped-adrenal-insufficiency-consensus-guidelines/.

BSPED (2021). Guideline: GnRH Analogue Stimulation Testing to Investigate Precocious Puberty. https://www.bsped.org.uk/media/1907/gnrh-analogue-stimulation-testing-in-cpp.pdf (accessed 14 February 2026).

Casar-Borota, O., Burman, P., & Lopes, M.B. (2025). The 2022 WHO classification of tumors of the pituitary gland: an update on aggressive and metastatic pituitary neuroendocrine tumors. *Brain Pathology* 35(1), e13302 https://doi.org/10.1111/bpa.13302.

Child Growth Foundation (2025). Hypopituitarism. https://childgrowthfoundation.org/conditions/hypopituitarism/ (accessed 14 February 2026).

Children's Cancer and Leukaemia Group (2021). Craniopharyngioma: Guideline for the management of children and young people (CYP) aged <19 years with craniopharyngioma. https://www.cclg.org.uk/sites/default/files/2025-03/craniopharyngioma-oct21.pdf (accessed 14 February 2026).

Christ-Crain, M., Bichet, D.G., Fenske, W.K., *et al.* (2019). Diabetes insipidus. *Nature Reviews. Disease Primers.* 5(1), 54 https://doi.org/10.1038/s41572-019-0103-2.

Cole, T. (2022). Genetic aspects of endocrine disease. In: Wass, J.A.H., Stewart, P.M., Amiel, S.A., & Davies, M.E. (eds). *Oxford Textbook of Endocrinology and Diabetes*, 3rd edn. Oxford: Oxford University Press.

Dack, R., & Garstang, J.J. (2022). Use of melatonin: a single-centre audit. *BMJ Paediatrics Open* 6(1), e001349 https://doi.org/10.1136/bmjpo-2021-001349. PMID: 36053610; PMCID: PMC8852702.

D'Alessandri-Silva, C., Carpenter, M., Ayoob, R., *et al.* (2019). Diagnosis, treatment, and outcomes in children with congenital nephrogenic diabetes insipidus: a pediatric nephrology research consortium study. *Frontiers in Pediatrics* 7, 550.

Daniel MS (2023). Congenital hypothyroidism. https://emedicine.medscape.com/article/919758-overview?form=fpf

Davies, K., & Bryan, S. (2022). Biological basis of child health 12: the endocrine system and common childhood endocrinopathies. *Nursing Children and Young People* 34(1) https://doi.org/10.7748/ncyp.2021.e1342.

Delahoyde, M.K., Tyack, C., Kugarajah, S., & Joseph, D. (2024). Insomnia and other sleep disorders in adolescence. *BMJ Paediatrics Open* 8(1), e001229.

Di Pietro, G., Forcucci, F., & Chiarelli, F. (2023). Endocrine disruptor chemicals and children's health. *International Journal of Molecular Sciences* 24(3), 2671. https://doi.org/10.3390/ijms24032671.

Dwyer, A.A., & Greenspan, D.L. (2021). Endocrine nurses society position statement on transgender and gender diverse care. *Journal of the Endocrine Society* 5. https://doi.org/10.1210/jendso/bvab105.

El Sayed, S.A., Fahmy, M.W., & Schwartz, J. (2019). *Physiology, Pituitary Gland.* StatPearls Publishing, Available at: https://www.ncbi.nlm.nih.gov/books/NBK459247/.

Endocrine Society (2024). Hypopituitarism. Endocrine Society, 22 July 2024, https://www.endocrine.org/patient-engagement/endocrine-library/hypopituitarism.

Esposito, D., Olsson, D.S., Ragnarsson, O., *et al.* (2019a). Non-functioning pituitary adenomas: indications for pituitary surgery and post-surgical management. *Pituitary* 2019 22(4), 422–434.

Esposito, S., Laino, D., D'Alonzo, R., *et al.* (2019b). Pediatric sleep disturbances and treatment with melatonin. *Journal of Translational Medicine* 17, 77 https://doi.org/10.1186/s12967-019-1835-1.

Feldt-Rasmussen, U., Effraimidis, G., & Klose, M. (2021). The hypothalamus-pituitary-thyroid (HPT)-axis and its role in physiology and pathophysiology of other hypothalamus-pituitary functions. *Molecular and Cellular Endocrinology* 525, 111173.

Gandhi, K., Tosur, M., Schaub, R., *et al.* (2017). Racial and ethnic differences among children with new-onset autoimmune Type 1 diabetes. *Diabetic Medicine* 34(10), 1435–1439 https://doi.org/10.1111/dme.13408.

Gebauer, J., Higham, C., Langer, T., *et al.* (2019). Long-term endocrine and metabolic consequences of cancer treatment: a systematic review. *Endocrine Reviews* 40(3), 711–767.

Gherbon, A. (2025). *Epidemiology of Type 1 Diabetes.* IntechOpen, https://doi.org/10.5772/intechopen.1009817.

Gibney, J., Banerjee, I., & Ho, K.K.Y. (2022). Hormones across the lifespan'. In: Wass, J., Arlt, W., & Semple, R. (eds). *Oxford Textbook of Endocrinology and Diabetes*, 3rd edn. Oxford: Oxford Academic https://doi.org/10.1093/med/9780198870197.003.0005 (accessed 1 June 2025).

Haddad, R.A., Giacherio, D., & Barkan, A.L. (2019). Interpretation of common endocrine laboratory tests: technical pitfalls, their mechanisms and practical considerations. *Clinical Diabetes And Endocrinology* 24(5), 12 https://doi.org/10.1186/s40842-019-0086-7.

Hannema, S.E., Busiah, K., Butler, G., *et al.* (2024). Endocrine management of transgender and gender diverse adolescents: expert opinion of the ESPE working group on gender incongruence and the Endo-ERN main thematic group on sexual development and maturation. *Hormone Research in Pædiatrics*, 1–41.

Hinson, J.P., Raven, P., & Chew, S.L. (2022). *The Endocrine System: Systems of the Body Series*, 3rd edn. Churchill Livingstone, Edinburgh.

Hoang, T.D., Stocker, D.J., Chou, E.L., & Burch, H.B. (2022). Update on clinical management of Graves disease and thyroid eye disease. *Endocrinology and Metabolism Clinics of North America* 2022 51(2), 287–304 https://doi.org/10.1016/j.ecl.2021.12.004.

Hoffman, L.S., Fox, T.J., Anastasopoulou, C., *et al.* (2023). Maturity onset diabetes in the young. [Updated 2023 Aug 14]. In: *StatPearls [Internet].* Treasure Island (FL): StatPearls Publishing Available from: https://www.ncbi.nlm.nih.gov/books/NBK532900/.

Hui, C., Khan, M., Khan Suheb, M.Z., *et al.* (2024). Arginine Vasopressin Disorder (Diabetes Insipidus) [Updated 2024]. In: StatPearls [Internet]. Treasure Island (FL): StatPearls Publishing. https://www.ncbi.nlm.nih.gov/books/NBK470458/ (accessed 14 February 2026).

Human Growth Foundation (2025). Pediatric growth hormone deficiency. https://www.hgfound.org/pediatric-growth-hormone-deficiency (accessed May 2025).

Iglesias, P. (2024). An Update on Advances in Hypopituitarism: Etiology, Diagnosis, and Current Management. *Journal of Clinical Medicine.* 13(20), 6161 https://doi.org/10.3390/jcm13206161.

Jacobsen, L.M., Bruggeman, B.S., & Winter, W.E. (2024). *Quick Guide to Endocrinology-The Pediatric Version.* Elsevier.

Jameson, J.L., & De Groot, L.J. (2022). *Endocrinology: Adult and Pediatric*, 8th edn. Saunders, Philadelphia.

Jeesuk, Y. (2014). Endocrine disorders and the neurologic manifestations. *Annals of Pediatric Endocrinology & Metabolism* 19(4), 184–190.

Jouinot, A., Bonnet-Serrano, F., & Bertherat, J. (2022). Common features of endocrine tumours. In: Wass, J., Arlt, W., & Semple,

R. (eds). *Oxford Textbook of Endocrinology and Diabetes*, 3rd edn. Oxford: Oxford Academic https://doi.org/10.1093/med/9780198870197.003.0008.

Kaplowitz, P.B. (2024). Precocious puberty, *Medscape*. http://emedicine.medscape.com/article/924002-overview ().

Khanolkar, A.R., Amin, R., Taylor-Robinson, D., *et al.* (2016). Ethnic minorities are at greater risk for childhood-onset type 2 diabetes and poorer glycemic control in England and Wales. *The Journal of Adolescent Health* 59(3), 354–361 https://doi.org/10.1016/j.jadohealth.2016.05.012.

Khardori, R. (2024). Diabetes insipidus. *Medscape*. https://emedicine.medscape.com/article/117648-overview (accessed May 2025).

Knight, J. (2021). Endocrine system 1: overview of the endocrine system and hormones. *Nursing Times* 117(5), 38–42.

Knowles, R.L., Ridout, D., Crowe, S., *et al.* (2017). Ethnic and socioeconomic variation in incidence of congenital heart defects. *Archives of Disease in Childhood* 102(6), 496–502 https://doi.org/10.1136/archdischild-2016-311143.

Knowles, R.L., Oerton, J., Cheetham, T., *et al.* (2018). Newborn screening for primary congenital hypothyroidism: estimating test performance at different TSH thresholds. *Journal of Clinical Endocrinology & Metabolism* 103(10), 3720–3728 https://doi.org/10.1210/jc.2018-00658.

Lackey, A.E., & Muzio, M.R. (2025). DiGeorge syndrome. In: *StatPearls [Internet]*. Treasure Island (FL): StatPearls Publishing. Available from: https://www.ncbi.nlm.nih.gov/books/NBK549798/.

Levy, M., Prentice, M., & Wass, J. (2019). Diabetes insipidus. *British Medical Journal* 364 https://doi.org/10.1136/bmj.l321.

Lima, L.M.T. (2019). Insulin resistance underlying type 2 diabetes. *The Lancet Diabetes & Endocrinology* 7(6), 424.

Marquez, R.R.C. (2024). Hypopituitarism (Panhypopituitarism). Medscape. http://emedicine.medscape.com/article/122287-overview#a4 (accessed June 2025).

Mathew, P., Kaur, J. & Rawla, P. (2023). Hyperthyroidism. StatPearls [Internet]. Treasure Island (FL). StatPearls Publishing. https://pubmed.ncbi.nlm.nih.gov/30725738 (accessed 14 February 2026).

Molina, P. (2023). *Endocrine Physiology*, 6th edn. McGraw-Hill Medical, New York.

Molitch, M.E. (2017). Diagnosis and treatment of pituitary adenomas: a review. *Journal of the American Medical Association* 317(5), 516–524.

Murray, P.G., & Clayton, P.E. (2022). Disorders of growth hormone in childhood. [Updated 2022 Mar 9]. In: Feingold, K.R., Ahmed, S.F., Anawalt, B. *et al.* (eds). *Endotext [Internet]*. South Dartmouth (MA): MDText.com, Inc. Available from: https://www.ncbi.nlm.nih.gov/books/NBK278971/.

Nallagonda, S., Inusa, A., Gupta, R., & Nallagonda, M. (2023). Thyroid disorders in neonates: a practical approach to congenital hypothyroidism & thyrotoxicosis. *Paediatrics And Child Health* 33(6), 149–153.

National Institute for Health and Care Excellence (NICE) (2015; updated 2023). Diabetes (type 1 and type 2) in children and young people: diagnosis and management. NICE guideline [NG18]. Available at: https://www.nice.org.uk/guidance/ng18 (accessed June 2025).

National Institute for Health and Care Excellence (NICE) (2025). Hyperthyroidism. https://cks.nice.org.uk/topics/hyperthyroidism/ (accessed 14 February 2026).

National Organization for Rare Disorders (NORD) (2024). Hypoparathyroidism. https://rarediseases.org/rare-diseases/hypoparathyroidism/ (accessed 14 February 2026).

NICE (2023). Thyroid disease: assessment and management. National Institute for Health and Care Excellence. https://www.nice.org.uk/guidance/ng145 (accessed 14 February 2026).

NICE (2024a). Addisons disease. https://cks.nice.org.uk/topics/addisons-disease/ (accessed 14 February 2026).

NICE (2024b). Diabetes type 1. https://cks.nice.org.uk/topics/diabetes-type-1/ (accessed 14 February 2026).

NICHD (2021). Puberty and precocious puberty. https://www.nichd.nih.gov/health/topics/puberty (accessed 14 February 2026).

Ohanenye, C., Zakria, D., & Golant, A.K. (2024). Atopic dermatitis in skin of color. In: Brownstone, N., Liao, W., & Bhutani, T. (eds). *Clinical Cases in Atopic Dermatitis. Clinical Cases in Dermatology*. Cham: Springer https://doi.org/10.1007/978-3-031-52147-8_2.

Orphanet (2022). Classic congenital adrenal hyperplasia due to 21-hydroxylase deficiency. https://www.orpha.net/en/disease/detail/90794 (accessed 14 February 2026).

Park, H.K., & Ahima, R.S. (2023). Endocrine disorders associated with obesity. *Best Practice & Research Clinical Obstetrics & Gynaecology* 90, 102394.

Patil, N., Rehman, A., Jialal, I., & Saathoff, A.D. (2023). Hypothyroidism (Nursing). In: StatPearls. StatPearls Publishing, Treasure Island (FL). PMID: 33760505. https://europepmc.org/article/NBK/nbk568746#__NBK568746_dtls__ (accessed 14 February 2026)

Paton, C., Gringras, P., Ruan, A., *et al.* (2024). Quality of melatonin use in children and adolescents: findings from a UK clinical audit. *BMJ Mental Health* 27(1).

Petersenn, S., Fleseriu, M., Casanueva, F.F., *et al.* (2023). Diagnosis and management of prolactin-secreting pituitary adenomas: a Pituitary Society international Consensus Statement. *Nature Reviews. Endocrinology* 19, 722–740 https://doi.org/10.1038/s41574-023-00886-5.

Petty, J. (2021). Chapter 11: The endocrine system. In: Peate, I. & Gormley-Fleming, E. (eds). *Fundamentals of Children's Anatomy and Physiology*, 2nd edn. Oxford: Wiley.

Pinhas-Hamiel, O., & Zeitler, P. (2023). Type 2 diabetes in children and adolescents – a focus on diagnosis and treatment. [Updated 2023 Nov 7]. In: Feingold, K.R., Ahmed, S.F., Anawalt, B. *et al.* (eds). *Endotext [Internet]*. South Dartmouth (MA): MDText.com, Inc. Available from: https://www.ncbi.nlm.nih.gov/books/NBK597439/?utm_source=chatgpt.com.

Russ, S., Anastasopoulou, C., & Shafiq, I. (2023). Pituitary adenoma. [Updated 2023 Mar 27]. In: *StatPearls [Internet]*. Treasure

Island (FL): StatPearls Publishing. Available from: https://www.ncbi.nlm.nih.gov/books/NBK554451/.

Shaikh, M.G., Lucas-Herald, A.K., Dastamani, A., *et al.* (2023). Standardised practices in the networked management of congenital hyperinsulinism: a UK national collaborative consensus. *Frontiers in Endocrinology* 14, 1231043.

Sharma (2023). Pituitary adenoma. https://bestpractice.bmj.com/topics/en-gb/1030 (accessed 14 February 2026).

Sharma, L., Momodu, I.I., & Singh, G. (2025). Congenital adrenal hyperplasia. [Updated 2025 Jan 27]. In: *StatPearls [Internet]*. Treasure Island (FL): StatPearls Publishing. Available from: https://www.ncbi.nlm.nih.gov/books/NBK448098/.

Simpson, J.L., & Rechitsky, S. (2019). Prenatal genetic testing and treatment for congenital adrenal hyperplasia. *Fertility and Sterility* 111(1), 21–23.

Sinha, S. (2022). Pediatric hypothyroidism. *Medscape* http://reference.medscape.com/article/922777-overview (accessed June 2025).

Stoupa, A., Carré, A., Polak, M., *et al.* (2025). Genetics of primary congenital hypothyroidism: three decades of discoveries and persisting etiological challenges. *European Thyroid Journal* 14(2), e240348 https://doi.org/10.1530/ETJ-24-0348.

Syeda, U.A., Battillo, D., Visaria, A., & Malin, S.K. (2023). The importance of exercise for glycemic control in type 2 diabetes. *American Journal of Medicine Open* 9, 100031.

Tidy, C. (2023a). Pituitary Tumours. https://patient.info/doctor/pituitary-tumours (accessed 14 February 2026).

Tidy, C. (2023b). Hyperparathyroidism. https://patient.info/hormones/thyroid-and-parathyroid-glands/hyperparathyroidism (accessed 14 February 2026).

Tong, C.V., & Ooi, X. (2021). Addison's disease presenting with hyperpigmentation. *BMJ Case Reports* 14, e245610.

van Trotsenburg, P., Stoupa, A., Léger, J., *et al.* (2021). Congenital hypothyroidism: a 2020-2021 consensus guidelines update-an ENDO-European reference network initiative endorsed by the European society for pediatric endocrinology and the European society for endocrinology. *Thyroid* 31(3), 387–419. https://doi.org/10.1089/thy.2020.0333.

Vakharia, K. (2022). Childhood ketoacidosis. https://patient.info/doctor/childhood-ketoacidosis (accessed 14 February 2026).

Waugh, A., & Grant, A. (2022). *Ross and Wilson Anatomy and Physiology in Health and Illness*, 14th edn. Churchill Livingstone, Edinburgh.

West, M. (2023). What is the thymus gland?. https://www.medicalnewstoday.com/articles/thymus (accessed 14 February 2026).

Yau, M., Gujral, J., & New, M.I. (2016). Congenital adrenal hyperplasia: diagnosis and emergency treatment. [Updated 2019 Apr 16]. In: Feingold, K.R., Ahmed, S.F., Anawalt, B. *et al.* (eds). *Endotext [Internet]*. South Dartmouth (MA): MDText.com, Inc. Available from: https://www.ncbi.nlm.nih.gov/books/NBK279085/.

Yu, J. (2014). Endocrine disorders and the neurologic manifestations. *Annals of Pediatric Endocrinology & Metabolism* 19(4), 184–190.

CHAPTER 14

Disorders of the digestive system

Elizabeth Gormley-Fleming

AIM

The aim of this chapter is to provide an overview of the anatomy and physiology of the digestive system. Disturbances to the pathophysiology and impact on the growth, development and well-being of the child and young person will be outlined.

LEARNING OUTCOMES

On completion of this chapter, the reader will be able to:

- Describe the general function of the gastrointestinal system.
- Discuss the pathological processes of disorders of the gastrointestinal system.
- Identify structural defects in the newborn.
- Identify signs and symptoms indicating gastrointestinal disorders.
- Be familiar with the management of disorders in infants, children and young people.

KEYWORDS

- oesophagus
- motility
- inflammation
- obstruction
- structural defects
- malabsorption

Test your prior knowledge

1. What structures and organs make up the gastrointestinal system?
2. What function does the gastro-oesophageal sphincter have?
3. What is meconium and when would you expect to see it?
4. At what stage of embryonic/foetal development is the palate and mouth formed
5. What is the function of bile and where is it produced?
6. What function do intestinal villi play in digestion and absorption?
7. Label the following diagram.
8. How does food move through the gastrointestinal system from the mouth to the anus?
9. Where is the appendix located?
10. Why do infants regurgitate milk and when does it become of concern?

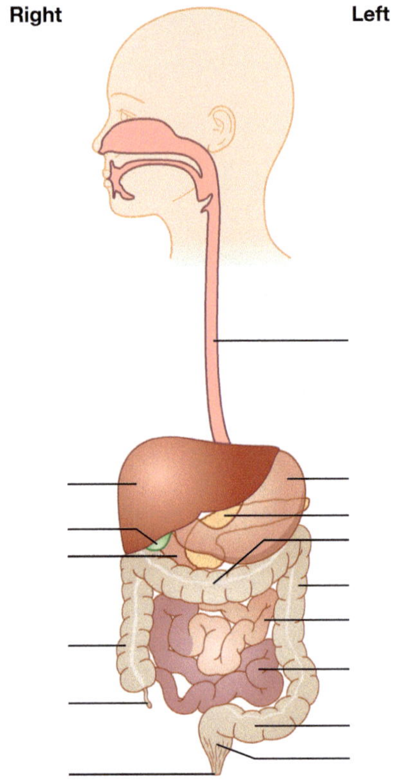

Introduction

The gastrointestinal (GI) system includes the mouth, pharynx, oesophagus, stomach and intestines, ending at the anus; in total, it measures approximately 10 m in length. Supporting structures include accessory organs necessary for digestion, such as salivary glands, liver, pancreas and gallbladders. The function of the GI tract is to digest and absorb nutrients and then eliminate waste products.

In this chapter, some of the most common GI disorders in infants, children and young people will be presented. Nursing care of the infant, child or young person and management of these disorders will be considered within the context of a family-centred approach to care. The chapter is organised under the main headings of motility disorders, inflammatory conditions, obstructive disorders, malabsorption disorders, structural defects and hernias.

Motility disorders

Motility disorders include all those affecting the normal movement of matter through the GI system. Any condition that slows or speeds the movement of matter through the GI system alters the absorption rate of fluids and nutrients. Symptoms may include diarrhoea and vomiting, resulting in fluid and electrolyte disturbances.

Gastroenteritis (diarrhoea)

Gastroenteritis is an acute or chronic inflammation of the stomach and intestines, often accompanied by vomiting and diarrhoea. It can affect any part of the GI tract and may be caused by a viral, bacterial or parasitic infection. This condition is common in toddlers and pre-school-age children, with rotavirus being more common in children under 2 years of age (Winter, 2021). Frequent episodes of diarrhoea, especially if accompanied by vomiting, can lead to severe dehydration in infants and young children, putting them at risk for hypovolaemic shock if fluid and electrolytes are not replaced. This may necessitate a hospital admission for intravenous fluids.

Diarrhoea can be acute or chronic. Acute diarrhoea is defined as a sudden increase in frequency and change in consistency of stools, often caused by an infection. This is usually self-limiting and may or may not be severe enough to cause dehydration. Chronic diarrhoea occurs over more than 14 days and is often caused by chronic conditions, such as inflammatory bowel disease (IBD), malabsorption syndromes, food allergies or non-specific causes. Causes of acute and chronic diarrhoea are presented in Table 14.1.

Diarrhoea can be mild, moderate or severe. This is determined by the number of stools and how liquid they are. In addition, the severity of other accompanying symptoms, such as irritability, anorexia, nausea and vomiting and electrolyte imbalance, determines the severity and subsequent treatment.

Diagnosis is based on history, physical examination and laboratory results. A thorough history should include questions about recent travel, day-care attendance and recent medications or dietary changes. Questions should also be asked about the frequency and character of stools, urinary output and intake of food and fluids and the presence of fever or vomiting. Physical examination gives an

TABLE 14.1 Possible causes of acute and chronic diarrhoea

Acute diarrhoea	Chronic diarrhoea
• Bacterial, viral and parasitic infections • Associated conditions, such as upper respiratory tract infections, urinary tract infections and otitis media • Dietary causes, such as overfeeding, incorrect formula reconstitution or excess sugar • Medications: iron and antibiotics • Ingestion of a toxin, such as lead or organic phosphates • Irritable bowel syndrome and Hirschsprung disease • Colon disease: necrotising enterocolitis and colitis	• Malabsorption causes: coeliac disease, short-bowel syndrome, lactose intolerance, pancreatic or enzyme deficiency • Allergies • Immunodeficiency conditions • Inflammatory bowel diseases: ulcerative colitis and Crohn's disease • Endocrine causes: hyperthyroidism, adrenal hyperplasia, Addison's disease • Motility disorders: Hirschsprung disease, intestinal obstruction • Parasitic infestations • Abdominal tumours

indication of the severity of the dehydration. Laboratory evaluation of blood and urine gives an indication of electrolyte imbalance, and stools can be examined for the presence of infectious organisms, viruses, parasites, ova, fat and undigested sugars.

An infant or child who presents with gastroenteritis but is responding normally to social cues, is content/smiling, is awake or awakens quickly, has a strong cry with normal skin colour and turgor, is passing urine and has moist mucous membranes is at low risk of clinical dehydration and shock.

Medical management depends on the clinical features the child presents with, suggesting if they are systemically unwell, the level of dehydration and the degree of shock. Rehydration with an intravenous solution chosen to correct the specific dehydration will be used in those children with severe diarrhoea and accompanying dehydration. Oral rehydration solution (ORS) should be administered in accordance with published guidelines (NICE CSK, 2024a). Clear oral fluids or breast milk will be introduced as soon as possible, and then progression to a normal diet. Fruit juice and carbonated drinks should be discouraged. Hand hygiene advice should be given to parents and carers. If the diarrhoea is caused by bacteria or parasites, antibiotics may be prescribed. The local health protection team should be notified when there is confirmation of a notifiable disease.

Medication alert

Because of the risk of masking the signs and symptoms of more serious illnesses, anti-emetics and anti-diarrhoeal medications are not generally used in children.

Constipation

Constipation is a common problem in childhood; depending on the criteria used to diagnose the condition, the prevalence may be as high as 30%, and in one-third of those, the condition becomes chronic (NICE, 2017).

The exact cause of constipation is not fully understood, but it may be dietary, an underlying disease, psychological factors, or it may be idiopathic and therefore have no known cause. It may also be because of defects in filling or emptying of the rectum, such as in Hirschsprung disease (Mueller and Goldstein, 2022), stricture or stenosis. Constipation in infancy is uncommon and most often associated with changes of diet, such as from breastfeeding to cow's milk, due to the protein content. The most common time for the condition is during toddler and childhood years, when withholding of stool may be the cause because of the unpleasant sensations associated with defecating. In the older child, it is more commonly associated with a lack of fibre in the diet and a sedentary lifestyle. Children and young people with physical disabilities and associated impaired mobility are more prone to constipation.

Delayed passing of meconium (> 48 hours of birth in a term baby), abdominal distension with vomiting, and new/undiagnosed weakness in legs should have urgent referral to a paediatrician.

Signs and symptoms may include abdominal pain, abdominal distension, hard and painful stools, a decrease in stool frequency, excessive flatulence, lack of appetite, general malaise, constipation with faecal soiling (encopresis) and irritability. Diagnosis is made on a thorough history of stool frequency and consistency and a physical examination. Early diagnosis and treatment of an acute episode of constipation is important in order to prevent the condition from becoming chronic. Early identification of constipation and effective treatment can improve outcomes for children and young people (NICE CSK, 2025a).

If children present with evidence of faltering growth, developmental delay or concerns about their well-being, which may indicate systemic disease, then they should be referred for specialist assessments for testing GI disorders such as coeliac disease.

The first line of treatment for constipation that has no underlying pathological cause is dietary management. However, for children with impacted faeces, an enema and/or laxatives will be administered, accompanied by both behavioural interventions and dietary modification to ensure a balanced diet and adequate fluid intake. The goals for management are to restore and maintain regular toileting routines and evacuation of stool. Nursing care focuses on teaching parents about normal bowel patterns in children and the appearance of normal stool. Families need reassurance that establishing normal patterns can take time, and they need to be persistent and consistent and provide the child with positive reinforcement.

A balanced diet with adequate fluid and fibre intake, along with daily physical activity, is essential in maintaining regular bowel movements.

Vomiting

Vomiting is one of the most common symptoms in childhood. In infants, it is normal to regurgitate small amounts of milk, called posseting, but in childhood, it is often due to gastroenteritis. It may also be associated with other conditions; see Table 14.2 for some of the causes. The history of vomiting and associated symptoms may help identify the cause. Vomiting in childhood is usually self-limiting with no treatment required; however, complications can occur, and these may include: dehydration, electrolyte imbalances, aspiration or malnutrition.

The vomiting reflex is under the control of the central nervous system, specifically the medulla. Nausea, meaning the desire to vomit, is a sensation that may be induced by a number of causes, including inner ear, visceral or emotional stimuli. It may lead to retching due to the contraction of the abdominal muscles.

A thorough history should be taken to ascertain the underlying cause, alongside a physical examination to identify any abdominal pain or dehydration. The type of vomitus and its relation to meals or specific foods, behaviour and any accompanying pain need to be ascertained. It is also important to assess for the presence of constipation, diarrhoea or jaundice. Other causes, such as urinary infections, brain tumour and any anatomic abnormalities, need to be ruled out with diagnostic tests, such as blood and urine analysis, X-ray and brain scan. If a cyclic vomiting pattern is present, it may indicate an eating disorder such as bulimia, and therefore, a psychiatric assessment may be needed.

If the vomiting persists for more than 24 hours, parenteral fluids may need to be considered in order to correct or prevent dehydration. Anti-emetic drugs are usually only administered in cases of extensive post-operative vomiting, chemotherapy-induced vomiting or

TABLE 14.2 Possible causes of vomiting

Newborns and infants	Older children and adolescents
• Overfeeding • Gastro-oesophageal reflux • Pyloric stenosis • Whooping cough • Small bowel obstruction • Constipation • Systemic infection	• Gastroenteritis • Migraine • Raised intracranial pressure • Toxic ingestion or medication • Pregnancy • Stress

for travel sickness. Nursing care is determined by the cause of the vomiting but, in general, includes observing the type of vomit, placing the infant or child who is vomiting in a position to prevent aspiration, cleaning the mouth after vomiting to prevent the acid from damaging teeth, assessing for dehydration, carrying out routine observations and encouraging small amounts of fluid regularly when tolerated. Once vomiting has ceased, fluids and small amounts of diet can be encouraged.

TABLE 14.3 Possible complications of gastro-oesophageal reflux disease (GORD)

- Reflux oesophagitis due to acid irritation of the membranes
- Recurrent aspiration pneumonia due to the risk of aspiration
- Frequent otitis media
- Dental erosion in a child or young person with neuro-disability, in particular, cerebral palsy
- Faltering growth

Source: Adapted from NICE (2019).

Gastro-oesophageal reflux disease

Gastro-oesophageal reflux (GOR) refers to the return of gastric contents into the oesophagus and is a normal physiological process occurring several times a day. GOR disease (GORD) occurs when the effects of GOR lead to symptoms that are severe and require medical treatment. It is difficult to differentiate between GOR and GORD, and both terms may be used interchangeably. The cause of GORD is a poorly functioning GO sphincter, which normally prevents stomach contents from regurgitating back into the oesophagus.

Some posseting of milk is considered normal in newborns following a feed; however, regurgitation that continues or increases requires further investigation. Infants with reflux are at risk of aspiration and apnoea, particularly if lying down.

Simple GOR is characterised by effortless regurgitation, and this is usually mild and transient, usually begins before the infant is 8 weeks old, and may occur several times a day, but this lessens in frequency over time. It is important to reassure parents that in well infants, with no symptoms other than effortless regurgitation, 90% of cases usually resolve before they are 1 year old and do not require further investigation (NICE, 2019). There is an increased prevalence of GORD in premature infants, children or young people with obesity, hiatus hernia, diaphragmatic hernia or oesophageal atresia (OA) repair, and children with a neuro-disability.

Other symptoms include heartburn, regurgitation, epigastric and retrosternal pain and weight loss, and most sufferers are irritable. Feeding difficulties with associated reduced intake, arching of the back and irritability are seen in infants during feeding. Sandifer syndrome – spasmodic torsional dystonia with arching of the back and opisthotonic posturing is observed in severe cases of GORD. Infants with GORD, particularly premature infants, are at risk for aspiration and apnoea. Diagnosis is made on the symptoms, and an upper GI contrast study is performed for those with persistent or recurring symptoms. In infants with unexplained bile-stained vomiting, an upper GI contrast study will be done urgently in order to rule out more serious disorders, such as intestinal obstruction (NICE, 2019).

Treatment depends on the severity and cause of GORD. Initially, in infants, feeding with thickened feeds and upright positioning may be enough for milder cases. Feeding smaller amounts more often may help reduce abdominal distension and associated reflux. Frequent winding throughout a feed also helps prevent the build-up of abdominal wind associated with feeding. Depending on the healthcare provider, pharmacological treatment may be administered; this would depend on the cause of the problem and the severity.

In some cases, where there is failure to thrive or persistent weight loss, enteral tube feeding may be considered. Surgery for GORD is only performed when medical therapy has failed and complications develop (Table 14.3).

Nursing management focuses on ensuring the infant or child receives adequate nutrition. Daily weights and plotting infant or child weight and height on a percentile chart will monitor growth. Communication with the parents and carers is essential in the long-term management of GORD.

Infant positioning

Infants must always be put to sleep on their back in order to reduce the risk of sudden infant death syndrome (SIDS), and this is still the case if they have GOR. Infants can be fed in a more upright position to help prevent regurgitation.

(NICE, 2019)

Inflammatory conditions

Inflammatory disorders may be acute or chronic and can occur anywhere in the GI tract. Causes may include injuries, foreign bodies, surgery, microorganisms or chemicals. Included here are appendicitis and IBD.

Appendicitis

Appendicitis is an inflammation of the vermiform appendix, which is a blind sac located near the end of the caecum. Appendicitis is the most common cause of acute abdominal surgery in children and can occur at any age, although it is most often seen in children over 9 years of age and peaking in the second decade of life (CKS NICE, 2025b). Appendicitis is rare before the age of 2 years of age and peaks at ages 15–19 years (Gil *et al.*, 2023).

Appendicitis results from an obstruction in the lumen of the appendix, usually by a faecalith, which is a hardened faecal mass. It can also be caused by a parasitic infestation, stenosis of lymphoid tissue or a tumour. The tissue becomes swollen due to the continuing production of mucus secretions, causing build-up and pressure within the lumen, which results in compression of blood vessels. This compression can lead to ischaemia, tissue death and necrosis. The appendix may perforate or rupture, allowing faecal matter and bacteria to be released into the peritoneal cavity. This then spreads rapidly throughout the abdomen, causing peritonitis. Progressive peritoneal infection can lead to small bowel obstruction, septicaemia, electrolyte imbalance and hypovolaemic shock.

Early abdominal symptoms of appendicitis include tenderness, colicky cramping pain around the umbilicus, anorexia, nausea and fever. The pain experienced around the umbilicus is known as referred pain. The pain often begins in the epigastric area or periumbilical area and then migrates to the lower right quadrant over 24–48 hours. Focal abdominal tenderness occurs at the site of McBurney's point, which is located two-thirds along the line between the umbilicus and the left anterosuperior iliac spine (see Fig. 14.1). Rebound tenderness, guarding and rigidity may also be present.

Appendicitis pain

Any sudden relief of pain may indicate a ruptured appendix. The initial pain relief is due to the release of pressure.

Diagnosis can be difficult as children often present with appendix symptoms when they have other conditions, such as Meckel diverticulum, gastroenteritis, pelvic inflammatory disease and mesenteric adenitis. Delaying treatment can result in the appendix rupturing. Blood

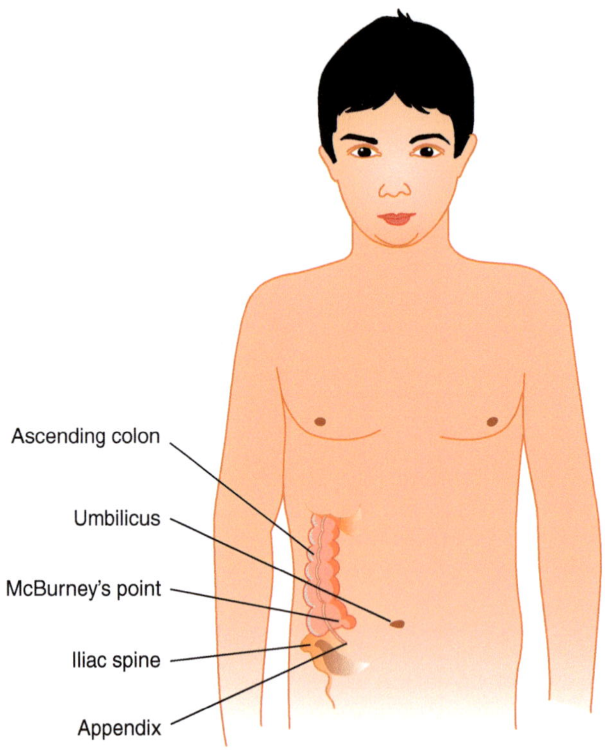

FIGURE 14.1 Common location of pain in children and adolescents with appendicitis.
Source: Ball *et al.* (2015)/with permission of Pearson.

analysis for white cell count and a CT scan may assist with the diagnosis, although this is mainly done based on the symptoms and physical examination. The treatment is surgical removal of the inflamed appendix, and the child can generally be discharged fairly quickly following surgery if they have an uncomplicated recovery. Laparoscopic appendectomy is the preferred choice of surgical procedure as the child will have less pain, a lower incidence of surgical site infections and a decreased duration of hospital stay, so recovery is quicker.

Children with a ruptured appendix will need intravenous antibiotic therapy and fluids prior to surgery. Irrigation of the peritoneal cavity during surgery will be performed to remove any infected exudate, and subsequent abdominal drainage may continue for a few days post-operatively. Oral fluids are slowly introduced, and diet is not commenced until bowel sounds are active due to the risk of a paralytic ileus.

Pain management is essential and should be assessed using a pain assessment tool; however, pain is to be expected following any abdominal surgery and the nurse should anticipate this and treat accordingly. A sudden admission for an acute condition is very worrying for both the child and parents, and they will need to be reassured. On discharge, parents will need to be advised on the signs of infection and when their child will be able to return to normal activities.

Inflammatory bowel disease

IBD includes both Crohn's disease and ulcerative colitis (UC) and is a chronic relapsing immune-related disorder (Long *et al.*, 2024). These are both long-term conditions that often begin in childhood, so they have implications that are far reaching. However, these two distinct long-term disorders have similar aetiologies and clinical features, even though their histology differs. Both disorders have the potential to negatively affect growth, normal development and well-being, so they can have a significant impact on the child and family. Onset is before age 20 years, with the majority diagnosed around 12 years, although there is an increasing incidence in the under 5 years of age group. Globally, the incidence and prevalence of IBD are rising, with the most significant increase in East Asia (Long *et al.*, 2024). Environment and lifestyle factors have been listed as potential causes.

Crohn's disease occurs commonly in the ileum, colon and rectum, whereas ulcerative colitis is limited to the colon. Crohn's disease can affect any part of the digestive tract, from the mouth to the anus. Crohn's disease is thought to be an immune-mediated condition caused by environmental triggering events (NICE, 2024a). Extra-intestinal manifestations such as eye, liver, skin and joint abnormalities have been reported in people who have been diagnosed with Crohn's disease. There may be a genetic association, which is more common in children with Crohn's disease. There is also a link between developing IBD and limited exposure to GI pathogens in early childhood (Winter, 2021).

Although many symptoms are shared between Crohn's disease and ulcerative colitis, there are differences illustrated in Table 14.4. Diagnosis of IBD may be made initially on history and blood testing; however, further tests, such as endoscopy, biopsy and radiological tests, are needed to confirm the diagnosis.

Management of the two conditions differs slightly, although the aim is to induce and maintain remission and reduce the incidence of flare-ups while still promoting normal growth and development, controlling inflammation and reducing or eliminating symptoms (Winter, 2021). Curative therapy is not yet available. Treatment includes medical treatment with 5-aminosalicylates (5-ASAs) to support remission induction. Corticosteroids are used in moderate to severe disease, but long-term use may cause side effects, and they are therefore limited to short periods of treatment. Immunosuppressive drugs and biological therapy may also be used to induce and maintain remission.

TABLE 14.4 Clinical manifestations of inflammatory bowel diseases (IBD)

Characteristics	Ulcerative colitis	Crohn's disease
Rectal bleeding	Common	Uncommon
Diarrhoea	Often severe	Moderate to severe
Pain	Less frequent	Common
Anorexia	Mild or moderate	May be severe
Weight loss	Moderate	May be severe
Growth retardation	Usually mild	May be severe
Anal and perianal lesions	Rare	Common
Fistulas and strictures	Rare	Common
Rashes	Mild	Mild
Joint pain	Mild to moderate	Mild to moderate

A vaccination history should be obtained, and vaccinations updated for all patients with Crohn's disease, those with moderate to severe ulcerative colitis at diagnosis, and prior to commencing immunomodulator or biologics in all patients.

Body image, self-esteem and well-being: UC and Crohn's disease can lead to significant weight loss and delays in growth and physical development, along with episodes of hospitalisation and the requirement to take medication. As a result, CYP with either disease may have reduced school attendance and participation in social events. This can lead to them feeling different from their peers, socially isolated and may impact their ability to form healthy relationships with peers.

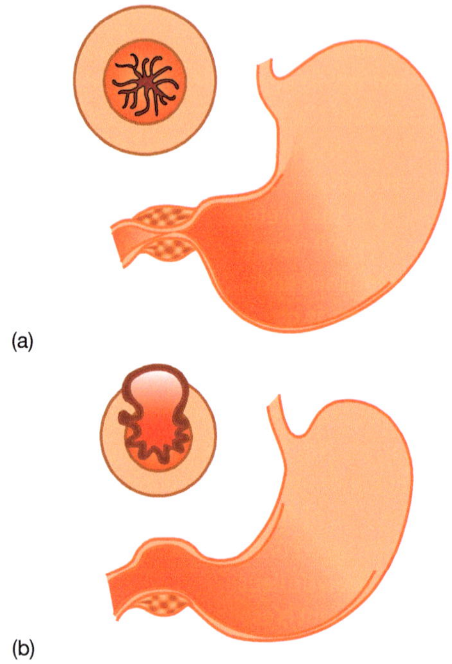

FIGURE 14.2 Hypertrophic pyloric stenosis. (a) Enlarged muscular tumour nearly obliterates pyloric canal. (b) Longitudinal surgical division of muscle down to submucosa establishes adequate passageway.
Source: Hockenberry and Wilson (2024) / with permission of Elsevier.

Surgery is more of an option in ulcerative colitis because it is limited to the colon. Crohn's disease is more disabling and may result in more serious complications (Chiarello *et al.*, 2021). Long-term complications of IBD include the need for a permanent ileostomy or colostomy, an ileo-anal pouch formation and possible colorectal cancer.

Nutritional support is needed, and a nutritionist will be involved in planning the dietary needs of the child (NICE, 2024b). The emotional impact of the disease on the child and family requires support both during exacerbations when hospitalised and in the community, where most of the management occurs.

Frequent absences from school can affect a child's self-esteem and cause social isolation from their peers. Body image is a concern for children, particularly adolescents and with prolonged corticosteroid treatment, delayed sexual maturation and growth retardation may result. In cases where an ostomy has been performed, the child and family will need support and encouragement for the child to lead as normal a life as possible.

Obstructive disorders

Pyloric stenosis is a hypertrophic obstruction caused by hyperplasia and hypertrophy of the circular pyloric muscle at the lower opening of the stomach. It may also be referred to as infantile hypertrophic pyloric stenosis (IHPS) (pyloric stenosis [Fig. 14.2]). This thickened muscle results in narrowing of the pyloric canal, leading to an outlet obstruction. It is more common in firstborn babies, with boys being affected 4–6 times more frequently than girls. The condition is more common in Caucasians and more likely in full-term newborns, typically between 2 and 12 weeks of age. The exact cause is unknown, but there may be a family history of the disorder.

Manifestations include progressive vomiting, which may be projectile; this is non-bilious in the early stages but may become brown if gastritis develops. The thickened pylorus can be felt as an olive-like mass and may be palpable in the abdomen. Initially, the infant appears well with only slight regurgitation after feeds, but as the obstruction becomes worse due to swelling, causing increasing narrowing of the lumen, the vomiting becomes worse; this usually occurs at around 3 weeks. There may also be visible gastric peristalsis on the abdomen. The infant becomes increasingly irritable and fails to gain the expected weight.

A test feed may be performed: the baby is fed, and a doctor is palpating the abdomen so they can feel the lump and then witness the vomiting. Diagnosis is confirmed by an ultrasound and upper GI radiography with barium.

Pre-operatively, infants need intravenous fluids to correct any dehydration and electrolyte imbalance. A nasogastric tube will be inserted to remove any remaining fluids prior to surgery. Treatment is a surgical pyloromyotomy, which consists of an incision in the pyloric muscle to expand the opening. Feeds are recommenced according to the surgeon's protocol, but usually commence 4–6 hours following surgery with clear fluids unless breastfeeding (Garfield & Sergent, 2023). Intravenous fluids may be necessary until adequate amounts of fluid are taken orally in order to maintain fluid and electrolyte balance. Some vomiting may still occur following surgery, and parents need to be reassured that this is normal. Parents also need reassurance that the treatment is usually successful with no reoccurrence in the affected infant. It is unusual for subsequent infants to be affected with the condition.

Intussusception (Fig. 14.3)

Intussusception is a common cause of intestinal obstruction in infants and young children, usually before the age of 3 years, but most commonly around the age of 6 months. It is more common in males than in females. Generally, the cause is unknown; however, it is common in children with cystic fibrosis. It may also follow a recent infection or be caused by a polyp, lymphoma or Meckel diverticulum.

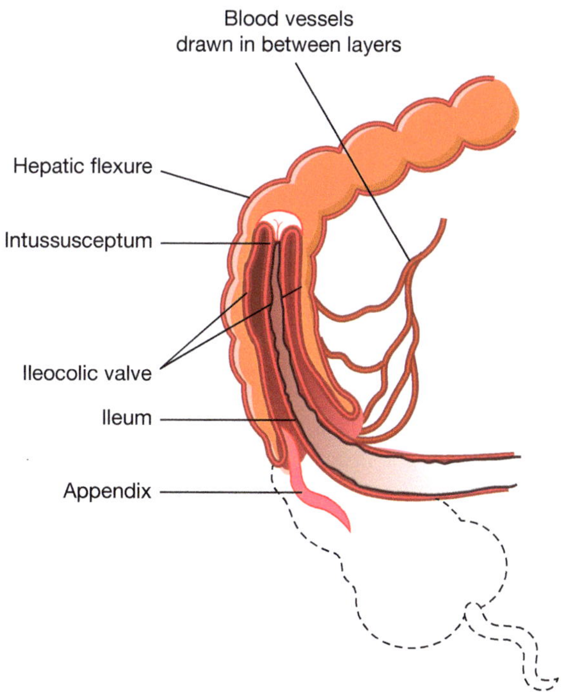

FIGURE 14.3 Ileocaecal valve (ileocolic) intussusception.
Source: Hockenberry and Wilson (2024) / with permission of Elsevier.

Intussusception occurs when one portion of the bowel telescopes into a more distal portion of the bowel, propelled by continuing peristalsis, the most common site being the ileocaecal valve. The mesentery is still attached to the telescoped portion of the bowel and is compressed, causing lymphatic and venous obstruction. Mucus production is increased, producing jelly-like stools. This results in oedema and pressure causing obstruction, which can also lead to ischaemia.

Manifestations include sudden onset of colicky pain, inconsolable crying and drawing up of the knees to the chest in a previously healthy infant or child. This is usually accompanied by vomiting that contains bile or faecal material. Electrolyte imbalance and dehydration can develop. On palpation, the abdomen is tender with a palpable sausage-shaped mass. Continuing symptoms may include fever, shallow respirations, rapid pulse and decreased blood pressure. If not treated, ischaemia can lead to necrosis, perforation and peritonitis.

Ten percent of children may have a spontaneous reduction of the vaginated bowel (Devitt & Thain, 2011). This may be indicated by the passage of a normal brown stool and will need reporting immediately, as the course of treatment may be altered. Treatment of pain and hypovolaemic shock MUST precede any investigation. Management of the condition is determined by the condition of the child and whether there is evidence of bowel perforation or not. Non-surgical management involves an air enema which is the administration of air rectally to reverse the telescopic segment of the bowel; the success rate is 80–90% (Oxford University Hospital, 2024). Surgery is indicated if manual reduction fails. If this is unsuccessful or if the affected portion of bowel is gangrenous or strangulated, then resection is performed.

Nursing considerations

Because this is a potentially fatal condition, nurses need to be alert to older children presenting with a more chronic picture of diarrhoea, anorexia, weight loss, periodic pain and vomiting.

Nursing management includes monitoring and correcting any imbalance in fluid and electrolytes by administering intravenous fluids. Post-operative care focuses on observing the child for infection, maintaining patency of the naso-gastric tube and controlling pain. The presence of bowel sounds is important prior to commencing any oral intake in order to prevent the development of a paralytic ileus. Clear fluids or breastfeeding may then be commenced and slowly increased according to the practitioner's protocol.

Malabsorption syndromes

Coeliac disease

Coeliac disease (gluten-sensitive enteropathy) is an autoimmune disorder characterised by intolerance to dietary gluten, the protein present in wheat, rye, oats and barley. This protein causes damage to the villi in the small intestine, leading to malabsorption of nutrients. The incidence is 1 in 100 people in the United Kingdom (NICE, 2025c) and is usually diagnosed between 6 and 18 months of age, when these proteins are first introduced in the diet. It is more common among family members of the same family and in children with Down syndrome, Turner syndrome, type 1 diabetes and autoimmune thyroid disease (NICE, 2025c). Coeliac disease is less prevalent in countries where gluten-containing foods do not form part of the staple diet, e.g., Vietnam and Japan.

Coeliac disease can present with several symptoms, both GI and non-GI (see Table 14.5). Diagnosis is confirmed through serological testing (NICE, 2019b). If serology testing is equivocal, then intestinal biopsy may be indicated along with additional serology testing.

TABLE 14.5 Symptoms of coeliac disease

Gastrointestinal symptoms	Non-gastrointestinal symptoms
• Indigestion • Diarrhoea • Abdominal pain • Bloating • Distension • Constipation	• Fatigue • Dermatitis • Herpetiformis • Anaemia • Osteoporosis • Reproductive problems • Neuropathy • Ataxia • Delayed puberty • Growth delay • Weight loss or static weight

Source: Adapted from NICE (2025b).

If not detected and properly treated, coeliac disease can cause serious malnourishment and debilitation. The complications of coeliac disease may include anaemia, small bowel ulcerations, bleeding disorders, malignancy (intestinal lymphoma), osteoporosis, vitamin D and iron deficiencies and lactose intolerance. Treatment is a lifelong elimination of gluten from the diet and dietary supplements such as calcium and vitamin D. Dietician input is required to provide information and ongoing support. Many of the problems with the disease are due to poor compliance with a gluten-free diet.

Nursing care priorities focus mostly on helping the child and family adhere to a dietary regimen and providing them with information on the disease. It is difficult for a child to understand that they need to adhere to the restricted diet when they have no symptoms. This may lead to exacerbation of symptoms due to non-compliance with the dietary requirements.

The maintenance of a gluten-free diet is a nutritionally safe intervention that will enable remission. The need for nutritional supplements should not be routinely recommended unless clinically indicated in children and young people with coeliac disease.

Structural defects

Tracheoesophageal fistula (TOF) and oesophageal atresia (OA)

Tracheoesophageal fistula (TOF) and oesophageal atresia (OA) are congenital malformations of the oesophagus. In TOF, the oesophagus fails to develop in the foetal stage as one continuous passage and either results in a blind end known as OA or connects to the trachea via a fistula. See Fig. 14.5 for the most common formations. The most common manifestation is when the oesophagus ends in a blind end, and the distal section attached to the stomach inserts into the trachea (example (c) in Fig. 14.4) (Durkin & De Coppi, 2022).

The incidence is one in 3000–4500 live births, with a slightly higher in males than in females, and these infants usually have lower birth weights with a higher incidence of pre-term births than average (Durkin & De Coppi, 2022). Associated anomalies may include GI abnormalities, including imperforate anus, urinary tract anomalies, vertebral defects and cardiac defects.

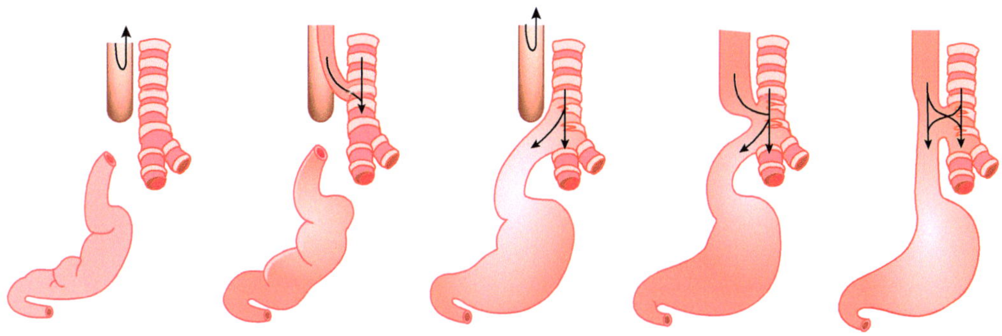

(a) (b) (c) (d) (e)

FIGURE 14.4 (a)–(e) Five most common types of oesophageal atresia (OA) and tracheoesophageal fistula (TOF). (See text for discussion).
Source: Hockenberry and Wilson (2024) / with permission of Elsevier.

Pre-natal diagnosis is dependent on the type of OA and the presence of a fistula or not (Durkin & De Coppi, 2022). Post-natal diagnosis will usually present in the first hours of birth. Newborns with the defect will present with frothy saliva and drooling from the mouth and nose, and choking and coughing with associated respiratory distress. This may be mild or more serious, depending on the type of defect present. On feeding, the infant may begin coughing and gagging despite swallowing normally, and fluid will return through the nose and mouth. Due to milk aspiration, apnoea and cyanosis may result. In mild cases, diagnosis may not occur until later in life when the child has experienced chronic respiratory problems and oesophageal reflux. A distended stomach may also be evident due to inspiratory air entering the stomach via a fistula. The type of defect is confirmed by the presenting signs and symptoms and by radiographic studies.

The priority for treatment is to maintain a patent airway, necessitating nil by mouth to prevent aspiration and intravenous solutions to maintain fluid and electrolyte balance. Accumulated secretions will be removed by suction if there is an oesophageal pouch. A permanent sump pump (Replogle tube) may be inserted to allow a continuous low suction pressure to prevent the build-up of secretions. A naso-gastric tube may be inserted into type E (see Fig. 14.5) or a gastrostomy tube to remove air from the stomach. Surgical correction of the malformation will be performed in one or two stages. Success is dependent on the type of defect and an early diagnosis.

Prior to surgery, these infants should be nursed with the head of the bed slightly elevated in order to reduce aspiration. Airway, respirations, oxygen saturation and colour should be continuously monitored for any deterioration. Suction equipment should be at hand, and no oral fluids should be given. Infants should not be given a dummy (pacifier) pre-surgery, as this increases the production of secretions. Following surgery, the secretions from the low-suction naso-gastric tube need to be monitored, noting the volume, viscosity and colour. Respiratory function needs close monitoring, and nurses should be alert to any signs of infection. Gastrostomy feeds may be given until the surgical site is healed. Oral feeds with sterile water may follow, and then increase to feeding as per practitioner protocol. Sucking on a pacifier post-surgery prevents oral aversion. Parents need reassurance and should be encouraged to participate in the care of their infant.

Long-term follow-up is advocated as the incidence of dysphagia, GOR disease, asthma and other respiratory conditions is noticeably higher in patients with OA (Krishnan *et al.*, 2016).

Cleft lip and cleft palate (Fig. 14.5)

Cleft lip (CL) with or without cleft palate (CP) is a common birth defect. The combination of CL and CP occurs in 1 : 940 births and is more common in male infants, whereas CP alone occurs in 1574 births, with this being more common in female infants (Frederick *et al.*, 2022). The exact cause is unknown, but it is thought to be a combination of both genetic and environmental factors (Zajac & Vallino-Napoli, 2026). There is an increased incidence in families

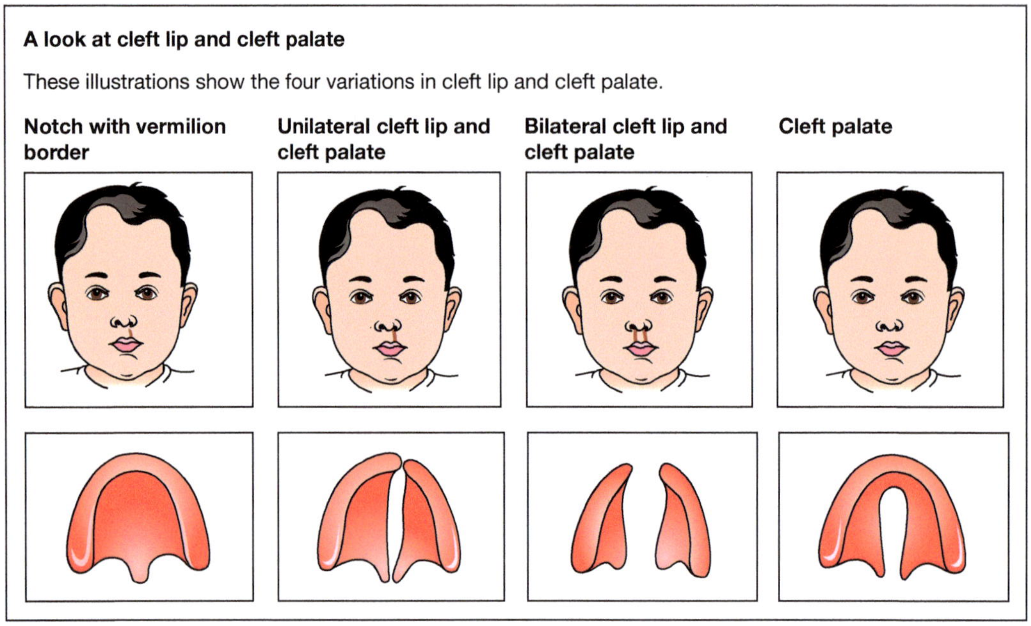

FIGURE 14.5 Cleft lip (CL) and cleft palate (CP).
Source: Devitt and Thain (2011)/with permission of Lippincott Williams & Wilkins.

with a history of CL and CP. Environmental factors or teratogens during the first trimester of pregnancy may include alcohol consumption, ingestion of some medications, such as anticonvulsants, retinoids, steroids or illegal drugs such as cocaine, and smoking. However, folic acid supplements during pregnancy are known to have a protective action against the condition.

The variations seen in the defect are due to the different stages in palatine development (see Fig. 14.6). Interruption in any of these stages can result in the defect. The earlier the interruption is, the greater the severity of the cleft. A CL and CP may occur together or alone and may be bilateral or unilateral. It may involve both the soft and hard palates and, depending on severity, may extend up into the floor of the nasal cavity. It is usually diagnosed antenatally at birth; however, a small CP without involvement of the lip may not be diagnosed immediately.

Treatment consists of surgical repair to the lip (cheiloplasty) and palate (palatoplasty). CL repair usually occurs when the infant is around 3 months old; further aesthetic surgery is sometimes needed when the child is older. CP repair usually occurs later, between 6 and 12 months of age, again with the possibility of further surgery as the child grows and develops (CLAPA, 2025).

For pre- and post-operative nursing care, see Table 14.6. There are a number of specialist feeding devices available to assist with feeding prior to repair. Mothers need to be alerted to the fact that infants and children with a CP are at increased risk of otitis media due to the altered position of the Eustachian tubes. On discharge, parents should be taught how to care for the suture line and monitor the child's feeding to maintain a healthy weight gain. Further surgery may be necessary as the child matures.

Nursing considerations

Following surgery, nothing (such as tongue depressors, suction tubes, spoons or straws) should be inserted into the mouth in order to prevent compromising the suture line.

Hernias

A hernia is a protrusion of an organ or part of an organ through an abnormal opening in the muscle wall. The abnormal opening may be a result of incomplete foetal closure or from musculature weakness. The organ

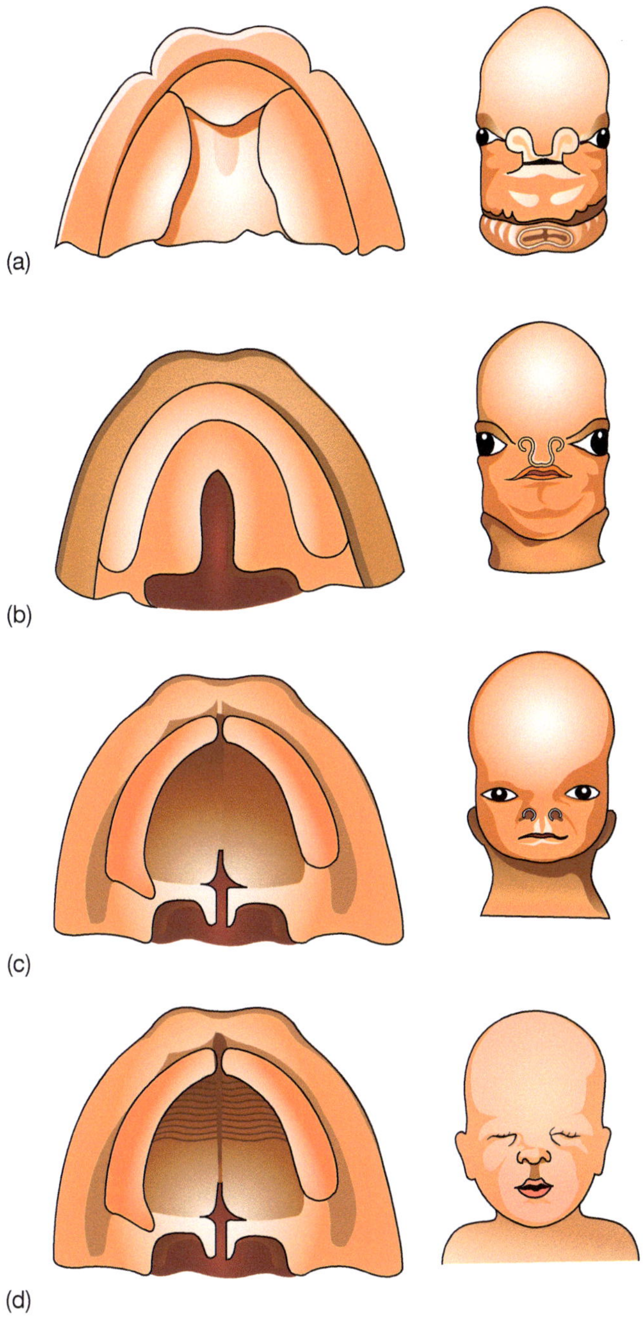

FIGURE 14.6 (a)–(d) Stages in palatine development (see text for discussion).
Source: Hockenberry and Wilson (2024) / with permission of Elsevier.

protrudes due to pressure, with the danger that it could lose function, or blood flow could be reduced, ultimately causing ischaemia. Two common hernias that present in infancy and childhood are the umbilical hernia and the inguinal hernia.

The umbilical hernia is common in infants and occurs when there is incomplete development of the umbilical ring. It may be associated with some congenital anomalies such as Down syndrome. Any abdominal pressure increases the size of the hernia, such as crying.

TABLE 14.6 Pre- and post-operative nursing care of the infant with a cleft lip and/or cleft palate

Pre-operative nursing care	Post-operative nursing care
Cleft lip • Provide parental emotional support • Feed the infant slowly to decrease aspiration risk • Small, frequent feeds and wind frequently • Promote sucking between feeds to aid speech development • Position upright to feed to aid swallowing and prevent milk from entering the nasal cavity	Cleft lip • Maintain a patent airway and observe for respiratory distress • Maintain a patent airway and observe for respiratory distress • Restrict hand-to-mouth movement in order to protect the suture line • Clean the wound following a feed • Keep the infant calm, as crying stresses the suture line • Use a syringe and soft tube to feed at the side of the mouth initially to protect the suture line • Monitor pain and administer analgesia • No soothers until the wound is healed
Cleft palate • Give a small amount of water after feeds to clean the palate • Wean onto a cup prior to surgery • Observe for fluids entering the nasal cavity and compromising respiration • Feed sitting up to aid swallowing and prevent aspiration	Cleft palate • Maintain a patent airway and observe for respiratory distress • Provide a clear drink following feeds to clean the suture line • Use a cup to feed • Start with clear fluids and increase up to soft foods • Monitor pain and administer analgesia • No soothers • Provide soft toys to prevent injury

The hernia usually resolves on its own within 3–5 years, but if it persists, elective surgery may be needed. If the hernia becomes incarcerated and is not reducible manually, then surgical intervention is indicated, as there is a danger of ischaemia.

Inguinal hernia is the most common and accounts for approximately 80% of all hernias in childhood (Hockenberry & Wilson, 2024). There is a strong gender predisposition, and males are 90% more likely to have an inguinal hernia than females (Morgado & Holland, 2024). It is more common in black children and very low birthweight infants. Children with a maternal history of inguinal hernia or connective tissue disorders have a higher risk of developing and inguinal hernia before the age of 13 years (Auger *et al.*, 2022). Inguinal hernia is caused by the persistence of the processus vaginalis, which is the tube preceding the testicle as it travels through the inguinal canal to reach the scrotum in boys, or the round ligament into the labia in girls. This occurs around 8 months' gestation. Normally, the upper portion atrophies, and the lower portion forms the tunica vaginalis, which encloses the testicle within the scrotum. When the upper portion fails to atrophy, abdominal fluid descends, creating a bulge or mass (see Fig. 14.7).

This defect may cause no symptoms and usually presents as a painless inguinal swelling. It can be reduced with gentle pressure and diminishes in size with rest. It becomes more prominent when the infant cries or when the child coughs, strains or is active. It becomes a problem if the herniated loop of intestine becomes compressed or partially obstructed. Symptoms then may include redness, oedema, tenderness, anorexia or abdominal swelling. Occasionally, strangulation occurs when there is a loss of blood supply, which can lead to necrosis. The treatment is surgical repair, usually elective unless strangulated, in which case it is a surgical emergency. Nursing management consists of early recognition of the hernia and post-operative care of the wound. This includes monitoring for normal bowel function and pain control (Table 14.7).

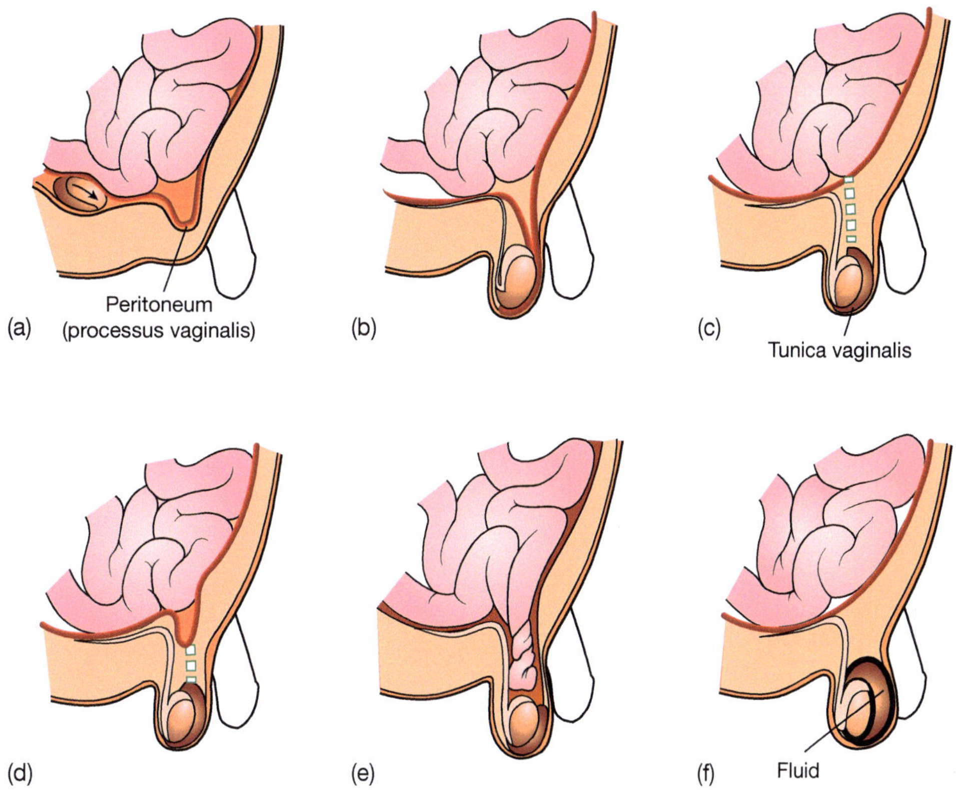

FIGURE 14.7 Development of inguinal hernias. (a) and (b), prenatal migration of processus vaginalis (c), Normal. (d), partially obliterated processus vaginalis. (e), Hernia, (f), Hydrocele.
Source: Hockenberry and Wilson (2024) / with permission of Elsevier.

TABLE 14.7 Causes of potential alteration in post-operative vital signs

Potential alteration	Potential causes
Heart rate	
Increase:	Pyrexia Pain Haemorrhage leading to decreased perfusion and shock Respiratory distress – early stage Medication
Decrease:	Hypoxia Respiratory distress – late stage Raised intracranial pressure Medication
Respiratory rate	
Increase:	Respiratory distress Pain Hypothermia Pyrexia Increase in circulating fluid volume – fluid overload

(Continued)

TABLE 14.7 (*Continued*)

Potential alteration	Potential causes
Decrease:	Medication including anaesthetic agents Pain
Blood pressure	
Increase:	Excessive intravascular volume Raised intracranial pressure Pain CO_2 retention Medication
Decrease:	Medication, especially opioids Anaesthetic agents – vasodilators
Temperature	
Increase:	Sepsis Shock – late sign Malignant hyperthermia Environmental factors – room, heating blankets
Decrease:	Anaesthetic agents – vasodilators Medication – muscle relaxants Cold intravenous fluids and/or blood Environmental factors – room too cold

Source: Hockenberry and Wilson (2024) / with permission of Elsevier.

Paediatric early warning system – related to a case study

Case study 14.1

7-year-old Paul's mother brings him into the emergency department with severe abdominal cramping pain. This pain started suddenly the evening before (24 hours ago) and has slowly worsened. Paul has a pyrexia of 38.5 °C and is now unable to keep any food or fluids down. He has diarrhoea. On palpation, the pain is worse, and he has rebound tenderness in the lower right quadrant. He is most comfortable with his knees drawn up to his chest. He is diagnosed with acute appendicitis and scheduled for an appendectomy. Paul is admitted to the ward awaiting surgery. He has an intravenous infusion in situ and has had intravenous paracetamol.

This is the first time Paul has been in hospital, and his parents are worried about how he will cope with the experience and the pain following surgery. Paul's observations have been recorded hourly (see the table) since he arrived.

- How would you prepare Paul for surgery?
- Activity: Access the national paediatric early warning system (PEWS) observation and escalation chart for Paul's age group here:https://www.england.nhs.uk/publication/national-pews-observation-and-escalation-charts/
- Plot his observations since he arrived. Calculate his PEWS. How would you construct your SBAR to escalate his current condition?

What actions might the nurse take based on the score on this chart?

Vital sign	2200 h	2300 h	2400 h	0100 h	0200 h	0300 h	0400 h	0500 h
Respiratory rate (breaths per minute)	24	24	26	30	30	28	32	36
Respiratory distress	None	None	None	None	None	None	None	None
Oxygen saturations	97	98	98	98	98	97	97	96
Respiratory support	None	None	None	None	None	None	None	None
Heart rate	110	131	124	128	128	126	130	142
Blood pressure	112/67			114/64			112/64	122/80
AVPU	A	A	A	A	A	A	A	A
Pain score (1–10 scale)	9	9	8	8	9	7	7	4
Temperature	38.1	38.2	37.9	38.0	38.1	38.1	38.2	38.8

Case study 14.2

James, a 6-week-old baby, is brought to the hospital by his parents with a history of worsening vomiting and failure to gain expected weight. On examination, James has been vomiting since he was 3 weeks of age and is hungry and irritable. He has mild dehydration and visible gastric peristalsis. An olive-shaped mass is palpable in the epigastrium, right of the umbilicus. James' mother describes his vomiting as forceful.

A diagnosis of pyloric stenosis is made, and James is nil by mouth in preparation for a pyloromyotomy surgical procedure. Intravenous fluids and electrolytes are commenced to correct any dehydration and restore the electrolyte balance.

James' parents are very upset as this is their first child, and they are worried that this could happen again with future children.

- What information would you give to James' parents about this condition?
- What post-operative care would you provide to James?

Conclusion

The GI system plays a vital role in sustaining health by enabling digestion, nutrient absorption and waste elimination. In infants, children and young people, disorders of the GI tract can have profound effects not only on physical well-being but also on growth, development and quality of life. This chapter has outlined common GI conditions across categories such as motility, inflammation, obstruction, malabsorption, structural anomalies and hernias, while emphasising the importance of accurate assessment and timely management. Central to effective care is a family-centred approach, which recognises the role of parents and caregivers in supporting the child's health journey. Integrating clinical knowledge with compassionate, developmentally appropriate nursing practice can help enhance outcomes and promote both recovery and resilience in young patients.

References

Auger, N., del Giorgio, F., Le-Nguyen, A., *et al.* (2022). Maternal risk factors for paediatric inguinal hernia. *British Journal of Surgery* 109(1), 129–135.

Ball, J., Bindler, R., & Cowen, K. (2015). *Principles of Pediatric Nursing: Caring for Children*, 6th edn. Pearson, New York.

Chiarello, M.M., Cariati, M., & Brisinda, G. (2021). Colonic Crohn's disease - decision is more important than incision: a surgical dilemma. *World Journal of Gastrointestinal Surgery* 13(1), 1–6.

Cleft Lip & Palate Association (CLAPA) (2025). What is cleft lip and palate? Available at: https://www.clapa.com/what-is-cleft-lip-palate/ (accessed 2 August 2025).

Devitt, P., & Thain, J. (2011). *Children's and Young People's Nursing Made Incredibly Easy.* Lippincott Williams & Wilkins, London.

Durkin, N., & DeCoppi, P. (2022). Management of neonates with oesophageal atresia and tracheoesophageal fistula. *Early Human Development.* 174.

Frederick, R., Hogan, A.C., Seabolt, N., & Stocks, R.M.S. (2022). An ideal multidisciplinary cleft lip and cleft palate care team. *Oral Diseases* 28, 1412–1417.

Garfield, K., & Sergent, S.R. (2023). Pyloric stenosis. In: *StatPearls [Internet].* Treasure Island (FL): StatPearls Publishing; Available from: https://www.ncbi.nlm.nih.gov/books/NBK555931/ (accessed 2 August 2025).

Gil, L.A., Deans, K.J., & Minneci, P.C. (2023). Appendicitis in children. *Advances in Pediatrics* 70(1), 105–122.

Hockenberry, M.J., & Wilson, D.. (eds) (2024). *Wong's Nursing Care of Infants and Children*, 12th edn. Elsevier.

Krishnan, U., Mousa, H., Dall'Oglio, L., *et al.* (2016). ESPGHAN-NASPGHAN guidelines for the evaluation and treatment of gastrointestinal and nutritional complications in children with esophageal atresia-tracheoesophageal fistula. *Journal of Pediatric Gastroenterology and Nutrition* 63(5), 550–570.

Long, D., Wang, C., Huang, Y., *et al.* (2024). Changing epidemiology of inflammatory bowel disease in children and adolescents. *International Journal of Colorectal Disease* 39, 73.

Morgado, M., & Holland, A.J. (2024). Inguinal hernias in children: update on management guidelines. *Journal of Paediatrics and Child Health* 60, 648–653.

Mueller, J.L., & Goldstein, A.M. (2022). The science of Hirschsprung disease: what we know and where we are headed. *Seminars in Pediatric Surgery* 31(2).

National Institute for Health and Care Excellence (NICE) (2017). Constipation in children and young people: diagnosis and management. NICE guideline [CG99]. Available at: https://www.nice.org.uk/guidance/cg99/chapter/Introduction (accessed 2 August 2025).

National Institute for Health and Care Excellence (NICE) (2019). Gastro-oesophageal reflux disease in children and young people: diagnosis and management. NICE guideline [NG1]. Available at: https://www.nice.org.uk/guidance/ng1 (accessed on 3 August 2025)

National Institute for Health and Care Excellence (NICE) (2019b). Coeliac disease: recognition, assessment and management. NICE guideline [NG20]. Available at: https://www.nice.org.uk/guidance/ng20 (accessed on 3 August 2025).

National Institute for Health and Care Excellence (NICE) Clinical Knowledge Summary (2024a). Gastroenteritis. Available at: https://cks.nice.org.uk/topics/gastroenteritis/ (accessed on 2 August 2025).

National Institute for Health and Care Excellence (NICE) Clinical Knowledge Summary (2024b). Crohn's Disease. Available at: https://cks.nice.org.uk/topics/crohns-disease/ (accessed on 2 August 2025).

National Institute for Health and Care Excellence (NICE) Clinical Knowledge Summary (2025a). Constipation in children. Available at: https://cks.nice.org.uk/topics/constipation-in-children/ (accessed on 2 August 2025).

National Institute for Health and Care Excellence (NICE) Clinical Knowledge Summary (2025b). Appendicitis. Available at: https://cks.nice.org.uk/topics/appendicitis/ (accessed on 2 August 2025).

National Institute for Health and Care Excellence (NICE) Clinical Knowledge Summary (2025c). Coeliac disease. Available at: https://cks.nice.org.uk/topics/coeliac-disease/ (accessed on 2 August 2025).

Oxford University Hospitals NHS Foundation Trust (2024). Intussusception. Available at: https://www.ouh.nhs.uk/media/sdncnqxu/65485intussusception.pdf (accessed 2 August 2025)

Winter, J.M. (2021). Caring for children with gastrointestinal problems. In: Glasper, A., Richardson, J., & Randall, D. (eds). *A Textbook of Children's and Young People's Nursing*, 3rd edn. London: Churchill Livingstone Elsevier.

Zajac, D.J., & Vallino-Napoli, L.D. (2026). *Evaluation and Management of Cleft Lip and Palate. A developmental Perspective*, 2nd edn. Plural Publishing, San Diego CA.

CHAPTER 15

Disorders of the renal system

Cathy Poole

AIM

The aim of this chapter is to help the reader develop an understanding of renal diseases diagnosed in children and young people.

LEARNING OUTCOMES

On completion of this chapter, the reader will be able to:

- Distinguish between upper renal tract and lower renal tract disorders.
- Identify a selection of renal anomalies.
- Describe a renal disorder-focused nursing assessment.
- Describe some of the more common medical and surgical renal disorders, and identify key care interventions.

KEYWORDS

- upper and lower renal tract
- congenital anomalies
- hypovolaemia
- preservation of kidney and bladder function
- renal investigations
- haematuria
- proteinuria
- assessment

Test your prior knowledge

1. What does the urinary system consist of?
2. At what point during pregnancy is a detailed ultrasound scan done of the unborn foetus?
3. Describe CAKUT.
4. Describe the nursing care of a child with nephrotic syndrome.
5. What is the treatment for vesicoureteric reflux?

Introduction

Some renal system disorders are common, such as urinary tract infections (UTIs), while others, like bladder exstrophy and nephropathic cystinosis, are rare. This chapter focuses on the disorders most frequently seen in children's nursing and introduces some of the more complex or uncommon conditions. When discussing renal disorders, the entire urinary tract – including kidneys, ureters, bladder and urethra – should be considered (Fig. 15.1). Urinary system disorders are often classified as upper or lower tract disorders (Peate & Gormley-Fleming, 2015). Accordingly, this chapter is organised into upper and lower urinary tract disorders. Management may be medical, surgical or a

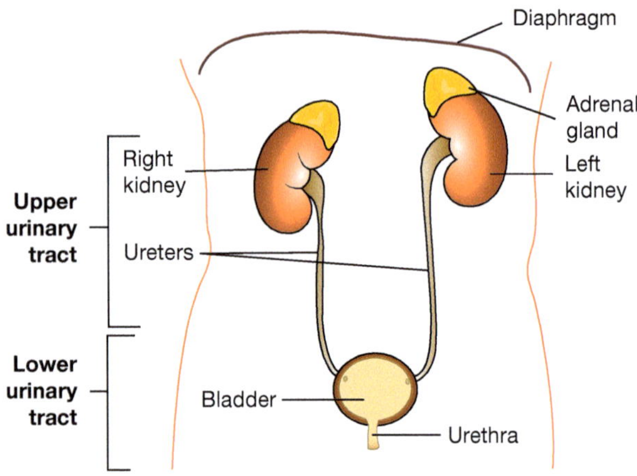

FIGURE 15.1 Upper and lower urinary tracts.

combination, and the chapter will outline nursing care for infants, children and young people with these conditions.

Before routine antenatal ultrasound screening, many congenital renal malformations were not diagnosed until symptoms appeared in infancy, childhood or adulthood. Early diagnosis is now recognised as important, and a section of this chapter covers renal anomalies detectable during the antenatal period. The chapter also highlights the value of a focused renal nursing assessment (Table 15.1).

Renal anomalies detected or suspected antenatally

Congenital abnormalities of the kidney and urinary tract (CAKUT) are among the most commonly diagnosed antenatal conditions (Walker et al., 2023). CAKUT can range from mild pelvic dilatation of the kidney (hydronephrosis) to dysplastic kidneys (abnormally developed kidneys). Some antenatally detected abnormalities have little or no impact on renal function, while others may have serious consequences, potentially leading to chronic kidney disease (CKD), kidney failure and the need for dialysis or transplantation.

The UK Kidney Association (2021) reports that CAKUT occur in 4.2–30 per 10 000 live births, representing 20–30% of anomalies detected on antenatal scans. They are the leading cause of CKD in children, accounting for around half of those needing dialysis or transplantation.

Advances in ultrasound allow foetal kidneys to be visualised from 9 weeks' gestation, though routine scans occur between 18 and 20 weeks (Walker, Winyard & Marlais, 2023). Dilatation of the urinary tract is the most common anomaly. Foetal kidney scans measure the renal pelvis diameter (RPD), with an RPD >10 mm at 26 weeks suggesting significant dilatation requiring postnatal follow-up. RPD may indicate either upper or lower urinary tract flow impairment, or lower urinary tract obstruction (LUTO).

Early identification of renal anomalies is important, as they may be associated with abnormal kidney development and function (Katsoufis *et al.*, 2019). Early detection allows timely intervention, potentially preventing progressive damage. However, minor anomalies, most commonly RPD, are often detected. RPD rarely requires intervention but does need antenatal follow-up and possibly postnatal investigations, which can cause parental anxiety. LUTO affects an estimated 2.2–3.3 per 10 000 births and is more common in boys (Walker et al., 2023). Table 15.1 summarises these anomalies.

TABLE 15.1 Antenatal urinary tract

Antenatal anomaly detected	Brief description of anomaly
Renal agenesis (Classic Potter Syndrome)	Absence of both kidneys, associated with reduced volume of amniotic fluid (oligohydramniosis), lung hypoplasia, low-set ears, beaked nose, downward eye slants and limb abnormalities. Incompatible with life. Affects 1 in 4000–10 000 births.
Solitary kidney	Solitary kidney is a condition in which children have a single kidney instead of two kidneys.
Horseshoe kidney	During embryonic development, the kidneys fuse together to form a horseshoe shape. Incidence of 1 in 400 to 500 births.
Duplex kidney	Children with a duplex kidney (also called a duplicated collecting system) have two ureters coming from a single kidney. Duplex kidneys can occur in one (unilateral) or both (bilateral) kidneys (Fig. 15.2).
Ectopic kidney (or renal ectopia)	An ectopic kidney does not grow in the proper location. It occurs in about 1 in 1000–5000 births. Infants, children and young people with an ectopic kidney usually have no symptoms, but sometimes it may cause urinary problems, e.g., urine blockage, infection or urinary stones.

TABLE 15.1 *(Continued)*

Antenatal anomaly detected	Brief description of anomaly
Hydronephrosis	One or both kidneys are stretched and swollen (dilated). It is quite common, affecting about 1 in 100 pregnancies. Most cases are not serious.
Multicystic dysplastic kidney (MCDK)	The kidneys have bundles of cysts in them, which are like sacs filled with liquid. MCDK can be unilateral or bilateral. The cysts can be very large initially; however, over time, they become smaller, and the kidney gradually shrinks. It is estimated that 1 in 4300 babies is born with unilateral MCDK. Bilateral MCDK is much rarer.
Posterior urethral valves (PUVs)	PUVs affect only boys, causing extra urethral tissue that can block urination before and after birth. Incidence is 1 in 1300–8000 male births.

Source: Adapted from infoKID; https://infokid.org.uk/ (accessed 22/01/2025).

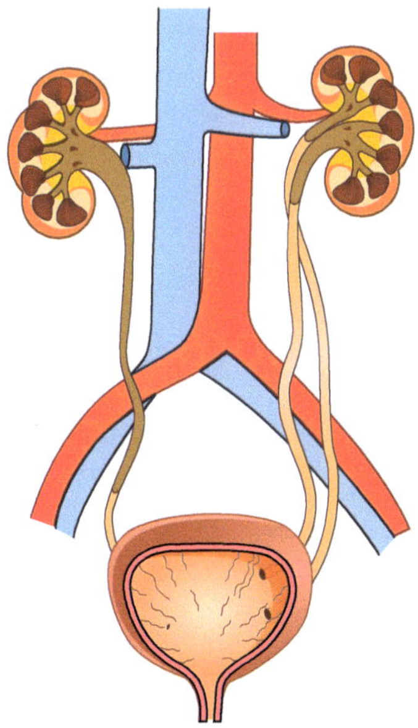

FIGURE 15.2 Duplex left kidney.

In summary, kidney and urinary tract anomalies are the most common antenatal abnormalities. Routine ultrasound enables early detection, guiding postnatal care to protect renal function.

Case study 15.1

Katie, aged 35 years, attended her local hospital for a routine antenatal ultrasound scan (USS) of her baby at 34 weeks' gestation, as a previous USS had raised concerns about the appearance and measurement of the right kidney. This USS identified that there was evidence of pelvic dilation of the right kidney, as set out here.

- Left kidney normal
- Right kidney abnormal
- Ureters: normal/not visible
- Bladder: normal
- Hydronephrosis, right side: mild dilatation, normal cortex
- In today's USS, the foetal growth, liquor and Doppler appear normal
- The right renal pelvis is mildly dilated at 8.8 mm, the renal cortex has a normal appearance and the ureter is not visible.

The outcome of this USS was discussed with Katie, who was informed that she would be referred to the neonatal team.

- What information about CAKUT would you provide for Katie?
- What follow-up advice would you provide for Katie?
- What resources could you signpost Katie to?

Assessment of the renal system

Nursing assessment is central to planning and delivering patient- and family-centred care. The Nursing and Midwifery Council (NMC, 2018) emphasises that nurses must 'make sure that people's physical, social and psychological needs are assessed and responded to'. Therefore, holistic assessments should include criteria specific to the renal system (see Table 15.2).

Herbal and dietary supplements are widely promoted on social media for their purported benefits. However, some pose hidden risks to kidney health (Claure-Del Granado & Chavez-Iniguez, 2024). Examples of supplements implicated in kidney syndromes are listed herewith (Claure-Del Granado & Chavez-Iniguez, 2024).

- Willow bark
- St. John's wort
- Liquorice
- Horsetail
- Ginseng
- Dandelion
- Stinging nettle

TABLE 15.2 Assessment of the renal system

Urinary symptoms: Enuresis (bedwetting), new-onset incontinence, frequency, urgency, quantity, dysuria and its timing during voiding (at beginning or end, throughout), change in colour and odour of urine, haematuria, presence of stones or sediment in the urine, toilet-training problems and reduced urine output.
Hydration status, including blood pressure, fluid balance, and weight, ankle and eye oedema (periorbital oedema) and sunken fontanelle in babies.
Growth and feeding, diet or fluid restrictions and sudden weight loss.
Urine output (neonates 1–3 mL [kg/h]; children 2 years 0.5–1 mL [kg/h]).
Urinalysis (pH, ketones, protein, blood, leukocytes, nitrite, glucose and specific gravity). Proteinuria and haematuria are early signs of disorders of the renal system.
Blood chemistry (urea, creatinine, electrolytes, albumin and haemoglobin).
Skin condition: Temperature, turgor (hydration assessment) and moisture, colour, evidence of any rashes and enlarged and painful nodes (axilla and groin).
Inexplicable crying, holding genitalia, discolouration of external genitalia, pain or swelling of the testicles, penile discharge, itching or swelling of the genitalia and urethral or vaginal discharge.
Location of pain: Flank, suprapubic, genital, groin or low back pain.
Medication: Prescribed, over-the-counter (OTC) or herbal remedies and supplements.

Source: Adapted from The Royal Children's Hospital Melbourne (2014) (Accessed 20/01/2025).

Families should always be advised to discuss the use of such treatments with their doctors, renal nurse specialists or pharmacists, as these may also interfere with the pharmacodynamics of prescribed treatments.

Infants, children and young people presenting with urinary tract symptoms often require further tests to confirm a diagnosis (Viteri *et al.*, 2020). Common renal investigations include:

- **Renal ultrasound:** Non-invasive assessment of urinary tract anatomy.
- **Three-dimensional ultrasound and elastography:** Emerging techniques providing sharper images, sometimes reducing the need for CT or dimercaptosuccinic acid (DMSA) scans.
- **CT scan:** Detailed X-ray imaging of internal structures; used less frequently in children due to lower incidence of renal stones and tumours.
- **DMSA scan:** Radioisotope scan showing functional and damaged kidney areas, often after infections.
- **Intravenous urogram:** Detailed view of renal calyces and ureters.
- **Voiding cystourethrography (VCUG):** X-rays of the bladder and urethra during urination to detect vesicoureteric reflux (VUR).
- **MAG3 scan:** Assesses kidney function, urine drainage and obstruction using injected mercaptoacetyltriglycine.
- **Kidney biopsy:** Tissue sampling to examine kidney structure under a microscope.

Blood tests are also routinely performed to support diagnosis and management, including urea, creatinine, electrolytes, albumin, haemoglobin and estimated glomerular filtration rate (eGFR). Understanding normal results allows nurses to explain tests and results to children and families effectively.

For a successful outcome of these specialist investigations, the child and family need full preparation, explanation and, where required, provide informed consent.

Medical disorders of the upper urinary tract

Proteinuria

Proteinuria is the leakage of protein from the blood into the urine. Normally, proteins are too large to pass through the glomeruli, but kidney damage can allow them to do so. Most cases are detected by dipstick urinalysis. Small amounts of protein may appear during febrile illnesses and, if it resolves when the child recovers, it is not a concern and does not require specialist referral (Schulga & McKie, 2024). Persistent proteinuria warrants further investigation, as management depends on the underlying cause (Table 15.3).

TABLE 15.3 Some causes of proteinuria

Nephrotic syndrome
Glomerulonephritis
Renal dysplasia
Vesicoureteric reflux (VUR)
Vasculitis
Orthostatic proteinuria
Acute kidney injury (AKI)
Renal tubular diseases – very rare in children
Hypertension
Diabetes – rare in children, very common in adults (diabetic nephropathy)

Source: Adapted from infoKID; https://infokid.org.uk/conditions/proteinuria/causes-of-proteinuria/ (accessed 29/01/2025).

Nephrotic syndrome

Nephrotic syndrome is the most common glomerular disease in children, though it remains rare, affecting fewer than 5 in 100 000 children worldwide annually (Vivarelli *et al.*, 2023; Downie *et al.*, 2017). It can occur at any age, most often between 2 and 7 years, and is more common in boys (Wang & Greenbaum, 2019). A very rare congenital form, Finnish-type nephrotic syndrome, appears in the first year of life. The condition is more frequently reported in children of Asian descent, though reasons for this are unclear (NHS, 2022). Nephrotic syndrome is classified by response to steroid treatment or underlying cause, and the specific type may only be identified after a course of steroids.

Children with nephrotic syndrome typically present with periorbital oedema, particularly in the morning, generalised oedema affecting the legs, ankles, scrotum or vulva, and breathlessness due to pleural effusions or abdominal distension from ascites. Urine may appear frothy, rich in albumin, resembling whipped egg white.

For 85–90% of children, proteinuria resolves with corticosteroid therapy, termed steroid-sensitive nephrotic syndrome. Complications such as hypovolaemia, thrombosis and infection require careful monitoring. Nursing assessment should include temperature, pulse, respirations and BP at least every 4 hours, with weight usually measured twice daily. Vital signs may need to be checked more frequently depending on the child's condition.

Hypovolaemia in children with nephrotic syndrome is a common but serious complication which can be overlooked. It can manifest as abdominal pain, high or low BP, cold hands and toes, a prolonged capillary refill time (CRT), ongoing tachycardia or symptoms of renal failure (Smith, 2017). Laboratory tests suggesting hypovolaemia include elevated urea or haemoglobin.

Nursing consideration

Children with nephrotic syndrome require careful hydration assessment, as generalised oedema can give the false impression of hypervolaemia, while they are often hypovolaemic. Heavy protein losses (proteinuria) reduce osmotic pressure, causing fluid to shift from the intravascular to the interstitial space.

Glomerulonephritis

Glomerulonephritis is a kidney disease affecting the glomeruli within the Bowman's capsule (Fig. 15.3). Inflammation of the glomeruli impairs the kidney's ability to filter urine. Causes include:

- Acute glomerulonephritis, often post-streptococcal infection (APSGN), the most common cause of acute nephritis in children worldwide (Alhamoud *et al.*, 2021).

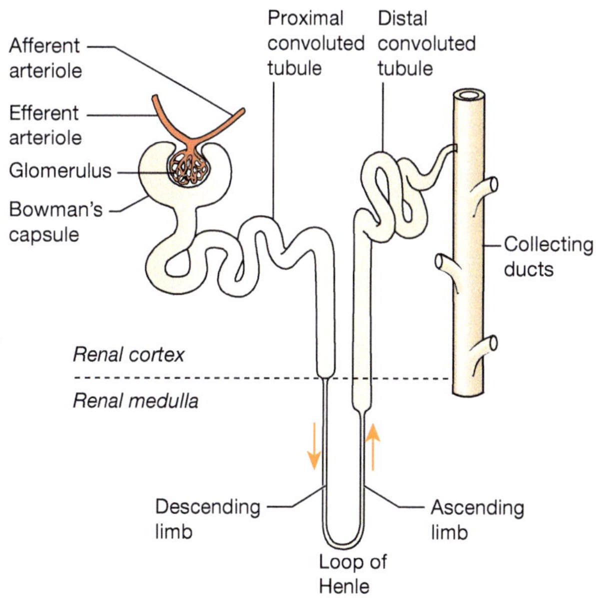

FIGURE 15.3 The nephron.
Source: Peate & Gormley-Fleming (2015)/John Wiley & Sons.

TABLE 15.4 Possible signs and symptoms of glomerulonephritis

Haematuria and proteinuria	Urine looks dark brown in colour
Fluid overloaded	Hypertensive Increase in body weight Oedema Headaches Seizures Reduced urine output (oliguria) Increased respiratory rate
Changes in physical appearance	Pale skin colour Skin rash, especially over the buttocks and legs Lethargic
Other	Sore throat Decreased appetite

Source: Adapted from Children's Hospital of Philadelphia (2025) (accessed 2 May 2025).

- Systemic immune diseases, such as systemic lupus erythematosus (SLE), which are very rare in children.
- Other rare systemic conditions, including polyarteritis nodosa, Wegener vasculitis and Henoch–Schönlein purpura (HSP).
- Inherited disorders, such as Alport syndrome.

APSGN predominantly affects children aged 5–12 years, with males affected approximately twice as often as females. Over 95% of cases occur in low- and middle-income countries (Miller & Beneden *et al.*, 2022).

Children who present with glomerulonephritis can have a wide variety of signs and symptoms. The most common are listed in Table 15.4.

Diagnosis of glomerulonephritis is based on history and physical examination, supported by investigations such as:

- Urinalysis to assess infection, measure proteinuria and in haematuria, count and classify blood cells.
- Blood tests, including full blood count, urea and electrolytes, antibody detection, complement levels and eGFR.
- Renal ultrasound to assess kidney size and structure.
- Chest X-ray if respiratory symptoms are present.

Management and nursing care depend on symptoms and the underlying cause. A healthy diet is important, with reduced salt and, if necessary, potassium intake; dietary adjustments may also be needed to increase calories during illness. Dietitians provide essential guidance (McDonald, 2022). Additional management may include antibiotics, antihypertensives, diuretics, or, rarely, immunosuppressive therapy or dialysis.

There are several causes of glomerulonephritis, the most common of which is associated with a streptococcal infection of the throat. For most children, the disease is mild, responds well to treatment and does not cause any long-term renal disease.

Henoch–Schönlein Purpura

HSP can affect all ages but is most common in children aged 2–11 years, occurring twice as often in boys (Great Ormond Street Hospital, 2019). It is more frequent in winter and often follows an upper respiratory tract infection. HSP causes inflammation and damage to capillaries, producing a characteristic rash.

Children with HSP typically present with a purple-red purpuric rash, symmetrically distributed over the buttocks, feet, ankles, backs of the legs, lower back and arms; joint pain (usually knees and ankles); abdominal colic-like pain; and sometimes proteinuria. Renal involvement is common but often resolves as the child recovers.

Most children require only symptomatic treatment, such as analgesia for joint pain and can be managed as outpatients. Symptoms usually resolve within days to weeks. HSP can recur within a few months, and a small number of children, particularly those with kidney involvement, may require specialist paediatric nephrology follow-up.

> Non-steroidal anti-inflammatory drugs (NSAIDs), for example, ibuprofen (e.g., Brufen®) are known to cause kidney damage and should be avoided as an analgesic in children with renal disease.

Haematuria

Haematuria is the presence of red blood cells (RBCs) in the urine. Population studies suggest that about 1% of school-aged children have two or more dipstick-positive tests for microscopic haematuria, but only a third persist at six months (Dalrymple, 2019). Normally, RBCs are too large to pass through the glomerular filters, but kidney damage can allow blood to enter the urine.

Microscopic haematuria is only detectable under a microscope, whereas gross haematuria causes visibly red urine. In healthy children, microscopic haematuria usually does not require investigation unless it is detected in at least three tests over several months. However, further investigation is needed if other symptoms, such as hypertension or proteinuria, are present.

Haematuria is a common finding in children and has many causes, which include the following:

- abnormal structures in the urinary tract (renal cysts)
- inherited diseases (Alport syndrome)
- mineral imbalances in the urine (hypercalciuria causing renal stones – calculi)
- glomerulonephritis
- idiopathic, where no cause of haematuria is found.

Growth and development – adolescent girls may have haematuria related to menstruation, so it is important to ask about menstrual history when haematuria is detected.

Chronic kidney disease

CKD is very rare in children, with hospital-based prevalence of 0.3–1 per 10 000 and population-based estimates of 1–10 per 1000, suggesting over 2 million affected worldwide (Harambat & Madded, 2023). In the United Kingdom, 110 children under 16 began long-term CKD treatment, about 9 per million, with 60% male (UK Kidney Association and UK Renal Registry, 2021). Of these, 25% were aged 0–4 years, 15% 4–8 years, 26% 8–12 years and 35% 12–16 years. Nearly half had congenital upper or lower urinary tract conditions, highlighting the importance of detailed antenatal scanning. By the end of 2021, 842 children under 16 were receiving long-term kidney failure treatment.

CKD in children involves permanent loss of kidney function, gradually progressing to end-stage renal disease (ESRD). Causes are detailed in Table 15.5. According to the UK Kidney Association and UK Renal Registry (2021), over 400 children had received a living donor kidney transplant, just over 200 a deceased donor transplant, just under 100 were on haemodialysis (HD) and just over 100 on peritoneal dialysis (PD). These forms of renal replacement therapy (RRT) are discussed in detail later in this chapter.

Understanding normal renal function (Peate & Gormley-Fleming, 2015) helps in recognising the physiological consequences of CKD (Table 15.6) and the need for specialist paediatric nephrology care. CKD is classified into five stages (Table 15.7) based on eGFR, which

TABLE 15.5 Causes of CKD in children

Causes of CKD in children
Conditions affecting structure of kidney or urinary tract
Glomerular conditions
Familial/inherited conditions
Miscellaneous
Multi-organ disease affecting the kidney
Non-congenital tubulointerstitial conditions

Source: UK Kidney Association and UK Renal Registry (2021)/with permission of The UK Kidney Association.

TABLE 15.6 Consequences of CKD

Functions of the kidney	Clinical consequence of CKD
Fluid balance	Reduced/no urine output (oliguria/anuria) leading to fluid overload, peripheral oedema, pulmonary oedema, shortness of breath.
Removal of waste	Uraemia which causes nausea, vomiting and loss of appetite. Persistent itchy skin (pruritus) due to uraemia.
Renin and angiotensin secretion	Reduced blood supply (hypoperfusion) to damaged nephrons causes increased secretion of renin, angiotensin and aldosterone causing hypertension.
Erythropoietin (EPO) secretion	Reduced production of EPO and the circulation of toxic waste substances cause renal anaemia. Anorexia and lethargy, failure to thrive.
Vitamin D synthesis	Without vitamin D synthesis, phosphate is retained, and calcium levels drop (hypocalcaemia), which results in secondary hyperparathyroidism. If left untreated, bones become painful, brittle and are prone to fracture (rickets and renal bone disease). Red eyes of uraemia, due to high plasma phosphate levels.
Acid–base balance	Reduction in the secretion of hydrogen ions culminates in metabolic acidosis.
Electrolyte balance	Hyperkalaemia causing heart arrhythmia. Kidneys normally excrete 90% of daily potassium intake.

TABLE 15.7 Stages of CKD and GFR

Stage	eGFR	Kidney function	What this means
1	90 or higher	Normal	Normally no symptoms
2	60–89	Mildly reduced	Normally no symptoms
3a	45–59	Moderately reduced	Normally no symptoms
3b	30–44	Moderately reduced	Symptoms of CKD may begin to be seen
4	15–29	Severely reduced	More symptoms of CKD are seen. Need to start to discuss and plan treatment options for stage 5
5	Less than 15	Very severely reduced and cannot support the body	This is also called end-stage renal failure (ESRF) or established renal failure. Treatments, including dialysis and kidney transplantation, have to commence

Source: Adapted from infoKid; www.infokid.org.uk/ (accessed 19th January 2025).

TABLE 15.8 Special considerations in CKD management for in children and young people

Growth	Children and young people with CKD often have reduced growth and require dietetic support to optimise nutrition. Dietitians monitor growth, provide renal dietary advice to ensure adequate energy and protein intake and manage fluid restrictions. Growth hormone therapy may also be prescribed.
Language development	Those diagnosed often require enteral feeding via gastrostomy or nasogastric tube, which can affect oral motor development. Hearing loss is also more common in children with CKD than in the general population.
Education	Children receiving RRT have been shown to have low average cognitive abilities and lower performance in literacy and numeracy compared to the general population. This is thought to be due to a combination of reasons. • Age at diagnosis of CKD • Duration of time on dialysis • Absence from school • Speech delay • Impact of biochemical imbalance (uraemia)

Source: Haffner (2020), Kim *et al.* (2022), and Kim *et al.* (2020).

measures the millilitres of blood filtered by the kidneys per minute. In children, eGFR is adjusted for a standard adult body surface area of 1.73 m^2.

There is no cure for CKD. In the United Kingdom, 58% of young people starting treatment were male, with most being White (67%), followed by Asian (25%) and other ethnicities (8%) (UK Kidney Association and UK Renal Registry, 2021). While dialysis and transplantation are the main treatments, several age-specific considerations are critical in managing this population (Table 15.8).

Treatment options include the following:

- **Peritoneal dialysis (PD):** Uses the peritoneal membrane to filter blood. Dialysate fluid is introduced into the peritoneal cavity for several hours, then drained and replaced. PD is typically performed at home, either several times a day or overnight (Fig. 15.4).
- **Haemodialysis (HD):** Blood is pumped through a dialyser ('artificial kidney') via a central venous catheter or arteriovenous fistula to remove waste and excess fluid. Sessions last 3–4 hours, three or

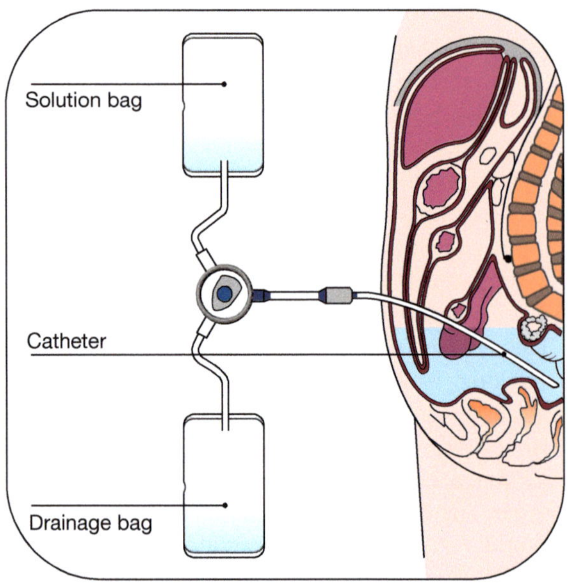

FIGURE 15.4 Peritoneal dialysis (PD).

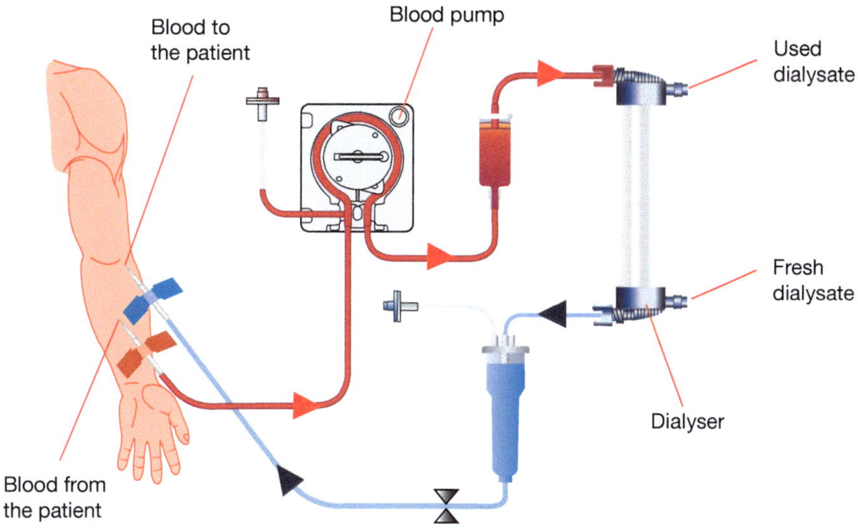

FIGURE 15.5 Haemodialysis (HD).

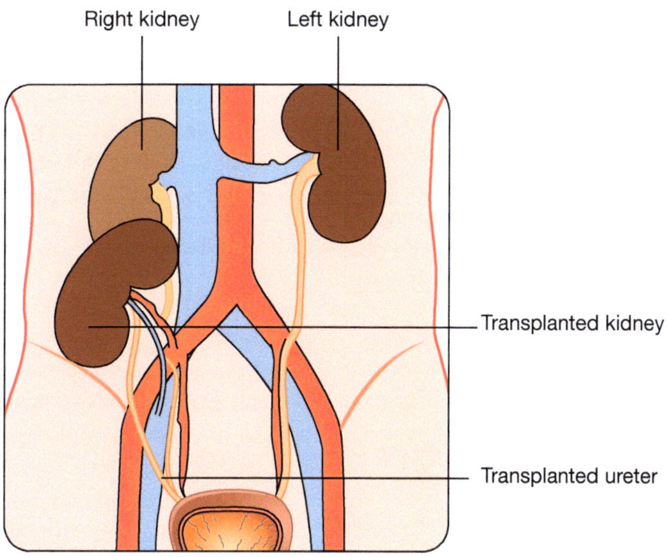

FIGURE 15.6 Renal transplantation.

more times a week, usually in a specialist unit, though some older children may do HD at home with support (Fig. 15.5).

- **Renal transplantation:** The preferred treatment, allowing children a more normal life without dialysis (Fig. 15.6). Types include deceased donor, living related donor or altruistic living donor. Living related donors are the most common in the United Kingdom.
- **Supportive care:** For some children and families, dialysis or transplantation may not be chosen. Supportive care focuses on managing symptoms of end-stage renal failure and providing medical, psychological and practical family-centred support.

CKD is rare in children and most commonly caused by structural congenital malformations, requiring specialist paediatric renal teams for holistic, family-centred care. While there is no cure, dialysis and transplantation allow many children to transition to adult renal services in their late teens.

Acute kidney injury

Acute kidney injury (AKI) is an abrupt decline in renal function, causing disturbances in water, electrolytes, acid–base balance, nitrogenous waste and BP. Understanding normal renal function (Peate & Gormley-Fleming, 2015) is key to recognising these consequences. In children, AKI is linked to prolonged hospitalisation, increased risk of CKD and mortality. Prompt recognition and management in paediatric emergency settings can reduce the risk of harm.

Like CKD, AKI is staged, though there is no universal definition. The pRIFLE (paediatric Risk, Injury, Failure, Loss, End-stage) and KDIGO (Kidney Disease Improving Global Outcomes) systems are commonly used (Table 15.9). AKI is more common in children than CKD and has multiple causes:

- **Pre-renal:** Most common, due to reduced renal perfusion from hypovolaemia (haemorrhage and dehydration), hypoxia, low cardiac output, vasodilation (warm shock) or sepsis.
- **Intrinsic (intrarenal):** Direct nephron damage, e.g., acute tubular necrosis, acute glomerulonephritis, uric acid nephropathy (tumour lysis syndrome), renal vein thrombosis, haemolytic uraemic syndrome (HUS) or pyelonephritis.
- **Post-renal:** Urinary tract obstruction, congenital or acquired, e.g., posterior urethral valves (PUVs), neurogenic bladder, phimosis, renal stones, blood clots or blocked urinary catheter.

When caring for children with a urinary catheter, a drop in hourly urine output should not be assumed to be absolute until catheter patency is checked. A catheter flush may be required to confirm patency (MSD Manual, 2025).

Medication alert

Several drugs are known to cause AKI, for example:

- prostaglandin synthetase inhibitors (ibuprofen)
- angiotensin-converting enzymes (ACEs) inhibitors (lisinopril and enalapril)
- angiotensin receptor blockers (losartan)
- diuretics
- antibiotics (vancomycin)
- calcineurin inhibitors (cyclosporine A, tacrolimus)

During assessment, take note of the medication that the child has been prescribed or which has been bought over the counter.

Children with AKI may be cared for in paediatric intensive care, high-dependency or renal units, depending on severity and multi-organ involvement. Nursing focuses on an ABC approach, addressing life-threatening issues first, including hydration, oxygenation, electrolyte imbalances, oedema and BP, alongside close monitoring of weight, hourly input and output, hourly PEWS and 6-hourly capillary blood glucose. While dialysis may be part of management, it is invasive and carries risks, so careful consideration is required before initiating specialist dialysis therapies.

Clinical status

- hyperkalaemia > 6.5 mmol/L
- urea > 40 mmol/L (> 30 mmol/L in neonates)
- severe hypo-/hyper-natraemia or acidosis
- uraemia with bleeding and/or encephalopathy
- anticipation of prolonged oliguria (i.e., HUS)
- intoxications
- inborn errors of metabolism (IEM)
- need for nutritional support

TABLE 15.9 Classification of AKI

AKI Stage	Serum Creatinine	Urine Output
1	Increase in serum creatinine by ≥ 0.3 mg/dL from baseline (≥ 26.5 µmol/L) within 48 h orincrease in serum creatinine to ≥ 1.5 times baseline within the prior 7 days	Urine volume ≤ 0.5 mL/kg/h for 6 h
2	Increase in serum creatinine to 2–2.9 times from baseline	Urine volume < 0.5 mL/kg/h for 12 h
3	Increase in serum creatinine to > 3 times from baseline or creatinine concentration > 353.6 µmol/L (4 mg/dL) or initiation of RRT or estimated GFR < 35 mL/min/1.73 m^2	Urine volume < 0.3 mL/kg/h for 24 h or anuria for at least 24 h

Abbreviations: AKI, acute kidney injury; GFR, glomerular filtration rate; RRT, renal replacement theory.
Source: KDIGO (2012)/with permission of NHS.

- degree of fluid overload
- involvement of multiple organ systems
- metabolic/electrolyte imbalance.

The decision to commence invasive dialysis treatment is supported by the classic mnemonic 'AEIOU'

Acidosis
Electrolyte disturbances (i.e. hyperkalaemia)
Ingestions
Overload (fluid)
Uraemia

AKI in children is increasingly well defined and common in critically ill patients, raising morbidity and mortality, particularly with sepsis, multi-organ involvement or fluid overload. Research focuses on improving awareness, diagnosis, care and outcomes (Yonekawa et al., 2022).

Haemolytic uraemic syndrome

HUS is a rare, severe and life-threatening condition that can cause AKI. Around 90% of cases occur in children, and up to 85% of those with typical HUS (tHUS) recover full kidney function. tHUS is usually caused by Shiga toxin-producing *Escherichia coli* (STEC-HUS or eHUS), which damages small kidney blood vessels and causes haemolysis. Other triggers include certain medications or underlying cancers, though less common. Additional enteric pathogens, such as *Shigella dysenteriae* and Campylobacter, have also been linked to tHUS (Byrne *et al.*, 2023).

Atypical HUS (aHUS) is familial, suggesting a genetic link, while pneumococcal-associated HUS (pHUS) arises from *Streptococcus pneumoniae* infection. HUS is most common in children under 5, with a UK incidence of 0.78 per 100 000 person-years, varying by age, gender, ethnicity and country. Children aged 1–4 years are most affected.

STEC resides in the gastrointestinal tract of asymptomatic ruminants, particularly cattle and sheep, and spreads via the faecal–oral route through direct animal contact, contaminated food or water, and person-to-person transmission in households or institutions (Sawyer *et al.*, 2021). HUS is, therefore, more frequent in summer and can occur in outbreaks, including nursery schools, farm visits or from undercooked beef burgers.

Children with HUS often present with symptoms lasting over 2 weeks, including profuse bloody or watery diarrhoea, vomiting, severe dehydration, acute abdominal pain, fever, irritability, fatigue and pale or yellowish skin (more noticeable on lighter skin due to haemolysis). Small oral bruises may also appear from altered clotting caused by bacterial toxins.

As the kidneys become involved, symptoms of AKI develop, for example, hypertension, raised urea, creatinine and potassium levels, and reduced urine output leading to fluid overload (oedema). Diagnosis is made using a combination of tests:

- blood samples for urea and electrolytes and full blood count and clotting screen
- stool culture
- abdominal X-ray
- urinalysis to assess for haematuria and proteinuria.

Management of HUS involves close monitoring, maintaining hydration, controlling BP, preventing infection, correcting anaemia with transfusions, managing electrolyte imbalances, ensuring adequate nutrition and, if needed, HD. Children are treated by paediatric nephrologists in specialist renal units and may require care in paediatric intensive care depending on illness severity.

- Good hand hygiene with soap and water, as hand gels or wipes do not remove *E. coli* O157.
- Strict hygiene when visiting farms, parks or camping sites.
- Cook meats thoroughly, especially on barbecues, and wash salads carefully; follow safe food storage and preparation guidelines.

Wilms' tumour

Wilms' tumour (nephroblastoma) is the most common childhood kidney cancer, affecting around 80 children annually in the United Kingdom. It is more common in Black children for unknown reasons and arises from immature embryonic cells that grow into a tumour. Most cases occur in children under five, particularly ages one to three, and usually affect one kidney, though both can be involved. Treatment typically combines surgery and chemotherapy, with around 10 children dying from the disease each year in the United Kingdom (Children with Cancer UK, 2016).

The most common symptom of a renal tumour is a painless abdominal swelling. Other possible signs include haematuria, hypertension, fever, diarrhoea, vomiting, weight loss or loss of appetite.

TABLE 15.10 Staging Wilms' tumour

Stage	Invasion/spread of the tumour
I	Tumour is only affecting the kidney and has not begun to spread. It can be completely removed with surgery.
II	Tumour has begun to spread beyond the kidney to nearby structures, but it is still possible to remove it completely with surgery.
III	Tumour has spread beyond the kidney, with lymph node involvement or tumour is confined to the abdomen; complete removal is not possible.
IV	Tumour has spread (metastasised) to other parts of the body, such as the lungs or liver.
V	Tumours in both kidneys (bilateral Wilms' tumour) and, therefore, each kidney requires individual staging.

Source: Adapted from Worsley *et al.* (2022) Wilms' tumour (staging).

A variety of tests and investigations will be undertaken, which will include the following:

- urine and blood samples to check kidney function
- an abdominal USS and CT
- scans of the chest and liver may be undertaken to check for any spread of the disease
- a biopsy of the tumour will be performed to assist in determining the type and stage (Table 15.10) of the tumour. This will help the paediatric oncologists decide on the most suitable treatment.

Treatment for Wilms' tumour depends on histology and stage. Surgery, either nephrectomy or partial nephrectomy, may be performed at diagnosis or after chemotherapy to shrink the tumour. Radiotherapy may also be used depending on the tumour stage. In bilateral cases, surgery aims to remove as much tumour as possible while preserving healthy kidney tissue (Cancer Research UK, 2023).

General medical renal nursing principles

Caring for children with renal disorders requires a holistic, family-centred approach, with attention to specific renal considerations:

- **Hypertension:** Use the correct BP cuff size, document it in the care plan and administer antihypertensives as prescribed.
- **Fluid balance:** Monitor for fluid overload due to reduced urine output by weighing twice daily and recording intake and output. Administer IV fluids and follow fluid restrictions, noting 'hidden fluids' in foods. Watch for dehydration as renal function recovers and obtain urine samples for urinalysis or lab assessment.
- **Infection risk:** Record and document vital signs accurately; isolation may be required.
- **Medications:** Children may require multiple drugs, including diuretics, antibiotics, antihypertensives and corticosteroids. Ensure correct timing, administration and monitor for complications.
- **Dietary management:** Liaise with dietitians for renal-specific diets (low sodium, low potassium, reduced protein or high-calorie). Reinforce adherence with the child and family.
- **Skin integrity:** Oedema or poor nutrition increases the risk of skin damage; perform meticulous care using local tissue viability scales.
- **Communication:** Effective skills are essential to engage children, young people and their families in care.

Surgical disorders of the upper urinary tract

Hydronephrosis

Hydronephrosis, which can occur prenatally, involves dilation of the kidneys due to urine accumulation. Refer to the earlier section on antenatal ultrasound scanning. In mild to moderate cases, kidney function is often preserved. Various tests may be performed to confirm the diagnosis:

- Ultrasound scan
- Blood and urine tests
- Nuclear medicine tests such as MAG-3 and DMSA scans
- Micturating cystogram (MUCG)

The need for surgery in hydronephrosis depends on its cause and severity, with monitoring via ultrasound and sometimes radioisotope scans. Treatment varies by underlying conditions:

- **Vesicoureteric reflux (VUR):** Usually managed with antibiotics.
- **Urinary tract obstruction:** May require pyeloplasty to correct the narrowing between the kidney and the ureter.

- **Neurogenic bladder:** Complex surgery, such as a Mitrofanoff procedure, may be needed to achieve continence.
- **Multicystic kidney disease:** The affected kidney typically shrinks and requires no removal, though severe cases causing symptoms like hypertension may need nephrectomy.

Ureteropelvic junction obstruction

The ureteropelvic junction (UPJ), where the kidney pelvis meets the ureter, can become obstructed, blocking urine flow to the bladder and causing hydronephrosis (Fig. 15.7) (Sezer, 2023). UPJ obstruction is a common congenital anomaly, occurring in 1 in 750–1000 live births.

Severe obstruction requires surgery – pyeloplasty – where the blocked segment is removed, and the ureter reconnected to the kidney, often via minimally invasive (keyhole) surgery. Advantages include smaller incisions, less pain and faster recovery. A stent may be placed to aid urine flow and healing. The primary goal is to restore drainage, reduce hydronephrosis and prevent renal damage.

Nursing care focuses on safe pre- and post-operative management, including infection prevention, adherence to fasting, maintaining hydration, reintroducing oral intake and careful monitoring of urine output, especially noting the first urine passed after surgery.

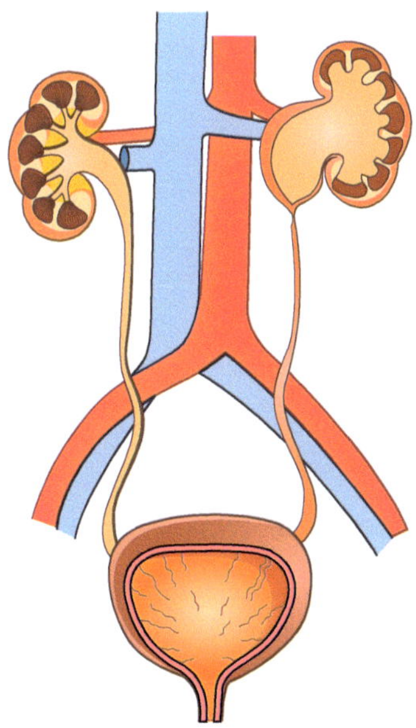

FIGURE 15.7 Ureteropelvic junction (UPJ) obstruction.

Nephrectomy

Nephrectomy is a surgical procedure to remove all or part (heminephrectomy) of a kidney:

- complete (radical) nephrectomy – the entire kidney is removed;
- partial nephrectomy – only diseased tissue is removed, leaving healthy kidney tissue in place.

There are many reasons why kidneys may need to be removed, for example:

- cancer of the kidney, i.e., Wilms' tumour
- kidney that has no remaining renal function and is causing symptoms of illness, i.e., pyelonephritis or hypertension
- donor kidney for transplantation.

Most nephrectomies are performed laparoscopically (keyhole surgery), though open surgery may be required for very large or infected kidneys. In either approach, the surgeon ligates the blood vessels and removes the kidney through the incision.

Post-nephrectomy nursing care focuses on strict fluid balance, monitoring urine volume and colour. If a wound drain is in place, its output must be carefully recorded. A urethral catheter is usually removed 2 days post-operation before discharge.

General surgical renal nursing principles

A holistic, family-centred approach is essential for children with renal surgical disorders, with particular attention to:

- **Dehydration risk:** Adhere to evidence-based preoperative fasting guidelines (RCoA, 2020) and liaise with theatre staff if surgery is delayed to protect renal function.
- **Pre-operative UTI exclusion:** Obtain a clean-catch urine sample, perform urinalysis and send for microscopy and culture as indicated.
- **Post-operative UTI risk:** Monitor children with catheters, nephrostomy tubes or stents according to local guidelines, including vital signs and urine testing.
- **Urinary retention:** Document and report the first urine passed post-theatre and monitor all urinary output.

- **Communication:** Keep the child and family fully informed about care and provide opportunities to ask questions.

Medical disorders of the lower urinary tract

Urinary tract infection

UTI is a common bacterial infection in the urinary tract and is classified as either:

- Lower UTI (cystitis) – this affects the bladder and urethra
- Upper UTI (acute pyelonephritis) – this affects the renal pelvis and the kidneys
- Asymptomatic bacteriuria – this is the presence of bacteria in urine when the child/young person does not have any signs and symptoms of a UTI

UTIs affect around 1 in 10 girls and 1 in 30 boys by age 16 (NICE, 2024a). By age 7, approximately 2.7% of girls and 1% of boys in the United Kingdom will have experienced an upper UTI (acute pyelonephritis). Various factors increase the risk of UTI in children and young people (see Table 15.11).

The prognosis for childhood UTIs is generally good, but children with underlying renal tract abnormalities may develop renal dysfunction. Boys are less likely than girls to have recurrent UTIs, while girls experience more recurrences, increasing with age. Infants and children with intrarenal or bilateral VUR are at higher risk of recurrent UTIs (NICE, 2024a).

Diagnosing UTIs in infants and children can be challenging because symptoms are often non-specific (Table 15.12). Confirmation requires a clean, uncontaminated urine sample, which is particularly difficult to obtain from young children.

The following methods of urine collection are recommended:

- **Clean-catch urine (CCU) sample:** Collected by holding a sterile container beneath the urethra with the nappy removed until urination begins, taking care to avoid skin contact with the container. This method is also suitable for older children.

TABLE 15.11 UTI risk factors in children and young people

Risk Factor	
Under 1 year of age	More common in boys under 3 months old and baby girls less than 1 year old
Females	But in the first 3 months of life, UTI is more common in boys than it is in girls
Infant boys who are not circumcised	Boys under 12 months old who are not circumcised have an increased risk of UTI
Previous UTI	Approx. 78% of girls and 71% of boys less than 1 year of age have a recurrence of UTI. This reduces to 45% of girls and 39% of boys with UTI after the age of 1 year
Voiding dysfunction	For example, children with structural abnormalities of the urinary tract, neurogenic bladder, voluntary withholding of urine or chronic constipation
Vesicoureteral reflux (VUR)	Family history of renal disease or VUR, which can affect one or both ureters and is graded I to V
Sexual activity	Adolescent girls have an increased relative risk in response to increased frequency of sexual intercourse
Formula-fed babies	Breastfeeding has a protective effect, which is more noticeable in girls, depending on the length of the time breastfeeding
Treatment with immunosuppressant drugs	Immunosuppression increases the risk of bacterial and fungal infections

Source: Adapted from NICE (2024a).

TABLE 15.12 Symptoms and signs of UTI in infants and children

Age group	Common signs and symptoms	Less common signs and symptoms
Infants younger than 3 months	Fever Vomiting Lethargy Irritability Poor feeding Failure to thrive	Abdominal pain Jaundice Haematuria and/or malodorous urine
Infants and children, 3 months or older	Fever Frequency of micturition, dysuria, abdominal pain, vomiting, poor feeding, dysfunctional voiding or changes in continence	Lethargy Irritability, haematuria, malodorous urine, failure to thrive, malaise and cloudy urine

Source: Adapted from NICE (2024a).

If a CCU sample is not possible, urine can be collected using:

- **Non-invasive urine collection pads:** Special absorbent pads (e.g., Newcastle pads) are placed in the nappy and urine is aspirated after voiding. Follow manufacturer instructions carefully. Cotton wool, gauze or sanitary towels should not be used, as bactericidal agents can cause false negatives.
- **Catheter or suprapubic aspiration (SPA):** Used when non-invasive collection is impractical or in emergencies, with SPA performed under ultrasound guidance (Diviney & Jaswon, 2020).

For infants and toddlers, suprapubic stimulation with cold-soaked gauze may aid urination and properly cleaned potties can be used to collect a clean-catch urine sample (NICE, 2022).

Urine bag sampling, where an adhesive sterile bag is placed on the perineum of non-toilet-trained infants, is not recommended because it has a high risk of contamination and false-positive results.

Urine samples should ideally be examined microscopically and cultured immediately. If this is not possible, refrigerate the sample to prevent bacterial overgrowth. Samples preserved with boric acid can be stored at room temperature for up to 96 hours, but boric acid may inhibit some organisms and leukocyte esterase tests. Always follow the manufacturer's instructions for sample volume (NICE, 2024a).

Urinalysis is a fundamental nursing skill, and dipstick testing must follow the manufacturer's guidelines. Key results for UTI detection are leucocyte esterase and nitrite reactions. Treatment with antibiotics depends on the causative organism, and further investigations may be required for infants and children, such as:

- renal USS
- DMSA scan
- micturating cystourethrogram.

Bacterial causes of UTI in children and young people include (BMJ Best Practice 2023):

- *Escherichia coli* – thought to cause 85–90% of paediatric UTIs.
- *Proteus mirabilis* – associated with uncircumcised males.
- *Staphylococcus saprophyticus* – associated with adolescent females.
- Pseudomonas species, *Klebsiella aerogenes* and Enterococcus species.
- *Serratia marcescens*, *Citrobacter* species and *Staphylococcus epidermidis* – may cause low-virulence infections if there is urinary tract malformation or dysfunction.
- Candida species can cause UTI in children who are immunosuppressed.

UTIs are common in childhood. Nursing management depends on collecting a clean, uncontaminated urine sample and promptly sending it to the laboratory to avoid false results. Parents should receive clear instructions for sample collection and be reminded to ensure their child completes the full course of antibiotics.

Growth and development

- By 2 years of age, some children will be dry during the day – but this is quite early
- By 3 years of age, 9 out of 10 children will be dry most days, but may still have the occasional accident
- By 4 years of age, most children will be consistently dry during the day
- It normally takes longer for children to be dry throughout the night

Daytime urinary incontinence (enuresis)

Daytime urinary incontinence (DUI) is involuntary urine leakage during the day in children aged five and older (ICCS). ERIC reports it affects 1 in 75 children in this age group. While occasional wetting is normal in younger children, DUI can become socially and academically challenging as children grow. It is more common in girls and younger children, and usually has no serious underlying cause. Several subtypes of DUI are described (Niuewhof-Leppink *et al.*, 2022; Table 15.13).

Nursing assessment of children with DUI is essential for planning appropriate management. Treatment is based on urotherapy, which encompasses all non-surgical and non-pharmacological interventions aimed at normalising micturition and often bowel habits. Urotherapy is either standard (SU), involving education, lifestyle advice and behavioural strategies, or specific (SU), including biofeedback, pelvic floor training, alarms and neuromodulation (Nieuwhof-Leppink *et al.*, 2021).

Nursing care for children with DUI typically includes:

- Excluding or managing UTIs and constipation.
- Advising on appropriate daily fluid intake (up to 1.5 L/7 glasses).
- Teaching regular voiding and correct toilet posture (feet on the floor or a footstool).
- Using a bladder diary for motivation and self-monitoring.

Parents should be reassured that daytime wetting is common, treatable, and requires consistent adherence to urotherapy.

> Children and young people with other comorbid behavioural problems, such as attention-deficit/hyperactivity disorder (ADHD), may struggle with understanding and following instructions.

TABLE 15.13 Subtypes of DUI

Subtypes	Symptoms
Overactive bladder (urge incontinence)	Frequency of micturition Voiding urgency Incontinence Constipation – due to the close proximity of the bowel to the bladder, a full bowel pressing on the bladder can prevent the bladder from emptying completely Enuresis
Dysfunctional voiding (micturition)	Failure to relax the bladder sphincter during micturition Normal micturition frequency Incontinence Constipation – as above UTIs – can cause irritation of the bladder and urinary frequency. Sometimes the bladder does not empty completely, which perpetuates the problem Enuresis
Underactive bladder	Low micturition frequency Incontinence Constipation – as above UTIs – as above
Micturition (voiding) postponement	Low micturition frequency Incontinence

Source: Adapted from Niuewhof-Leppink *et al.* (2022).

On rare occasions, children and young people with a DUI may need to be referred to a nephrologist or urologist if urotherapy has not been successful. In these cases, further investigations may be needed, for example, urodynamic studies and the prescription of oxybutynin, an anticholinergic drug.

Nocturnal enuresis (bedwetting)

NICE (2010) defines nocturnal enuresis as involuntary wetting during sleep, which is generally normal in children under 5 years. Bedwetting affects 5–10% of 7-year-olds and 1–2% of adolescents, and is twice as common in boys (NICE, 2024b). Risk factors include family history, male sex, developmental delay, constipation, DUI, ADHD, autism, and sleep apnoea. Diagnosis is based on three criteria.

1. bedwetting occurs at least twice weekly for 3 consecutive months or

2. bedwetting causes clinically significant distress or
3. bedwetting leads to impaired social, academic or other important areas of functioning

Nocturnal enuresis is categorised into two types (EAU, 2024):

1. Primary bedwetting **without** daytime symptoms – child has never achieved consistent night-time dryness and does not have any daytime symptoms.
2. Primary bedwetting **with** daytime symptoms – the child or young person has never achieved sustained continence at night and has daytime symptoms, for example, urgency, frequency, daytime wetting, abdominal straining or poor urinary stream.
3. Secondary bedwetting – bedwetting occurs when the child/young person has previously been dry for at least 6 months.

Most children and young people who have bedwetting without any daytime symptoms gain night-time continence by adolescence. However, the EAU (2024) reports that 7 out of 100 children with bedwetting at 7 years of age will continue to have this into their adult life.

A comprehensive nursing assessment should include the frequency and volume of night-time wetting, any identifiable patterns and whether the child wakes after wetting. Daytime continence should be established, as children who are continent during the day typically achieve night-time continence. Other relevant factors include constipation, soiling, developmental delays, behavioural issues and pain during urination. Although rare, the possibility of child maltreatment or female genital mutilation should also be considered if indicated.

Nursing management is similar to that for daytime enuresis. Strategies include encouraging the child to empty their bladder before bed, ensuring easy access to the toilet at night and taking the child to the toilet if they wake. Positive reinforcement, such as rewards for drinking appropriate amounts during the day and using the toilet before bed, can also be helpful.

Balanitis

Balanitis is inflammation of the glans penis, often involving the foreskin (NICE, 2024c). It affects around 4% of uncircumcised boys aged 2–5 years. Although it may recur, episodes usually become less frequent with age as the foreskin matures (BAPU, 2013).

It can be acute, chronic or recurrent and can be caused by:

- trauma
- skin conditions
- exposure to irritants – soap and bubble bath, for example
- infection – *Candida* (thrush), *Streptococcal* infection.

Nursing management involves identifying the cause through a full history. Parents or carers should be advised to clean the penis with lukewarm water and dry gently, avoiding retraction of an unfixed foreskin. Soap, bubble bath and baby wipes should be avoided. Nappies should be changed frequently. If infection is present, appropriate topical antibiotics, antifungals or steroid creams may be prescribed, and oral antibiotics may be needed for bacterial infections.

Case study 15.2

Vasil, a 10-month-old, arrived in the United Kingdom with his parents as asylum seekers 1 week ago. They speak little English and are living in government-provided accommodation. His mother reports that the tip of his penis is swollen, red and has some discharge. Vasil appears to have pain when urinating. Concerned, his parents brought him to the local children's emergency department.

On arrival, Vasil is crying and flushed, while his parents are anxious and trying to comfort him.

- What are your priorities in meeting this family?

Having contacted the hospital translation service, you have been able to reach out to a translator.

- How would you explain what observations/nursing care you need to do for Vasil?
- What children's nursing skills could you use to help calm Vasil?

You manage to undertake vital sign recordings for Vasil and establish that he is pyrexial with a temperature of 39.3 °C, his respiratory rate is 25 breaths per minute and his heart rate is 150 beats per minute. You attempt to record Vasil's BP, but he is too distressed for you to complete a successful BP recording. His oxygen saturation level is 99% in air and CRT is $\leq$ 2 seconds.

- If you were to record your findings on the national paediatric early warning system observation and escalation chart (PEWS), what would your escalation level be?

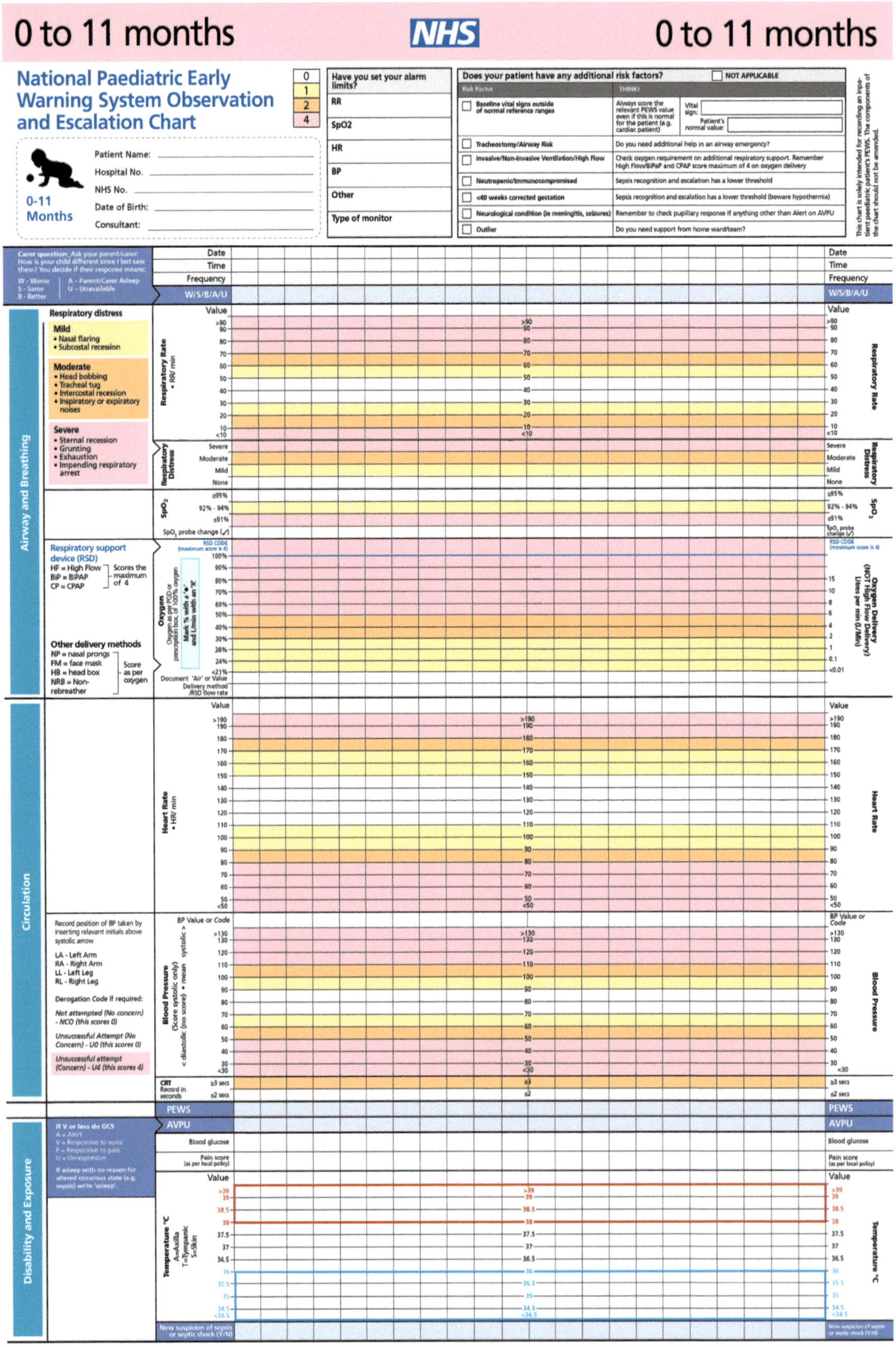
0 to 11 months
NHS
0 to 11 months
National Paediatric Early Warning System Observation and Escalation Chart
0
1
2
4
Patient Name:
Hospital No.
NHS No.
Date of Birth:
Consultant:
0-11 Months
Have you set your alarm limits?
RR
SpO2
HR
BP
Other
Type of monitor
Does your patient have any additional risk factors?
NOT APPLICABLE
Risk Factor
THINK!
Baseline vital signs outside of normal reference ranges
Always score the relevant PEWS value even if this is normal for the patient (e.g. cardiac patient)
Vital sign:
Patient's normal value:
Tracheostomy/Airway Risk
Do you need additional help in an airway emergency?
Invasive/Non-invasive Ventilation/High Flow
Check oxygen requirement on additional respiratory support. Remember High Flow/BiPaP and CPAP score maximum of 4 on oxygen delivery
Neutropenic/Immunocompromised
Sepsis recognition and escalation has a lower threshold
<40 weeks corrected gestation
Sepsis recognition and escalation has a lower threshold (beware hypothermia)
Neurological condition (ie meningitis, seizures)
Remember to check pupillary response if anything other than Alert on AVPU
Outlier
Do you need support from home ward/team?
This chart is solely intended for recording an inpatient paediatric patient's PEWS. The components of the chart should not be amended.
Carer question: Ask your parent/carer: How is your child different since I last saw them? You decide if their response means:
W - Worse
S - Same
B - Better
A - Parent/Carer Asleep
U - Unavailable
Date
Time
Frequency
W/S/B/A/U
Airway and Breathing
Respiratory distress
Mild
• Nasal flaring
• Subcostal recession
Moderate
• Head bobbing
• Tracheal tug
• Intercostal recession
• Inspiratory or expiratory noises
Severe
• Sternal recession
• Grunting
• Exhaustion
• Impending respiratory arrest
Value
Respiratory Rate • RR/ min
>90
90
80
70
60
50
40
30
20
10
<10
Respiratory Distress
Severe
Moderate
Mild
None
SpO2
≥95%
92% - 94%
≤91%
SpO2 probe change (✓)
Respiratory support device (RSD)
HF = High Flow
BiP = BiPAP
CP = CPAP
Scores the maximum of 4
RSD CODE (maximum score is 4)
Oxygen
100%
90%
80%
70%
60%
50%
40%
30%
28%
24%
<21%
Document 'Air' or Value
Delivery method /RSD flow rate
Other delivery methods
NP = nasal prongs
FM = face mask
HB = head box
NRB = Non-rebreather
Score as per oxygen
Oxygen Delivery (NOT High Flow Delivery) Litres per min (L/Min)
15
10
8
6
4
2
1
0.1
<0.01
Circulation
Heart Rate • HR/ min
>190
190
180
170
160
150
140
130
120
110
100
90
80
70
60
50
<50
Record position of BP taken by inserting relevant initials above systolic arrow
LA - Left Arm
RA - Right Arm
LL - Left Leg
RL - Right Leg
Derogation Code if required:
Not attempted (No concern) - NCO (this scores 0)
Unsuccessful Attempt (No Concern) - U0 (this scores 0)
Unsuccessful attempt (Concern) - U4 (this scores 4)
BP Value or Code
Blood Pressure (Score systolic only)
>130
130
120
110
100
90
80
70
60
50
40
30
<30
CRT Record in seconds
≥3 secs
≤2 secs
PEWS
AVPU
Disability and Exposure
If V or less do GCS
A = Alert
V = Responsive to voice
P = Responsive to pain
U = Unresponsive
If asleep with no reason for altered conscious state (e.g. sepsis) write 'asleep'.
Blood glucose
Pain score (as per local policy)
Temperature °C
A=Axilla
T=Tympanic
S=Skin
>39
39
38.5
38
37.5
37
36.5
36
35.5
35
34.5
<34.5
New suspicion of sepsis or septic shock (Y/N)

284

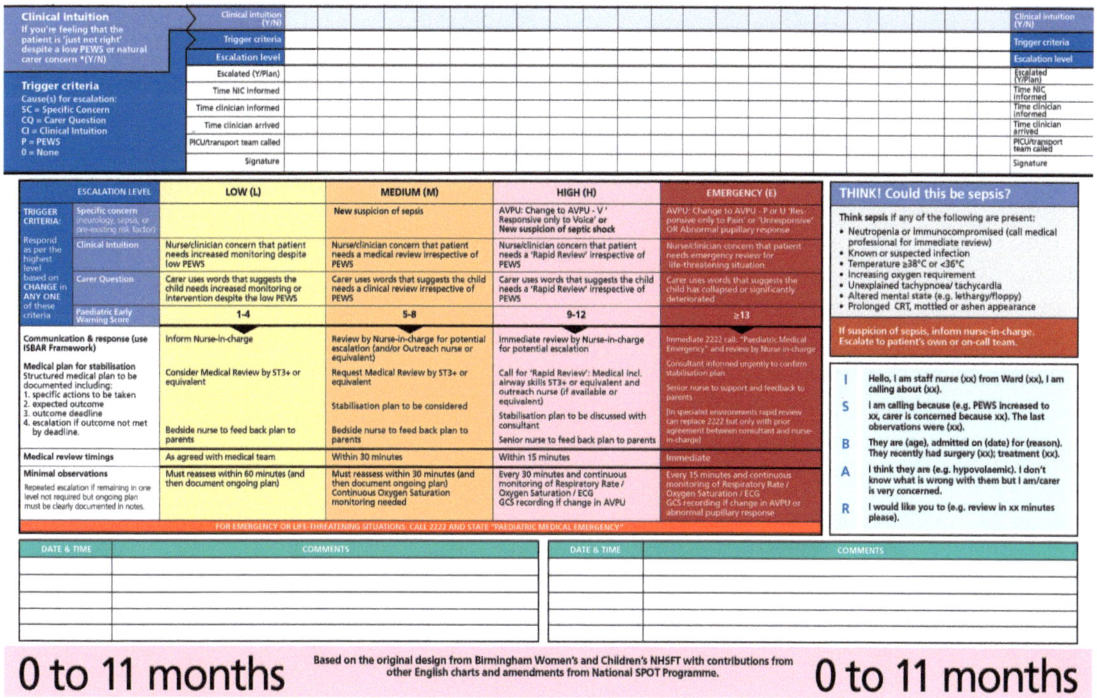

Clinical intuition
If you're feeling that the patient is 'just not right' despite a low PEWS or natural carer concern *(Y/N)

Trigger criteria
Cause(s) for escalation:
SC = Specific Concern
CQ = Carer Question
CI = Clinical Intuition
P = PEWS
0 = None

Clinical intuition (Y/N)																								Clinical intuition (Y/N)
Trigger criteria																								Trigger criteria
Escalation level																								Escalation level
Escalated (Y/Plan)																								Escalated (Y/Plan)
Time NIC informed																								Time NIC informed
Time clinician informed																								Time clinician informed
Time clinician arrived																								Time clinician arrived
PICU/transport team called																								PICU/transport team called
Signature																								Signature

ESCALATION LEVEL		LOW (L)	MEDIUM (M)	HIGH (H)	EMERGENCY (E)
TRIGGER CRITERIA: Respond as per the highest level based on CHANGE in ANY ONE of these criteria	Specific concern (neurology, sepsis, or pre-existing risk factor)		New suspicion of sepsis	AVPU: Change to AVPU - V 'Responsive only to Voice' or New suspicion of septic shock	AVPU: Change to AVPU - P or U 'Responsive only to Pain' or 'Unresponsive' OR Abnormal pupillary response
	Clinical Intuition	Nurse/clinician concern that patient needs increased monitoring despite low PEWS	Nurse/clinician concern that patient needs a medical review irrespective of PEWS	Nurse/clinician concern that patient needs a 'Rapid Review' irrespective of PEWS	Nurse/clinician concern that patient needs emergency review for life-threatening situation
	Carer Question	Carer uses words that suggests the child needs increased monitoring or intervention despite the low PEWS	Carer uses words that suggests the child needs a clinical review irrespective of PEWS	Carer uses words that suggests the child needs a 'Rapid Review' irrespective of PEWS	Carer uses words that suggests the child has collapsed or significantly deteriorated
	Paediatric Early Warning Score	1-4	5-8	9-12	≥13
Communication & response (use ISBAR Framework)		Inform Nurse-in-charge	Review by Nurse-in-charge for potential escalation (and/or Outreach nurse or equivalent)	Immediate review by Nurse-in-charge for potential escalation	Immediate 2222 call: "Paediatric Medical Emergency" and review by Nurse-in-charge
Medical plan for stabilisation Structured medical plan to be documented including: 1. specific actions to be taken 2. expected outcome 3. outcome deadline 4. escalation if outcome not met by deadline.		Consider Medical Review by ST3+ or equivalent Bedside nurse to feed back plan to parents	Request Medical Review by ST3+ or equivalent Stabilisation plan to be considered Bedside nurse to feed back plan to parents	Call for 'Rapid Review': Medical incl. airway skills ST3+ or equivalent and outreach nurse (if available or equivalent) Stabilisation plan to be discussed with consultant Senior nurse to feed back plan to parents	Consultant informed urgently to confirm stabilisation plan Senior nurse to support and feedback to parents [In specialist environments rapid review can replace 2222 but only with prior agreement between consultant and nurse-in-charge]
Medical review timings		As agreed with medical team	Within 30 minutes	Within 15 minutes	Immediate
Minimal observations Repeated escalation if remaining in one level not required but ongoing plan must be clearly documented in notes.		Must reassess within 60 minutes (and then document ongoing plan)	Must reassess within 30 minutes (and then document ongoing plan) Continuous Oxygen Saturation monitoring needed	Every 30 minutes and continuous monitoring of Respiratory Rate / Oxygen Saturation / ECG GCS recording if change in AVPU	Every 15 minutes and continuous monitoring of Respiratory Rate / Oxygen Saturation / ECG GCS recording if change in AVPU or abnormal pupillary response

FOR EMERGENCY OR LIFE-THREATENING SITUATIONS: CALL 2222 AND STATE "PAEDIATRIC MEDICAL EMERGENCY"

THINK! Could this be sepsis?

Think sepsis if any of the following are present:

- Neutropenia or immunocompromised (call medical professional for immediate review)
- Known or suspected infection
- Temperature ≥38°C or <36°C
- Increasing oxygen requirement
- Unexplained tachypnoea/ tachycardia
- Altered mental state (e.g. lethargy/floppy)
- Prolonged CRT, mottled or ashen appearance

If suspicion of sepsis, inform nurse-in-charge. Escalate to patient's own or on-call team.

I	Hello, I am staff nurse (xx) from Ward (xx), I am calling about (xx).
S	I am calling because (e.g. PEWS increased to xx, carer is concerned because xx). The last observations were (xx).
B	They are (age), admitted on (date) for (reason). They recently had surgery (xx); treatment (xx).
A	I think they are (e.g. hypovolaemic). I don't know what is wrong with them but I am/carer is very concerned.
R	I would like you to (e.g. review in xx minutes please).

DATE & TIME	COMMENTS

DATE & TIME	COMMENTS

0 to 11 months Based on the original design from Birmingham Women's and Children's NHSFT with contributions from other English charts and amendments from National SPOT Programme. **0 to 11 months**

Following review by a member of the medical staff, a diagnosis of balanitis is made for Vasil. He is prescribed some analgesia and an antibiotic ointment.

- What discharge advice would you provide for Vasil's mum and dad?

Vesicoureteric junction obstruction

A narrowing or blockage where the ureter meets the bladder is called a vesicoureteric junction obstruction (VUJO) (Fig. 15.8). This obstruction hinders urine flow to the bladder, causing urine to back up, dilating the ureter (megaureter) and kidney (hydronephrosis). VUJO affects roughly 1500–2000 children, usually involves only one kidney and is rarely associated with other abnormalities.

VUJO typically develops during foetal life and can often be detected on a routine antenatal ultrasound. The obstruction is usually caused by a narrowing at the ureter–bladder junction, but can also result from scar tissue, infection or kidney stones. Diagnosis is confirmed using radiological investigations, such as a renal ultrasound, DMSA scan or MAG3 scan (mercaptoacetyltriglycine).

The surgical correction of VUVJ obstruction depends upon the cause and severity of obstruction. There are three surgical approaches for VUJO:

1. Stent insertion
2. Ureteric re-implantation
3. Urinary diversion/cutaneous distal ureterostomy

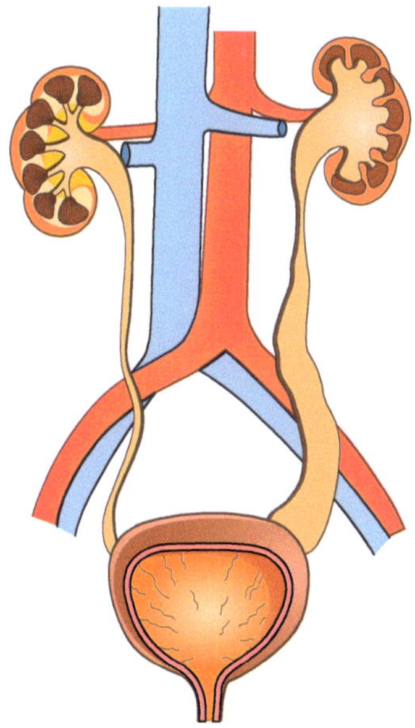

FIGURE 15.8 Vesicoureteric junction obstruction.

All the surgical approaches allow the affected kidney and ureter to decompress and have the potential to preserve upper renal tract function, which is a key priority in this surgery.

Vesicoureteral reflux

Vesicoureteral reflux (VUR) is a common condition in infants and young children where urine flows backwards from the bladder towards the kidneys, and can be unilateral or bilateral. It increases the risk of UTIs and may require continuous prophylactic antibiotics. VUR results from structural or functional ureter–bladder junction abnormalities or increased bladder pressure (e.g., neurogenic bladder and PUVs). Boys are affected earlier and more severely, while girls typically develop milder VUR later. VUR occurs in 30% of children with UTIs and 17% with normal kidneys, and should be suspected with recurrent febrile UTIs or lower urinary tract symptoms, regardless of bladder–bowel disorders (Chirico *et al.*, 2023).

It is diagnosed by undertaking a voiding cystourethrogram (VCUG). This test is considered to be the 'gold standard', which allows grading of the VUR from I to V (Fig. 15.9), by identifying the extent of reflux and whether it is unilateral or bilateral. Grades I and II are mild and grades III, IV and V are more serious.

There are two surgical approaches:

1. Endoscopic surgery
2. Ureteric reimplantation

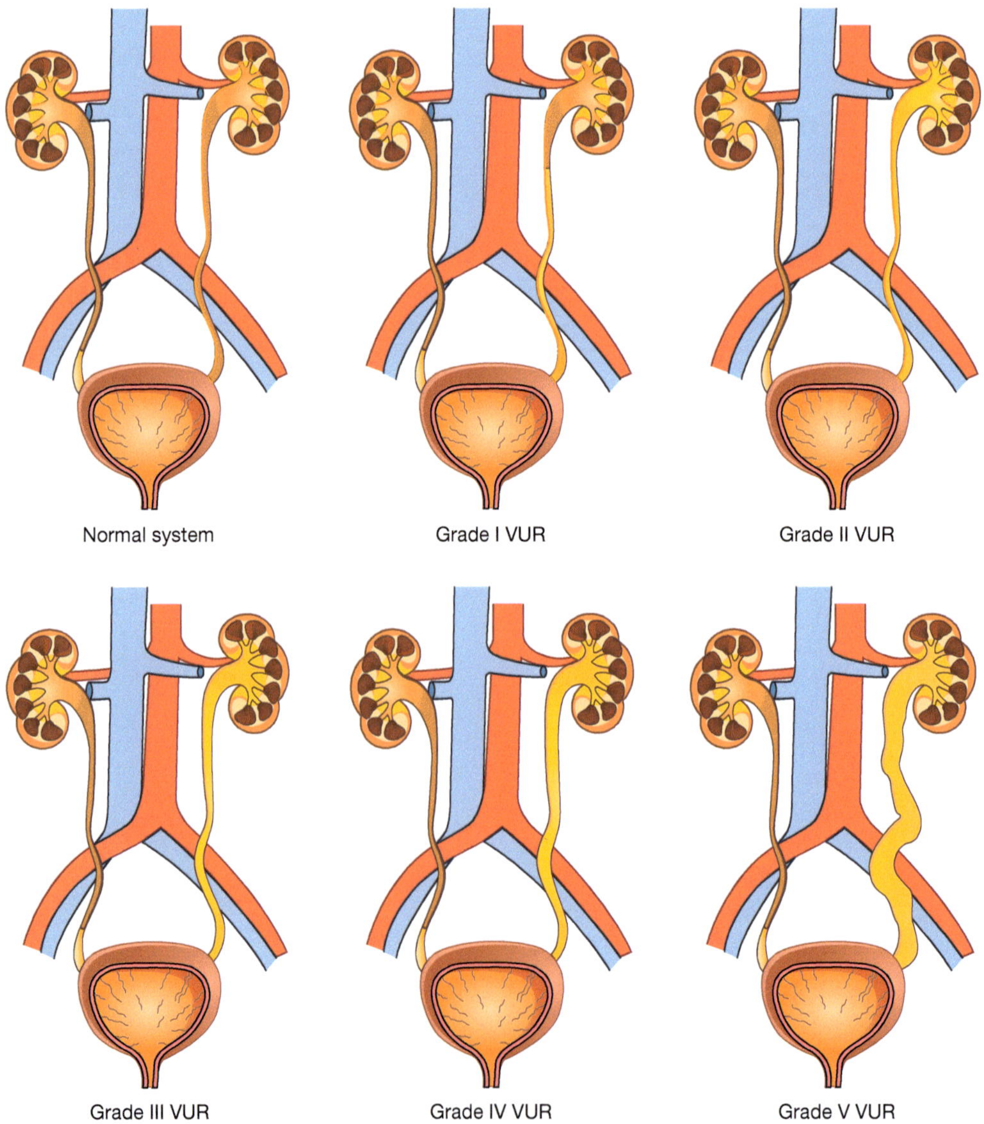

FIGURE 15.9 Stages of vesicoureteric reflux (VUR).

Conclusion

The renal system consists of the upper and lower urinary tract: kidneys, ureters, bladder and urethra. Many renal system anomalies are detected during the antenatal period through detailed ultrasound scanning. Some renal diseases are treated medically, some surgically and some require a combination of both. It is essential that the nursing care and management of infants, children and young people with renal disorders are embedded in a family-centred approach, and that as a paediatric nurse, you are mindful of renal medical- and surgical-specific nursing assessment and care.

References

Alhamoud, M.A., Salloot, I.Z., Mohiuddin, S.S., *et al.* (2021). A comprehensive review study on glomerulonephritis associated with post-streptococcal infection. *Cureus* 13(12), e20212 https://doi.org/10.7759/cureus.20212.

BMJ Best Practice (2023). Urinary tract infections in children. BMJ Publishing Group. Available at http://www.bestpractice.bjm.com (accessed 3 April 2025).

Byrne L, Douglas A, Launders N, Godbole G, Lynn R, Inward C and Jenkins C (2023). Haemolytic uraemic syndrome in children England, Wales, Northern Ireland, and Ireland: a prospective cohort study. Epidemiology and Infection, 151, e160, 1–9 https://doi.org/10.1017/S0950268823001413

Cancer Research UK (2023). Treating Wilms' Tumour. https://www.cancerresearchuk.org/about-cancer/childrens-cancer/wilms-tumour/treatment (accessed 19 February 2025).

Children with Cancer UK (2016). https://www.childrenwithcancer.org.uk/childhood-cancer-info/we-fund-research/projects-we-fund/molecular-evolution-wilms-tumour/ (accessed 19 February 2025).

Children's Hospital of Philadelphia (2025). Epididymitis.. https://www.chop.edu/conditions-diseases/epididymitis (accessed 4 Mar 2025).

Chirico, V., Tripodi, F., Lacquaniti, A., Monardo, P., Conti, G., Ascenti, G., and Chimenz, R. (2023) Therapeutic management of children with vesicoureteral reflux. Journal Of Clinical Medicine 2024, 13, 244. /10.3390/jcm13010244

Claure-Del Granado, R., & Chávez-Íñigue, J. (2024). Herbal and dietary supplements: hidden dangers to kidney health. *ASN Kidney News*, 30 August 2024.

Dalrymple, R. (2019). Haematuria, management and investigation in paediatrics (145) NHS Greater Glasgow and Clyde Paediatrics for Health Professionals. https://clinicalguidelines.scot.nhs.uk/ggc-paediatric-guidelines/ggc-paediatric-guidelines/emergency-medicine/haematuria-management-and-investigation-in-paediatrics-145/ (accessed 2 May 2025).

Diviney, J., & Jaswon, M.S. (2020). Urine collection methods and dipstick testing in non-toilet-trained children. *Pediatric Nephrology* 36, 1697–1708 https://link.springer.com/article/10.1007/s00467-020-04742-w (accessed 3 April 3035).

Downie, M.L., Gallibois, C., Parekh, R.S., & Noone, D.G. (2017). Nephrotic syndrome in infants and children: pathophysiology and management. Paediatrics and International Child. *Health* 37(4), 248–258.

EAU (2024). Paediatric urology. European Association of Urology. https://uroweb.org (accessed 3 April 2025).

Garriboli, M., Clothier, J., Selvaggio, G., & Harper, L. (2023). Editorial: Posterior urethral valves: advances in diagnosis, management, and long-term follow up. *Frontiers in Pediatrics* 19 July 2023 Sec. Pediatric Urology 11 https://doi.org/10.3389/fped.2023.1252048 (accessed 23 March 2025).

Great Ormond Street Hospital (2019). Henoch Schönlein Purpura (HSP). https://www.gosh.nhs.uk/conditions-and-treatments/conditions-we-treat/henoch-sch-nlein-purpura-hsp/ (accessed 2 May 2025).

Haffner, D. (2020). Strategies for optimizing growth in children with chronic kidney disease. *Frontiers in Pediatrics* 8, 399 https://pmc.ncbi.nlm.nih.gov/articles/PMC7406572/.

Harambat, J., & Madded, I. (2023). What is the true burden of chronic kidney disease in children worldwide? Paediatric. *Nephrology* 38, 1389–1393, 38, 1389.

infoKid (2024). PUV treatment. https://infokid.org.uk/conditions/posterior-urethral-valves-puv/puv-treatment/

Katsoufis, C.P., DeFreitas, M.J., Infante, J.C., *et al.* (2019). Risk assessment of severe congenital anomalies of the kidney and urinary tract (CAKUT): a birth cohort. *Pediatrics* 7. https://doi.org/10.3389/fped.2019.00182.

Kidney Disease: Improving Global Outcomes (KDIGO) (2012). Acute Kidney Injury Work Group KDIGO Clinical Practice Guideline for Acute Kidney Injury. Kidney International. Supplement 2012;2:1–138

Kim, J.H., *et al.* (2020). Renal syndromic hearing loss is common in childhood-onset chronic kidney disease. *Journal of Korean Medical Science* 35(44) https://pmc.ncbi.nlm.nih.gov/articles/PMC7669456/.

Kim, S., Van Zwieten, A., Lorenzo, J., *et al.* (2022). Cognitive and academic outcomes in children with chronic kidney disease. *Pediatric Nephrology* 37, 2715–2724 https://link.springer.com/article/10.1007/s00467-022-05499-0.

McDonald, C. (2022). Patient advice sheet Acute Glomerulonephritis in Children and Young people (<16 years. https://www.buckshealthcare.nhs.uk/wp-content/uploads/2022/05/Nephritis-in-Children-and-Young-people.pdf (accessed 2 May 2025).

Miller, K.M., Beneden, C.V., *et al.* (2022). Standardization of epidemiological surveillance of acute poststreptococcal glomerulonephritis. *Open Forum Infectious Diseases* 9(Suppl 1) https://wrap.warwick.ac.uk/id/eprint/170243/1/WRAP-Standardization-of-Epidemiological-Surveillance-of-Acute-Poststreptococcal-Glomerulonephritis-Seale-2022.pdf.

MSD Manual (2025). Some causes of Oliguria. https://www.msdmanuals.com/professional/multimedia/table/some-causes-of-oliguria

NHS (2022). Nephrotic syndrome in children. https://www.nhs.uk/conditions/nephrotic-syndrome/ (accessed 2 May 2025).

NICE (2010). CG111: Bedwetting in under 19s. National Institute of Health and Care Excellence. https://www.nice.org.uk (accessed 3 April 2025).

NICE (2022). Urinary tract infection in under 16s: diagnosis and management. National Institute for Health and Care Excellence. https://www.nice.org.uk (accessed 3 April 2025).

NICE (2024a). Urinary tract infection – children. Available at; https://cks.nice.org.uk/topics/urinary-tract-infection-children/ (accessed 3 April 2025).

NICE (2024b). Bedwetting enuresis. https://cks.nice.org.uk/topics/bedwetting-enuresis/ (accessed 3 April 2025).

NICE (2024c). Balanitis. https://cks.nice.org.uk/topics/balanitis/ (accessed 3 April 2025).

Nieuwhof-Leppink, A.J., Hussong, J., *et al.* (2021). Definitions, indications and practice of urotherapy in children and adolescents: standardization document of the International Children's Continence Society (ICCS). *Journal of Pediatric Urology* 17(2), 172–181.

Niuewhof-Leppink, A., Larsson, J., Holmdahl, G., and Goyal, A. (2022) Urotherapy book a case-based approach. https://www.espu.org/e-books/Urotherapy_book/ (accessed 3 April 2025).

Nursing and Midwifery Council (NMC) (2018). The Code. Professional standards of practice and behaviour for nurses, midwives and nursing associates. NMC, London.

Peate, I., & Gormley-Fleming, E. (2015). *Fundamentals of Children's Anatomy and Physiology*. Wiley, Oxford.

RCoA (2020). Preoperative care 4th Edition. https://rcoa.ac.uk/sites/default/files/documents/2020-08/21075%20RCoA%20Audit%20Recipe%20Book_10%20Section%20B.1_p62-100_AW_0.pdf

Sawyer C *et al.* (2021). Epidemiological investigation of recurrent outbreaks of haemolytic uraemic syndrome caused by Shiga toxin-producing *Escherichia coli* serotype O55:H7 in England, 2014–2018. Epidemiology and Infection 149, e108, 1–9. https://doi.org/10.1017/S0950268821000844

Schulga, P., and Mckie, A. (2024). Proteinuria in children: advice for referrers. Paediatrics for Health Professionals. NHS greater Glasgow and Clyde. https://clinicalguidelines.scot.nhs.uk/rhc-for-health-professionals/guidelines/primary-care-referral-guidelines/medical-paediatric-pre-referral-guidance/proteinuria-in-children-advice-for-referrers/ (accessed 2 May 2025).

Sezer, B.T. (2023). Ureteropelvic junction obstruction. In: Abdel-Gawad, M., Ali-El-Dein, B., Barry, J., & Stenzl, A. (eds). *The Ureter*. Cham: Springer https://doi.org/10.1007/978-3-031-36212-5_4.

Smith, G. (2017). Guidelines for the management of nephrotic syndrome in children. Children's Kidney Centre University Hospital of Wales. https://cavuhb.nhs.wales/files/welsh-clinical-network-for-paediatric-nephrology/guidelines-for-the-management-of-nephrotic-syndrome-in-children-pdf/ (accessed 05 February 2025).

The Royal Children's Hospital Melbourne (2014). Clinical Guidelines (Nursing). https://www.rch.org.au/rchcpg/hospital_clinical_guideline_index/nursing_assessment/#Renal (accessed January 2025).

UK Kidney Association and UK Renal Registry (2021). UK Renal Registry Annual Report Summary analyses of data for children and young people under 18 years to the end of 2021. UKKA.

Viteri, B., Calle-Toro, J.S., Furth, S., *et al.* (2020). State-of-the-art renal imaging in children. *Pediatrics* 145(2), e20190829.

Vivarelli, M., Gibson, K., Sinha, A., & Boyer, O. (2023). Childhood nephrotic syndrome. *Lancet* 402(10404), P809–P824.

Walker, E.Y., Winyard, P., & Marlais, M. (2023). Congenital anomalies of the kidney and urinary tract: antenatal diagnosis, management and counselling of families. *Pediatric Nephrology* (2024) 39, 1065–1075 https://doi.org/10.1007/s00467-023-06137-z.

Wang, C.S., & Greenbaum, L.A. (2019). Nephrotic syndrome. *Pediatric Clinics Of North America* 66(1), 73–85.

Worsley C, Hacking C, Qaqish N, *et al.* (2022). Wilms tumour (staging). Reference article, Radiopaedia.org (Accessed 19 Feb 2025). https://doi.org/10.53347/rID-2294

Yonekawa, K.E., Barreto, E.F., & Sutherland, S.M. (2022). *Pediatric Nephrology*, 8th edn. Springer Nature, Cham, Switzerland, pp. 1554–1676.

CHAPTER 16

Disorders of the reproductive systems

Michele O'Grady

AIM

This chapter provides understanding and insight into the disordered pathophysiology of male and female reproductive systems, which is required for safe, high-quality and effective informed care.

LEARNING OUTCOMES

On completion of this chapter, the reader will be able to:

- Describe common conditions in both boys and girls.
- Consider the psychological distress caused by reproductive ill health.
- Consider the role of the paediatric nurse in assessing reproductive health/ill health.
- Discuss and consider common conditions related to both the male and female reproductive systems.

KEYWORDS

- reproductive health
- male genitalia
- female genitalia
- female genital mutilation
- torsion
- psychological care
- sexually transmitted infection

Test your prior knowledge

1. In male foetal development, when do testes descend down the inguinal canal into the scrotal sac?
2. Spermatogenesis is the term for the production of what?
3. What does the male Tanner scale measure?
4. What shape are the ovaries?
5. What is the age range of female puberty?

Introduction

There are a vast number of disorders of the reproductive systems of both boys and girls, and it would be difficult to include all of them in a single chapter. However, common presentations have been chosen, and an attempt has been made to select the common conditions that are likely to present throughout your career.

> Throughout the chapter, there will be conditions common in girls and, to a lesser extent boys, which may be a symptom of sexual abuse, although this will be a rare cause of the complaint. It is essential that whenever a gynaecological examination takes place, it is carried out by a professional trained to diagnose sexual abuse. History taking and systematic assessment are vitally important in conditions of the reproductive system in order to identify possible signs of abuse.

Why is dealing with the reproductive system more difficult than any other system in the body? The short answer is that adults are often embarrassed to talk about or even consider that their children are developing into sexual human beings.

The use of language when dealing with children and young people can be challenging and depends on the conversations that parents may or may not have had with their children (Rogers *et al.*, 2015). What children call their genitalia can be varied, and in fact, some girls do not have a name for their vagina, so taking a history can be tricky. Throughout the chapter, this issue will be highlighted with helpful tips to overcome language difficulties. However, you, as the practitioner, need to be comfortable discussing matters affecting reproductive health, as children and young people will sense your discomfort, which will affect your therapeutic relationships.

Parents often struggle to talk to their children about sex, finding it difficult to know how much information to impart to their children and young people (Holman *et al.*, 2023). Easterbrook *et al.* (2022) comment on the limited research on Lesbian, Gay, Bisexual, Transgender, Queer (or questioning), Intersex, Asexual (LGBTQ+) parents talking to their children about sex, but think that these parents may be better at talking about sex than heterosexual parents; more research is required. Parents from different cultures and religions may also experience difficulties in navigating these difficult conversations, but research into this needs to be increased, with Solomon *et al.* (2022) commenting that there is a higher incidence of gonorrhoea infections among black women when compared to their white counterparts in England.

This poses a challenge to nurses caring for children and young people who may have a varied understanding of their own sexuality, and may be curious about their sexuality or may have never considered themselves and their sexuality.

Special considerations

Currently, over 6000 children and young people, aged four to 18 years, have been on the waiting list for over 3 years to be seen at the specialist gender identity service for children and young people (National Health Service England, 2024). In line with the NMC Code (NMC, 2018), these individuals deserve to be treated with respect and dignity; therefore, the recognition of their gender identity and specific health needs is vital. A survey of trans people's experience of accessing healthcare services within the United Kingdom said that NHS staff had no understanding of trans-specific language or healthcare needs (Stonewall, 2018).

Precise terminology in healthcare

Language is a dynamic and ever-evolving system, constantly adapting to reflect the changes in society, culture and human understanding. Inclusive and precise terminology matters significantly in healthcare as it will improve clinical accuracy. Relying on the binary notion of gender can result in misdiagnosis or inadequate treatment, leaving patients at risk.

It is important to become familiar with the terms related to gender and sexuality so that young patients feel that those offering care and support are comfortable and knowledgeable about them (see Table 16.1).

TABLE 16.1 Definitions of key terms related to gender and sexuality

Sex	The categories of male and female based on various biological and physiological traits of individuals, including chromosomes, hormones and reproductive organs. Sex is normally assigned at birth.
Intersex	A term used to describe a person who may have biological attributes of both sexes or whose biological attributes do not fit into the binary of male or female.
Gender	The socially constructed characteristics of women, men, boys and girls.
Gender identity	A person's sense of self and their own gender.
Gender incongruence	This is the clinical diagnosis used by the NHS for someone who is transgender.
Cisgender	A term used to describe a person whose gender identity aligns with their sex assigned at birth.
Transgender	An umbrella term used to describe a person whose gender identity does not align with their sex assigned at birth. This umbrella term may also encompass people who identify as non-binary, i.e., someone whose gender identity does not fit into the binaries of men or women.
Transitioning	The steps a trans-person takes to live their gender identity, and this will be different for each individual. For the majority, transitioning can be split into two aspects: social – such as name changes and using different pronouns; and medical – such as hormone therapy and surgical care.
Sexual orientation	A term used to describe a person's sexual attraction to others, or lack thereof.
Heterosexual	Refers to a person who is attracted to someone of the opposite sex or gender.
Bisexual	A term used to refer to a person who is attracted to more than one sex or gender.

The male reproductive system

One of the characteristics of the male reproductive organs is that most of the organs are outside the body. The reproductive system is closely linked with the neuroendocrine system, which produces hormones that are required for development and sexual maturation. The urinary system and the reproductive system are collocated. The testes are located in the scrotum outside the body because sperm production and storage need to be 3° cooler than body temperature. For an in-depth examination of the anatomy and physiology, please see Peate and Gormley-Fleming (2025). See Fig. 16.1 for an overview of the male reproductive system (see also Chapter 15 of this text).

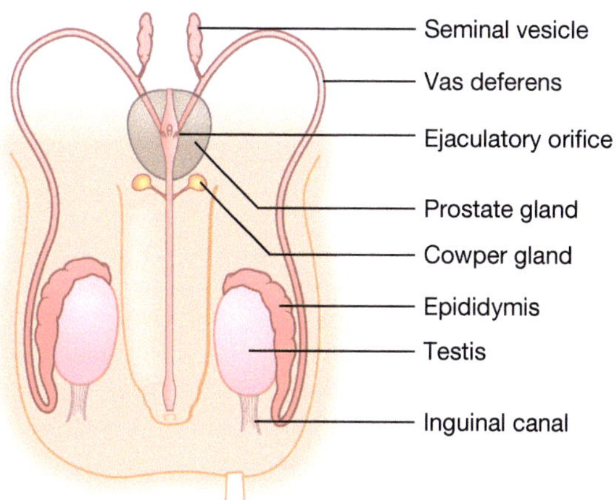

FIGURE 16.1 The male reproductive system.
Source: Reproduced with permission of Peate & Gormley-Fleming 2015/John Wiley & Sons.

TABLE 16.2 Some common male reproductive conditions

- Hydrocele
- Epididymitis
- Torsion of the testes
- Undescended testes
- Priapism
- Balanitis
- Inguinal hernia
- Hypospadias

Male reproductive issues

There are several common male reproductive issues that boys may experience. The healthcare worker is likely to see many of these during their career. Common problems affecting the male reproductive tract are shown in Table 16.2.

It is highly likely that boys who have a problem with their genitalia may be embarrassed and reluctant to tell their parents or health professionals about their concern. In an ideal world, boys could choose if they want to be examined by a female or male nurse/doctor, but often there is no option. Top tips for examination of boys' genitalia:

- Always take a detailed history first – it is important to use terminology that the child or young person is comfortable with, and not to portray any embarrassment.
- Carefully consider their choice of words.
- If an examination is required, try to minimise the number of people and occasions involved. This may mean doctors and nurses doing a first examination jointly.

There are several conditions relating to male reproductive health, but this chapter will consider cryptorchidism and testicular torsion, which is a surgical emergency.

Cryptorchidism (also known as undescended testes)

Cryptorchidism refers to the absence of one or both testes from the scrotum. It occurs in about 1% of infants over 3 months (Fawzy *et al.*, 2015). The precise cause is unclear. See Fig. 16.2 for a depiction of the development of the male reproductive tract.

Classification

Classification of undescended testes is based on testicular location, which may be either along the normal line of descent (abdomen, inguinal canal, external ring, prescrotal and upper scrotal) or in an ectopic position.

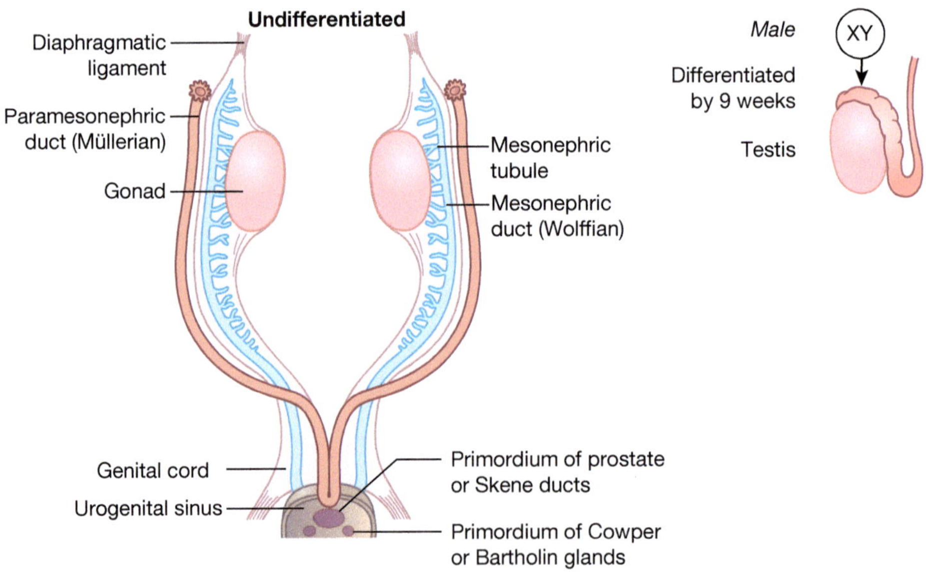

FIGURE 16.2 The development of the male reproductive tract.
Source: Reproduced with permission of Peate & Gormley-Fleming 2015/John Wiley & Sons.

- **True undescended testes:** The testes lie along the normal path of descent in the abdomen or inguinal region but do not reach the scrotum.
- **Ectopic testes:** The testes lie outside the normal path, for example, the perineum or penile shaft.
- **Ascending testes:** The testes have descended but are lying outside the scrotum.
- **Causes:** Not generally understood, but there are some risk factors:
- father or sibling who has had undescended testes
- low birthweight
- small for gestational age
- preterm delivery
- another genital abnormality, e.g., hypospadias.

Diagnosis

- Wash and warm hands prior to examination
- Examine the child lying down in a warm room, maintaining privacy and dignity
- Visual inspection
- Palpation by a qualified practitioner, e.g., general practitioner (GP), surgeon
- Screening within 72 hours of birth (National Institute for Health and Care Excellence [NICE], 2021), at 6–8-week check-up and at 3 months if undescended testes discovered.

Treatment

Surgical intervention is the treatment option. The surgical procedure undertaken brings the testis into the scrotum and anchors it to the wall of the scrotal sac.

Potential complications

- .Impaired fertility (Kolon *et al.*, 2014)
- Testicular cancer
- Testicular torsion
- Surgical complications, e.g., vascular damage

Psychological care

Several factors may lead to parental distress when treating this condition. Usually, it is diagnosed in young babies, and surgical intervention in a young baby is very traumatic for parents. Minimising distress is as important as treating the problem. Families require adequate explanations, detailed information and constant reassurance. Occasionally, an older child will present with one or both testes undescended. This can be very traumatic for all concerned, and the outcome for future fertility may not be positive.

Case study 16.1: testicular torsion

Ahmed is a 10-year-old boy who presents to the emergency department with a history of sudden pain in his left testicle. Ahmed and his mother are asylum seekers from Sudan who have only been in the country for a few weeks. His mother is concerned as he never complains of pain, so she has brought him to the hospital, and she is very anxious. Ahmed speaks very good English, and with a combination of a nurse with some Arabic, Language Line and Ahmed, a history was obtained.

Ahmed is triaged by the nurse. He has a PEWS score of zero, but he is complaining of moderate pain and is given analgesia of paracetamol 500 mg orally and ibuprofen 300 mg orally, having checked that he has no allergies and has not had any analgesia today. An urgent call is made to the surgeons, and they attend the department 10 minutes later.

The surgeons advise mum that Ahmed needs to go to the theatre for a surgical exploration of the testes to rule out testicular torsion, and he might lose the testicle if untreated. A tearful Ahmed is transferred to the theatre, promptly accompanied by his mum.

Ahmed had a testicular torsion, which was released, and the blood supply was restored to the testicle. Ahmed makes an unremarkable post-operative recovery with no complications and is discharged home that evening.

Investigations: Obtaining a urine sample

NICE (2022) recommends that a clean-catch specimen of urine is required from all children when ruling out a urinary tract infection (UTI), and a midstream specimen from older children.

In Ahmed's case, it is important to explain what is meant by a midstream urine sample. Many departments have a urine collection kit with a funnel attached to a sterile container.

Advise Ahmed to wash his hands.

Connect the funnel to the sterile container without contaminating the inside of the pot or funnel.

Explain to Ahmed that he should first wash the tip of his penis with the cotton wool balls and water provided, and pat dry. As he starts to pass urine, he should allow a small amount of urine to pass into the toilet before using the container to collect urine.

The nurse should be close by, wearing gloves, to take the container from Ahmed, removing the funnel and placing the cap on the bottle.

During urinalysis, the nurse should carefully follow the protocol depending on the urinalysis machine used in their department, provided they are trained to do so. Ahmed's name and details are entered into the machine, and a printout can be obtained. After the urinalysis is completed, local protocols will indicate whether the sample needs to be sent to the laboratory. Results must be documented in Ahmed's notes.

NB: Ahmed's parent will be anxious to know the result of the urine test, and provided you are competent to do so, or in discussion with a more senior practitioner, it is important to discuss the findings with Ahmed and his mother with the help of an interpreter.

Medication alert

Ibuprofen combines anti-inflammatory analgesic and antipyretic properties. It has fewer side effects than other non-steroidal anti-inflammatory drugs (NSAIDs); however, its anti-inflammatory properties are weaker.

Ibuprofen is generally well-tolerated, and the majority of people do not experience any side effects. The most common side effects are related to stomach irritation and include abdominal pain, indigestion and nausea. These can mainly be avoided by taking ibuprofen with food. Rarely, serious side effects, e.g., ulceration or bleeding of the stomach or intestines, may occur. If the child experiences any sign of bleeding from the stomach or bowels after taking this medicine, e.g., vomiting blood and/or passing black/tarry/blood-stained stools, consult a doctor immediately.

Special considerations

Working in the Emergency Department poses a problem for practitioners when faced with a surgical emergency and a family who requires help with communication, which can include a lack of English but also other disabilities such as hearing and sight problems. Nurses must develop an ability to develop a range of coping strategies to communicate effectively before a translator can be summoned.

Testicular torsion

The principal cause of testicular torsion is when the tunica vaginalis fails to encase the testicle, and the testis hangs free from the vascular structures, leading to a partial or complete venous occlusion. This can lead to ischaemia (tissue death) and could result in a loss of one or both testicles. It is estimated that the annual incidence of testicular torsion is 3.8 per 100 000 in young people under 18 years or 4 per 100 000 (Dam *et al.*, 2025). There are several predisposing factors relating to testicular torsion. Often it is spontaneous, but it can sometimes follow direct trauma.

Testicular torsion is a surgical emergency and requires urgent surgical intervention. Most hospital trusts will have a protocol, and nurses must ensure that surgeons are informed immediately when a child/young person attends with testicular pain. It is important that the parent and child are warned that the surgeons may react very quickly if torsion is suspected. In Ahmed's case, he was in the emergency department for less than 20 minutes before he was transferred to the theatre.

Signs and symptoms

- Testicular or lower abdominal pain – in young boys, always consider testicular symptoms (Dam *et al.*, 2025).
- A recent pain in the testicles that resolved – there may have been an episode of testicular pain, which may indicate an episode of spontaneously resolving testicular torsion.
- Pain is severe, often associated with vomiting, and the child can exhibit signs of shock.
- May or may not have been associated with trauma, e.g., kicked in the testicles.

Physical examination

- The initial examination is carried out by a senior A&E doctor, Emergency or Advanced Nurse Practitioner, with an urgent referral to the Surgical team once testicular torsion is suspected.

- **Ultrasound:** It does not provide adequate information and should not be used to diagnose torsion. The use of colour Doppler ultrasound (CDUS) or high-resolution ultrasonography (HRUS) may well diagnose torsion or rule it out, but it is important that the technology is used and interpreted by an expert (Dam *et al.*, 2025).
- Testicle may or may not appear swollen, hot or hard.
- PEWS may be normal, or a tachycardia and hypotension may indicate early shock. Pyrexia may be present.
- Urinalysis should be performed to rule out infection, but should not delay surgery if required.

Where possible, the examination should be carried out by a male member of the team to reduce embarrassment and distress to the young adolescent.

Treatment options

- **Orchiopexy:** This is carried out on a viable testicle, i.e., one where the blood supply is intact. The testicle is released and fixed to the inner scrotal wall.
- **Orchiectomy:** The testicle is removed, and a prosthetic implant is inserted later.

The physical care required to treat the patient is essential, and any delay in providing surgical intervention can have serious repercussions in the post-operative period. The importance of psychological care associated with an emergency surgical intervention is outlined in the following box.

Psychological care

- Rapid assessment and move to the operating theatre
- Scar on scrotum
- Possible loss of testicle
- Possible further surgery
- Reduced fertility

The speed of the assessment and the need for rapid surgery can be very traumatic for the child/young person and their families. In Ahmed's case, his time in the emergency department was less than 20 minutes. Because the time from diagnosis is so short, there is little opportunity to discuss theatre and pre- and post-operative care with the young person or the parent.

The removal of a testicle can cause both physical and psychological trauma to the young man and his family. Apart from the physical difference in his scrotum, there are also psychological effects. Although a prosthetic can be fitted so the scrotum looks normal, there is the undecided issue of future fertility.

Many sexual health services focus solely on women, but there are some local services, and nationally, the Brook Centres offer counselling around a range of sexual issues.

The stress and psychological trauma can impede healing and can affect the young person's mental health and well-being.

Female reproductive health issues

The female reproductive system is more complex than the male reproductive system. Similarities exist between both systems, with the endocrine system producing hormones required for biological development, sexual arousal and puberty. The female reproductive system is predominantly hidden inside the body, and the urinary system is collocated but not a part of the sexual organs. The female reproductive system is made up of the ovaries, fallopian tubes, uterus, vagina and external genitalia (see Figs 16.3 and 16.4). The breasts are also part of the female reproductive system.

The function of the female reproductive system is to produce ova and allow fertilisation of the ova to take place and the foetus to grow inside it. After birth, the reproductive system also prepares the breasts to feed the infant.

As with the male reproductive system, it is expected that the reader has an in-depth knowledge of the anatomy and physiology of the system, including the issues of puberty and menstrual cycle.

There is a range of conditions affecting female reproductive health, and this chapter will concentrate on some of the most common (see Table 16.3).

Menstrual disorders

Menarche, or the first period, has been described in the literature as a major milestone in a girl's life and many cultures celebrate the transition into womanhood (Pitangui *et al.*, 2013;

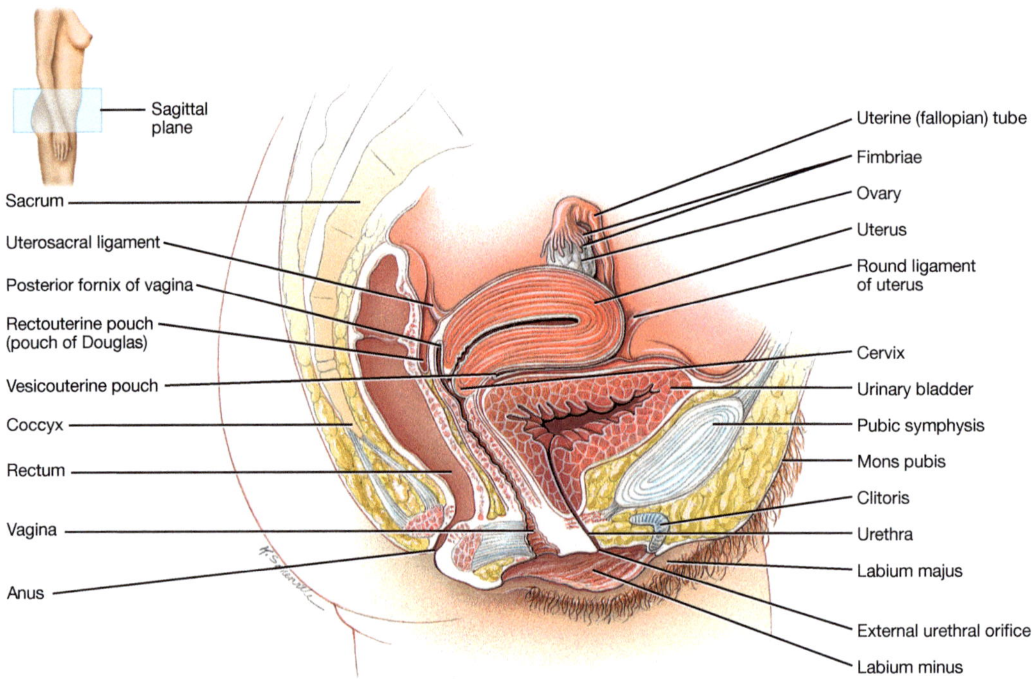

FIGURE 16.3 The female reproductive system.
Source: Reproduced with permission of Peate & Gormley-Fleming 2015/John Wiley & Sons.

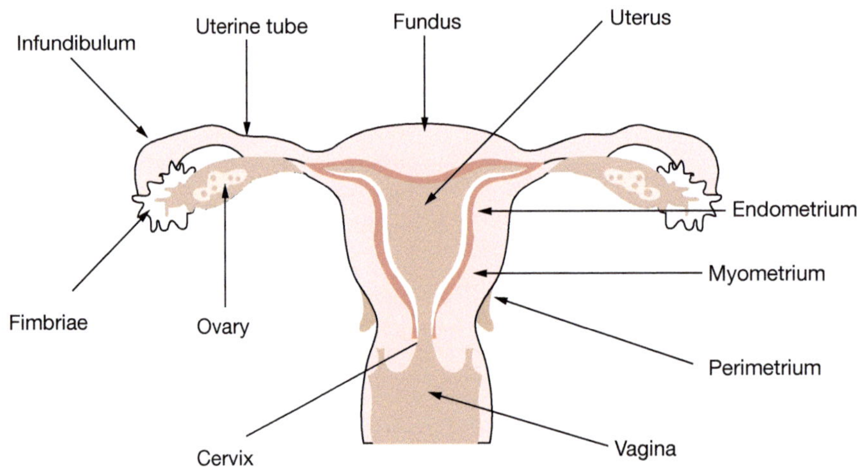

FIGURE 16.4 The uterus and associated structures.
Source: Reproduced with permission of Peate & Gormley-Fleming 2015/John Wiley & Sons.

TABLE 16.3 Some common female reproductive conditions
• Menstrual disorders • Abdominal pain • Vulvovaginitis • Sexually transmitted infections • Unprotected sexual activity • Female genital mutilation

Pateriya & Kanhere, 2014). Considered a normal part of life, Kcuik and Kives (2021) suggest that problems in menstruation are responsible for loss of education, as girls frequently do not seek medical help with significant health problems relating to abnormalities. Early menarche has been associated with depressive symptoms and antisocial behaviours in adulthood (Jiang *et al.*, 2025).

Guimarães *et al.* (2020) describe dysmenorrhea or pain during menstruation as the most common gynaecological complaint of young women. Primary dysmenorrhea can be described as painful menstruation in women with a normal pelvic anatomy. Secondary dysmenorrhea refers to pain due to a disorder in the pelvis. The physiology behind dysmenorrhea is an increased production of the hormone prostaglandins by the endometrium, causing uterine contraction and pain. It is thought that 50% of females may experience dysmenorrhoea at some point in their life, with 40–60% of young women experiencing dysmenorrhea, which impacts their lives (Ummah & Ismarwati, 2024).

Complementary therapies can be as effective as pharmacological treatment to alleviate the symptoms of dysmenorrhea, and young women are most likely to use a variety of alternative therapies (Ummah & Ismarwati, 2024).

Pain begins shortly before menstruation commences and can last 1–3 days. The pain can be associated with cramps, nausea and vomiting, and syncope (fainting). It can be very debilitating for some women and has been associated with missed days in school and educational deficit (Kcuik and Kius, 2022). Girls and adult women are unlikely to seek medical help and endure symptoms that may indicate an underlying pathology.

Menstruation is a normal part of everyday life for women. However, it appears that girls do not always discuss problems with their parents, and nurses need to use opportunities to take a menstrual history from girls whenever an overall health history is taken and encourage girls and their parents to discuss issues relating to dysmenorrhea.

Abdominal pain in girls

Almost all girls will have abdominal pain at one time or another. The pain can be anywhere between the chest and groin. Most of the time, it is not caused by a serious medical problem; however, sometimes abdominal pain may be a sign of something serious.

Abdominal pain in adolescent girls can be difficult to diagnose, as there are several causes, some of which are gynaecological, which can lead to a severe onset of abdominal pain (see Table 16.4).

Abdominal pain presentations in adolescent girls are outlined in Table 16.4.

Girls with abdominal pain require a thorough examination, and history taking is key. The history involves asking personal questions in a manner that is both respectful and non-judgemental. It is important to establish a rapport, and it may be advantageous to have time alone with the young person to allow them to give you information that they may not want shared with their parent. History should include:

- description and location of pain, including timing and any repetitive history
- urinary history
- bowel history
- menstrual history
- stress
- sexual activity.

TABLE 16.4 **Examples of abdominal pain presentation in adolescent girls**

	Acute	Chronic
Gynaecological	Ectopic pregnancy Miscarriage Pelvic inflammatory disease Ovarian cyst rupture Ovarian torsion	Dysmenorrhea Endometriosis Pelvic inflammatory disease Adhesions
Gastrointestinal	Gastroenteritis Appendicitis Perforation Bowel obstruction	Constipation Irritable bowel syndrome Lactose intolerance Coeliac disease
Urological	Pyelonephritis Cystitis Urethritis UTI (urinary tract infection)	Chronic cystitis
Other		Abdominal migraine

With pre-pubescent and pubescent girls, a urine test for urinalysis and a pregnancy test are required to rule out infection and pregnancy. This can be a difficult subject to broach with both the girls and their parents as some parents feel it is totally unnecessary and insulting. It is particularly difficult in families where sex has never been discussed, and sex education in school has been denied on religious or moral grounds. In most cases, parents make a joke of it and give consent; however, some parents will try to refuse consent. Generally, medical staff will not be able to proceed with an exploration of the causes of abdominal pain without a pregnancy test, and most parents accept this.

Informed consent

Informed consent for treatment must be given serious consideration. The nurse and other members of the multidisciplinary team must understand the key issues associated with consent.

1. Who can give consent?
2. What age is a child considered to be Gillick competent?
3. What is the difference between the Fraser guidelines and Gillick competency?

It is essential that the nurse can provide answers to these three questions to provide safe and effective, patient-centred care. Informed consent is one aspect of a person's human rights.

Abdominal pain is not only a symptom of gynaecological ill health, but it is also important to understand that it will be one of the differential diagnoses to consider. Equally, it is important to highlight that it is not the only cause of abdominal pain in adolescent girls.

Vaginal discharge

A common presentation in both primary care and emergency departments is vaginal discharge in children aged 4–8 years (George, 2021), although it is also seen in younger and older children. Salim and Hajar (2018) commented that the anatomy and physiology of the prepubertal vagina offer some explanation for the causes of vaginal discharge.

- Vaginal mucosa has a neutral pH
- The vagina lacks antibodies to fight infection
- The vagina is short – 3–4 cm
- The labia minora are small
- Labial fat pads are not present to help combat infection
- The vagina lies in close proximity to the rectum.

Early childhood growth and development

Very often, children will present with this condition shortly after starting nursery or school. Their new-found independence, which is a normal part of child development, often results in poor technique in wiping their bottom, leading to an infection.

Signs and symptoms associated with vaginal discharge

- Discharge, which may be seen by parent on the person's underwear
- Discharge may be foul-smelling
- Discharge may look green or have a pus-like appearance
- Pruritus (itch)
- Erythema (redness)/irritation around the labia
- Urinary symptoms, such as dysuria or frequency

Causes of vaginal discharge

There are a wide variety of causes for vaginal discharge in children.

- **Idiopathic:** There is no known cause.
- **Vulvovaginitis:** Irritation around the vulval area, which may be exacerbated by obesity, tight-fitting underwear or irritants such as bubble bath.
- **Foreign body:** History taking is very important, as children may admit that they put something into their vagina, or they may not remember. It is not unusual to find Lego, plastic, tissues and other items as the cause for the discharge.
- **Infection:** Often due to poor hygiene. Often occurs when the child starts becoming independent with toileting.
- **Sexual abuse:** Sexual abuse should always be considered when a child presents with vaginal discharge, but it is rare.

There are several factors that predispose young girls to acquire vaginal infections:

- lack of labial fat pads and pubic hair
- neutral vaginal pH (6.5–7.5)
- epithelium is thin and dry in the pre-pubertal vagina.

Making a diagnosis

- History taking from parent and child is important. Obtaining a history from a child may be difficult, but it is important to include them in the discussions, particularly if an examination is required.
- History of toileting behaviour is vital, particularly when establishing if the child wipes their own bottom unsupervised.
- Swabs may be taken, but high vaginal swabs are rarely indicated.
- If discharge is bloodstained, this is an indication for a gynaecology referral (McGreal & Wood, 2013).
- Examination should be carried out by a paediatric specialist or a gynaecologist. If the child cooperates and will put their legs in the 'frog leg' position, that may allow a visual inspection of the perineum and may indicate a pooling of discharge that can be easily swabbed. A play specialist carrying out distraction therapy may mean the child will allow the doctor to separate the labia and visualise the lower vagina. This may reveal a foreign body, although this is unlikely to be successfully removed without sedation, such as ketamine or a general anaesthetic.
- Swabs are most likely to grow anaerobic bacteria, followed by group A beta-haemolytic streptococcus.

Medication alert

Ketamine sedation is used very successfully in emergency departments and day units to avoid full anaesthesia.

Route of administration: Intramuscular.
Dose: Refer to British National Formulary for Children (BNFC) – latest edition.
Caution: Ketamine must only be administered by senior medical or anaesthetic staff.
Contra-indications: Head trauma, hypertension and cardiac disease.
Side effects: Diplopia, hallucinations, nausea, nightmares, tachycardia, transient psychotic effects and vomiting.
Side effects (rare): Arrhythmias, bradycardia and respiratory distress.
Caution for administration: Nurses should note that ketamine is a controlled drug and should be stored appropriately.

There are different strengths of ketamine, and errors can occur.

- Children should be recovered in a dark and quiet area to reduce side effects.
- Children may be discharged once they have eaten and passed urine.
- Parents should be apprised of the likelihood of nightmares.
- Ketamine is an alternative to a general anaesthetic.

Treatment

- Treat cause
- **Antibiotics for infection:** Antibiotic regimens depend on the causative organism
- **Removal of foreign body:** Under sedation or general anaesthetic
- **Diagnosis of abuse:** Suspicion of abuse will result in safeguarding protocols being put into action and will involve police and social services. It is likely to be very upsetting for the child as they may be taken into care pending investigation.

Health promotion advice

For many children, vaginal discharge is due to poor hygiene or irritants and can be treated with advice about the contributing factors. This is an important aspect of the nursing care of any child with vaginal irritation, regardless of the cause.

- Good toileting hygiene, always wipe from front to back after using the toilet.
- Encourage the child to sit on the toilet with their legs apart when urinating.
- Daily warm baths are very helpful, without the addition of scented bubble baths, and through gentle drying of the area is important.
- Wear cotton underwear that is not too tight.
- Avoid wearing pants in bed.

Psychological care

There is little written about the effect on parents of being asked if their child may have been sexually abused, but it is a question that may be asked during the investigation of vaginal discharge. Parents may feel very shocked and angry, especially when a cause other than abuse is found. It is important to acknowledge to parents that they are no longer suspected. Children who have had an intimate examination may also feel very vulnerable and upset. However, with treatment for the discharge, this is usually short-lived. All nurses must be aware of the effects of hospitalisation on families, and they must strive to make a hospital admission as pleasant as it can be.

Health promotion advice in this case is extremely important. There are many advice leaflets available, which are produced either nationally or locally.

Sexual health advice

There is a wealth of literature addressing issues regarding sexual health or sexual ill health. It is important to recognise some of the issues:

- Young people are having sex
- Sex education may not always adequately prepare young people for this stage in their lives
- Parents do not always want to accept their children as sexual beings
- Nurses are often perceived by young people as being uncomfortable around issues relating to sexual activity
- Discrimination towards LGBTQ+ young people is both common and unacceptable for nurses (Nursing & Midwifery Council [NMC], 2018).

There is an overwhelming amount of literature looking at various aspects of young people and sexual behaviour; the rest of this chapter is an attempt to highlight some of the issues and to encourage you to read more widely around the subject. The following issues are discussed in more detail in this chapter: sexually transmitted infections (STIs), emergency contraception in the under-age teenager, and FGM.

Sexual activity

Sexual activity in young people is monitored statistically using two measures: the rate of STIs and the teenage pregnancy rate (Schalet, 2011). There is a flaw to this measurement as it is a 'guestimate' based on those two measures.

Teenage pregnancy rates

The United Kingdom still has the highest pregnancy rate in Europe, even though there has been a fall in rates. STIs continue to rise despite government screening and treatment campaigns aimed at the under-25s.

The conception rate for women aged under 18 years in England and Wales has more than halved since 2011, when it was 30.9 conceptions per 1000 women of the same age; in 2021, it was 13.2 per 1000 women of the same age (Office for National Statistics, 2023).

Contraception

There are several different methods of contraception available. For further details, please go to www.fpa.org.uk for an in-depth explanation of what is available.

Emergency contraception

This is a complex issue for children's nurses for many reasons. The philosophy of family-centred care with a partnership between parents and young people is integral to our way of working, but this is challenged when young people seek emergency contraception or if you must suggest emergency contraception following an assault.

Case study 16.2: emergency contraception

The following case study highlights many of the issues faced by children's nurses. Mary is a 15-year-old girl who arrives at a children's emergency department on a Sunday morning at 1000. She refuses to say why she is seeking medical help and says it is personal. Mary is seen by a staff nurse and is triaged; she asks for emergency contraception. The department has a nurse-led protocol, so the triage nurse carries out the first part of the protocol before she is seen by another nurse. A baseline set of observations is taken:

- Temperature: 36.5 °C
- Pulse: 100 bpm
- Respiration: 20 breaths per minute
- Blood pressure 90/60 mmHg
- PEWS score = 0

The nurse asks for a urine sample and asks for consent to carry out a pregnancy test; consent is given. A senior nurse interviews Mary and takes a full medical and sexual history:

Allergies = nil
Medication = nil
Medical history = nil

Sexual history

Mary has a 15-year-old boyfriend called Tom. They have been together for 6 months. They had not previously had sexual intercourse. Mary had discussed the idea of starting contraception with her mother, who told her father, and he was very angry and said that, as she was not 16, she could not have sex, and if she did have sex, Tom would go to prison.

Mary's parents went away for the weekend, and Mary was supposed to have a friend come to stay, but she became unwell, and Mary asked Tom to stay. They had not intended to have sex on this occasion, but 'it just happened' as they had drunk some cider. They tried to use a condom, but it fell off, and Mary is petrified of getting pregnant. She is adamant that her parents must never find out, and she wants emergency contraception. Mary said she wanted to have sex with Tom, and they had sex a few times. The nurse clarified if they meant to have sex, and what sexual activity took place; it was penetrative sexual intercourse. Mary refuses to discuss this with her mother. Mary is prescribed levonorgestrel as sexual intercourse took place less than 12 hours ago, and she is advised to attend the genito-urinary medicine clinic in 3 weeks for STI screening and a family planning clinic as soon as possible to acquire contraceptive advice.

Mary is required to take the drug in front of the nurse to avoid the risk of a young girl obtaining emergency contraception for another young person.

The side effects were discussed, and what to do in the event of her vomiting in the next hour. Mary leaves the department feeling happy.

The emergency contraception protocol must be adhered to. These protocols are generally developed in conjunction with emergency department consultants, paediatric consultants, genito-urinary medicine consultants, child protection police, named nurse for safeguarding, paediatric senior nurses and family planning nurse specialists.

Key assessment considerations

Emergency contraception for girls under the age of 16 may raise issues of both sexual health and child protection. As a result of this, a thorough assessment is required to rule out any exploitation (O'Grady, 2011).

Confidentiality

Explain to the young person that you may have to refer them to another agency or refer them to another specialist.

A letter will be sent to their GP, but GPs are bound by confidentiality, and this will not be revealed to parents/carers.

Ask about the age of the young person. If she is under 13 years old, she is deemed to have been raped in the eyes of the law, and regardless of the age of the partner is at risk. Emergency contraception can still be dispensed, but the safeguarding team/Children Schools and Families and Child Protection Police need to be contacted immediately.

Exploitation: Sole interview

Many young people are accompanied by their boyfriend or even an older man who may or may not be their parent/carer. It is important that you are able to interview your young patient alone, at least for part of the consultation, in case she is being coerced in some way. If the accompanying man does not want this to happen, insist on it, and if the young girl leaves the department, seek urgent advice from the police/Children's Schools and Family and report the action.

Fraser competent (often referred to as Gillick competent)

Fraser competent:

You need to be satisfied

1. That your young person, although under the age of 16 years, understands your advice.
2. That you cannot persuade her to tell her parents that she is seeking contraceptive advice.
3. That she is likely to continue having sexual intercourse with or without contraceptive treatment.
4. That unless she receives contraceptive advice/treatment, her physical or mental health or both, are likely to suffer.
5. That her best interests require contraceptive advice and treatment to be given without parental consent.

The young person turning up and asking for emergency contraception does not necessarily indicate understanding.

It is not enough to understand the nature of the treatment sought; you must be comfortable that she is mature enough to understand what is involved.

Talking to the young person will help you assess competence.

Sexual intercourse

Has sexual intercourse taken place?

- The young person needs to describe her sexual activity, which can be embarrassing for her, but you should remain professional and help her understand that you are not judging her.
- No emergency contraception is required for masturbation.
- The exact timing of the sexual intercourse is important as it will inform your choice.
- If sexual intercourse has taken place in less than 72 hours levonorgestral (Levonelle) needs to be prescribed.
- If sexual intercourse has taken place between 72 and 120 hours, ulipristal (ellaOne) needs to be prescribed.
- If more than 120 hours have passed, it is too late for emergency contraception and the young person should be referred to the gynaecology team.

Consensual sex

The following questions need to be asked:

- Did you intend to have sex?
- Where did you have sex?
- Do you remember having sex?
- Is your partner a boyfriend/known to you?
- Were you under the influence of any other substances, including drugs or alcohol?

Medical assessment

A pregnancy test is required, and consent should be obtained.

If it is negative, proceed with the medication, but remember to explain to the young person that a negative test does not mean they are not pregnant from a previous encounter, or indeed, emergency contraception does not always guarantee no pregnancy. Advice should be given about the action to take if their period is late.

If positive, give the young person time and space and provide information on services to help her, such as Brook Advisory Centre, or Family Planning or their GP. Try to persuade her to talk to her parents/carers.

Medication/treatment

There are two different medications available to young people:

1. **Levonorgestrel:** Effective up to 72 hours, but may have a lesser effectiveness up to 120 hours. Dose to be repeated if vomited within 2 hours.
2. **Ulipristal:** Effective up to 120 hours. Dose to be repeated if vomited within 3 hours.

The other alternative for emergency contraception is the insertion of an intrauterine device. However, this will not be done in the emergency department, but the young person could arrange to go to a local Family Planning Clinic.

Can a nurse refuse to dispense emergency contraception?

Under the Abortion Act 1967, all nurses and doctors can refuse to dispense emergency contraception if they feel it is morally wrong to do so. This has also been upheld by the NMC Code (2018).

However, remember that this may be a vulnerable young person, and there may be safeguarding concerns. As a result, all nurses can assess the young person, but are not required to dispense the medication. This can be delegated to another member of staff.

It is important to note that Gillick competency can be used to discuss a child or young person's competence to give consent, whereas Fraser guidelines can only be used in relation to sexual/contraceptive issues. Lord Fraser intended that nurses and doctors would always try to persuade young people to try to discuss this with their parents. The case study regarding emergency contraception highlights some of the issues for nurses faced with this dilemma. Nurses should also be aware that if a young girl has been assaulted or is found drunk and cannot remember if she had sex, it is recommended that emergency contraception be offered.

Special consideration

This can be a confusing aspect to move from family-centred care, where all decisions are in partnership with the child or young person and their parent, to an exclusion of the parent. It can feel very unsettling for nurses to work in this way, and all staff involved in assessing girls who have participated in unsafe sexual behaviour need to have training to enable them to give good care.

Female genital mutilation

The World Health Organization (WHO, 2025) defines FGM as: 'FGM comprises all procedures that involve partial or total removal of external female genitalia, or other injury to the female genital organs for non-medical reasons'. There is much written about the fact that FGM is a traditional rather than a religious practice. This has made it far more difficult to address. The reasons given by mothers for allowing this to happen to their daughters include:

- FGM is a social convention: Mothers are pressurised by their society and family to conform.
- It is part of raising a young girl.
- A belief that it reduces a girl's libido and prevents her from wanting sex before marriage.
- It increases marriageability: In some cultures, a man would not marry a girl who is not circumcised.
- FGM is associated with beauty and modesty, with the thought that the girl is more hygienic.
- Some religious leaders promote FGM while others oppose it, and others decline to be involved, as it is clearly not a religious practice.
- It is a cultural tradition: – Often an argument for its continuance.

FGM is classified into four types, see Table 16.5.

TABLE 16.5 Classification of female genital mutilation

- **Type I:** Also known as clitoridectomy, this type consists of partial or total removal of the clitoris and/or its prepuce.
- **Type II:** Also known as excision, the clitoris and labia minora are partially or totally removed, with or without excision of the labia majora.
- **Type III:** The most severe form, it is also known as infibulation or pharaonic type. The procedure consists of narrowing the vaginal orifice with the creation of a covering seal by cutting and appositioning the labia minora and/or labia majora, with or without removal of the clitoris. The appositioning of the wound edges consists of stitching or holding the cut areas together for a certain period (e.g., girls' legs are bound together), to create the covering seal. A small opening is left for urine and menstrual blood to escape. An infibulation must be opened either through penetrative sexual intercourse or surgery.
- **Type IV:** This type consists of all other procedures to the genitalia of women for non-medical purposes, such as pricking, piercing, incising, scraping and cauterisation.

Source: Adapted from Royal College of Nursing (RCN), 2023.

Consequences for girls who have undergone FGM

There are both short- and long-term consequences relating to FGM.

Short-term

- severe pain
- haemorrhage
- shock
- septicaemia

Long-term

Physical

- chronic pain
- chronic pelvic infections
- development of genital abscesses, cysts and genital ulcers
- excessive scar formation
- urinary tract infections
- problems in childbirth

Sexual

- decreased libido
- painful intercourse
- fertility issues

Psychological

- post-traumatic stress disorder.

In terms of the pathophysiology of FGM, the difficulties faced by the woman will be related to the type of FGM and the time since it occurred (WHO, 2025) and can result in shock due to pain and haemorrhage, and infection in the first 10 days. There are other issues facing women in the future.

Dysmenorrhea: This can be due to the inability of the blood to escape, leading to stagnation of blood, causing bacteria to spread into the vagina and reproductive tract.

Recurrent urinary infections are due to the flap of skin obstructing the urethra; this obstruction prevents normal micturition, leading to a stagnation of urine.

When the young woman marries, which is a common practice in many parts of the world, infibulation may prevent sexual penetration from occurring, which leads to painful sexual intercourse or further cutting to allow penetration to take place.

Scar tissues in the reproductive tract due to surgery and infection lead to painful sexual intercourse.

During pregnancy, an opening of the infibulation may be required to prevent complications during labour; for example, the midwife will be unable to assess dilatation of the cervix.

Women who have received no antenatal care may require a caesarean section due to the small infibulation opening.

During labour, the vaginal canal may have lost its elasticity, and pelvic floor muscles are rigid, prolonging the second stage of labour.

There are many other complications relating to safe delivery of a baby, and postnatal complications are common.

The psychological trauma inflicted on a young girl, whether she is 5 or 14 years old, is a very real issue. It is a traumatic event that some girls report causes them to relive the pain for years. Girls often describe the anger felt towards their mothers, who have persuaded them that this is a good thing. There may be a requirement for long-term counselling from a therapist who has some understanding of this issue. In addition, there is a requirement to identify and educate women who have undergone FGM to persuade them not to inflict it on the next generation.

FGM: The legal position

- FGM has been illegal in the United Kingdom since 1985.
- Legislation was further strengthened with the Female Genital Mutilation Act 2003.
- In 2015, *Female Genital Mutilation Risks and Safeguarding: Guidance for professionals* was published. Five further reports were published in 2015, and the following clarification was enacted:
  - FGM is a form of child abuse
  - Identification of women who have undergone FGM should be reported, as there is a risk to other girls within that family
  - Girls under 18 years who have undergone FGM are to be referred to the police
  - Women who have undergone FGM are victims of crime
  - Every case of FGM must be reported in the NHS, GP practice and mental health trusts.

No FGM by 2030

- The target to eradicate FGM by 2030 is a long way away, with 99% of all girls undergoing FGM in Somalia. UNICEF has stated that the target to eradicate FGM by 2030 will only happen with a rapid decrease in new cases.

The nurse and FGM

FGM is a global issue for women, and nurses in the United Kingdom should be vigilant for signs of girls who might be about to be abducted to their country of origin to be forced to undergo FGM. With an increase in the migrant population, it is important to consider an intensification of the problem in the United Kingdom. FGM is a complex cultural issue that some may feel is beyond their comprehension. FGM is so common in some countries that it has the same legitimacy as male circumcision. There is little doubt that nurses have a part to play in the global fight against a practice that has horrific consequences for its victims.

Conclusion

Reproductive health and ill health are a significant part of nursing children and young people. However, it is important to acknowledge that it is often difficult to treat reproductive health in the same way as other systems because of the sensitive nature of the conversations while trying to obtain a better picture of the health of your patient.

The area of reproductive ill health, particularly relating to sexual health, requires all practitioners to keep updated on the latest research and become comfortable in talking to both young patients and their parents and carers.

The challenges faced by children's nurses in dealing with the reproductive health and ill health of the patients and families in their care should be faced head-on to provide these people with the care and treatment they deserve.

References

Dam, S.P., Mondal, S., Saradar, T.K., *et al.* (2025). Testicular torsion in children: a series of seven cases. *Journal of Clinical and Scientific Research* https://doi.org/10.4103/jcsr.jcsr_28_24.

Easterbrook, R., van Rhijn, T., & Neustifter, R. (2022). Lgbtq+ parents' experiences talking with their children about sex and sexuality. *The Canadian Journal of Human Sexuality* 31(1), 130–142.

Fawzy, F., Hussein, A., Eid, M.M., *et al.* (2015). Cryptorchidism and fertility. *Clinical Medicine Insights: Reproductive Health* 2015(9), 39–43.

George, T. (2021) *Everything you wanted to know about vaginal discharges.* Don't Forget the Bubbles. https://doi.org/10.31440/DFTB.45655.

Guimarães, I., & Póvoa, A.M. (2020). Primary dysmenorrhea: assessment and treatment. *Revista Brasileira De Ginecologia E Obstetrícia / RBGO Gynecology and Obstetrics* 42(8), 501–507.

Holman, A., Holloway, M., Meinecke, K., *et al.* (2023). "Did I Say Too Much? Did I Say Enough?": balancing the competing struggles parents experience in talking to their children about sex-related topics. *Journal of Family Communication* 23(3–4), 335–346.

Jiang, L., Hao, Y., Wang, Y., *et al.* (2025). Is early menarche related to depression? A meta-analysis. *Journal of Affective Disorders* 369, 508–515.

Kciuk, O., & Kives, S. (2021). Painful periods in adolescents. *Canadian Medical Association Journal (CMAJ)* 193(16), E560–E556.

Kolon, T.F., Herndon, C.D.A., Baker, L.A., *et al.* (2014). Evaluation and treatment of cryptorchidism: AUA guideline. *Journal of Urology* 192(2), 337–345.

McGreal, S., & Wood, P. (2013). Recurrent vaginal discharge in children. *Journal of Pediatric and Adolescent Gynecology* 26(4), 205–208.

National Health Service England. (2024). *Referral pathway for Children and Young People's Gender Services.* Retrieved from November 11th, 2024, from https://www.england.nhs.uk/long-read/referral-pathway-for-children-and-young-peoples-gender-services-community-and-hospital-paediatric-services/.

National Institute for Health and Care Excellence (NICE) (2021). Postnatal care. Clinical Guideline (NG194). NICE. London.

National Institute for Health and Care Excellence (NICE) (2022). Urinary tract infections in under 16s: diagnosis and management. Clinical guideline [NG224]. NICE, London.

Nursing and Midwifery Council (NMC) (2018). The Code: Professional standards of practice and behaviour for nurses and midwives and nursing associates. NMC, London.

O'Grady, M. (2011). Renal and reproductive problems. In: Glasper, A., McEwing, G., & Richardson, J. (eds). *Emergencies in Children's and Young People's Nursing.* Oxford: Oxford University Press.

Pateriya, P., & Kanhere, A. (2014). A study of menstrual patterns in adolescent girls. *Journal of Evolution of Medical and Dental Sciences* 3(23), 6345–6351.

Peate, I., & Gormley-Fleming, E. (2025). *Fundamentals of Children's Anatomy and Physiology*, 3rd edn. Wiley, Oxford.

Pitangui, A.C.R., Gomes, M.R.A., Lima, A.S., *et al.* (2013). Menstruation disturbances: prevalence, characteristics, and effects on the activities of daily living among adolescent girls from Brazil. *Journal of Pediatric and Adolescent Gynecology* 26(3), 148–152.

Rogers, A.A., Ha, T., Stormshak, E.A., & Dishion, T.J. (2015). Quality of parent-adolescent conversations about sex and adolescent sexual behaviour: an observational study. *Journal of Adolescent Health* 57(2), 174.

Royal College of Nursing (RCN) (2023). Female Genital Mutilation. An RCN REsource for Nursing and Midwifery Practice, RCN, London.

Salim, F., & Hajar, S. (2018). Pediatric vaginal discharge. *The International Journal of Tropical Veterinary and Biomedical Research* 2(2), 28–33.

Schalet, A. (2011). *Not Under My Roof: Parents, Teens, and the Culture of Sex.* University of Chicago Press, Chicago.

Solomon, D., Gibbs, J., Burns, F., *et al.* (2022). Sexual health inequalities among women aged 16-24. *European Journal of Public Health* 32(Supplement_3), ckac129.158 https://doi.org/10.1093/eurpub/ckac129.158.

Stonewall (2018). *LGBT in Britain, Trans Report.* Retrieved November 12th, 2024, from https://files.stonewall.org.uk/production/files/lgbt_in_britain_-_trans_report_final.pdf?dm=1724230505.

Ummah, T., & Ismarwati (2024). The impact of complementary therapies on dysmenorrhea in young women. *Majalah Obstetri & Ginekologi* 32(1), 29–38.

World Health Organization (WHO) (2025). Female genital mutilation. Fact sheet. WHO, Geneva. Available at: https://www.who.int/news-room/fact-sheets/detail/female-genital-mutilation (accessed April 2025).

CHAPTER 17

Disorders of the musculoskeletal system

Elizabeth Gormley-Fleming

AIM

The aim of this chapter is to enable the readers to develop their understanding and knowledge of the musculoskeletal system. This will include understanding the function and malfunction of the system.

LEARNING OUTCOMES

On completion of this chapter, the reader will be able to:

- Identify the structure of a bone and understand the mechanism of bone healing.
- Describe the key functions of the skeleton.
- Discuss the normal and abnormal pathophysiological changes that occur in the child's musculoskeletal system.
- Be conversant with a number of common disorders of the child's musculoskeletal system.
- Articulate the stages of healing in a bone fracture.
- Care for children with a range of musculoskeletal disorders.

KEYWORDS

- dysplasia
- fracture
- epiphysis
- metaphysis
- diaphysis
- subluxation
- traction
- cartilage
- abduction
- adduction
- rotation

Test your prior knowledge

1. List the bones of the upper extremity.
2. List the bones of the lower extremities.
3. Describe the developments that occur within the bone from birth to adolescence.
4. Describe the six types of bones that are found in the human skeleton.
5. How many bones are there in a baby's skeletal system?
6. Discuss the function of the various types of joints found in the human body.
7. What are the functions of the epiphysis and metaphysis, and where are they located?

Introduction

Musculoskeletal disorders of childhood occur as a result of trauma, infection, malignancies or are congenital in nature. Some may occur for no known reason. Bone disorders can range from those that cause extreme pain and restrict mobility to those that have little effect on the child's life. Musculoskeletal injury is common due to the active nature of children and their associated developmental stage.

The skeleton of the child continues to develop post birth and will do so until adulthood is reached. This series of adaptations is essential to facilitate walking and ossification of the bones. Bone growth occurs from the growth plates. This is a vulnerable area of the bone, so any interference with this process can have lifelong consequences. Hence, an understanding of this is important for the healthcare professional when undertaking a physical assessment of the child who presents with a potential musculoskeletal disorder.

The child's skeleton is more pliable and elastic than that of an adult. The bones have a greater tolerance and permit a greater degree of deformity, so they may simply bend or buckle (torus fracture), making diagnosis challenging.

The periosteal sleeve is greater in diameter than that of an adult, so the child's bone has the ability to remodel; the child's skeleton has the innate ability to heal itself. Remodelling of the bones leads to old bone being removed, which is replaced by new bone. During this process, other bone disorders may occur, which can either improve or remain constant as the child grows. It is these distinguishing features of the child's musculoskeletal system that lead to the distinct musculoskeletal conditions that are unique to childhood.

This chapter provides an outline of a number of musculoskeletal conditions, and the associated care is discussed. For detailed revision of the anatomy of the child's skeleton and muscles, please refer to Chapters 16 and 17 in Peate and Gormley-Fleming (2025).

Fractures

A fracture is a break or discontinuity in the bone. In children, the management and diagnosis of fractures are distinct from those of adults due to the uniqueness of the anatomy of their bones. In children, bones heal more rapidly than those of adults, as bone growth is more rapid. Fractures are very common in children and account for 25% of all childhood injuries, with a fractured radius and ulna being the most common type of injury. Typically, the incidence of fractures between males and females is slightly higher in males, with almost 2% of males sustaining a distal forearm fracture at the age of 13 years (Korup *et al.*, 2022).

Fractures in children usually occur as a result of a traumatic incident and tend to be age-related, for example, toddlers from falls, running into objects or climbing; school-age children – falls from bicycles, skateboards, scooters or motor vehicle accidents, and from climbing; young people – motor vehicle accidents, skateboarding and sports injuries. As the child matures, the incidence of fractures peaks at the 10–16 year age group.

Case study 17.1

Ross is a 9-year-old boy who is normally fit and well. He enjoys school life and has a range of interesting hobbies. He plays ice hockey and is very good at it. During a match, he is pushed over by an older player at high speed and crashes to the floor. He cries very loudly and shouts, 'my leg, my leg'. The first aider arrives. Ross is unable to move his right leg; it is abducted and there is a swelling in the mid-thigh. He is screaming in pain. An ambulance arrives, and Ross, following a full assessment, is given Entonox®, with very good effect. He has his leg placed in a splint for transport to the nearest Children's Emergency Department (CED).

On arrival at the CED, and following assessment, insertion of a cannula and administration of morphine and intravenous fluids, he is X-rayed. A fractured midshaft of the femur is confirmed. He is initially placed in simple traction and transferred to the children's ward while awaiting surgical fixation in theatre the following day. He is refusing to wriggle his toes for you and is complaining of pins and needles in his foot. His foot is pale and cool to touch.

What support do you think Ross will need over the coming weeks?

What support will his family need at the time of injury and surgery?

Vital signs

On admission to CED, Ross's vital signs were recorded. They were:

Vital sign	Observation	Normal value
Temperature	35.7 °C	36.0–37.2 °C
Heart rate	118 beats per minute	80–120 beats per minute
Respiratory rate	28 breaths per minute	20–25 breaths per minute
Blood pressure	96/57 mmHg	90–110 mmHg
Oxygen saturation	97% in air	98–100% in air
Level of consciousness	Alert on AVPU scale	Alert on AVPU scale
Pain score (1–5)	4	1 (no pain)

Ross's PEWS score is 1. Why do you think his temperature was 35.7 °C? His heart rate was 118 beats per minute. What explanation can you give for this? In view of his neurovascular status, how would you use the SBAR tool to escalate your concerns?

Access a PEWS chart here and calculate his PEWS.

https://www.england.nhs.uk/wp-content/uploads/2023/11/pews-observation-and-escalation-chart-5-12-years-updated.pdf

Types of fractures

When a bone fractures, it consists of fragments of bone. These fragments will either lie *distally* (further from the midline) or *proximally* (closer to the midline) to the middle of the bone. If the fragments are separated, it will be a *complete* fracture or an *incomplete* fracture when the fragments remain partially attached.

Fractures are either simple or complicated, open or closed. A complicated fracture will have bone fragments that may damage underlying organs, for example, lungs. An open fracture will have exposed bone visible through a wound in the skin. This is usually a result of high-impact trauma and will necessitate surgical intervention.

If the fracture is across the bone, it is called a *transverse* fracture. An oblique fracture is slanting but straight. A *spiral* fracture is slanting and circular twisting around the shaft of the bone (Fig. 17.1). A spiral fracture may result from physical abuse as a result of twisting a limb and will always warrant further investigation.

A *comminuted* fracture occurs when small fragments of bone from the fractured shaft lie in the surrounding tissues.

A *greenstick* fracture occurs when the bone is angulated beyond its capacity to bend and is an incomplete

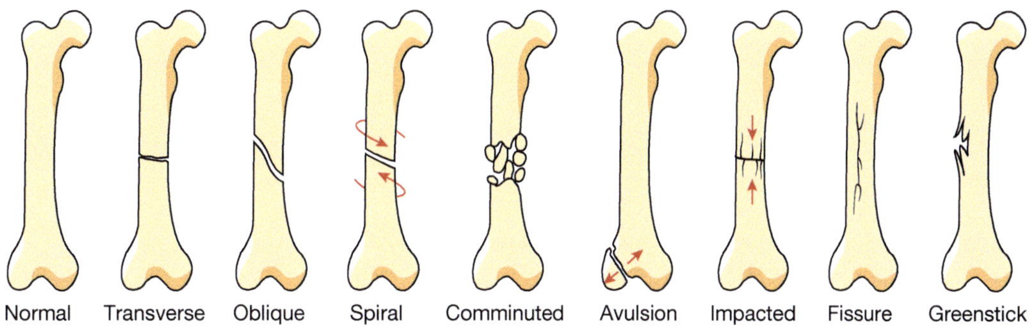

FIGURE 17.1 Fracture types.

fracture. This is common in young children due to the pliability of their bones.

Torus or *buckle* fractures occur when one side of the bone buckles on itself without disrupting the other side. They heal more quickly than greenstick fractures.

An *impacted* fracture occurs when a fragment of bone is firmly driven into the other. This is usually a result of landing feet first from a height.

A *fissure* is a crack on the surface of a bone, but not extending through the bone.

An *avulsion* fracture is the separation of a small segment of bone from the cortex at the insertion site of a ligament or tendon.

Fractures in infancy and early childhood are rare and are usually the result of a fall from a height or from a motor vehicle accident. Bone injury in an infant or young child will always require further investigation. Physical abuse will need to be excluded (NICE, 2017). Detailed radiological imaging will be required.

Osteogenesis imperfecta should be considered a possible diagnosis if multiple fractures are identified. Other associated features, e.g., blue sclera and hearing loss, may also be present.

Features of fractures in children

Table 17.1 outlines the types, causes and features of fractures in children in relation to their location.

Diagnosis of a fracture

In addition to the history taken and systematic assessment, radiological imaging will be required. This is normally an X-ray in the first instance, and in the case of serious trauma, a CT scan will be performed (NICE, 2025, 2022). The signs of a fracture include:

- deformity that is visible or palpable
- swelling at the fracture site
- abnormal movement and impaired function in the affected limb
- tenderness over the fracture site
- crepitus or grating between the bone ends
- bruising around the fracture
- pain on any movement, bending or compression.

Certain age groups and fractures may not necessarily display classic signs and can be missed. The young

TABLE 17.1 Location and features of fractures

Location of fracture	Features
Skull and facial bones	Requires a significant impact to fracture the skull. Types of fractures include: Linear: straight line fracture Depressed: bone is pushed inwards towards the brain (may require surgical involvement) Diastatic: a fracture that has spread to more than one bone of the skull, as they are not yet fused properly Basilar: a fracture in the base of the skull; can lead to spinal cord damage. Facial bone injury is usually a result of high-energy trauma
Wrist and forearm	Common injury in the over-5 age group Usually resulting from a fall on an outstretched arm Midshaft and distal fractures of radius usually; ulna frequently involved Majority are simple transverse fractures requiring immobilisation in a cast or splint for 4–6 weeks
Epiphyseal injuries	Accounts for up to a quarter of all skeletal injuries Radius and ulna are the most frequent sites of injury 10–15-year age group most affected Usually resulting from a fall on an outstretched arm

TABLE 17.1 (*Continued*)

Location of fracture	Features
Clavicle fracture	Shaft of clavicle usually affected Common injuries from falls and sport injury as a result of excessive compression to the shoulder Treatment is supportive in the form of analgesia and application of a sling to immobilise Reduction is required in extreme cases of displacement only Can occur during the birth process if baby is large and mother has small pelvis
Humerus	Supracondylar fractures are the most common, usually as a result of impact to the elbow from a fall; can lead to significant vascular injury and compromise 10% of humeral fractures occur at the shaft – in the infant and young child, this may be as a result of twisting, so it requires detailed investigation. In the older child, it may be as a result of direct trauma The mechanism of injury in fractures of the humerus is usually a fall onto an outstretched hand Proximal humeral fractures are rare, with distal humeral fractures involving the lateral epicondyle more than the medial Treatment will depend on the injury, with supracondylar fractures usually requiring open reduction
Rib cage	Rare but could occur as a result of high-energy impact or direct physical trauma (physical abuse)
Spinal fractures	Rare in childhood Resulting from significant trauma: fall from a height, motor vehicle accidents, diving, and sports injury Cervical spine most likely to be injured
Pelvis	Rare but associated with crush injury (horse-riding fall) and motor vehicle accidents Expect damage to associated organs: bladder, bowel and blood supply
Hip	Rare but may occur as a result of motor vehicle accidents or a fall from a height Can lead to avascular necrosis of the femoral head and damage to the growth plates
Femur	Common site of injury in young children. Peaks at 2–3 years of age. Usually femoral shaft involved. Motor vehicle accident or fall from a significant height is the usual cause. Management will depend on the age of the child and the type of injury and fracture
Patella	Rare but may occur as a result of high-energy trauma May be a single crack or multiple cracks, which is called a 'stellar' fracture More common in males than females
Tibia and fibula	Most common lower extremity fracture is midshaft of tibia and fibula Majority are non-displaced and will be managed in a cast and non-weight-bearing Tibia fractures in preschool children are commonly as a result of a rotating mechanism injury to the lower limb
Ankle	Young people are most likely to fracture ankles Growth plate involved in 1 of every 6 fractures Males more likely to fracture ankles Direct trauma (sport) is the most common cause
Foot	Metatarsals account for 50% of fractures of the foot. Most are non-displaced Mechanism of injury is as a result of direct and indirect trauma, falls and jumping from a height and twisting injuries

Source: Nettina (2018)/Wolters Kluwer Health.

child may not be able to communicate their injury, so signs of injury need to be considered, for example, refusal to use a limb. In cases of physical abuse, the parents/carers may not volunteer information or may give false information in relation to the presenting signs and symptoms. Equally, the older child may not identify the exact mechanism of injury if risk-taking behaviour has been involved.

An undisplaced fracture may have no evidence of a deformity; a fracture within a capsule may not have any sign of bruising. Some fractures, such as those of the radial head and scaphoid, are difficult to diagnose, so MRI should be performed if there is any doubt, as they are often associated with poor long-term outcomes (NICE, 2025). Non-verbal children will be unable to report pain, so changes in behaviour should not be ignored. Untreated fractures can lead to life-changing consequences.

Pathophysiology of a fracture

A bone fractures when a force is applied to it, and the bone is unable to absorb the force. Once the fracture has occurred, the muscles immediately contract in an attempt to splint the injured area (Hockenberry & Wilson, 2024). A result of this is deformity of the bone produced secondary to the muscles pulling the bone out of place. Bleeding occurs at the site of injury, resulting in haematoma formation, which is essential to healing.

Healing occurs in three or four distinct but overlapping stages (Fig. 17.2):

1. Early inflammatory stage
2. Repair stage (fibrous)
3. Bony callus formation
4. Remodelling stage.

Early inflammatory stage

In the inflammatory stage, a haematoma develops from the fracture site in the immediate aftermath of the fracture. Macrophages, monocytes, lymphocytes, polymorphonuclear cells and fibroblasts infiltrate the bone under prostaglandin mediation (Waters *et al.*, 2025). Granulation tissue forms and mesenchymal cells arrive at the injured site. Nutrients and oxygen supply are provided by the exposed cancellous bone and muscle.

Repair stage (Fig. 17.2)

Vascular ingrowth is supported by the presence of fibroblasts. A collagen matrix is laid down, and osteoid is secreted and mineralised with calcium salts, which leads to the formation of a very soft callus around the fracture. On X-ray, this has a cloud-like appearance. The callus is very weak and needs to be protected during this stage, which usually takes 4–6 weeks by internal fixation,

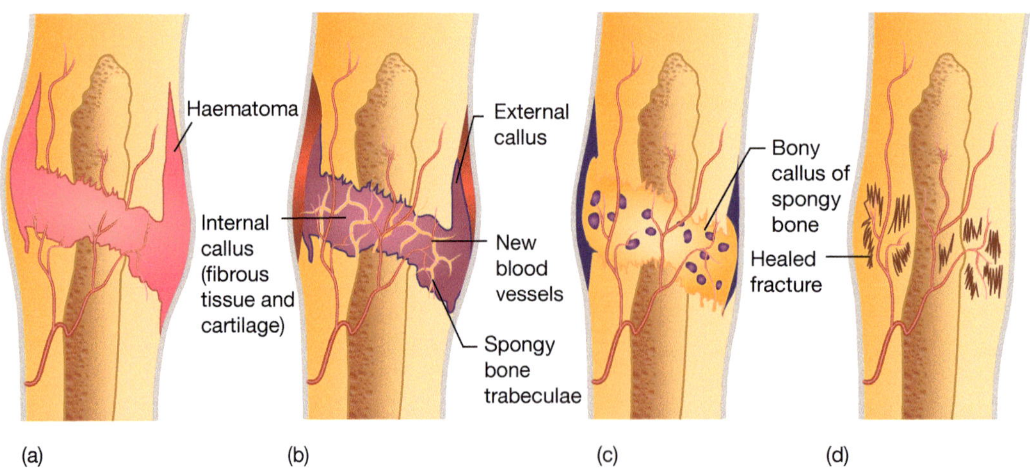

FIGURE 17.2 Stages in bone healing. (a) Haematoma formation. (b) Fibrocartilaginous callus formation. (c) Bony callus formation. (d) Bone remodelling.

traction or a cast. Failure to protect the newly formed callus could result in unstable fibrous union, leading to deformity. The callus then ossifies and a bridge of woven bone is formed between the ends of the fracture fragments.

Remodelling

Remodelling is when the fractured bone has healed to its original shape, structure and strength (Waters *et al.*, 2025). This is a slow process and takes place over a period of months to years. The amount of stress placed on the bone during this phase is important in remodelling. Bone is laid down where it is required as the fracture site is exposed to the axial loading force. Adequate strength is normally achieved within 3–6 months.

Traction

The use of traction has somewhat gone into demise as technology has evolved to produce fixation devices that allow partial or full mobility. Surgical interventions are now used more frequently, further reducing the length of time and use of traction, although outcomes have been shown to be no different in terms of mobility (Wang & Su, 2023 & Wright, 2023). Therefore, it is important that the healthcare professional understands the principles of traction to be able to provide appropriate care for children who may still be required to be immobilised by this method. It is often used in the early stages of fracture management to realign the bones, thus preventing loss of blood flow, damage to the nerves and pain reduction.

Traction means to pull, and in order to be effective, there must be a counter-traction (pull in the opposite direction) (Fig. 17.3).

The general purpose of traction is to provide rest to a limb, treat a dislocation or correct a deformity, immobilise a specific area of the body or promote alignment either pre- or post-operatively.

Traction can be applied to the upper extremities, lower extremities or to the cervical area (Table 17.2). It can be applied manually by hand, directly to the skin surface via adhesive bandages, or to the skeleton by wire, pins or tongs inserted through the diameter of the bone (Royal College of Nursing, 2021).

The care of a child in traction includes:

- Checking the traction system daily to ensure weights are hanging freely, cords and knots are intact, pulleys are working effectively, that counter-traction is being maintained, and the end of the bed is elevated.
- Outer bandages should be removed at least daily; limb inspected, washed and dried; and outer bandage reapplied.

TABLE 17.2 **Types of traction and examples of each**

Traction	Type
Upper extremity	Overhead/halter neck Dunlop traction
Lower extremity	Gallows/Bryant Bucks or Pugh's Thomas splint Russell 90/90 Balanced Skeletal (Denham or Steinmann pin)
Cervical	Halo brace Halo vest Crutchfield tongs

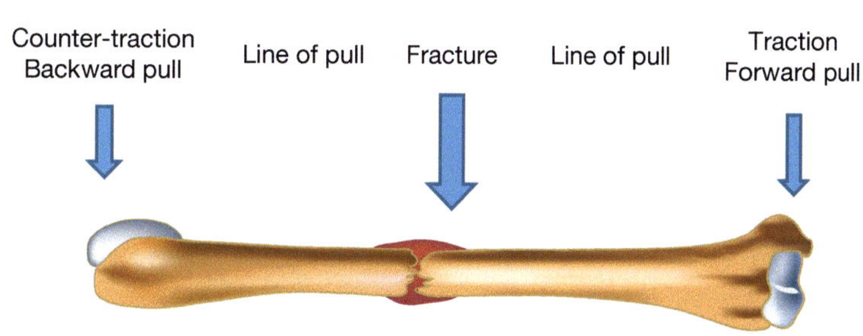

FIGURE 17.3 Application of traction to maintain bone alignment.

- Neurovascular status should be assessed and documented.
- Pressure area care administered.
- Passive and active exercises performed along with breathing exercises, e.g., blowing bubbles, a balloon, to prevent chest infections.
- General physical and personal care needs will be delivered in conjunction with parental/carer involvement.
- Relief of boredom is also an important aspect of care, as is maintaining educational needs.

External fixation

If a fracture cannot be reduced and managed by traction or the application of a cast, then external fixation may be used. This is now common when there is associated soft tissue involvement and bone loss. The external fixator holds the bone in alignment as the bone and bone fragments are held in place by metal pins, which are attached to an external metal frame. This frame can be in situ for a number of months, thus restricting mobility and activity. An important aspect of caring for a child with an external fixator in place is to ensure their neurovascular status is intact and that the pin sites are inspected and cleaned as per local policy. Early detection of pin-site infection will need prompt treatment. Management of pain is essential, as is the provision of psychological care, as acceptance of the external frame and the altered body image associated with this may take some time for the child and family.

Pharmacology

The use of non-steroidal anti-inflammatory drugs (NSAIDs) is a much-debated topic. NSAIDs are very good for pain relief, reduce swelling and inflammation and have less side effects than opioids. They are thought to impede healing, and the evidence has shown that their use for more than three days in high doses can delay union and therefore increase the rate of non-union in children over 11 years of age, but they do not appear to delay fracture healing in children younger than 11 years of age (Mullen *et al.*, 2022). Rates of non-union are rare, and other evidence purports that the benefits of NSAIDs outweigh the evidence on non-union (Briggs, 2023).

Distraction

Distraction is the process of separating opposing bone to encourage regeneration of new bone. Distraction osteogenesis is used to treat non-union of fractures, for limb lengthening and malalignment. The bone is surgically 'broken', K wires are inserted proximally and distally to the fracture. Manual distraction is achieved by adjusting the telescopic rods on the rings to increase the distance between the rings. A percutaneous ostomy is performed to create a false growth plate at the same time. Histogenesis of muscle, nerves and skin occurs simultaneously with the development of the new bone (Guan *et al.*, 2024). The Ilizarov frame (Fig. 17.4) has been used since the 1960s, and its use has been extended to manage acute trauma to the limb where skin integrity has been reduced.

Scrupulous pin care is essential, and the child and family will often assume responsibility for this once the child has recovered post-operatively. There are inherent risks for the child who has an external fixation device. These include pin site infection, increased length of hospital stays, pain and delays in fracture healing. The child/young person and their family will need to be taught to recognise signs of infection (Campbell & Watt, 2020; Walker *et al.*, 2018) and for loosening of the pins. The child and family will also learn how to adjust the frame to achieve distraction. The child will be able to mobilise partially weight-bearing on crutches. As the Ilizarov frame will

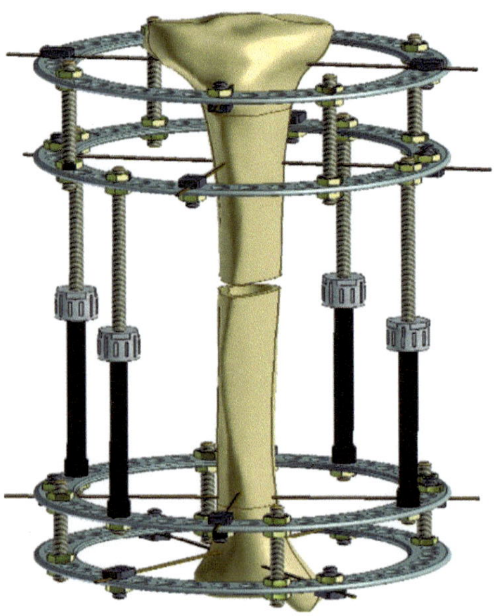

FIGURE 17.4 Ilizarov frame.

be in situ for months, the child will need support to return to their normal activities of living. Significant support is often required as the device is obvious; thus, body image and self-esteem are challenged. The Ilizarov frame is removed under general anaesthetic, and the child will need to carry on using crutches post removal for up to 4–6 weeks.

Care and management

A systematic and holistic assessment is required, and initial interventions are directed at assessing and managing airway, breathing, circulation, disability and exposure prior to dealing with the fracture (NICE, 2022, 2025). Once the child is stable, the fracture can be assessed.

The extent of the injury may be assessed using the 5 Ps to identify vascular compromise. These are:

- **P**ain – administer analgesia
- **P**ulse – palpate pulses distal to the fracture
- **P**allor – the limb
- **P**araesthesia – sensation distal to the fracture site
- **P**aralysis – movement distal to the fracture site.

Neurovascular status should be rechecked on a frequent basis.

The principles of management are the same for all fractures:

- Reduction – to restore normal alignment
- Immobilisation – to promote healing of the bone
- Rehabilitation – to normal function or to assist with impaired mobility.

Any alteration to the neurovascular status of a limb must be escalated, and prompt medical attention must be sought.

Open wounds should be covered with a sterile dressing initially. It is likely that open wounds will require surgical intervention. Antibiotics will need to be administered to prevent infection and the development of osteomyelitis.

Avoid moving the affected limb if possible, particularly if it has not been splinted. Soft splints, such as folded towels, may be used until a more definitive splint is applied. The child may require sedation prior to the application of any splinting device and will need continuous cardiovascular monitoring during this procedure.

The child and family are likely to be very anxious and traumatised by the events that have brought them to the hospital, and they will need reassurance and an explanation of the plan of care. Once the plan of care is established, it is likely that parental involvement will be significant in relation to personal care, play and passive exercises of the limbs. Education in the use of mobility aids will be required, as will preparation for discharge.

Growth and development

Musculoskeletal disorders in children can impact their growth and development. Muscle atrophy, loss of muscle strength, and changes in bone density are all recognised consequences even after relatively short periods of time. In addition, the critically unwell child who requires periods of sustained hospitalisation is also at risk of muscle atrophy in addition to other systemic impacts. It has been shown that children in intensive care have a decrease of > 10% of their muscle mass after a short period of time (Tume *et al.*, 2024).

To maintain muscle mass, there needs to be a balance between muscle protein synthesis and muscle protein breakdown and any imbalance in this will result in either muscle gain or muscle loss. Muscle protein synthesis is suppressed in the presence of immobilisation, so even after a short duration of immobilisation, muscle wasting will occur (Crossland *et al.*, 2019). There is a reduction in muscle fibre size and an accelerated reduction in type II, fast-twitching muscle fibres compared to type I, slow-twitching.

Children and young people who have an upper limb immobilised in a cast have been shown to have reduced physical activity and are at risk of increasing their body mass, as there is often no corresponding decrease in dietary intake (Maggio *et al.*, 2018). An increase in physical activity should be encouraged in the short term to compensate for their energy intake.

For healthy bone development and growth, movement is an essential activity. Changes to the mechanical load during periods of immobilisation lead to greater absorption of bone rather than bone formation. The net result of this is demineralisation, impacting mostly on trabecular bone.

Changes to the muscles occur more rapidly than changes to the skeletal integrity. When planning nursing care, active and passive exercises incorporated into daily care plans, along with the use of appropriate assistive technologies, need to be a primary consideration to maintain muscle strength and joint mobility.

Limping in childhood

There are a number of conditions that present with a limping child. Limps can be classed as either painful or painless (Lissauer & Carroll, 2021) and are generally categorised according to age (NICE, 2020). While most limps are usually not serious, the cause of the limp will need to be investigated to rule out serious disease. Limps can present at any stage in childhood from age 1 year up to adulthood, and Table 17.3 outlines some of the causes.

The following signs all require urgent assessment by a paediatrician: Children with a temperature >38.5 °C, unable to weight bear, night pain, weight loss, > 3 day history, or unexplained or patterned bruising. Pain with passive movement.

TABLE 17.3 **Some causes of limp in childhood**

Age	Painful limp	Painless limp
1–3 years of age	Trauma, both accidental and non-accidental Osteomyelitis Septic arthritis Transient synovitis	Developmental dysplasia of the hip Neuromuscular defects, e.g., cerebral palsy Juvenile idiopathic arthritis
3–10 years	Trauma, both accidental and non-accidental Osteomyelitis Septic arthritis Transient synovitis Perthes disease Malignant disease Juvenile idiopathic arthritis	Juvenile idiopathic arthritis Developmental dysplasia of the hip Neuromuscular defects – Duchenne's muscular dystrophy
11–18 years	Slipped capital femoral Epiphysis Trauma Juvenile idiopathic arthritis Osteomyelitis Septic arthritis Bone tumours	Juvenile idiopathic arthritis Slipped capital femoral epiphysis Dysplastic hip Neuromuscular defects, e.g., cerebral palsy

Transient synovitis

Commonly known as irritable hip, the onset of transient synovitis typically follows a viral infection and peaks in the 5–6 years age group and is less common in the under 3 years of age group. It is more common in boys than in girls. There is no systemic involvement, and there is no pain when resting. Pain is only present on passive movements at the extreme range of movement, so hip abduction, flexion and rotation. Usually, this is self-limiting.

A child who has a normal temperature, is limping but mobile and does not have any other symptoms is likely to have transient synovitis, which can be managed with oral analgesia and, as a safety net, reviewed in 48–72 hours or sooner if indicated.

Slipped upper femoral epiphysis

Slipped upper femoral epiphysis (SUFE) is a relatively common disorder of the child or young person's hip, but it is a condition where correct diagnosis and immediate treatment are critical if bone integrity is to be maintained (NICE, 2020). There is displacement of the epiphysis of the femoral head postero-inferiorly (Fig. 17.5) (Lissauer & Carroll, 2021). The metaphysis also slips downwards and backwards.

Occurrence is more common in boys than in girls, usually between 10 and 16 years of age. A downward trend in the age of occurrence has been reported, and the suggested rationale for this is the phenomenon of children maturing at a younger age (Tucker *et al.*, 2019). The risk of SUFE is increased in children who are obese. Children with Down syndrome, adiposogenital syndrome, hypothyroidism, pituitary tumours and decreased growth hormone levels are also more predisposed to developing SCFE.

One hip or both may be involved, with 20% of children having bilateral involvement. Of the children who present with one-sided SUFE initially, 20–30% will develop a contralateral SCFE within 12–18 months (Nettina, 2018).

The child may present with hip pain; mid-thigh pain; knee pain; a sudden, insidious onset of a limp; and a decreased range of motion in the hip.

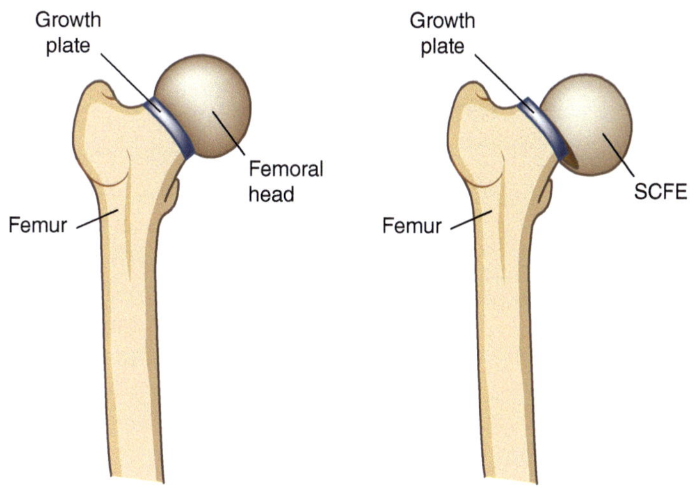

FIGURE 17.5 Normal femur and femur with slipped capital femoral epiphysis.

The goal of treatment is to prevent complications, e.g., avascular necrosis and necrosis of cartilage. Accurate diagnosis is paramount, and prompt treatment is essential. Delay in diagnosis and treatment can have life-changing effects.

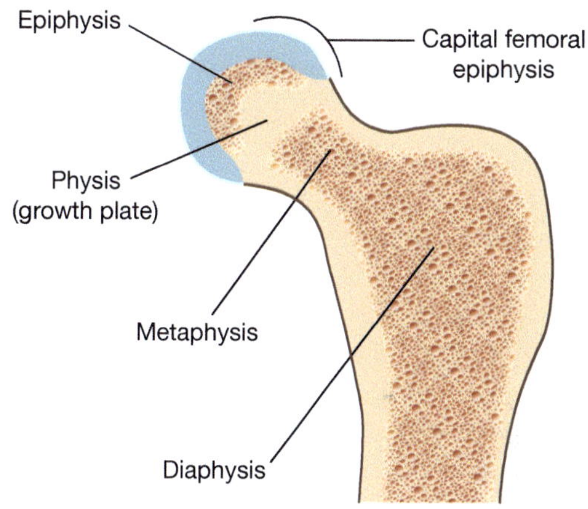

FIGURE 17.6 Growth plates of the femur.

Pathophysiology

The exact aetiology is unknown, but it is thought that there are predisposing risk factors such as inactivity, periods of rapid growth spurts and overweight.

The epiphyseal growth plate widens unusually, and there is a zone of hypertrophy. In addition to this, there is abnormal cartilage maturation, endochondral ossification and instability of the perichondral ring. This leads to inadequate organisation of the cartilage columns. Slippage then occurs through this weakened area. During adolescence, the proximal physis changes from horizontal to oblique. This redirects the forces felt through the hip from compression to shear (Chatterton & James, 2024). In children who present with SUFE, a disorganisation of collagen fibrils and an accumulation of glycoproteins within the growth plates have been identified, but the exact role of this is unknown.

The femoral neck slips off the proximal femoral epiphysis, and it remains contained within the acetabulum. This is one of the few joints in the body where the epiphysis is within the joint capsule (Fig. 17.6). This is referred to as a Salter–Harris-type physeal fracture.

Classification

SUFE is classified by the duration of the symptoms. There are three elements to this:

1. Acute-sudden onset and symptoms have been present for less than 3 weeks.
2. Chronic – symptoms lasting 3 weeks or more with changes.
3. Sudden acute exacerbation of symptoms.

It is essential to determine if the child can bear weight with a stable hip or will be non-weight bearing with an unstable hip.

Classification identifies the percentage of displacement of the hip in relation to the neck of femur and radiological interpretation (Chatterton & James, 2024) (Table 17.4).

TABLE 17.4 Radiological classification of SUFE

Classification	% displacement
Type I	Less than 33% displacement
Type II	33–50% displacement
Type III	> 50% displacement

Diagnosis

Definitive diagnosis is confirmed by radiological evaluation, X-ray, CT scan, MRI and bone scan if avascular necrosis is suspected. A full physical examination of the child is required, including examination of the hip joint (Jani & McKay, 2024). There must be no passive manipulation of the hip until a diagnosis has been established.

Care and management

A detailed nursing assessment should be carried out, including the onset of symptoms along with the characteristics and location of pain. Hip movement and associated restrictions should be noted.

Control of pain is an essential aspect of nursing care. An age-appropriate pain assessment tool should be used, and analgesia administered as prescribed, with effectiveness monitored. This is a requirement in the pre- and post-operative period.

Immobilisation through bed rest will be required, and activity will be restricted as directed. This may include the application of skin traction. The provision of mobility aids, e.g., crutches or a wheelchair, should be considered.

The child and family should be prepared for surgery in accordance with local policy. Post-operative care will be determined by the procedure carried out.

Support for the child and family in following any pre- and post-operative restrictions is required in order to prevent lasting damage to the femur and hip joint (Nettina, 2018). Assistance with mobilisation will be needed, so early introduction to the physiotherapy team is recommended.

The management options for SUFE will be dependent on the severity of the slip. Surgical intervention will be required. Fixation permits early stabilisation of the slippage, preventing further slippage and amelioration of potential risks (Chatterton & James, 2024). For mild to moderate slips, percutaneous fixation is required, and there may be prophylactic pinning of the contralateral hip using either Kirschner wires or cannulated screws (NICE, 2015).

In severe cases, open fixation of the growth plate with a bone graft is required. The aim of this procedure is to relocate the capital femoral epiphysis to its central position in the acetabulum and preserve the blood supply to the epiphysis, thus reducing the risk of avascular necrosis. This may involve surgical dislocation of the hip, removal of bone from the metaphysis of the femoral neck, adduction and rotation of the limb or realignment of the epiphysis to its normal position within the acetabulum, which is kept in situ with cannulated screws or Kirschner wires.

Perthes disease

This is a self-limiting condition of the proximal femur characterised by interruption of the blood supply to the capital femoral epiphysis. This results in avascular necrosis. This loss of blood supply is temporary, and revascularisation and re-ossification occur over a period of 24–48 months (Beni *et al.*, 2025; Lissauer & Carroll, 2021).

Boys are five times more likely to be affected than girls, and it is more common in the 5–10-year age group. Ten to 20% of cases are bilateral. The exact aetiology of Perthes disease remains unknown, but early recognition and treatment are essential in preserving the femoral head deformation. There is a strong association between the disease and socio-economic deprivation; the north-west of England has nearly double the number of incidences compared to the southwest of England (Galloway *et al.*, 2024).

Pathophysiology

While the aetiology is unknown, it is known that there is an interruption to the vascular supply to the femoral head, leading to necrosis. Perthes disease has four identified stages:

- Stage 1 Avascularity
- Stage 2 Revascularisation
- Stage 3 Reossification
- Stage 4 Healing

Stage 1: Avascularity

Vascular occlusion is triggered spontaneously, and the capital femoral epiphysis is deprived of blood. This results in the osteoblasts in the epiphysis dying and a

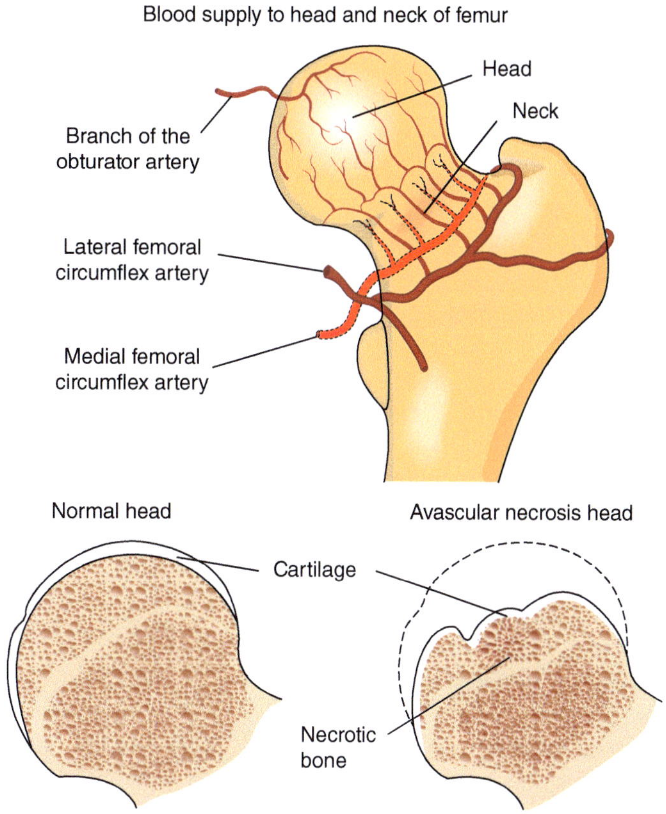

FIGURE 17.7 Avascularity of the femoral head.

cessation in bone growth, resulting in widening of the joint space. Synovitis, hypertrophy of the articular cartilage and hypertrophy of the ligamentum teres occur (Joseph *et al.* 2023). The soft tissue changes and muscle spasm result in the femoral head extruding from the acetabulum laterally. Weight bearing causes stress and further muscle contractions within the hip joint and onto the extruded part of the avascular femoral head. This results in the trabeculae collapsing, leading to an irreversible deformity of the femoral head (Joseph *et al.*, 2023) (Fig. 17.7). The greater the degree of extrusion of the femoral head, the greater the propensity for deformation. This stage may last for weeks to several months. The child may show signs of the disease at this stage by walking with a limp or altered gait.

Stage 2: Revascularisation

This stage may also be referred to as fragmentation. The X-ray appearance of the femoral head will show a flattened femoral head. Necrotic bone is reabsorbed and replaced with woven bone initially. The head of the femur is particularly vulnerable during this stage, as it is lacking in strength and is prone to pathological fractures. Any abnormal force to the weakened epiphysis can lead to progressive deformities (Nettina, 2018). If more than 20% of the width of the epiphysis extrudes outside the acetabulum, damage is likely to be irreversible (Joseph *et al.*, 2023). This stage may last for 1–2 years.

Stage 3: Reossification

The head of the femur gradually begins to reshape as new, stronger bone develops. The nucleus of the epiphysis breaks up into tiny fragments. New bone develops at the medial and lateral aspects of the epiphysis. All of the necrotic bone is now replaced, and this stage, the longest, lasts 2–4 years.

Stage 4: Healing

Bone regrowth is complete, and the femoral head will have reached its final shape. The reshaped femoral head may or may not resemble the desired spherical shape. This is dependent on a number of factors:

- extent of damage that occurred during the fragmentation stage;
- age of the child at the onset of the disease;
- instigation of treatment.

Treatment that is instigated after fragmentation or in the latter stages of fragmentation is likely to prevent further damage to the femoral head and is said to be remedial in nature (Joseph *et al.*, 2023).

Diagnosis

The child is likely to present with a history of limp or pain in their hip. This may have been present for a period of time and may worsen with activity. There may be referred pain in their knee, thigh or groin. On examination, the child will have limited abduction (Fig. 17.8) in the affected hip, and it will be internally rotated.

On examination of the hip joint, the child is likely to develop muscle spasm on internal rotation. Trendelenburg gait will be evident; when the child is weight-bearing on the affected limb, there will be a dip on the opposite side of the pelvis (Fig. 17.9).

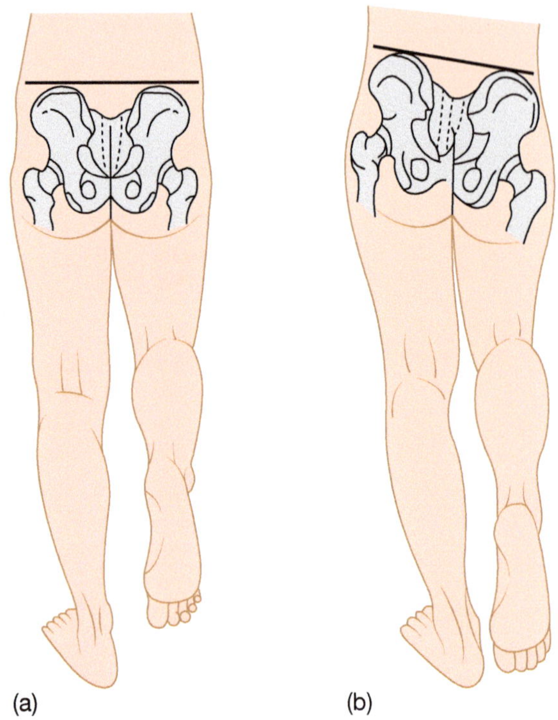

FIGURE 17.9 Trendelenburg gait. (a) Normal hip joints. (b) There is a dip on the opposite of the pelvis when weight bearing on the affected side.

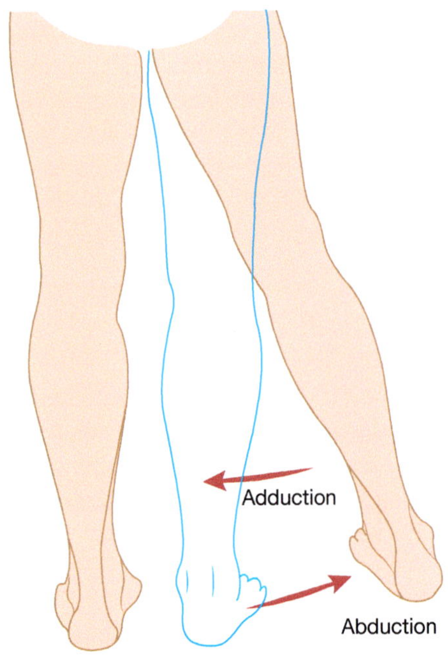

FIGURE 17.8 Abduction of the lower limb.

Investigations

An X-ray will be required following a full physical examination. The child with Perthes disease will need several X-rays during the course of treatment, which can last 2 years or longer. The X-ray required of the hip joint will be an anteroposterior view and a frog-leg lateral. It will identify the extent of epiphyseal involvement and its condition, and will enable the doctor to identify the stage of the disease. It is important to note that as the condition progresses, the X-rays of the hip joint may look worse before any improvement is seen. An early X-ray may not show any abnormality. The young child with Perthes disease who is being managed through observation will require an X-ray every 3–4 months to monitor the progress of the disease.

Magnetic resonance imaging (MRI) has limited use in the detection of infraction of the bone and is less beneficial in identifying the stages of healing.

Bone scanning may be required to confirm the diagnosis if the X-ray is questionable. Ultrasound may be useful if joint effusion is suspected in the early stages.

Care and treatment

The goal of treatment with Perthes disease is to relieve pain, protect the shape of the femoral head by containment and restore normal hip movement. Containment of the femoral epiphysis well into the acetabulum in order to protect the epiphysis is the desired outcome of any intervention (Perry *et al.*, 2022; Joseph *et al.*, 2023). Treatment early in the disease process is key to a positive outcome. If left untreated, the femoral head will be deformed and inadequately positioned with the acetabulum, leading to the likelihood of the early onset of arthritis. The child and family need to be aware that the treatment is long-term.

There are many treatment options for Perthes disease, and the plan of treatment will be dependent on the following factors:

- Age of child at the onset of the disease – younger children have greater potential for developing new bone;
- The degree of damage to the femoral head. If more than 50% of the femoral head has been affected by avascular necrosis, the prospect for bone regrowth and special shaping of the femoral head is diminished;
- The range of motion of the hip joint;
- The stage at which the disease is diagnosed. Ideally, this needs to be achieved early in stage 1.

Treatment is either non-surgical or surgical.

Non-surgical treatment will involve

- Observation entailing regular monitoring on an outpatient basis with X-ray of the hip. This will continue while the condition is stable and until the head of the femur has completely healed.
- Reduction of activity, such as running, jumping or any activity that has a high impact on the hip joint. This may include periods of bed rest and skin traction if the femoral head is not in a satisfactory position or if there is loss of function of the joint and muscle spasm. Braces and a cast may also be used to restrict movement. Parental involvement in the care of the child will be required, as one of the challenges with caring for the child with Perthes disease is that they are well and active, but need to have their activity restricted.
- Analgesia, NSAID medication to reduce inflammation of the hip joint.
- Physical therapy to restore the range of movement in the hip joint. This may include hip abduction and exercises to promote internal rotation of the hip joint and hydrotherapy.

Surgical treatment will be required to re-establish the alignment of the femoral head in the acetabulum and thus the function of the hip joint. It may be required if non-surgical interventions have been unsuccessful or the child meets the criteria set out earlier. It includes:

- **Soft tissue release:** This will improve movement within the hip joint as the tight muscles within the groin are released.
- **Shelf acetabuloplasty:** For example, a bone graft is used to enlarge the acetabulum so the femoral head will fit more securely into the newly formed acetabulum.
- **Pelvic osteotomy:** The acetabulum is reoriented, so it covers the anterolateral aspect of the femoral epiphysis.
- **Femoral osteotomy:** The head of the femur is repositioned in the acetabulum by cutting through the femur. The alignment is secured with a plate and screws until after the healing stage of the disease has occurred.

Post-surgery (osteotomy), the child is usually placed in a cast to protect the alignment for 6–8 weeks. In the initial post-operative period, opioid analgesia will be required, so close monitoring of the child's condition is necessary. Blood transfusion may be required (Hockenberry & Wilson, 2024).

Healthcare professionals need to be aware that some children may not be able to take non-steroidal anti-inflammatory medication (NSAIDs). Examples of these are: ibuprofen, naproxen, indomethacin and diclofenac acid. As an effective analgesic in musculoskeletal disorders, the lowest dose of NSAID should be used (BNFC, 2025). NSAIDs have both analgesic and anti-inflammatory effects. The relief of pain is usually within a short time frame once the NSAID has been consumed, but the anti-inflammatory effect may not be achieved for up to 3 weeks. This can be longer in some conditions, e.g., juvenile idiopathic arthritis.

NSAIDs reduce the production of prostaglandins, which inhibit the enzyme cyclo-oxygenase. There are different types of cyclo-oxygenase, and inhibition of cyclo-oxygenase 2 will reduce gastrointestinal intolerance. Gastrointestinal symptoms are unusual with short-term use of NSAIDs (BNFC, 2025).

NSAIDs should be used with caution in children with asthma, angioedema, urticaria, rhinitis and allergic disorders. For children with renal, cardiac or hepatic impairment, caution is required when prescribing NSAIDs.

NSAIDs are contraindicated in children with severe heart failure and gastric ulceration. However, children do appear to tolerate NSAIDs better than adults and gastrointestinal side effects are less commonly reported.

While there is no consensus on treatment for Perthes disease, treatment should aim to prevent the deformation of the femoral head in order to minimise the risk of secondary arthritis, which might necessitate hip replacement at a later stage. Activity should be encouraged, and a multidisciplinary approach to caring for the child and family is required, as implications on education and wellbeing can be significant.

Developmental dysplasia of the hip

Developmental dysplasia of the hip (DDH) is a spectrum of disorders relating to abnormal development of the hip. These can range from dysplasia to subluxation to complete dislocation of the hip (Table 17.5). The incidence of DDH in the United Kingdom is 0.5–1 in 1000 newborns having a unilateral, irreducible hip dislocation (Nicholson *et al.*, 2023). DDH is more common in girls and in the left hip (Paton, 2017). Bilateral involvement is evident in 50% of cases, and it is more common in Caucasians (Nettina, 2018).

Neonatal screening identifies the majority of babies with DDH, but not all, as it may not be possible to detect if the acetabulum is only mildly shallow. In the United Kingdom, all infants should be screened within 72 hours of birth (National Health Service England [NHSE], 2025, NICE, 2021a, 2021b). The rapid referral to ultrasound has led to speedy and accurate diagnosis in the neonatal period. Not all dysplastic or unstable hips will require treatment.

TABLE 17.5 Key terms associated with DDH

Instability: a diagnosis made on examination where passive manipulation caused the hip to subluxate or dislocate.
Subluxation: partial dislocation of the femoral head from the acetabulum. There is incomplete contact between articular surfaces of the femoral head and acetabulum. Usually diagnosed by ultrasound.
Dysplasia: an abnormality of the development of the acetabulum. This usually results in a shallow and dysmorphic acetabulum.
Dislocation: complete loss of contact between the articular surfaces of the femoral head and acetabulum.

A number of risk factors are known, and these include:

- breech birth
- first born
- large baby
- oligohydramnios
- positive family history of DDH
- intrauterine malposition that leads to other musculoskeletal disorders, e.g., tortocolis, metatarsus adductus
- cultural swaddling of babies where legs are adducted
- underlying neuromuscular disorders.

Diagnosis

Neonatal screening for DDH will detect the majority of cases, but not all. Both the Ortholani and Barlow tests should be performed (NHSE, 2025). Diagnosis in the older infant and child can be challenging, as the disorder can be advanced by the time the condition is suspected (Nicholas *et al.*, 2023). Unilateral DDH is more likely to be detected early, as asymmetry of the lower limb will be more obvious and likely to concern the parents/carers. Other signs that may be apparent in the older infant and child are:

- limited abduction
- limb length discrepancy
- asymmetries of the thigh skin folds
- asymmetry of buttocks
- unequal knee heights (Galeazzi sign)
- crawls with difficulty
- delayed walking
- difficulty sitting astride an adult's legs or a bicycle
- stands or walks with external rotation
- trunk tilts towards the affected hip when walking (Trendelenburg gait)
- limp evident if able to walk, or a waddling gait (Bi-lateral DDH).

Radiological diagnosis with ultrasound is the recommended imaging modality to diagnose and to monitor possible DDH if there is uncertainty about the position of the femoral head in relation to the acetabulum.

Care and treatment

The primary aim of treatment is to achieve reduction of the hip, which will increase the chances of having a functioning hip joint and therefore a normal range of movement.

Early diagnosis is likely to, but may not, necessarily avoid the need for surgical intervention.

Splinting is usually the initial treatment modality, and the infant will be placed in a Craig splint or Pavlik harness (Fig. 17.10). If hip reduction can be maintained, the acetabulum appears to be able to develop around the head of the femur. This results in improved stability of the hip and associated dysplasia (Paton, 2017). The splint may be in situ for a number of months. The position of the infant in the splint is important as the blood supply to the femoral head is easily compromised and could lead to avascular necrosis or deformity of the femoral head. The straps of the harness prevent the hips from abducting beyond the midline, and flexion is maintained between 90° and 100°. Close monitoring will be required, and the infant will need to have an ultrasound to monitor their progress and for the development of complications. For hips that are severely subluxed and not reducible, the infant will require weekly ultrasound scanning while the splint is in situ. The infant with a dysplasia of the hips will normally have an ultrasound every 3 weeks.

If the child's hip is not responding to treatment with a Pavlik harness, the Ifeld abduction orthosis may be used (Nicholson *et al.*, 2023). This is a more rigid form of hip abduction and has demonstrated comparable success rates with that of closed reduction and the application of a hip spica (Sanker *et al.*, 2015).

If diagnosis is delayed and the hip is unstable, a hip spica (Fig. 17.11) following closed reduction may be used (Lissauer & Carroll, 2021). The child may have a period of traction prior to this. The hip spica places the hip in a secure position, promoting good blood flow, thus avoiding the risk of avascular necrosis. An arthrogram and/or abductor tenotomy will often be performed at this stage, giving a more detailed picture of the hip. The hip spica will be in situ for 3 months, but it will be changed under general anaesthetic at 6-weekly intervals to examine the hip because the child will be growing, and the hip spica is likely to be soiled. Parental education and support will be needed to enable them to meet their child's care needs while h/she is in the hip spica.

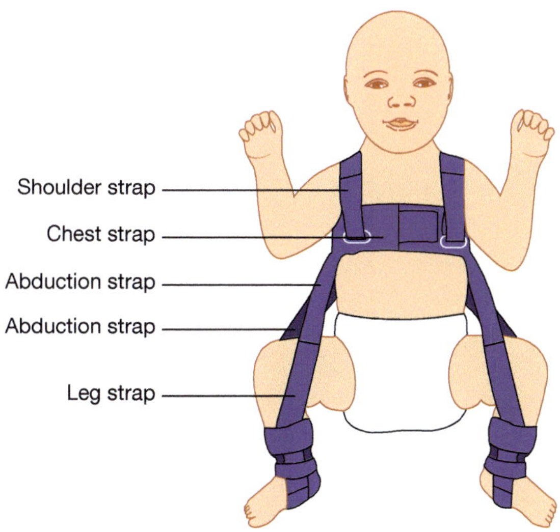

FIGURE 17.10 Pavlik harness.

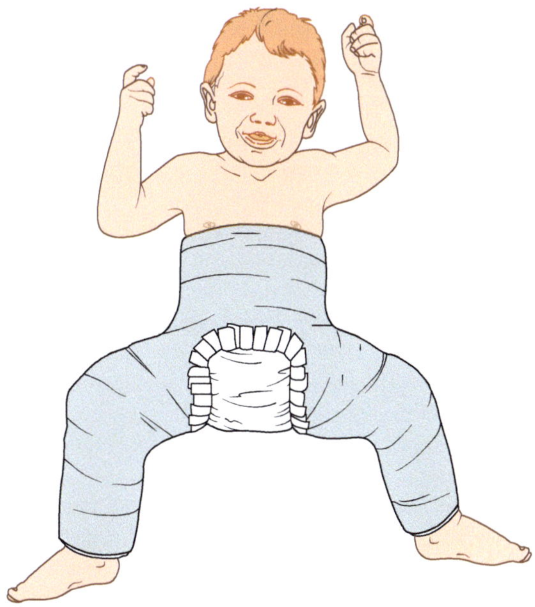

FIGURE 17.11 Hip spica.

If correction is not achieved by the aforementioned methods, the child will need an open reduction and femoral osteotomy at a later stage. Remodelling of the femoral head within the acetabulum occurs within 12–18 months following open reduction of the hip. Diagnosis after 24 months of age will require surgical treatment, and surgery is effective up to the age of 8 years.

In addition to the care the child requires pre- and post-surgery, nursing care interventions for a child with DDH should focus on skin integrity, mobility and family care. The parents/carers will need an explanation about the conditions and treatments. The parents/carers will need to be comfortable with applying the Pavlik harness. Competency in handling their child in a hip spica will be required before the child can be discharged. This will include transporting the child and attending to their personal hygiene needs. The mother may need assistance with breastfeeding, as positioning can be more difficult due to the weight of the cast.

Neurovascular status will need to be monitored, and this should be explained to the parents prior to discharge.

Good skin care is essential when caring for an infant or a child in a hip spica. Skin integrity is important, and normal hygiene habits should be maintained. Pressure points should be checked while the child is in the Pavlik harness. The condition of the skin in the perineal area, abdomen and lower limbs should be checked for developing pressure ulcers. The condition of the hip spica around the perineal area should be checked, as it can get soggy from urine if the correct size nappy is not used. Additional padding may be required overnight to avoid urine leaking into the cast.

Parents and carers will need to be helped and advised on how to maintain skin integrity, when to change the plastic coverings around the edge of the spica and how to position their child throughout the day. Referral to community nursing teams should be made, and out-of-hours contact advice provided.

The child in a hip spica will need assistance to turn, as they will be unable to do this themselves initially. Tummy time is also important for those under 6 months to assist with developing their head control. They will be unable to crawl while in their hip spica, so activities that encourage foot action and upper body engagement will be beneficial. Safe transportation of the child in a hip spica must be a priority.

Investigations

Barlow test: The hip is adducted and gentle pressure is applied to the hips. A 'clunk' will be felt as the hip subluxes out of the acetabulum (Fig. 17.12). This is a positive test.

Ortolani test: The thumb is placed over the inner thigh and the index is placed on the greater trochanter. The hip is then abducted and gentle pressure is placed on the greater trochanter. A 'clunk' will be felt when the hip is reduced (Fig. 17.13). This is a positive test.

Both tests are only suitable for infants younger than 6 weeks of age. The fingers should not leave any marks on the infant's skin, and the test should be performed gently. One hip at a time should be tested. The Barlow test should be performed first and then the Ortolani test.

If either test is positive, then the baby must be referred for an ultrasound to confirm the diagnosis.

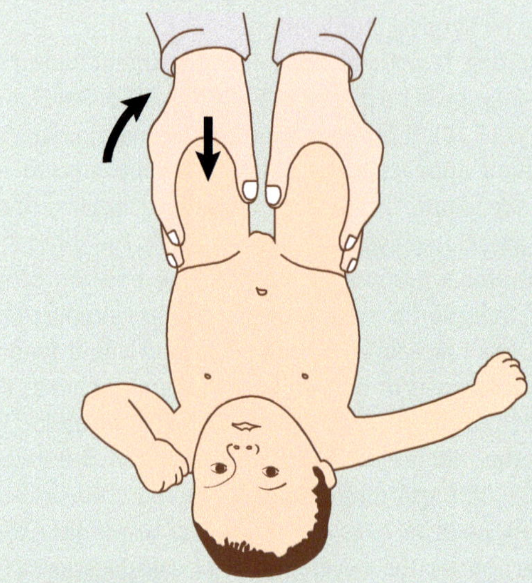

FIGURE 17.12 Barlow test.

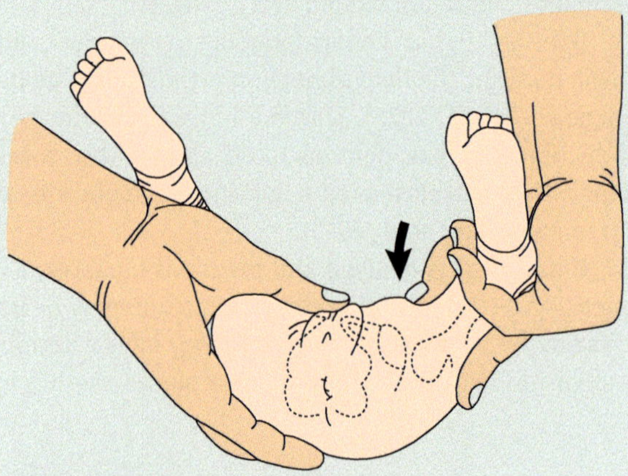

FIGURE 17.13 Ortolani test.

Conclusion

This chapter has provided an insight into the anatomy and pathophysiology of a number of musculoskeletal conditions that are common in childhood. The focus has been on providing information that is pertinent for the delivery of effective care by enhancing the reader's understanding of the pathophysiological changes that occur either as a result of injury or those due to abnormal development, and the impact that this has on the child and family or carers. It is by no means exhaustive, as the range of musculoskeletal conditions in childhood is vast.

References

Beni, R., Sabba, M., Hussain, A., *et al.* (2025). Management of Legg-Calve-Perthes disease: a scoping review with advice on initial management. *Archives of Disease in Childhood* 110, 341–346.

Briggs, B. (2023). No good evidence proves that NSAIDs hinder fracture healing. *Emergency Medicine News* 45(7), 4.

British National Formulary for Children (BNFC) (2025). [online] Available at: https://bnf.nice.org.uk/ (accessed July 2025).

Campbell, F., & Watt, E. (2020). An exploration of nursing practices related to care of orthopaedic external fixators (pin/wire sites) in the Australian context. *International Journal of Orthopaedic and Trauma Nursing* 36.

Chatterton, B.D., & James, K. (2024). Slipped capital femoral epiphysis: diagnosis, classification and controversies in management. *Orthopaedics and Traumatology* 38(6), 365–370.

Crossland, H., Skirrow, S., Puthucheary, Z.A., *et al.* (2019). The impact of immobilisation and inflammation on the regulation of muscle mass and insulin resistance: different routes to similar end-points. *The Journal of Physiology* 597(5), 1259–1270.

Galloway, A.M., Keene, D.J., Anderson, A., *et al.* (2024). Clinical consensus recommendations for the non-surgical treatment of children with Perthes' disease in the UK. *The Bone & Joint Journal* 106-B, 501–507.

Guan, S., Du, H., Wu, Y., & Qin, S. (2024). The Ilizarov technique: a dynamic solution for orthopaedic challenges. *Orthopaedic Surgery* 16, 2111–2114.

Hockenberry, M.J., & Wilson, D. (eds) (2024). *Wong's Nursing Care of Infants and Children*, 12th edn. Elsevier.

Jani, S., & McKay, D. (2024). Orthopaedics and rheumatology. In: *Textbook of Paediatric Emergency Medicine*. Oxford: Wiley Blackwell.

Joseph, B., Shah, H., & Perry, D.C. (2023). Epidemiology, natural evolution, pathogenesis, clinical spectrum, and management of Legg–Calvé–Perthes. *Journal of Children's Orthopaedics* 17(5), 385–403.

Korup, L.R., Larsen, P., Nanthan, K.R., *et al.* (2022). Children's distal forearm fractures: a population-based epidemiology study of 4,316 fractures. *Bone & Joint Open* 3(6), 448–454.

Lissauer, T., & Carroll, W. (2021). *Illustrated Textbook of Paediatrics*, 6th edn. Mosby/Elsevier, London.

Maggio, A.B.R., Martin, X.E., Tabard-Fougère, A., *et al.* (2018). What is the real impact of upper limb cast immobilisation on activity-related energy expenditure in children? *BMJ Open Sport & Exercise Medicine* https://bmjopensem.bmj.com/content/4/1/e000359 (accessed on 27 May 2025).

Mullen, R., Cogburn, J., & Desanto, K. (2022). NSAIS use and effects on bone healing. *American Family Physician* 2022, 106(5), 578–579.

National Health Service England (NHSE) (2025). Newborn and infant physical examination (NIPE) screening programme handbook. Availableat:https://www.gov.uk/government/publications/newborn-and-infant-physical-examination-programme-handbook/newborn-and-infant-physical-examination-screening-programme-handbook (accessed May 31 2025).

National Institute for Health and Care Excellence (NICE) (2017). Child abuse and neglect. NG76. Available at: https://www.nice.org.uk/guidance/ng76 (accessed on 30 May 2025).

National Institute for Health and Care Excellence (NICE) (2022). Fractures (complex): assessment and management. (NG37). Available at: https://www.nice.org.uk/guidance/ng37 (accessed 30 May 2025)

National Institute for Health and Care Excellence (NICE) (2025). Fractures (non-complex): assessment and management (NG38). Available at: https://www.nice.org.uk/guidance/ng38 (accessed 30 May 2025).

National Institute for Health and Care Excellence (NICE) CKS. (2020). Acute childhood Limp. Available at: https://cks.nice.org.uk/topics/acute-childhood-limp/ (accessed 26 May 2025).

National Institute for Health and Clinical Excellence (NICE) (2015). Open reduction of slipped capital femoral epiphysis. Interventional procedures guidance [IPG511] Available at: https://www.nice.org.uk/guidance/ipg511 (accessed 31May 2025).

National Institute for Health and Clinical Excellence (NICE) (2021a). Pregnancy and neonates: hip screening. Available at: https://www.nice.org.uk/indicators/ind77-pregnancy-and-neonates-hip-screening/IND77-20250313.pdf (accessed on 31 July 2025).

National Institute for Health and Clinical Excellence (NICE) (2021b). Postnatal care. NG194. Available at: https://www.nice.org.uk/guidance/ng194/chapter/Recommendations#postnatal-care-of-the-baby (accessed 30 May 2025).

Nettina, S. (2018). *Lippincott Manual of Nursing Practice*, 11th edn. Wolters Kluwer/Lippincott Williams & Wilkins, Philadelphia.

Nicholson, A., Dunne, K., Taaffe, S., *et al.* (2023). Developmental dysplasia of the hip in infants and children. *BMJ (Clinical Research Ed.)*, 383–387.

Paton, R.W. (2017). Screening in developmental dysplasia of the hip (DDH). *Surgeon* 15(5), 290–296.

Peate, I., & Gormley-Fleming, E. (eds) (2025). *Fundamentals of Children's Anatomy and Physiology*, 3rd edn. Wiley, Oxford.

Perry, D.C., Arch, B., Appelbe, D., *et al.* (2022). The british orthopaedic surgery surveillance study: slipped capital femoral epiphysis: the epidemiology and two-year outcomes from a prospective cohort in Great Britain. *Bone & Joint Journal* 104-B(4), 519–528.

Royal College of Nursing (RCN) (2021). *Traction Principles and Application. Clinical Professional Resources.* Royal College of Nursing, London.

Sankar, W.N., Nduaguba, A., & Flynn, J.M. (2015). Ilfeld abduction orthosis is an effective second-line treatment after failure of

Pavlik harness for infants with developmental dysplasia of the hip. *The Journal of Bone and Joint Surgery. American Volume* 97(4), 292–297.

Tucker, A., Ballard, J., & Cosgrove, A. (2019). Temporal changes in slipped upper femoral epiphysis at a regional level: a declining incidence and literature review. *Journal of Children's Orthopaedics* 13(5), 445–456.

Tume, L.N., Simons, C., Latten, L., *et al.* (2024). Association between protein intake and muscle wasting in critically ill children: a prospective cohort study. *Journal of Parenteral and Enteral Nutrition* 48(5), 615–623.

Walker, J.A., Scammell, B.E., & Bayston, R. (2018). A web-based survey to identify current practice in skeletal pin site management. *International Wound Journal* 15(2), 250–257.

Wang, M., & Su, Y. (2023). Suitability of skin traction combined with braces for treating femoral shaft fractures in 3–5 years old children. *Journal of Orthopaedic Surgery and Research* 18(63).

Waters, P.M., Skaggs, D.L., & Flynn, J.M. (2025). *Rockwood and Wilkins' Fractures in Children*, 10th edn. Lippinott. Wolter Kluwer, Philadelphia.

Wright, E. (2023). Fracture Management in the infant, child and young person. In: Clarke, S. & Drozd, M. (eds). *Orthopaedic and Trauma Nursing: An Evidence-based Approach to Musculoskeletal Care*, 2nd edn. Oxford: Wiley Blackwell.

CHAPTER 18

Disorders of the skin

Elizabeth Gormley-Fleming

AIM

The chapter introduces the reader to altered pathophysiology and the impact this may have on the child, young person and family. The skin can often be the first sign of an underlying health issue.

LEARNING OUTCOMES

On completion of this chapter, the reader will be able to:

- Describe the anatomy of the skin.
- Accurately describe a skin condition/rash.
- Outline the care of children with a wound.
- Articulate the difference between healing by primary intention and secondary intention.
- Understand the physiological changes that occur during wound healing.
- Explain the physiological change that occurs when a child has eczema.
- Understand the body's response to a burn injury, identify the classification of a burn injury and know how to calculate.

KEYWORDS

- integument
- epidermis
- dermis
- epithelialisation
- inflammatory
- proliferation
- maturation
- keloid
- hypertrophic scar

Test your prior knowledge

1. Describe the functions of the skin.
2. List the layers of the epidermis.
3. Identify the different types of glands and their location.
4. List the accessory organs of the skin.
5. Discuss how wounds heal.
6. Discuss the mechanism of injury in relation to burns.
7. Highlight the impact burns can have on a child physically and psychologically.
8. Discuss the life cycle of head lice.
9. Describe the role of the healthcare professional when providing care to a child with a disorder of skin.

Introduction

The skin is the largest organ in the human body. It has several vital functions that are essential to sustain life. The skin, also known as the integumentary system, is a complex organ that is essential for human survival due to its physiological functions. It undergoes significant changes from birth to adulthood, such as thickening of the dermis and increased activity of the sebaceous glands. The most dynamic changes occur within the first 3 months of life (Visscher *et al.*, 2015). At birth, the skin of a term baby is developed sufficiently to cope with extra-uterine life.

As a system, the skin has contributions from basic germ layers: the ectoderm and the mesoderm. The ectoderm forms the surface epidermis and the associated glands, while the mesoderm forms the underlying connective tissue of the dermis and subcutaneous layer (Carlson, 2019). It is also populated with melanocytes and sensory nerve endings. These different tissues perform many specific functions: thermoregulation, synthesis of vitamin D, excretion and immunity.

Frequently referred to as the largest organ in the body, the skin covers all of the body's external surfaces and is approximately 10% of the body mass. By adulthood the skin will be almost 2 m^2. The ratio of skin surface to body weight is highest at birth, and this will decline progressively during infancy. At birth, the surface area is nearly three times greater than that of an older child, whereas at 37 weeks' gestation or less, it is proportionally five times greater than that of a term baby (Peate & Gormley-Fleming, 2025).

The skin is the first line of defence against the environment. Skin disorders of childhood vary greatly in both symptoms and severity. They can be permanent or temporary, painful or painless, minor to life-limiting. They are frequently associated with viral or bacterial infections, for example, slapped cheek syndrome and meningococcal septicaemia. Some of the more common conditions are identified in Table 18.1. Empirical evidence has demonstrated that loss of skin integrity in infants and children is most commonly attributed to wounds secondary to congenital conditions, thermal injury, extravasation injury, epidermal stripping and pressure ulcerations (Baranoski & Ayello, 2020).

Disorders of the skin are normally described by the type of lesions that appear on the skin, the shape of the lesion, the colour and the configuration. Noting the type, shape, location and colour of the lesion is an essential component of obtaining a history of the rash or skin condition. Therefore, it is important to be able to describe accurately the details of any rash an infant or child presents with, for example, a generalised, macular erythematous rash, hot to touch.

TABLE 18.1 Skin conditions of childhood

Congenital/ present at birth	Infections	Acquired/ trauma
Epidermolysis bullosa	Cellulitis	Surgery
Haemangioma	Herpes simplex	Burns
Eczema	Rubeola (measles)	Epidermal stripping
Café au lait spots	Verrucas	Pressure ulcerations
Port wine stains	Necrotising fasciitis	Blunt force trauma
Mongolia blue spots	Impetigo	Nappy rash
Lymphatic malformations, e.g., cystic hygroma	Molluscum contagiosum	Melanoma
Albinism	Pilonidal sinus	Acne
Vitiligo	Shingles	Urticaria
	Ringworm	Friction
	Chicken pox	Sunburn

Types of lesions

Lesions may be described as either primary or secondary.

Primary lesions

- Macule – flat, distinct, discoloured area usually < 1 cm in diameter.
- Papule – a solid raised lesion, distinct border < 1 cm in diameter.
- Pustule – a small raised area of skin containing cloudy, purulent fluid.
- Wheal – a raised (itchy) area of the skin.

- Nodule – a solid raised area under the skin that is filled with fluid or tissue.
- Vesicle – small fluid-filled sacs.
- Petechiae – non-raised red-brown non-blanchable lesions.
- Bulla – vesicle or blister > 1 cm in diameter.
- Plaque – solid and elevated lesion on the skin > 1 cm in diameter.
- Cyst – soft, firm mass in the skin that will be filled with fluid or semi-solid material in a sac.

Secondary lesions

- Crusts – covering formed by drying serum, blood or pus.
- Scales – excessive dead cells that are produced due to an abnormality or inflammatory change.
- Lichenification – thickening of the skin.
- Fissures – cracks in the skin as a result of prolonged drying of the skin.
- Ulcer – destruction of the epidermis and part of the dermis.

Colour

- White – leukoderma and hypomelanosis
- Red – erythema
- Pink – hypermelanosis
- Brown
- Blue
- Grey
- Black

Shape

- Round
- Oval
- Annular – ring-shaped
- Irregular
- Guttae – drop-like

Arrangement

- Grouped – clustering of lesions
- Disseminated
- Generalised – widespread
- Discrete – lesions remain separate
- Linear – in lines
- Multiformed – more than one type of lesion
- Telangiectasia – dilated cutaneous vessels that are thread-like or lines

Epidermolysis bullosa

Epidermolysis bullosa (EB) is an inherited disorder that occurs in 1 : 17000 children in the United Kingdom. It is a group of skin-blistering conditions, and it is characterised by blisters, skin breakdown, pain, deformity and infection that can lead to secondary complications and an increased risk of squamous cell carcinoma (Watson, 2016). The epithelial lining of other organs may also be affected and blister as a result of minimal trauma. A lifelong condition, the child with EB will require lifetime healthcare input.

EB is generally an inherited autosomal dominant disorder in that it relies on only having one affected parent for transmission. If a parent is a carrier, there is a 50% chance of having a child from each pregnancy who will inherit EB. Males and females are affected equally.

It may also be autosomal recessive, so each parent would carry the affected gene, and the risk of having a child born with EB would be 25% for each pregnancy.

It may occur by genetic mutation, with neither parent carrying an affected gene.

Diagnosis

Diagnosis is by immunohistochemistry (Tenedini *et al.*, 2015). A definitive diagnosis will require a skin biopsy, possibly imaging and endoscopy if there is thought to be involvement of the gastrointestinal tract (Bruckner-Tuderman *et al.*, 2014). This is essential even in the presence of a complete history and assessment in order to prescribe the correct plan of treatment. Blood sampling for genetics is obtained. Amniocentesis may be performed for prenatal diagnosis as early as the 10th week of gestation (National Institute of Arthritis and Musculoskeletal and Skin Diseases [NIAMS], 2013).

Types of epidermolysis bullosa

There are various types of EB, ranging in severity from mild to life-limiting. Currently, there are more than 30 types of EB, so categorisation is ongoing as research develops in this area. An International consensus was reached in 2008 on the currently used names. Classification is dependent on the layer of skin at which blistering occurs (Fig. 18.1), as follows:

- Epidermolysis bullosa simplex (EBS)
- Junctional epidermolysis bullosa (JEB)
- Dystrophic epidermolysis bullosa (DJB)
- Multiple levels of blistering – Kindler syndrome.

Epidermolysis bullosa simplex

EBS is a generalised form and is usually present at birth, with blisters occurring primarily on the hands and feet. Blistering may be more widespread in subtypes of EBS. The cells of the epidermis are normally supported by keratins, which give the cells their shape and support. The keratin, usually type 5, type 14 or rarely plectin, is absent or present in insufficient amounts. In the presence of friction, the cells rupture, causing fluid to leak, which forms a blister. Finger and toenails may be absent. Blisters may occur inside the mouth. There may be thickening of the skin on the palms of the hands and soles of the feet. Anaemia may be present. In general, the blisters are small but plentiful and approximately 2 cm in size. EBS accounts for 70% of cases (British Association of Dermatologists [BAD], 2015).

Junctional epidermolysis bullosa

Junctional epidermolysis bullosa (JEB) is usually severe, and the child will have large blisters on its face, trunk and legs. It can be life-threatening because of the risk of infection and fluid loss. Blisters may also be present in the upper airway, oesophagus, lower intestinal system and urogenital system. This may lead to life-threatening episodes.

Absent finger and toenails may be in evidence, and the skin may have a very thin appearance (atrophic scarring). Alopecia may occur following blistering of the scalp. The child will have delayed growth secondary to malnutrition. Anaemia is common. Involvement of soft tissues of the nose and mouth will be identified. JEB accounts for 5% of all cases (BAD, 2015).

Dystrophic epidermolysis bullosa

Dystrophic epidermolysis bullosa (DEB) occurs in approximately 25% of cases (BAD, 2015). This may be either the autosomal dominant or recessive forms of DEB. In the dominant and mild recessive forms, blisters will be present on the hands, feet, elbows and knees. There will be milia present on the trunk and limbs. The oesophagus is usually affected. Nails will be present but misshapen.

In severe DEB, there will be blisters over large areas of the body surface. In addition, there will be loss of nails, pruritus, scarring, anaemia and delayed growth. There may be inflammation of the eyes and corneal erosion. The gastrointestinal tract and the oral cavity are likely to be affected. Early loss of permanent teeth occurs.

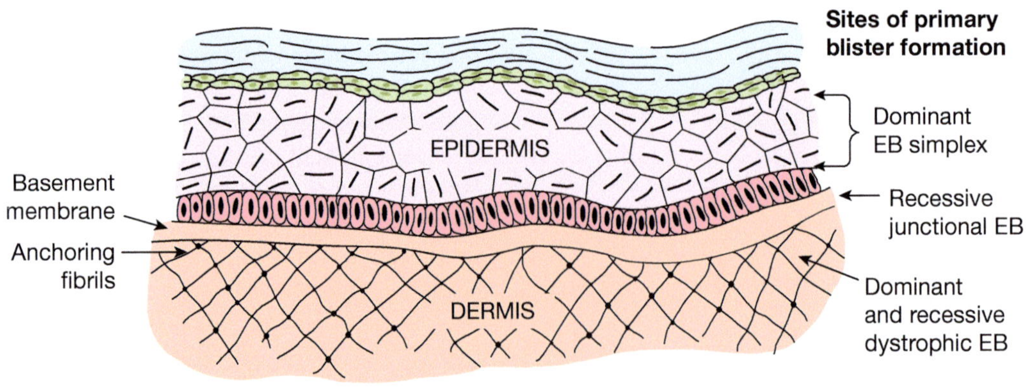

FIGURE 18.1 Cross-section of the skin and primary sites of blister formation.

Pseudosyndactyly – fusion of the fingers and toes – will affect most sufferers of this type of DEB. Squamous cell carcinoma has been reported in young people with recessive DEB (NIAMS, 2013).

Kindler syndrome

Kindler syndrome is a rare type of EB. In addition to blistering, there are changes to the appearance of the skin – poikiloderma (breakdown of the skin) – and involvement of the gastrointestinal tract and the eyes. Hyperkeratosis of the soles of the feet and the palms of the hands will occur.

Kindler syndrome is usually diagnosed by the age of 1 year, with the presence of blisters on the hands and feet being the initial cause of concern. By the age of 5 years, the skin will be considerably thinner and more wrinkled than that of an unaffected child. It occurs as a result of a defect in the gene *KIND1* (also called the *FERMT1* gene) and is an autosomal recessive disorder (Genetic Reference, 2016). Children with Kindler syndrome are more susceptible to skin damage from sunlight, so treatment plans and education on safety in the sun need to be provided.

Pathophysiology

Cytolysis, which is the destruction of cells by either rupture or disintegration, occurs. This causes blisters to form in the epidermis or basement membrane. It is the result of a genetic mutation, which affects the protein at the epidermal–dermal junction.

In EBS, cytolysis leads to blister formation in the basal or spinous layers of the epidermis. The keratinocytes have abnormal keratin filaments, and they may also be structured inadequately. In JEB, there is a separation of the epidermis from the basal lamina. The protein structures, hemidesmosomes, which are thread-like fibres, are absent or reduced; thus, the epidermis is not firmly anchored to the base membrane. As a result of this, the tissues separate, and blistering occurs in the upper area of the base membrane, the lamina lucida. In cases of DEB, the basal lamina and the epidermis are attached, but a blister cavity forms below the lamina densa of the dermo–epidermal junction (Nettina, 2010). The hemidesmosomes (anchoring fibrils) are abnormal, reduced in number, or completely absent.

Case study 18.1

Harry is 8 years old and has EBS, which was diagnosed when he was an infant. He has a severe form of EBS. As a baby and toddler, he had frequent admissions to hospital. He attends his local lower school and tries his best to get involved in a range of activities, as he dislikes not being able to participate. His mum has requested that he does not play football during the lunch break but Harry does not want to feel left out. He borrows some trainers and develops even more blisters on his feet. Harry has multiple blisters at the moment as the weather has become warmer. These are located on his hands, feet, trunk, legs, arms, face and in his mouth. He does not want to tell his mum about these new blisters. His mum normally bursts new blisters to reduce the risk of infection.

After a few days, he is complaining of a lot of pain in his feet, and when his mum takes his socks off to look at his feet, she notices that the skin is red, hot, and there is yellow/greenish fluid draining from the lateral malleolus on his left foot and from the dorsum of his right foot. He is not eating or drinking very much at the moment either, and is generally not himself. His mum knows that he needs to be seen by a doctor and takes him to the local hospital. He is also a patient at a specialist centre for EB and has regular appointments there with a dermatologist and an EB nurse specialist.

A full history is taken, and his vital signs are recorded (Table 18.2). He is pyrexial and the paediatrician arranges to have blood tests, a full blood count (FBC) and a C-reactive protein (CRP) (Table 18.3).

TABLE 18.2 Harry's vital signs

Vital sign	Harry's observations	Normal range
Temperature	38.5 °C	36.0–37.2 °C
Pulse	130 bpm	80–120 bpm
Respiration	20 breaths per minute	20–25 breaths per minute
Blood pressure	100/60 mmHg	90–110 mmHg
Oxygen saturation	97%	98–100%
Pain score (1–5)	3	0

TABLE 18.3 **Harry's blood test results**

Test	Harry's results	Normal range
White blood cells (WBCs)	16.4	4.5–13.5 WBC × 10^9/L
Neutrophils	9 × 10^9/L	1.5–8 × 10^9/L
Lymphocytes	8.4 × 10^9/L	1.5–7.0 × 10^9/L
Red blood cells (RBCs)	4.8 × 10^{12}/L	4.0–5.2 × 10^{12}/L
Haemoglobin (Hb)	11.1 g/100 mL	11.5–15.0 g/100 mL
Platelets	240 × 10^9/L	150–450 × 10^9/L
C-reactive protein	25 mg/L	< 5 mg/L

Care and management

A holistic, systematic assessment is required based on the individual's needs. Care will be planned and implemented in accordance with findings. In addition to treating any infections, the aim of care should be to prevent any further trauma and blistering to the skin by any of the care interventions.

Pain

The pain score will indicate the type of analgesia required. This will need to be reassessed on a regular basis and the appropriate analgesia administered as required. Opiates are frequently used to control pain prior to the change of dressings. Appropriate monitoring will need to be considered to ensure the safety of the child.

Infection

There is a very high probability that a secondary infection is present, so antibiotics will need to be prescribed. These may be oral, usually a penicillin-based antibiotic or clarithromycin if there is a known allergy to penicillin (BNFC, n.d.), or topical antibiotics may be prescribed. The choice of oral or topical antibiotics will be determined by the clinical assessment. A swab of the infected area is required for culture and sensitivity. This will identify the organism and indicate if the antibiotics prescribed are suitable.

Hydration and nutrition

Hydration is important when there is a loss of skin integrity and fluid loss from blisters. Oral fluids should be encouraged. A petroleum-based product should be used to protect the lips. If oral hydration is not possible, intravenous fluids will be required. Utmost care is required when inserting a cannula; use of a tourniquet is not recommended. Adhesive dressing must not be used to secure the cannula once in situ.

Because of the presence of blisters in the mouth and oesophagus, oral intake may be insufficient. A naso-gastric tube should not be used. The presence of a naso-gastric

Medicines management

- Topical medications may be antibiotics, anti-fungal, analgesics, steroids or anaesthetics. These are applied directly to the affected area. They include creams, ointments, sprays, lotions and patches.
- Care must always be taken when applying topical medication to protect both the child and the nurse/parent. The manufacturer's instructions should be followed. The dose to administer must be checked carefully.
- The wearing of gloves is normally advised, so adherence to local policy is essential. Gloves can potentially drag the skin of a child with EB, so sprays are preferable as they will reduce the risk of further trauma to the child's skin.
- Most topical medication is provided in tubes. These do not have child-proof caps, so safe storage in the home needs to be discussed with parents/carers.

tube will cause additional blistering both on insertion and while in situ. The dietician is an integral member of the care team and will usually suggest high-calorie and protein-fortified drinks and food. These will replace the protein lost from the fluid that drains from the blisters. Nutritional supplements may also be prescribed, such as minerals and vitamins. The dietician can also advise on foods and fluids that will prevent and assist with constipation.

Blisters and skin care

The objective of care is to reduce pain and prevent discomfort, excessive loss of body fluid and infection, and to promote healing. Careful skin and wound assessments must be undertaken frequently, and management tailored for the type of EB and the wound(s).

If not lanced, blisters will continue to enlarge (Denyer, 2010). Apply very gentle pressure with soft gauze to the blister. A sterile hypodermic needle, 14 or 16 gauge, is inserted at the lowest point of the blister and passed through it to create an exit point. Fluid will then drain from the blister. Heavy drainage from the blisters can irritate the skin further, so it is important that this is absorbed and removed. If the roof of the blister is intact, then leave it exposed. The needle should not be resheathed prior to disposal. Parents/carers are generally educated to pierce their child's blisters in the home environment.

Daily cleaning of the skin is important. The skin should be patted, not rubbed. Using antiseptic washes is thought to help reduce the risk of contracting skin infections (BAD, 2015).

Clothing should be soft, loose and made of natural fibres. Overheating should be avoided. Shoes should be well-fitting and made of natural material.

Dressings must be non-adherent (silicone-based) and cut to size. Hydrogel dressing will assist with cooling blistered areas. Dressings should be secured using a tubular bandage or silicone-based tape. Dressings must be changed when strike-through occurs. If silicone tape is in situ, it should be rolled back. An appropriate dressing removal spray should be used, or the dressing should be soaked off in a bath. Fingers and toes should be dressed individually (Denyer & Murrell, 2010).

Atopic eczema

Atopic eczema usually develops in early childhood and often has a genetic predisposition. It is a chronic inflammatory pruritic condition which follows a pattern of acute episodes and periods of remission. It is often erratic and varies in severity. The skin's natural barrier is broken down, which makes it susceptible to trigger factors, such as allergens, chemicals and irritants. While rarely serious, it does have a significant impact on the child's and parents'/carers' quality of life.

Pathophysiology

There is a genetic predisposition to developing atopic eczema. If both parents have the condition, there is an 80% chance that one of their children will be affected. However, the aetiology is multifactorial with the environment, immunological and physical factors all possibilities in its development.

Immunoglobulin IgE will be elevated. An increased amount of histamine is released from the basophils, and hyper-reactive T cells secrete proinflammatory cytokines.

Various dendritic cells, such as Langerhans cells, inflammatory epithelial cells or plasmacytoid cells, all play a role in determining the impact of the underlying mechanism. Corneocytes separate in the epidermis and reduce the epidermal lipids. It is thought that this disruption to the epidermal barrier is a result of a mutation in the *FLG* gene (filaggrin). Filaggrin is found in the upper layers of the stratum corneum.

The epidermis already has an inability to retain water so fluid leaks from the cells. This makes the skin dry and the skin barrier is now less effective (Burns et al. 2004). Bacteria can penetrate, which results in an inflammatory response. As a result of the inflammatory response, erythema and oedema occur in the epidermis. There is increased blood flow, which in turn causes the white blood cells (WBCs) to leak into the dermis. This causes vesicles and blistering of the epidermis. When this is scratched and the skin breaks, weeping occurs.

Itching is an important factor in diagnosing eczema (Rudolf *et al.*, 2020), it is referred to as the 'itch that becomes a rash'.

Diagnosis

There is no single marker that will definitely diagnose atopic eczema. It is a clinical diagnosis based on the evaluation of signs, symptoms and history. It is diagnosed when the child presents with an itchy skin condition and three of the following (NICE, 2023):

- Visible flexural dermatitis in the skin creases, or in the case of a child < 18 months of age, dermatitis on the cheeks and/or extensor surfaces.
- History of flexural dermatitis or dermatitis on the cheeks and/or extensor surfaces in a child < 18 months of age.

- Dry skin in the last 12 months.
- Personal history of asthma, allergic rhinitis or positive family history of atopic eczema in children < 4 years of age; family in this case refers to parents and/or siblings.
- Onset of symptoms before 2 years of age.

Children of Asian, Black African or Black Caribbean ethnicity may present with eczema on the extensor surfaces rather than the flexures, and follicular and discoid patterns may be more prevalent.

Assessment

A holistic approach must be taken when assessing a child with atopic eczema. This includes noting the severity of the eczema and the impact of this on the child's quality of life. The impact on the parents/carers should also be assessed. A range of quality of life scoring tools for infants and children with eczema is available, and an age-appropriate tool should be utilised.

Trigger factors

A range of triggers has the potential to irritate the skin and lead to an exacerbation of eczema. With atopic eczema likely triggers are:

- food allergens (eggs, milk and fish)
- contact allergens (wool, synthetic fabrics, house dust mite, animal dander and heat/cold)
- inhalant allergens (dust and trees)
- irritants (soaps)
- skin infections.

Treatment

The goals of treatment are to improve skin integrity, identify and eliminate trigger factors, control pruritus and prevent infection. A stepped care plan is recommended so treatment is adjusted up or down according to the severity of the eczema (NICE, 2023). Emollients, followed by topical steroids, are the predominant treatment agents. Topical calcineurin inhibitors are recommended if topical steroids do not control the atopic eczema. Occlusive dressing-bandages are recommended for short-term use. These are applied over an emollient or topical steroid cream.

Phototherapy may be recommended in severe cases when quality of life is severely impacted. Antihistamines are not recommended for routine use. They may have a role to play when sleep disturbance is significant or when itching is severe. Bacterial infections will require systemic antibiotics, and herpes infections will require systemic acyclovir.

Infected eczema or eczema herpeticum requires urgent medical treatment. Red 'punched' out lesions are present in eczema herpeticum and must be treated with antiviral medications.

Growth and development

Good sleeping habits are essential for normal growth and development. Children with eczema have shown to have increased incidence of sleep deprivation and fatigue and this also impacts negatively on maternal health (Bawany *et al.*, 2021). The cumulative effect of sleep loss can affect bonding, relationships and maternal mental well-being as mothers are notably the main caregivers at night (British Association of Dermatologists, 2024). It is well recognised that eczema often flares up at night (Afzal & Ali, 2023). Five factors are thought to contribute to this:

1. Skin temperature increase as core temperature decreases due to surface vasodilatation resulting in increased itching.
2. The relationship between the immune system and our body clocks. Cytokines are proteins that act as signals between the immune cells and other cells. Some cytokines, such as gamma interferon, are sleep-promoting but also switch on inflammatory signals. The level of cytokines peaks at night-time as the immune system is rejuvenating cells. Perversely, eczema may worsen at night-time as the inflammatory response in the skin is increased. The sleep cycle is dependent on cortisol level dropping at night, which is lowest at midnight and peaks an hour after waking (O' Byrne *et al.*, 2021). Recognised as a stress hormone, it also has an anti-inflammatory action. The sleep cycle is

dependent on the level of cortisol dropping. Collaboration between cytokines and cortisol levels may exacerbate eczema symptoms at night.

3. Eczema is itchy and this leads to inflammatory cytokines being released. The immune system reacts and inflammation increases the need to scratch/itch, so a vicious itch-scratch cycle occurs. As itching often occurs when sleeping, it is very difficult to avoid, which is why keeping nails short and wearing mitts at night can avoid skin damage from itching and scratching.
4. *Exposure to allergens:* Children with eczema may have a protein deficit called filaggrin in their skin. The main function of this protein is to act as a barrier and protect the skin, retain moisture and prevent toxins from entering. At night, dust mites are active in the presence of body temperature, and they feed on dead skin. Their habitat is usually beds and bedding, and eczema is associated with dust mite allergy (Bumbacea *et al.*, 2020). When the skin is damaged, immune cells are exposed to dust mite, stimulating an allergic response, causing inflammation, itching and redness. Hypoallergenic bedding made from natural fibres is advised along with frequent cleaning.

Wounds

A wound is a breach in the surface of the skin necessitating the healing process to commence. The majority of wounds in children are relatively minor, and healing occurs without significant impact on the child. Today, the increasing complexity of medical and surgical care provided to infants and children has resulted in an increase in the risk of complications from wounds that may be non-healing, and also from pressure ulcers, intravenous extravasation injury and moisture-associated skin damage. The extremely low-birthweight neonate is at significant risk of skin breakdown because of the fragility of their skin. Life-threatening sepsis secondary to wound infection is a further potential risk. Wounds may be caused by trauma, surgery, friction, pressure, chemical injury, biological injury and infection.

Revisit Chapter 19 in Peate and Gormley-Fleming (2025) to revise the anatomy and physiology of the skin.

Age-dependent factors need to be considered in wound care as the physiology of the skin (Table 18.4) alters significantly over the period from newborn to young person.

TABLE 18.4 Age-related factors to consider in skin care

Age	Factors to be considered
Premature infant	• Impaired epidermal barrier resulting in trans-epidermal water loss and electrolyte imbalance • Thermoregulation • Immature immune system • Potential to absorb topical agents as the body surface area to weight ratio is greater • Enhanced susceptibility to irritants
Term infant	• Fragile skin • Thermoregulation • Immature immune system • Potential to absorb topical agents as body surface area to weight ratio is greater
Toddler	• Potential to absorb topical agents as body surface area to weight ratio is greater • Possible removal of dressings • Contamination of wounds and dressings through normal activities and exploring environment • May not cooperate at dressing changes, making assessment and care planning more difficult due to fear and anxiety
Child	• Possible removal of dressings • Contamination of wounds and dressings through normal activities and exploring environment • Developmental delay may compound wound healing • May not cooperate at dressing changes, making assessment and care planning more difficult due to fear and anxiety

Source: King *et al.* (2014)/with permission of Sage Publications.

Case study 18.2

Kate, aged 10 years, was climbing over a fence at her grandparents' farm and sustained a laceration to her right thigh (10 cm) from some barbed wire that was not visible to her. Following first aid, she is brought to her local minor injuries unit. In triage, a complete assessment is undertaken, and her vital signs are normal. A 'TIME' clinical decision support tool was utilised (see Box 18.1). This is a 5-step clinical decision support tool that enables a holistic patient and wound assessment and selects appropriate treatment and identifies short-term goals. Her wound is exposed, and it is noted that she has an 'L'-shaped laceration on the medial aspect of her thigh and it is deep. Following analgesia, the wound is irrigated with sterile water to remove the dressing that was applied at school. It is decided that this wound should be sutured because of its location and depth. Kate is a cheerleader and needs to get back to training soon. She is anxious about having a scar. Consent is obtained from Kate and her mum. Following the instillation of local anaesthetic, 12 absorbable sutures are inserted using a septic non-touch technique. Entonox® is administered during the procedure.

BOX 18.1 **Time Acronym**

T-Tissue
I-Inflammation or infection
M-Management of exudate

Source: Adapted from Garten *et al.* (2020).

The vaccination status of all children and young people should be checked in the event of traumatic wounds. Vaccination status worldwide has decreased in recent times.

Wound healing

Wound healing is a complex and dynamic process and occurs by either primary intention (healing) or secondary intention. In children, wound healing tends to occur more rapidly than in young people and adults because of the numbers of neutrophils, lymphocytes and monocytes present in the inflammatory phase (Baranoski & Ayello, 2020).

Wound healing involves four stages:

1. coagulation and haemostasis
2. inflammation
3. proliferation
4. maturation/regeneration.

A series of overlapping stages and complex processes will occur during healing, and its duration is variable. There are a number of factors that will determine this: general health, nutritional status, ischemia and infection.

Primary healing (intention)

Primary healing occurs when the wound repairs following minimal destruction of the tissues, the edges of the wound are in close apposition, for example, a surgical incision (Waugh & Grant, 2023) and the healing process is generally unremarkable. The wound edges are normally sterile, there is minimal tissue damage and the wound edges are routinely sutured (Fig. 18.2). Scar formation is typically minimal, but a keloid may develop.

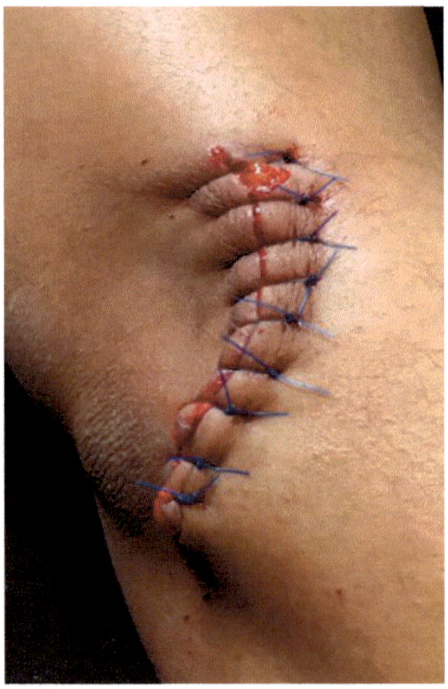

FIGURE 18.2 Wound healing by primary intention.

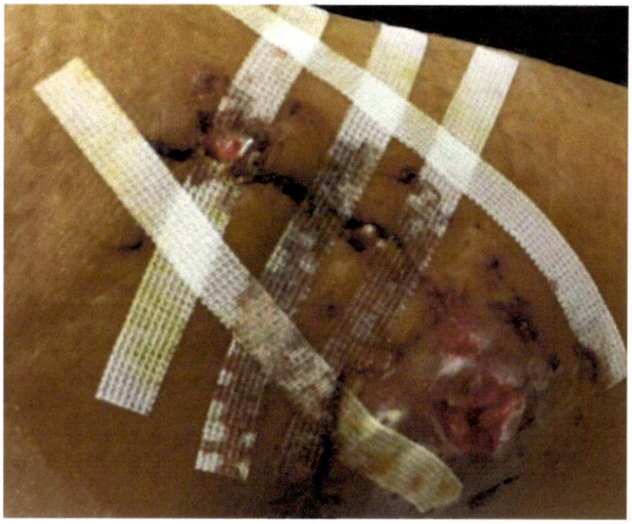

FIGURE 18.3 Healing by secondary intention-infected wound.

Secondary healing (intention)

The wound is left open, so healing can occur spontaneously or the wound may be sutured at a later date. A burn injury, trauma injury, pilonidal sinus, ulcer or infected wounds (Fig. 18.3) are examples of wounds that would be allowed to heal by secondary intention. The cavity fills with granulation tissue, and eventually, closure will be achieved by the formation of a scar. Scars tend to be wider in wounds that heal by secondary intention.

Wound swab

A wound swab will identify the causative organism of infection and will indicate the antibiotic required based on sensitivity. Wound swabs should not be done routinely. Clinical judgement should be exercised to determine the need for the swab, as microbiological assessment alone may not confirm the diagnosis of a wound infection (International Wound Infection Institute, 2022). A holistic assessment of the child and their wound(s) is essential for signs of infection (Bryant and Nix, 2023). Prior to taking a swab, the child's level of pain should be assessed and analgesia administered as prescribed. A detailed explanation of the procedure should be given to the child and parents/carers.

Two techniques are practised when performing a wound swab: the Levine method and the 'Z' technique.

Technique	Description	Considerations
Levine method	The swab should be rotated back and forth over a 1 cm^2 area of the wound. There should be sufficient pressure applied to express fluid from the wound bed. This should be repeated in other areas of the wound if required.	Thought to be more effective than other methods (Copeland-Halperin *et al.*, 2016). More painful for the child as pressure needs to be applied to the wound bed. Excessive pressure may cause trauma to the wound bed.
Z technique	The swab should be moved in a zig-zag pattern across the wound while being gently rotated between the fingers.	More comfortable for the child More risk of contamination when a large area of a wound requires swabbing.

Inflammatory stage

This is a non-specific local reaction to tissue damage as a result of trauma or infection. As an essential part of wound healing, the body's defence mechanism is activated at the time of injury. Vascular and cellular activity is immediately initiated. Vasoconstriction occurs, and this is transient, lasting for 5–10 minutes. This reduces the blood flow and is followed by a release of von Willebrand factor from the platelets and endothelial cells. After this, a fibrin platelet clot is formed. This assists with control of bleeding and is part of the clotting cascade (Deely, 2012). The complement and the kinin systems are triggered by the release of the Hageman factor during the clotting cascade (Marieb & Keller, 2022).

Growth factors are involved in the healing process, and they are released from the platelets. The role of growth factor is to stimulate cell proliferation (Deely, 2012).

The kinin system is activated and kininogen is converted to bradykinin. Dilatation of the microcirculation follows with RBCs, leukocytes (neutrophils), plasma proteins and plasma fluids leaving the microcirculation. They permeate the injured area to cause redness, warmth, oedema and pain (Soley *et al.*, 2018). Following this, neutrophils and monocytes enter the wound and begin to destroy the wound debris. They are attracted to the wound by kinins. Neutrophils squeeze through the capillary walls into the tissues and can be found at the wound site within half an hour of sustaining the injury. Once they have destroyed any bacteria present by phagocytosis, the neutrophils decay, as they are unable to regenerate.

Macrophages will be evident at the injured site, and they will also be involved in digesting the debris and decaying neutrophils, as they have a longer life span than phagocytosis. Oxygen is required for both macrophages and neutrophils to function at their optimum (Barysch & Läuchli, 2020). T lymphocytes migrate to the wound, and their role is to influence the activity of the macrophages. They produce colony-stimulating factor, which encourages the macrophages to produce cytokinins and enzymes.

The activation of the plasma protein leads to the release of histamine, prostaglandins and serotonin from the mast cells. This results in vasodilation and an increase in capillary permeability. Fluid then flows into the injured area, and this is referred to as exudate.

Inflammation will continue for 4–5 days. It requires energy and nutrition. The sensation of pain in the wound is often absent at the time of injury, but once the kinin system becomes activated, pain will be experienced. The presence of prostaglandins, which causes chemical irritation, will also enable the sensation of pain to be felt (Deely, 2012). If the inflammatory stage is prolonged, the risk of hypertrophic scarring is increased. This stage may continue into the proliferation stage.

Proliferation stage

This stage is characterised by the development of granulation tissue. Fibroblasts multiply and migrate across the fibrin strands. This serves as a matrix. Angiogenesis is an essential component of wound healing and is controlled by the action of the chemical mediators, physical factors, the extracellular matrix and metabolic factors (Libby *et al.*, 2024). Endothelial budding occurs on the blood vessels, which are in close proximity, and angiogenesis occurs. These then penetrate and supply nourishment to the injured tissue.

Collagen is synthesised by the fibroblasts on days 2–7 post injury. Macrophages produce various growth factors, including fibroblast growth factor. These then stimulate fibroblasts production, which later divide and produce collagen fibres (Deely, 2012). Type III collagen can be found in the wound in the early stages of wound healing; this will later change to Type I.

Fibroblasts are essential to the proliferation stage of wound healing. They also produce a cellular matrix, which is visible in the wound bed as granulation tissue. The fibroblasts are responsive to the localised oxygen levels. Poor vascularisation will delay wound healing. The surface of the wound will have a low oxygen tension that encourages the macrophages to produce growth factors, and this will initiate the angiogenesis process. Capillary loops are formed from the undamaged capillaries beneath the wound, which form buds that project towards the surface of the wound. Collagen is required for the formation of these capillary loops (Soley *et al.*, 2018). The wound gains tensile strength, and by week 3 post injury, it will have recovered 30% of its pre-injury tensile strength.

The process of contraction is enabled by the role of the fibroblasts and occurs at day 5 post injury. This involves the rearrangement of the extracellular matrix. The exact mechanism is unknown. The surface area of the wound is reduced by the contraction, and this accounts for the closure of a large amount of the cavity wounds. The risk of the contraction process is that it may lead to contracture development from shallow wounds. This process is more apparent in wounds that heal by secondary intention.

The number of macrophages and fibroblasts decreases as the capillary network is formed and the wound fills with granulation tissue.

Maturation/remodelling stage

This is the final stage. The wound's vascularity is reduced, as there is no longer a need to transport cells to the wound site. Collagen fibres undergo a process of lysis and regeneration. They become more organised, align more closely to each other and thus increase tensile strength. This process peaks at 14–21 days. Collagen production slows down, and the wound site matures. Its appearance will change from red, raised and hard to a flat, soft and pale scar. The scar will only ever have a tensile strength of 70–80% of normal tissue.

Complications of wound healing

The majority of wounds heal effectively and within normal time frames. However, healing may be impaired. This can result in:

- Hypertrophic scars – excessive fibrous tissue response leading to excessive collagen being deposited and to a larger scar forming.
- Keloid – excessive fibrous response, may take time to form, more common in children and dark skin. They do not flatten out and need further treatment.
- Contractures – wound contraction that continues after re-epithelialisation has occurred, leading to loss of function, appearance and mobility. Will require additional treatment.
- Acute to chronic wound – delayed healing due to underlying aetiology.

Epidermal stripping

Epidermal stripping is a common form of iatrogenic skin injury in neonates and children. This can be a result of their fragile skin or because of an impaired epidermal barrier. The neonate has attenuated rete ridges, so adhesive products adhere more forcefully to the epidermis (Baranoski & Ayello, 2020). Not only can this lead to an increase in discomfort, but it can also lead to an increase in morbidity. The correct dressing choice must be made, for example, soft silicone to avoid epidermal stripping in the first instance. Once it has occurred, it is necessary to consider how epithelialisation can be promoted, so careful choice of dressing is essential.

Burns

Burns are a common cause of damage to the skin and underlying tissues and can have devastating life-changing consequences for a child and their family. A burn is an injury caused by energy transfer from a heat source to the body (Stylianou *et al.*, 2015). Heat sources may be from thermal, radiation, chemical or electrical sources. A scald is a burn that occurs as a result of steam or liquid coming into contact with the skin.

The severity of the burn injury correlates with the rate of heat transferred to the skin. This also depends on the mechanism of transfer, the duration of transfer of heat and the conductivity of heat through the tissues. When the skin is burnt or scalded, continuity is lost, damage to the stratum corneum will permit entry of micro-organisms and damage to the Langerhans cells will diminish the immune response, making the child susceptible to serious infection. Thus, any burn of size has the ability to make the child seriously ill.

Incidences

The incidence of burns and scalds in the United Kingdom remains high. Approximately 250 000 people will sustain a burn injury per annum in the UK. A significant amount of these will be as a result of thermal injury and scalds. Children aged 1–4 years account for 20% of this total, and 70% of these will be due to scalds. It is estimated that 30 children per day will be seen in A & E in the United Kingdom following a hot drink burn injury (Children's Burns Trust, 2025). Each year, 500 children are admitted to hospital following scalds, with 2000 attending A& E as a result of bath water scalds (Royal Society for the Prevention of Accidents, 2025). Most burns occur in the kitchen in the early evening. Boys are more at risk than girls.

Flame-retardant bed wear and bedding have seen a reduction in the number of burn injuries due to flames. The 5–12-year age group accounts for 10% of the total population of burn injury patients; this is most likely to be a flame injury, often as a result of using an accelerating agent (e.g., lighter fluid and aerosols).

Mechanism of injury

The mechanism of injury will be:

- *Thermal:* scalds, flames or contact heat, e.g., iron or cooker ring
- *Electrical:* domestic electricity, high-tension injury or flash injury
- *Chemical injury*

- *Non-accidental injury:* Three to 10% of burn injuries in infants and children are due to non-accidental injury. These are more common in the under 3 age group. The suspicion of non-accidental burn injury should lead to immediate safeguarding procedures being implemented.

Non-accidental injury should be suspected if the following injury pattern is present:

- Obvious patterns of burn injury from irons, cigarettes and cooker rings
- Burns to genitals, perineum, soles of feet and buttocks
- Uniformity of depth and symmetry
- No splash marks in a scald injury
- Absence of burn injury to flexion creases, as a child may be defending themselves by curling into a foetal position
- 'Doughnut' marks – absence of scald injury to an area that has been in contact with a surface as a result of the child being held down, e.g., in a bath of hot water. There may be an area of unaffected skin, as it was in direct contact with the bath.

The mechanism of injury will determine the treatment required. This may be resuscitation, analgesia, burn treatment and ongoing supportive treatment as indicated by the child's condition.

Classification of burns

The child's survival and outcome are dependent on the following factors: size and depth of burn, age, presence of inhalation injury and comorbidities. Burn injury is classified according to the depth of injury to the skin (Fig. 18.4) and the severity of injury (Table 18.5). The depth of the burn injury is classified in degrees.

Burn depth is related to the temperature of the source of the heat and the duration of contact with that source. The child's thin skin makes it more difficult to assess the depth of burn injury. A burn injury that may appear to be partial thickness may, in fact, be a full-thickness burn. A temperature below 44.4 °C will cause no local damage unless exposure is prolonged, whereas exposure to a temperature of 70.6 °C for less than one second will lead to a third-degree burn in a child. Burns may also be classified as minor, moderate or major. The percentage of injured

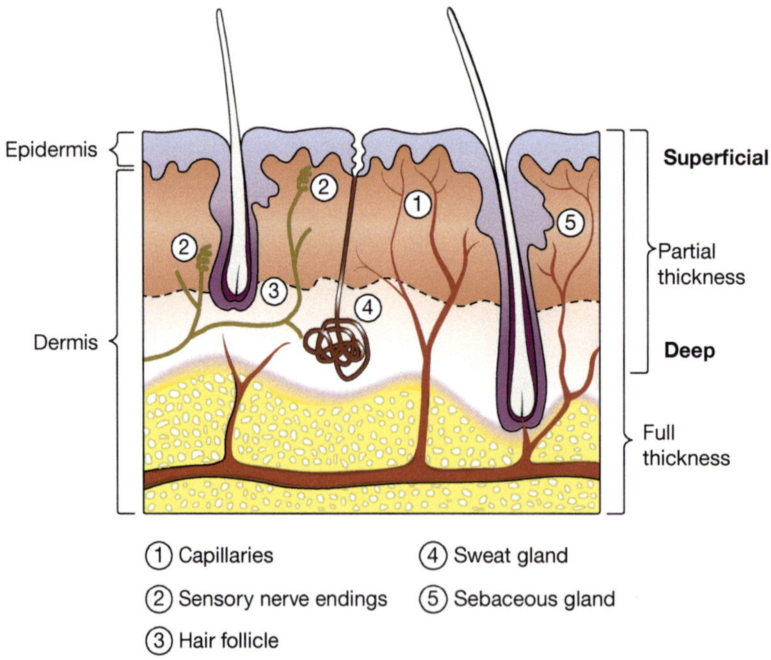

FIGURE 18.4 Degree of burn injury.

TABLE 18.5 Classification of burns and presentation of injury

Classification	Presentation
First degree Superficial	The burn injury only affects the epidermis, the skin will be red, and there are no blisters. An example of a first-degree burn is mild sunburn. Healing will occur in 7–10 days. There will be no scarring.
Second degree Partial thickness	The epidermis and some of the dermal layer will be injured. There will be blistering. Swelling and pain will be present. The appearance will range from pink to red to shiny to pale to mottled. Some of the dermal appendages will remain, and spontaneous epithelialisation will occur.
Third degree Full thickness	The dermis and epidermis are destroyed; underlying structures may also be destroyed, such as the subcutaneous layer. The injured area will appear white or charred. This is the core of the burn-zone of coagulation. Scarring will be significant, and skin grafting required.
Fourth degree	This will involve injury to ligaments, muscles and bones. As nerves will have been destroyed, sensation may be reduced or absent. Scarring and loss of function will be significant. Skin grafting required.

TABLE 18.6 Burn severity classification

Classification	Percentage of TBSA	Description
Minor	10%	First- and second-degree burn
Moderate	10–20% 2–5%	Second-degree burn Third-degree burn not involving ears, eyes, face, hands, feet or genitals. Excludes circumferential burns
Major	20% 5–10%	Second-degree burns Third-degree burns All burns involving face, eyes, hands, ears, feet and genitals All electrical burns Burns with other associated injuries, e.g., fractures, head injuries High-risk groups, e.g., diabetes

and lost skin is reported as total body surface area (TBSA). Burns severity classification is outlined in Table 18.6.

Calculation of the burn injury area

The TBSA is based on the age of the child, as this identifies the changes in body surface area, which alter as the child grows. In the young child, the head constitutes a greater proportion of the surface area compared to the lower limbs. As a rough estimate, the palm of a child's hand with the fingers extended can be considered equal to 1%. The 'rule of 9s' is not appropriate for use in young children, but may be acceptable for use with the child < 10 years of age. The Lund and Browder chart (1944) is a more accurate assessment tool to use for calculating the percentage of burn injury in children (Fig. 18.5).

Pathophysiology of burns

It is important to know the mechanism of burn injury in order to provide the correct treatment and to anticipate the physiological response that may occur.

All burn injuries will result in both a local and systemic response. The physiological reaction to a burn injury is very similar to the inflammatory process.

The intact blood vessels adjacent to the site of the injury dilate; this leads to redness, which will blanch on the application of direct pressure. Leukocytes and platelets adhere to the endothelium. There is an increase in the permeability of the capillaries, which results in oedema. Monocytes and polymorphonuclear leukocytes flood the site of injury. Immature fibroblasts, new capillaries and new collagen fibrils appear within the wound to form granulating tissue (Nettina, 2010).

AGE vs. AREA

Initial Evaluation

UMC.519a, Rev 3.99

Area	Birth–1 year	1–4 year	5–9 year	10–14 year	15 year	Adult	2"	3"	Total	Donor Area
Head	19	17	13	11	9	7				
Neck	2	2	2	2	2	2				
Art. Trunk	13	13	13	13	13	13				
Post. Trunk	13	13	13	13	13	13				
R. Buttock	2½	2½	2½	2½	2½	2½				
L. Buttock	2½	2½	2½	2½	2½	2½				
Genitalia	1	1	1	1	1	1				
R.U.Arm	4	4	4	4	4	4				
L.U.Arm	4	4	4	4	4	4				
R.L.Arm	3	3	3	3	3	3				
L.L.Arm	3	3	3	3	3	3				
R.Hand	2½	2½	2½	2½	2½	2½				
L.Hand	2½	2½	2½	2½	2½	2½				
R.Thigh	5½	6½	8	8½	9	9½				
L.Thigh	5½	6½	8	8½	9	9½				
R.Leg	5	5	5½	6	6½	7				
L.Leg	5	5	5½	6	6½	7				
R.Foot	3½	3½	3½	3½	3½	3½				
L.Foot	3½	3½	3½	3½	3½	3½				
						TOTAL				

Cause of Burn ______________________

Date of Burn ______________________

Time of Burn ______________________

Age ______________________

Sex ______________________

Weight ______________________

Height ______________________

Date of Admission ______________________

Signature ______________________

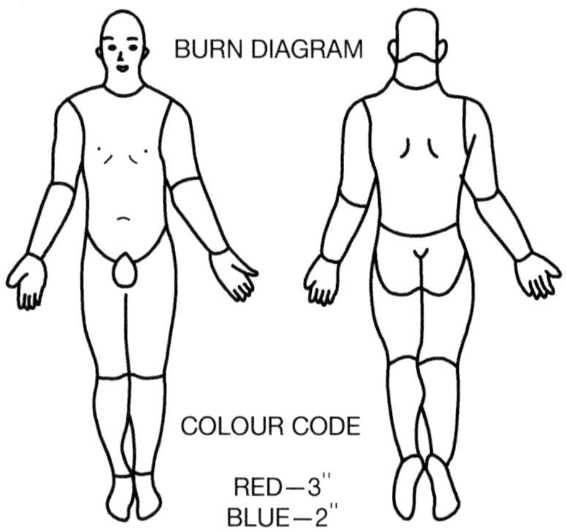

FIGURE 18.5 Chart to determine the extent of burn injury.

Once granulating tissue has begun to form, a skin graft can be placed on the wound.

Local response

There are three zones of burns (Fig. 18.6), and these are evident on the first day after the burn injury. First described by Jackson in 1947 (as cited by Hettiaratchy & Dziewulski, 2004) as:

- zone of coagulation
- zone of stasis
- zone of hyperaemia.

Zone of coagulation

The zone of coagulation is the central zone and has the most contact with the heat source and, therefore, the point of maximum damage. The centre consists of dead cells and damaged tissue. Tissue loss is irreversible as a result of coagulation of the constituent protein, so blood flow is absent. It usually appears white or charred.

Zone of stasis

The zone of stasis is usually red, and there will be decreased tissue perfusion. Balancing may be evident on the application of pressure initially, but this may not persist. Circulation through the superficial blood vessels may cease after a couple of days, leading to further loss of tissue if perfusion is not maintained. One of the aims of burns resuscitation is to increase tissue perfusion to prevent further tissue loss, so any challenge to this has the potential to result in more tissue loss (Zwierello *et al.*, 2023). Prolonged hypotension, oedema and infection will impact the zone of stasis and may lead to extensive tissue loss if not treated. Coagulation occurs, leading to vascular occlusion. Prostaglandins, histamine and bradykinins are the chemical mediators in this progressive vascular occlusion. Oedema occurs as the endothelial cells are altered, as is the basement membrane function, so permeability is increased. If ischaemia persists, the burn will become a full-thickness burn injury.

Zone of hyperaemia

This is the outermost zone and there is increased perfusion to the tissue. As long as this tissue remains free from infection and perfused, the likelihood of recovery is high.

Systemic response

If the burn injury is > 10% of the TBSA, there will be a systemic impact. This will involve the majority of body systems (Fig. 18.7).

Cardiovascular system

Children have almost three times the body surface area to body mass ratio of adults. This has significant implications as fluid loss will be greater in children than in adults, which is a major consideration in the resuscitation process (Suman & Owen, 2020).

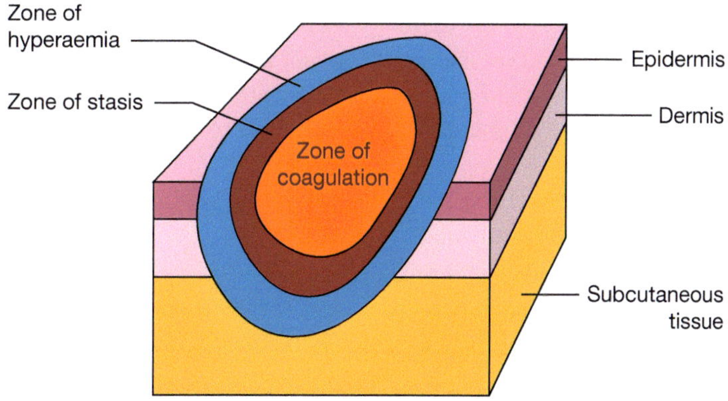

FIGURE 18.6 Jackson's burns zones.

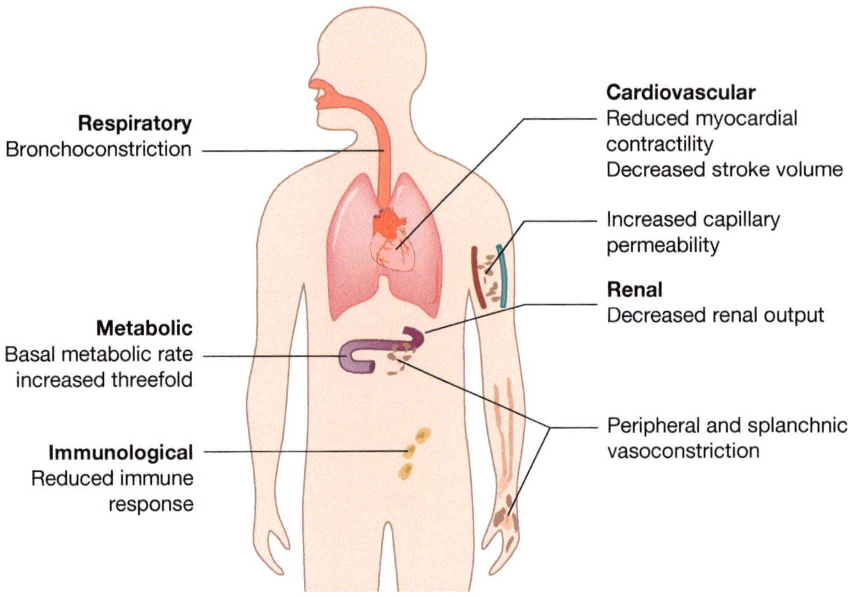

FIGURE 18.7 Systemic impact of burn injury.

A function of the epidermis is to act as a water-vapour barrier. If this is damaged, fluid may be lost from the non-functioning epidermis. The fluid volume deficit is directly proportional to the depth and extent of the burn injury. Capillary permeability is increased, resulting in a loss of intravascular protein and fluid into the interstitial compartments. This occurs in the first 24–36 hours. This protein-rich fluid will ooze from the injured site in the presence of second- and third-degree burns. Recognition and treatment of this fluid loss is essential as the intravascular volume is reduced. Hypovolemic shock will result if it is left untreated.

The protein that is lost to the interstitial space will remain there for a number of weeks before it returns to the intravascular space. When this happens, it will either result in a diuresis in children who have good cardiac and renal functions, or for those who have less than optimal cardiac and renal functions, there is a risk of pulmonary oedema and fluid overload.

Haemoviscosity occurs as a result of the red blood cell (RBC) mass reduced. This is due to the destruction of the RBC from the burn injury, which results in the blood becoming concentrated and fluid leakage from the capillary walls. The haematocrit rises, and the impact of this is a sluggish blood flow. This can result in capillary stasis, leading to tissue necrosis.

Decreased cardiac output occurs as a result of the reduced circulating blood volume. The child will have an increased heart rate. Stroke volume is decreased due to vasoconstriction in the peripheries, leading to a significant increase in peripheral resistance. There is a decrease in the contractility of the myocardium as a result of the release of tumour necrosis factor α. This, together with fluid loss, will lead to systemic hypotension and may result in end-organ hypoperfusion, i.e., renal failure (Zwierello *et al.*, 2023). The body will attempt to compensate for the loss of circulating volume by further constricting vessels and withdrawing fluid from undamaged tissues. This will present as thirst in the patient.

Electrolyte imbalance is probable, and hyponatremia will be present due to fluid shift from the intravascular to the interstitial space. Hyperkalaemia may result from initial cell destruction, but this may change to hypokalaemia as a result of fluid shifting and not being replaced (Pham *et al.*, 2008). Anaemia may result from the destruction of RBCs at the time of injury.

Thermoregulation

Hypothermia is likely because of the large BSA to body mass ratio in children. Children < 2 years of age lose heat more rapidly as they have thinner layers of skin and subcutaneous tissue than older children. In the very young child, thermoregulation is based on nonshivering thermogenesis. As a result, the metabolic rate will be increased, which makes additional demands on oxygen consumption, leading to the production of lactate.

Respiratory system changes

As this chapter is concerned with the skin, inhalation injuries will not be considered. However, the impact of major burn injury will lead to hyperventilation and, therefore, an increase in oxygen consumption. The outcome of this is respiratory alkalosis, which can change to respiratory acidosis due to pulmonary insufficiency. Bronchoconstriction may occur due to the release of inflammatory mediators.

Renal system changes

If blood flow to the renal system is compromised, the impact may be either diuresis or oliguria. Oliguria will result in decreased creatinine clearance. Glomerular filtration may also be decreased. The presence of haemoglobin (Hb) and possibly myoglobin (deep muscle damage) as a result of an electrical burn injury may lead to tubular necrosis. Monitoring of urine output is an essential aspect of nursing care.

Metabolic changes

The release of catecholamine is the primary mediator of the metabolic response in a child with a burn injury. Initially, the greater demand on the metabolic system is due to increased oxygen consumption (Zwierello *et al.*, 2023). Pyrexia is common in the days following a burn injury (moderate and major burns). The healing process also requires energy, so there will be an accelerated demand for glucose. However, total body stores of glucose are limited and glucose stored in the liver and muscles as glycogenesis is quickly exhausted, thus increasing gluconeogenesis in the liver.

Insulin levels decrease and hyperglycaemia ensues shortly after the burn injury. As a result of gluconeogenesis, hyperglycaemia will persist even after insulin levels increase. Protein is mobilised from visceral and skeletal sources. This will attempt to meet the increased demand for nutrition.

Initially, the child's weight may increase post-burn due to adequate fluid resuscitation; however, once the fluid begins to mobilise, weight will reduce, and nutritional support will be required to ensure metabolic demands are met to facilitate the healing process.

Gastrointestinal tract

The sympathetic nervous system response to the burn injury may result in a decrease in peristalsis, leading to vomiting and gastric distension. Gastric ulceration may also occur due to ischaemia of the gastric mucosa (Zwierello *et al.*, 2023).

Immunological system

Sepsis following a burn injury is a major threat to the long-term outcome and survival of the child. Burnt skin is sterile for approximately 24 hours (Marieb & Keller, 2022). Cell-mediated and humoral pathways are affected by alterations in the immune response (Zwierello *et al.*, 2023). The effectiveness of the immune system is reduced after 1–2 days post-burn injury. The removal of the skin as a barrier facilitates bacterial and fungal growth. The abnormal inflammatory responses following a burn injury lead to a reduction in the delivery of oxygen and WBCs to the injured area. Hypoxia, thrombosis and acidosis in the injured area further reduce resistance to pathogenic bacteria. Serum albumin, complement and other immunoglobulins are reduced after the burn injury, as is the number of lymphocytes, which may lead to lymphocytopenia. Susceptibility to fungi, viruses and gram-negative organisms is increased. This can lead to systemic septicaemia, which would require aggressive treatment to prevent loss of life.

Conclusion

Skin conditions can be listed as congenital, acquired through injury, surgery or infection, or as a result of non-accidental injury. Many of the congenital skin conditions will range in severity from life-limiting to minor birthmarks. Burn injury is common in the younger age group, and injury from trauma can also result in significant loss of skin integrity. Whatever the cause, recognition of the systemic impact of loss of skin integrity is of paramount importance when assessing the child. Understanding the physiological changes that occur is essential in enabling the healthcare professional to perform a holistic assessment and in planning appropriate treatment. Supportive care for the child and family is required as is ongoing education to enable self-care or care by family where possible.

References

Afzal, U.M., & Ali, F.R. (2023). Sleep deprivation and the skin. *Clinical and Experimental Dermatology* 48(10), 1113–1116.

Baranoski, S., & Ayello, E.A. (2020). *Wound care essentials: practice principles.* Wolter Kluwer, Philadelphia.

Barysch, M.J., & Läuchli, S. (2020). Oxygen therapy in wound healing. In: Alavi, A. & Maibach, H. (eds). *Local Wound Care for Dermatologists. Updates in Clinical Dermatology.* Cham: Springer.

Bawany, F., Northcott, C.A., Beck, L.A., & Pigeon, W.R. (2021 Apr). Sleep disturbances and atopic dermatitis: relationships, methods for assessment, and therapies. *The Journal of Allergy and Clinical Immunology. In Practice* 9(4), 1488–1500.

British Association of Dermatologist (2024) Mums of babies with eczema sleep less. https://www.bad.org.uk/mums-of-babies-with-eczema-sleep-less/ (accessed 2 April 2025).

British Association of Dermatologists (BAD) (2015). Epidermolysis bullosa simplex. Patient Information Leaflet. Last updated August 2015. Available at: http://www.bad.org.uk/for-the-public/patient-information-leaflets/epidermolysis-bullosa-simplex (accessed April 2018).

British National Formulary for Children (BNFC) (n.d.). [online] Available at: https://bnfc.nice.org.uk/ (accessed 2 April 2025).

Bruckner-Tuderman, L., Eady, R.A., Bauger, E.A., *et al.* (2014). Inherited epidermolysis bullosa: updated recommendations on diagnosis and classification. *Journal of the American Academy of Dermatology* 70(6), 1103–1126.

Bryant, R., & Nix, D. (2023). Acute and chronic wounds: intraprofessionals from novice to expert. In: *Acute and Chronic Wounds Current Management Concepts.* Missouri: Elsevier.

Bumbacea, R.S., Corcea, S.L., Ali, S., *et al.* (2020). Mite allergy and atopic dermatitis: Is there a clear link? (Review). *Experimental and Therapeutic Medicine* 20(4), 3554–3560.

Burns, T., Breathnach, S., Cox, N., & Griffiths, C. (eds) (2004). *Rook's Textbook of Dermatology*, Vol. *1*, 7th edn. Blackwell Science, Oxford.

Carlson, B. (2019). *Human Embryology and Developmental. Biology*, 6th edn. Elsevier, Philadelphia, PA.

Children's Burns Trust (2025). Burns database. Available at: http://www.cbtrust.org.uk/burns-database/ (accessed: 3 April 2025).

Copeland-Halperin, L.R., Kaminsky, A.J., Bluefeld, N., & Miraliakbari, R. (2016). Sample procurement for cultures of infected wounds: a systematic review. *Journal of Wound Care* 25(4), S4–6, S8-10.

Deely, C. (2012). *The Care of Wounds: A Guide for Nurses*, 4th edn. Wiley, Oxford.

Denyer, J. (2010). Wound management for children with epidermolysis bullosa. *Dermatologic Clinics* 28(2), 257–264.

Denyer, J., & Murrell, D.F. (2010). Wound management for children with epidermolysis bullosa: epidermolysis bullosa: part II – diagnosis and management. *Dermatology Clinic* 28, 257–264.

Garten, A., Bellingeri, A., Weir, D., *et al.* (2020). *Strategies to reduce practice variation in wound assessment and management: The T.I.M.E. Clinical Decision Support Tool.* World Union of Wound Healing Societies. Consensus Document.

Genetics Home Reference (2016). Kindler syndrome. [online] Available at: https://ghr.nlm.nih.gov/condition/kindler-syndrome (accessed June 2016).

Hettiaratchy, S., & Dziewulski, P. (2004). ABC of burns: introduction. *British Medical Journal* 328(7453), 1366–1368.

International Wound Infection Institute (2022). *Wound Infection in Clinical Practice. Best Practice*, 3rd edn.

King, A., Stellar, J.J., Blevins, A., & Shah, K.N. (2014). Dressing and products in pediatric wound care. *Advances in Wound Care* 3(4), 324–334.

Libby, J.R., Royce, H., Walker, S.R., & Li, L. (2024). The role of extracellular matrix in angiogenesis: beyond adhesion and structure. *Biomaterials and Biosystems* 15.

Lund, C.C., & Browder, N.C. (1944). The estimation of areas of burns. *Surgery, Gynaecology, Obstetrics* 79, 352–358.

Marieb, E.N., & Keller, S. (2022). *Essentials of Human Anatomy and Physiology*, 13th edn. Pearson Education Ltd, Harlow.

National Institute for Health and Care Excellence (NICE) (2023). Atopic eczema in under 12s: Diagnosis and management. Clinical guideline [CG57]. NICE, London.

National Institute of Arthritis & Musculoskeletal & Skin Diseases (NIAMS) (2013). Epidermolyosis bullosa. [online] Available at: https://www.niams.nih.gov/health-topics/epidermolysis-bullosa (accessed 25 April 2018).

Nettina, N. (ed) (2010). *Lippincott Manual of Nursing Practice*, 9th edn. Wolter Kluwer/Lippincott Williams & Wilkins, Philadelphia.

O'Byrne, N.A., Yuen, F., Butt, W.Z., & Liu, P.Y. (2021). Sleep and circadian regulation of cortisol: A Short review. *Current Opinion in Endocrine and Metabolic Research.* 18, 178–186.

Peate, I., & Gormley-Fleming, E.A. (2025). *Fundamentals of Children's Anatomy and Physiology*, 3rd edn. Wiley, Oxford.

Pham, T.N., Cancio, L.C., Gibran, N.S., & American Burn Association (2008). American Burn Association practice guidelines burn shock resuscitation. *Journal of Burn Care & Research* 29(1), 257–266.

Royal Society for the Prevention of Accidents (2025). Accidents to children. [online]. Available at: https://www.rospa.com/policy/home-safety/advice/accidents-to-children#scalds (accessed 3 April 2025).

Rudolf, M., Lauder, A.J., & K. (2020). *Essential Paediatrics and Child Health*, 4th edn. Wiley Blackwell, Oxford.

Soley, B.S., Horinouchi, C.S.D., Pawloski, P.L., *et al.* (2018). Kinin Receptors in Skin Wound Healing. In: Shiffman, M. & Low, M. (eds). *Chronic Wounds, Wound Dressings and Wound Healing. Recent Clinical Techniques, Results, and Research in Wounds*, Vol. 6. Cham: Springer.

Stylianou, N., Buchan, I., & Dunn, K.W. (2015). A review of the international burn injury database (iBID) for England and Wales: descriptive analysis of burn injuries 2003–2011. *British Medical Journal* 5(2), 1–10.

Suman, A., & Owen, J. (2020). Update on the management of burns in paediatrics. *BJA Education* 20(3), 103–110.

Tenedini, E., Artuso, L., Bernardis, I., *et al.* (2015). Amplicon-based next generation sequencing: an effective approach for the molecular diagnosis of epidermolysis bullosa. *British Journal of Dermatology* 173(3), 731–738.

Visscher, M.O., Adam, R., Brink, S., & Odio, M. (2015). Newborn infant skin: physiology, development, and care. *Clinics in Dermatology* 33, 271–280.

Watson, J. (2016). Diagnosis, treatment and management of epidermolysis bullosa. *British Journal of Nursing* 25(8), 428–431.

Waugh, A., & Grant, A. (2023). *Ross and Wilson Anatomy and Physiology in Health and Illness*, 14th edn. Churchill Livingstone, Edinburgh.

Żwierełło, W., Piorun, K., Skórka-Majewicz, M., *et al.* (2023). Burns: classification, pathophysiology, and treatment: a review. *International Journal of Molecular Sciences* 13, 24(4), 3749.

CHAPTER 19

Mental health difficulties in children and young people

Laura Lowe, Emily Burke, and Gemma Bush

AIM

Increase nursing students' understanding of mental health difficulties in children and young people.

LEARNING OUTCOMES

On completion of this chapter, the reader will be able to:

- Identify children in paediatric settings who might be struggling with their mental health.
- Differentiate between mental health difficulties.
- Begin to understand how to tailor your approach to meet the needs of children and young people who have experienced trauma.
- Understand the basics of communicating with children and young people who are autistic.

KEYWORDS

- mental health
- eating disorders
- neurodiversity
- trauma
- therapeutic approach
- self-harm
- anxiety
- psychosis
- depression
- autism

Test your prior knowledge

1. Which mental health problem is associated with hallucinations?
2. What needs to be considered if a young person is admitted with an eating disorder?
3. Can asking a young person if they are feeling suicidal be beneficial?
4. How might autistic girls differ in presentation from boys?
5. Is medication always the best approach to treat mental health problems?

Introduction

Prioritising the mental health of children and young people is everybody's business. It was estimated in 2023 that 20% of 8–16-year-olds in England were experiencing mental health problems (Newlove-Delgado *et al.*, 2023). Mental and physical health are closely linked and should not be viewed separately. Children and young people with long-term physical illnesses may be more likely to experience a mental health problem due to long-term stress of their illness, social isolation and other factors (Finning *et al.*, 2022). Some mental health problems, such as eating disorders, cause significant physical health problems. Therefore, partnership working between services is essential to meet the holistic needs of CYP (Health and Care Act, 2022). Children's nurses working in all clinical and community settings will encounter children and young people experiencing mental health problems. It is important to recognise when a young person might be struggling and understand a helpful response.

This chapter explores neurodivergence and different mental health challenges that young people can experience. It provides a brief overview of some therapeutic approaches to support children and young people living with mental health problems.

Child and young people's mental health services

Child and Young People's Mental Health Services (CYPMHS) is also known as Child and Adolescent Mental Health Services (CAMHS). CYPMHS are the specialist services working with young people who are experiencing mental health problems.

Diagnoses and formulation

Mental health difficulties and neurodiversity differ from physical health illnesses. Therefore, assessment skills and rating scales are used to try to understand the young person's individual experience rather than invasive tests (see Box 19.1). Sometimes diagnoses may change as understanding increases about what that young person is experiencing. While a diagnosis might help gain clarity about a particular treatment plan, there is debate about whether a formulation is a more helpful approach (Johnstone, 2018). Formulation refers to the process of understanding and exploring what has been going on for that young person and family, which has led to the difficulties they are currently experiencing, as opposed to basing an understanding of their difficulties on a broad diagnostic label.

In a formulation approach, the 4Ps can be used to help understand why a young person is experiencing a crisis at that time, and what might help recovery (see Box 19.1).

Formulation can be used alongside diagnosis, and for some young people and families, a diagnosis can be reassuring. It can help them put a name to what they are experiencing, find alternative support networks (e.g., charities and voluntary organisations) and access particular pathways of treatment. See Box 19.2 for a discussion concerning investigations and assessments associated with children and young people's mental health.

BOX 19.1 The 4 Ps of formulation

Predisposing factors: Factors which increase the likelihood of developing a mental health problem, e.g., family history, trauma.

Precipitating factors: Factors triggering the onset of the current problem, e.g., bullying, death of a family member.

Perpetuating factors: Factors preventing recovery, e.g., ongoing family situation.

Protective factors: Factors which decrease the likelihood of developing a mental health problem, or promote recovery, e.g., a good support network.

Source: Barker (1995).

Nature versus nurture

Often, people wonder if mental health difficulties are a result of nature (e.g., genetics – 'it runs in the family') or nurture (e.g., life experiences). The reason why people experience mental health problems is complex. Studies including family members do indicate that there is a genetic component to some mental health problems (Pettersson *et al.*, 2019). This genetic influence varies between disorders, with some seeming to have a stronger genetic element, but mental health problems are not

BOX 19.2 **Investigations and assessments used with children and young people**

Investigations and assessments in children and young people's mental health

A range of age- and presentation-appropriate assessments, including Routine Outcome Monitoring, can be used with young people. These include:

- Blood tests (e.g., to check for refeeding syndrome or medication levels)
- Physical assessment (e.g., physical observations)
- Strengths and Difficulties Questionnaire (SDQ)
- Children's Global Assessment Scale (CGAS)
- Revised Children's Anxiety and Depression Scale (RCADS)
- Autism Diagnostic Observation Schedule (ADOS)
- The Autism Diagnostic Interview-Revised (ADI-R)

The Child Outcomes Research Consortium (https://www.corc.uk.net/) outline other outcome measures.

solely genetic. It is believed that some young people may have a genetic predisposition to certain mental health problems; factors such as prenatal environment, upbringing, life events and environment influence whether they develop these problems.

The brain and mental health

Mental health problems may be linked to brain chemistry and structure, but it's unclear if these differences cause mental health issues, as symptoms often have multiple contributing factors. The brain is crucial for processing emotions, thoughts and general emotional regulation. Chapter 9 of this text provides further detail regarding the nervous system. As the brain develops throughout adolescence into adulthood, this can affect how young people process and manage emotions.

- **Frontal lobe:** Involved in emotions and problem-solving, not fully developed until the mid-20s, which impacts emotional regulation and impulsivity.
- **Temporal lobe:** Processes sensory information, emotions, memory and language.
- **Parietal lobe:** Processes sensory data, language, and spatial awareness.
- **Occipital lobe:** Responsible for visual processing and memory formation.

Neurotransmitters like serotonin, dopamine and noradrenaline play a role in mood regulation. Imbalances in these chemicals can contribute to mental health issues. While the serotonin theory of depression has been questioned, some medications work to change the levels of neurotransmitters in the brain. Some treatments target neurotransmitter levels, such as antipsychotics and antidepressants.

Development

Age and developmental stage are key when working with children and young people. Developmentally, certain behaviours, like fear of the dark or food preferences, are typical for younger children but may signal stress in older ones. It's important to consider these factors when assessing mental health.

Trauma

Trauma can be a contributing factor to a young person developing mental health problems. Trauma can describe the longer-term impact of a highly distressing event, or series of events, which has made someone feel unsafe, known as adverse childhood experiences. Young people can react differently to distressing events due to factors such as past experiences, emotional resilience and support. Trauma can affect them emotionally, physically and socially, often expressed through behaviour rather than words. Childhood trauma can be linked to later mental health issues, highlighting the importance of appropriate support and trauma-informed healthcare. Some children and young people experience complex trauma. The UK Trauma Council (UKTC) (2022) defines complex trauma as *'traumatic experiences involving multiple events with interpersonal threats during childhood or adolescence'* and young people who experience complex trauma can be at a much greater risk of developing mental health problems.

When working with children and young people who have experienced trauma, it is important to understand trauma-informed care. This involves being compassionate, focusing on the young person's strengths and offering choice to the young person. It is also important to recognise the impact of trauma on how they might be behaving. Staff should think about what practical support could help the young person feel safe (Davies, 2022).

It is essential to establish trust, as the children and young people may struggle to trust adults due to past experiences. Offering choices and control helps counter feelings of powerlessness. For example, when a young person with complex trauma needs a physical examination, explain the process, who will perform it and allow them to stop the examination if uncomfortable. Give them control over how they express discomfort (e.g., verbally/hand signal) and who is in the room, including preferences about the examiner's gender. This approach should be used with all young people, as trauma history may not be known.

It is also vital to care for your own well-being. Working with traumatised children and young people can be challenging, so reflection and supervision are crucial.

Language and mental health

The language used to discuss mental health problems is important as it can help tackle stigma and discrimination around mental health. It is important to use person-first language, e.g., in handover, 'Ed is a young person who hears voices' instead of 'Ed is the psychotic boy in the side room'. Language also impacts how we understand someone. You may hear nurses using phrases such as 'kicking off', but we should understand behaviour as a form of communication and understand that the young person was struggling to manage their emotions or became dysregulated. Similarly, if behaviour is viewed as 'attention seeking', then it can prevent people from trying to understand it. Instead, try to consider why they might have been struggling to talk about their feelings and instead expressed feelings through behaviour.

Activity

You are in handover and hear: *'Beth kicked off after her mum left and she didn't get her own way about having her friend visit. She started headbutting the wall, so security was called. It was a tough evening – she was really attention seeking and kept punching the wall and herself.'*

What was going on for Beth? How could the nurse have used more thoughtful language? What might this handover make other nurses feel about Beth?

Stigma and stereotypes

Stigma still exists around mental health problems and young people may be reluctant to seek help or talk about their experiences for fear of others' reactions. Common stereotypes or stigma around mental health are that individuals are 'dangerous', 'attention seeking' and 'being dramatic'. Some people feel that stigma is worse than their mental health problems (Thornicroft *et al.*, 2022). We can start to tackle stigma by ensuring our language doesn't perpetuate stereotypes, e.g., not describing someone who got angry as 'they went psycho', and challenging stigma or stereotyping of others and ourselves. Try the activity in Box 19.3.

Recovery-focused approach

A recovery-focused approach moves away from a deficit model of illness, which places professionals as the experts. Instead, a recovery approach focuses on the individual's strengths and resilience, understanding that individuals are unique. Through this understanding, we need to

BOX 19.3

Rate on a scale of 1–10 (1 being very comfortable, 10 being very uncomfortable) how comfortable you'd be spending time alone playing cards with a young person with each of the listed mental health problems. Reflect on why you rated it this way – are there stereotypes about the diagnosis, or is it due to lack of experience with it, and what can you do to become more comfortable?

Depression	1	2	3	4	5	6	7	8	9	10
Psychosis	1	2	3	4	5	6	7	8	9	10
Anxiety	1	2	3	4	5	6	7	8	9	10
Eating disorder	1	2	3	4	5	6	7	8	9	10
Autistic	1	2	3	4	5	6	7	8	9	10
Self-harm	1	2	3	4	5	6	7	8	9	10
Suicidal	1	2	3	4	5	6	7	8	9	10

empower young people and families to make choices about treatment and ensure we foster a sense of hope to facilitate recovery. It is important to note that recovery in mental health does not necessarily mean an absence of symptoms, but it might involve managing these symptoms and building on quality of life.

Mental health problems

Self-harm

The National Institute for Health and Care Excellence (NICE) (2022) defines self-harm as 'intentional self-poisoning or injury, irrespective of … purpose'. Prevalence rates vary around self-harm, as often young people do not present to services, but a large-scale study in England estimated that 7.5% of teenagers had self-harmed (Geulayov *et al.*, 2024). Rates have increased over the past 20 years, and more young people self-harm than adults, most commonly girls (Diggins *et al.*, 2024). Self-harm can include cutting, but also head banging, burning, hitting, and other methods.

While self-harm is a risk factor for suicide, not everyone who self-harms is suicidal. The reason people self-harm is highly individual and can include distraction or impulsivity. It can also become quite addictive, with people needing to self-harm more severely to get the same feeling. Professionals should assess risk and create a personalised safety plan.

It is important to listen and be non-judgemental if a young person says that they have self-harmed. Perry *et al.* (2020) found that young people wanted to be included in decisions and not be judged. When caring for a young person who has self-harmed, it is usually unhelpful to ask them to 'promise' not to self-harm again. They might not be able to keep that promise and may feel guilty admitting if they self-harm again. Instead, focus on practical support to help keep them safe for a period of time. This period of time might be small initially, e.g., the next hour. It can be helpful to plan what they can do if they do get the urge to self-harm until it reduces (Hetrick *et al.*, 2020). Box 19.4 provides an overview of strategies that may be helpful.

Depression

Feeling sad or occasionally low in mood is normal, but this is usually not enduring (long-lasting) and does not impact their daily life, so it would not be depression. Depression impacts a young person's ability to engage in their usual activities, and symptoms can include low mood, irritability, sleep and appetite changes, loss of interest in usual activities, lack of energy, struggling to concentrate, thoughts of suicide/self-harm, among other symptoms (Thapar *et al.*, 2022).

Depression is more prevalent in teenagers and may be linked to changes happening in puberty and the increase in societal and relationship expectations. Young people who are experiencing depression cannot simply 'cheer up'. Psychological therapies such as Cognitive Behaviour Therapy (CBT) are the best treatment approach (NICE, 2019).

Suicidal ideation

If a young person feels very low in mood, then they may feel suicidal. Sometimes people worry that if they ask about suicidal thoughts, they will put that idea in their head. However, this is not the case. It is important that you ask a young person about suicidal thoughts, as this gives them the chance to share how they are feeling. If a young person does have suicidal thoughts, ascertain whether they have a plan and what this involves, e.g., if they plan to take an overdose, have they got tablets and do they have a plan of when to do this? Risk assessments are essential for any child or young person who feels suicidal to help keep them safe. This may involve removing potential risks, such as ligature items or unswallowed medication, and ensuring they are not left alone if they are at high risk of acting on impulsive thoughts.

Anxiety

Feeling worried is an emotion that everyone feels and can help keep us safe, as it can warn us that something is unsafe. However, excessive anxiety can stop children and young people from engaging in their day-to-day activities and can cause considerable distress. Anxiety disorders can also be closely linked to other mental health problems, such as obsessive-compulsive disorder (OCD), and many autistic children and young people may also experience anxiety.

Symptoms of anxiety can include physical symptoms like stomach pains, struggling to sleep, a change in appetite and increased heart rate due to the fight, flight or freeze reaction. Other symptoms can include anger or irritability, being clingy, struggling to concentrate, worrying

BOX 19.4 Strategies for a young person who has the urge to self-harm

- Change of environment, e.g., if they self-harm in their bedroom, sit in the lounge.
- Go out in public.
- Write down feelings.
- Distraction (plan individually).
- Breathing exercises.
- Tear up paper – write down their feelings and then tear this up.
- Use their self-soothe box (see Fig. 19.1).

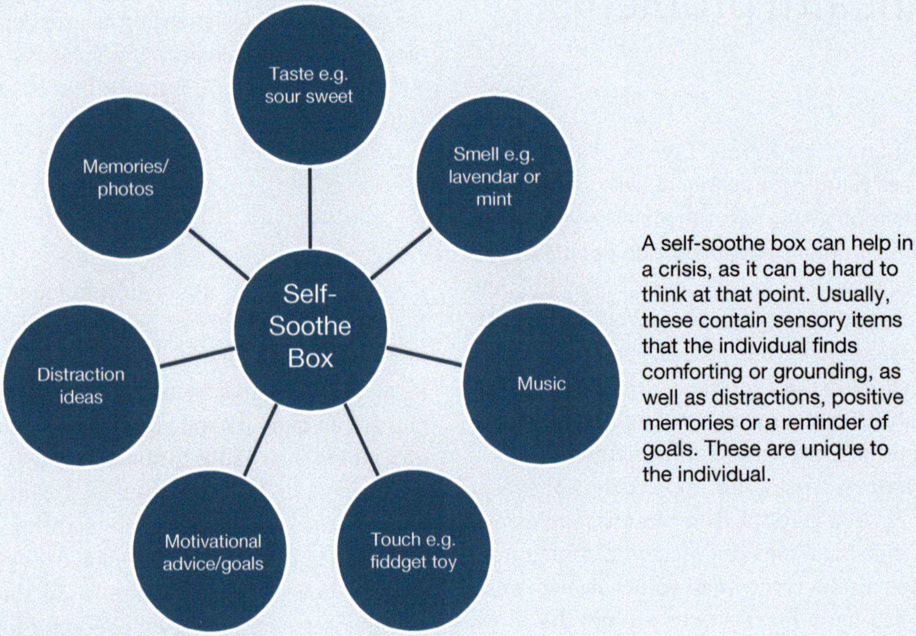

FIGURE 19.1 Self-soothe box.
Source: Adapted from YoungMinds, (2019).

excessively and being tearful (NHS, 2023). Techniques listed in Box 19.8 may help with anxiety, and CBT is a highly effective treatment (Schwartz *et al.*, 2019).

Fight, flight or freeze

When a CYP feels in danger, an innate physiological response occurs, releasing hormones, including cortisol and adrenaline. These cause physiological changes, including increased heart rate, rapid breathing and a heightened sense of alertness. This fight, flight or freeze response is how the body responds to danger as it prepares to fight or escape the danger. Often with anxiety or during a panic attack, there is a perceived threat, e.g., giving a presentation, but the body reacts as it would to a physical threat. So, the young person may want to run away from the situation or feel frozen and unable to participate. Techniques to help with anxiety can be found in Box 19.5.

Psychosis/schizophrenia

Psychosis is when people experience symptoms such as seeing, hearing or feeling things that are not there, these are called hallucinations, or they believe something which is not true, this is called a delusion. Auditory hallucinations are usually voices or sounds that cannot be heard by anyone else, but to the person experiencing them, they sound real. Young people may turn to see who spoke to them or answer the voice. This can make it hard to concentrate on a conversation as they may struggle to differentiate between what is and is not real. Similarly, visual hallucinations feel very real to the person experiencing them, and these are

BOX 19.5 **Techniques to help anxiety (Childline, 2025)**

- When they are calmer, talk about why they felt anxious and try breaking the situation down into smaller chunks to identify the cause and how to tackle this.
- Plan distraction activities in advance that can help to bring them back to the present when they are anxious (called grounding). For example, name 5 things they can see, 4 things they can hear, 3 things they can touch, 2 things they can smell and 1 thing they can taste. Or to look around for 3 items of each colour of the rainbow.
- At the moment of intense anxiety, reassurance that they are safe, and the feelings will pass.

Breathing Exercise

Often, if someone is panicking and highly anxious, they will be breathing too quickly, which can heighten anxiety, so slowing down their breathing is useful.

- For children, encourage them to slowly 'smell the flower' and 'blow out the candle' to calm their breathing.
- You can also encourage them to trace their finger up and down the fingers on their other hand, breathing in as they go up the finger and out as they go down.
- Ask the young person to breathe in through their nose slowly, counting to 3 and breathe out through their mouth slowly, counting to 3.

Activity: Try these breathing exercises.

often frightening. Young people may see scary images, such as someone in the shadows, or blood on the walls.

Some people experience fixed beliefs called delusions. Often persecutory, delusions can make young people feel unsafe – for example, believing they are being followed, or their food is poisoned. Delusions and hallucinations feel very real to the person, so it is unhelpful to deny or confirm them. Instead, acknowledge their experience, focus on helping them feel safe and try distraction techniques. Other symptoms include disorganised thoughts, making communication difficult. Be patient and offer alternative ways to communicate, such as writing or taking extra time to listen.

Reflect

Reflect on what it might feel like to experience hallucinations or delusions.

If you believed that plug sockets were being used to spy on you and your family was in danger, or if you believed the nurse doing a blood test was actually taking it for sinister reasons, how might you behave and feel?

Obsessive-compulsive disorder (OCD)

OCD affects approximately 1–2% of the population. It involves repetitive, distressing and intrusive thoughts (obsessions), and repetitive acts (compulsions) that temporarily reduce the anxiety or distress associated with the obsession. Obsessions differ between individuals and can change over time. Common themes include: a fear of something bad happening; intrusive thoughts about causing harm (*harm OCD*); persistent distressing doubts about relationships (*relationship OCD*); disturbing thoughts around religion/morality (*scrupulosity*); unwanted sexual thoughts causing feelings of disgust/guilt; and worries about germs (*contamination OCD*) (OCD UK, 2025).

Compulsions serve to neutralise thoughts and temporarily reduce anxiety. Common compulsions include thinking of a neutralising thought to counteract what their intrusive thought was; repeatedly checking bodily sensations; praying; mental acts, e.g., counting; cleaning or washing; hoarding; checking; tapping; and re-ordering. Compulsions are time-consuming and significantly interfere with life. CBT, exposure and response prevention therapy and medication are effective treatment options for OCD (NICE, 2005). Children should initially be offered psychological input.

Attention-deficit hyperactivity disorder (ADHD)

ADHD is a neurodevelopmental condition that affects hyperactivity, inattention and impulsivity. The DSM-5 (Diagnostic and Statistical Manual) lists three subtypes of ADHD – predominantly inattentive, predominantly hyperactive–impulsive and combined type. Symptoms must be present before 12 years and across multiple settings, such as home and school (American Psychiatric Association [APA], 2013).

Neurodiversity describes the natural variation of human brains. Neurodivergence refers to where someone's brain differs from what is considered 'typical', e.g., autism, ADHD, dyslexia, dyspraxia and OCD.

Approximately 5% of children have ADHD (NICE, 2024a), though girls are less likely to be diagnosed. Research suggests that girls are more likely to present with predominantly inattentive symptoms, such as daydreaming or internal restlessness, which are less

BOX 19.6 **Symptoms of ADHD**

- Difficulty sustaining attention
- Forgetfulness and losing things
- Difficulty staying organised
- Avoidance of tasks requiring sustained mental effort
- Easily distracted
- Frequent mistakes
- Difficulty following through on instructions
- Appearing fidgety
- Restlessness
- Difficulty playing quietly
- Excessive talkativeness
- Appearing to be 'driven by a motor'
- Often interrupting others
- Difficulty taking turns

Source: APA (2013)/with permission of the American Psychological Association.

visible. Diagnostic overshadowing, where symptoms are incorrectly attributed to another condition, is more common in girls (Martin, 2024).

Emotional dysregulation is very common in ADHD (van Stralen, 2016). Children with ADHD tend to struggle to regulate their emotions, so they can become overwhelmed quickly and react without thinking. Additionally, adolescents with ADHD are more likely to struggle with their mental health (Gnanavel *et al.*, 2019). See Box 19.6 for an overview of ADHD symptoms.

There can be an increased risk of accidental injury amongst children with ADHD, due to impulsivity and inattention (Ruiz-Goikoetxea *et al.*, 2018). Children with ADHD can be supported with strategies and environmental adaptations, for example, using fidget toys or movement breaks during appointments. They may need questions repeated or prompting to follow through on tasks.

ADHD medication may be prescribed where ADHD has a moderate to severe impact and if clinically indicated. There are two main types – stimulant medication and non-stimulant medication. Common side effects include appetite suppression and increased heart rate or blood pressure (or postural hypotension with Guanfacine) (NICE, 2018). If the child or family members have any new heart-related concerns, the prescriber should be informed.

Autism

Autism is a neurodevelopmental condition that impacts how an individual experiences, interacts and responds to the world around them. It is not a learning disability, though some people with a learning disability are also autistic (NHS, 2022).

Autistic people may communicate or interact differently (e.g., literal interpretation of language), have intense interests, find change or uncertainty difficult, have sensory sensitivities or sensory-seeking behaviour and find repetitive movements (stimming) self-regulating. Autistic children can find the world overwhelming and require additional support to navigate it (see Box 19.7). Every autistic person is different, and their needs will fluctuate depending on their environment and circumstances, but the following are usually helpful.

Official statistics state that 1 in 100 people are autistic (World Health Organization, 2023). However, statistics vary: US figures report 1 in 36 (Centers for Disease Control and Prevention [CDC], 2024) and Northern Ireland 1 in 20 (Autism Northern Ireland, 2023). Girls are less likely to receive a diagnosis than boys for various reasons. Their special interests tend to be more socially acceptable, diagnostic overshadowing/misdiagnosis, meaning that autistic traits are explained as symptoms of another condition; girls tend to mask their difficulties more, and girls may portray fewer repetitive behaviours. Autistic girls typically experience high levels of anxiety and may appear perfectionistic or rigid in their thinking. They may struggle

BOX 19.7 **Interventions that may help an autistic child**

- Clear, direct language
- Visual supports, e.g., visual timetables
- Social stories™ (Gray, 2015)
- Communication cards
- Advance notice of change
- Structure and routine (consider this with appointments)
- Preparation for transitions
- Consideration of the sensory environment
- Ear defenders/headphones
- Access to a quiet space
- Fidget toys

Source: NICE (2013) and Berkshire Healthcare (2025).

with their emotions more than peers and may find social situations and friendships challenging (Autistic Girls Network, 2022).

Links to other mental health problems and misdiagnoses

Autism and ADHD have historically been misunderstood. Childhood ADHD has only been recognised in the NICE guidelines since 2000 (entering the DSM in 1968 as 'Hyperkinetic Reaction of Childhood'), and autism was only introduced into the DSM in 1980 as 'Infantile Autism', so these diagnoses are relatively new (Lange *et al.*, 2010; Rosen *et al.*, 2021). Misdiagnosis continues to occur; for example, emotional dysregulation and anxiety may be seen as symptoms of a personality disorder. 25% of autistic patients felt they had been misdiagnosed prior to their autism diagnosis and 17.9% autistic women felt they had been misdiagnosed with a personality disorder (Kentrou *et al.*, 2024).

Autistic/ADHD people do develop certain conditions more frequently than others. These include Developmental Coordination Disorder (also known as Dyspraxia), gastrointestinal problems, anxiety disorders, epilepsy, eating disorders and sleep disorders.

Pathological demand avoidance

Pathological Demand Avoidance (PDA) is understood to be a profile within autism, in which a person avoids everyday demands to an extreme degree due to associated anxiety (National Autistic Society, 2025). Demands can be indirect, including questions, decisions, expectations or bodily demands such as hunger. Individuals may use strategies, including diversion techniques, to avoid the demand, may experience excessive mood swings and appear controlling (PDA Society, 2022).

PDA does not appear in diagnostic manuals or NICE Guidelines, so recognition of it varies. Where a child presents with a demand avoidant profile, the PDA Society (n.d.) advises that reframing/disguising requests or demands, anxiety management, negotiation and collaboration can help.

Emotionally based school avoidance

Emotionally Based School Avoidance (EBSA) describes children who face extreme distress and anxiety around school, usually resulting in prolonged school absence. This impacts around 1–5% of school children to varying degrees (Elliot & Place, 2019) and affects both genders. Neurodivergent children are overwhelmingly affected by EBSA. 92.1% of those with persistent school attendance difficulties were neurodivergent and 83.4% were autistic (Connolly *et al.*, 2023). Rather than viewing school distress as a problem with the child, the systemic failure of the education system to meet the needs of that child should be considered.

Further approaches that may help neurodivergent children and families

A needs-led approach is increasingly being implemented to support neurodivergent children and families. This approach identifies and supports a child's needs irrespective of a diagnosis (Coady *et al.*, 2024). For children with additional needs, reasonable adjustments should be made (Equality Act, 2010). This may include longer or differently timed appointments, quieter waiting areas and using visual aids.

My experience (anonymous)

I was sectioned (under the Mental Health Act) on a CAMHS unit. They diagnosed me with Emotionally Unstable Personality Disorder and anxiety, but I'm autistic and have ADHD, I just wasn't diagnosed then.

I remember feeling very scared and overwhelmed. I struggled meeting new staff, not knowing the timetable and the unpredictability of the environment. It felt very busy and loud, and I didn't always feel safe with new staff on shift.

When staff were patient and got to know me, this helped. Sometimes they talked to me about my interests, or their pets and I felt more comfortable and would open up to them. When they approached me with compassion and understood that I was trying my hardest even if it didn't look like it, this helped me. When they prepared me for changes to routine and explained what to expect (like in ward round), this reduced my meltdowns and anxiety. They also encouraged me to write down my feelings and gave me questions in advance of ward round. This helped me to communicate my needs.

Eating disorders

People experiencing an eating disorder can have a fear of gaining weight or might avoid particular foods or may need to eat food in a particular way. Treatment approaches will be specific to individual needs, so a full assessment is essential. Working with children and young people experiencing eating disorders is complex and requires excellent communication skills. Anyone can develop an eating disorder, regardless of age or gender, but eating disorders are generally more prevalent in teenagers, particularly girls. It is estimated that up to 4% of females and 0.3% of males will experience anorexia nervosa, and approximately 3% of females and 1% of males will experience bulimia nervosa (van Eeden *et al.*, 2021). Boys do develop eating disorders, but as these are typically seen as female disorders, it can take longer for them to receive support.

Anorexia nervosa

With anorexia nervosa, young people restrict their intake to lose weight. Anorexia nervosa often begins subtly, with young people gradually cutting out foods like carbohydrates or fatty foods. Over time, this can extend to most foods. Eating can cause intense distress, with feelings of guilt, shame and anxiety. Distressing feelings and a drive to burn calories can lead to compensatory behaviours like over-exercising, vomiting or misuse of laxatives. These actions may feel out of control and can seriously impact physical and mental health. Eating disorder behaviours are often hidden, so changes may go unnoticed initially. Young people might eat alone, hide food and avoid social eating. Some young people may obsess over weighing themselves multiple times a day, while others avoid it entirely.

Anorexia can affect cognitive functioning, leading to difficulty processing information, concentrating, irritability and rigid thinking, especially around food. They may also develop a strong focus on food-related activities, like baking or watching cooking shows, but restrict their own eating. Mealtimes can be challenging for families (St. Pe *et al.*, 2025), with children and young people refusing to eat. This can lead to significant tension, and parents often feel very anxious about how to manage mealtimes.

Physical symptoms (Box 19.6) such as gastrointestinal issues, muscle weakness and amenorrhoea (lack of menstruation) can occur, and anorexia has the highest mortality rate of mental health problems (NICE, 2024b). This is due to physical complications, significant weight loss and electrolyte imbalances (through vomiting or excessive laxative use), but also an increased risk of suicide.

Bulimia nervosa

Bulimia nervosa involves recurrent episodes of uncontrollable binge eating followed by compensatory behaviours to prevent weight gain. A binge eating episode is a compulsion to eat large quantities of food in a short period of time, and often this feels out of control and might be done mindlessly. These episodes often lead to feelings of distress and shame, which lead to compensatory behaviours, most commonly vomiting, but can include restricted eating and excessive exercise. Usually, young people with bulimia will have concerns about their shape or weight, and it is not uncommon for a young person to go on to develop bulimia nervosa after a period of anorexia nervosa, or vice versa.

During an eating disorder assessment, the binge-eating episodes and frequency of the binge-purge cycle are important to assess. More frequent binge-purge cycles can result in more serious physical complications, such as damage to the oesophagus, damaged tooth enamel and an imbalance of electrolytes, which, if severe, can cause cardiac arrest. They may also be at higher risk of self-harm and suicide (Wade, 2019), and, therefore, a thorough risk assessment is vital.

Avoidant restrictive food intake disorder

Avoidant restrictive food Intake disorder (ARFID) is characterised by:

1. Apparent lack of interest in food.
2. Fears of eating certain foods.
3. Sensory avoidance around food, e.g., texture.

ARFID is not 'picky eating'; they may be fearful of trying anything other than their 'safe' foods, and it is highly linked to Autism (Keski-Rahkonen & Ruusunen, 2023). While ARFID may result in weight loss or lack of weight gain, unlike anorexia or bulimia, children do not usually present with weight or shape concerns. Treatment approaches focus on family-based interventions and cognitive behavioural therapy (Marino *et al.*, 2024) to help them gradually expand the range of foods.

Treatment approaches in eating disorders

The treatment approach must be tailored to the type of eating disorder that a child or young person is experiencing. In outpatient services, the Maudsley Method (Le Grange, 2005) or family-based treatment approach (Lock and Le Grange, 2005) is advised for anorexia nervosa (NICE, 2020).

The Maudsley Model includes three phases:

1. **Weight restoration** – psychoeducation and supporting parents to take control of their child's eating with the aim of weight restoration.
2. **Returning control of eating** – slowly shifting responsibility for eating back to the child (age appropriately).
3. **Establishing a healthy identity** – age-appropriate independence and asserting healthy parental boundaries.

In inpatient services, staff usually take responsibility for eating, and over time, the responsibility is passed back to the family and young person in preparation for discharge (Hage *et al.*, 2015). Ideally, staff offer pre-meal support, which might involve deciding the meal (within parameters) and establishing boundaries around eating. Staff should offer support during the meal, such as encouragement to eat healthily, e.g., not smearing food, not hiding food. Support during the meal should not involve negotiation about food, as the focus should be on eating. Usually, meals have a clear time boundary, e.g., 45 minutes and a plan of what happens if they have not finished. This may allow the young person to feel safe to eat. Post-meal support is also essential as young people may feel distressed after, so support can enable the young person to talk through feelings.

Working with young people experiencing eating disorders can bring up challenging feelings in staff, and the risk of burnout can be high. So staff need to have opportunities to talk about their feelings in supervision

Case Study 19.1 Depression and anger

Dominic, 14 years old, the only child of Sandra. His Dad died in a motorbike accident when he was 2 years old, and his Mum has not had a relationship since. Dominic does not remember his Dad but has a good relationship with his grandparents and is close with his extended family. His maternal grandma moved in with them following the death of his Dad and lived with them for a while to support Dominic and his Mum. Dominic has a large extended family, and he used to see them all regularly.

Dominic has struggled in school from Reception onwards, often becoming angry and saying the work was too hard. He was diagnosed with dyslexia at 6 years old and received support. This helped; he engaged in primary school but found the transition to secondary school difficult. He became more disengaged with school when he transferred schools at 11 years old, saying he 'felt dumb' and started to get into trouble at school. He managed to go to school 2–3 days a week, but over the last year, he has refused to go more often, staying in his room, refusing to get up. His Mum says she feels powerless to help as he becomes aggressive and angry, punching the wall.

Dominic has always had a poor sleep routine, waking up at night and not falling asleep until 11 p.m. In the last year, he has particularly struggled to sleep at night, instead staying up late playing video games. His Mum has tried to get him into a better sleep routine, but he becomes angry and has threatened to kill himself when she removes his gaming system. His grandparents do offer support, and he has stayed overnight at both sets of grandparents on occasion.

He loves sports and used to compete in judo and rugby, but has not attended his clubs for the last few months as he 'can't be bothered'. His coaches are supportive and keen to have him back in the clubs. He has maintained contact with his friends and Snapchats and while gaming.

His mum took him to the GP a few months ago due to concerns about his mental health after he punched a wall in anger when she tried to get him to go to school. Dominic had become distressed, and he hurt his hand when he punched the wall. He said he felt like he could not control his anger, and he wanted to feel happy again, but felt this was not possible. The GP met with Dominic and diagnosed depression. She spoke to his school to refer him to a CYPMHS mental health support team that works with schools to help him get back into school more regularly and for support around his mood and anger.

Dominic did engage with the mental health support team and attended one-to-one support as well as a group focusing on anger management. His mood is still low, but slowly he is starting to see an improvement. He has regularly gone to school 3 days a week for the last month. This is his best attendance in years. School is working with him to gradually increase the time he has in school, and Dominic has said his aim is to go back to his rugby club next season. He plans to go back to Judo next month. He has learnt some techniques for managing when he feels angry and is starting to recognise when he feels anger building up and what he can do to manage that. He finds fidget toys helpful, and playing basketball helps him calm down. School and mum have supported this.

(Bommen *et al.*, 2023). Staff feelings can include frustration, anger and feeling stuck, which often reflects how that young person is feeling. Naming how hard it must be to eat and drink can be helpful in validating the experience for the young person. Sharing personal struggles with eating is not usually helpful, as it moves the focus away from the young person. Support and compassion towards the young person and family are crucial.

Other areas to consider when working with young people with an eating disorder

If a young person vomits as a compensatory behaviour, then ensuring someone is with them after eating can be useful to reduce the chance of vomiting. In addition, it is important that electrolyte levels are monitored as these can become imbalanced due to repeated vomiting or overuse of laxatives.

In treatment, it may be helpful to view the eating disorder as separate from the young person, recognising it as a controlling force rather than part of their personality. Staff should support the young person's autonomy, helping them challenge the eating disorder and work towards goals like returning to school, with support from staff and family.

If a young person is unable to eat or drink enough, then, depending on risk, they may need to be fed via a nasogastric tube. However, this should be a last resort. If a young person does not consent to a nasogastric tube, then the Mental Health Act, 1983 may need to be used so that they can be treated, but this should not be a common occurrence, as it is always better to work collaboratively with a young person.

The appropriate use of language is important when working with a young person with an eating disorder, as they may feel guilty for eating. The use of praise is often unhelpful (see Box 19.8).

Reflection

You are supporting James, 14 years old, to eat lunch. He has anorexia nervosa, was admitted 4 days ago and continues to lose weight (2 kg since admission). James is awaiting transfer to an eating disorders unit. He says he cannot eat lunch and appears tearful.

What might you say to James?

BOX 19.8 Helpful and unhelpful phrases when working with young people with eating disorders

Helpful phrases

- I can see how hard you're working.
- It's our decision that you eat this food.
- You have to eat this; there's no choice (if this is the clinical decision).
- I know it's not easy, keep going.

Unhelpful phrases

- Well done for eating everything!
- You don't have to eat it all.
- I wish I had your willpower!
- If you eat one more bite, you can exercise.
- You're looking healthy.
- I want to lose weight.
- I eat clean foods.
- I had an eating disorder.

Source: Adapted from Beat (2025).

The Medical Emergencies in Eating Disorders Guidance (MEED)

The MEED (Medical Emergencies in Eating Disorders) Guidance (Royal College of Psychiatrists, 2023) is an important tool in the management and assessment of risk in eating disorders. It is used by medical practitioners who encounter a person experiencing an eating disorder in their clinical setting and outlines a risk rating of red, amber and green, based on the assessment of physical and mental health symptoms. The MEED guidance must be considered when a young person presents with an eating disorder, and the risk checklist can be found in Box 19.9.

Refeeding syndrome

This is a dangerous condition that can affect young people with eating disorders, where there has been a period of starvation. syndrome can occur when food and nutrition are reintroduced too quickly. Changes in electrolytes (drop in potassium, magnesium and phosphate in particular) and fluid within the body can cause dangerous

BOX 19.9 MEED risk checklist for clinicians (Royal College of Psychiatrists, 2023)

Appendix 3: Medical emergencies in eating disorders risk checklist for clinicians

Assessing

Does the patient have an eating disorder?

Yes: Anorexia nervosa- Bulimia nervosa- Other

Not sure: **Request psychiatric review**

Is the patient medically compromised?

- ☐ BMI <13 (adults); m%BMI <70% (under 18)?
- ☐ Recent loss of >1kg for 2 consecutive weeks?
- ☐ Acute food or fluid refusal/intake <400kcal per day?
- ☐ Pulse <40?
- ☐ BP low, BP postural drop >20mm, dizziness?
- ☐ Core temperature <35.5°C?
- ☐ Na <130mmol/L?
- ☐ K <3.0mmol/L?
- ☐ Raised transaminase?
- ☐ Glucose <3mmol/L?
- ☐ Raised urea or creatinine?
- ☐ Abnormal ECG?
- ☐ Suicidal thoughts, behaviours?

Is the patient consenting to treatment?

Yes:

No: Mental health assessment requested

Refeeding

High risk for refeeding syndrome?

- ☐ Low initial electrolytes
- ☐ BMI <13 (adults) or %mBMI <70% (under 18s)
- ☐ Little or no intake for >4 days
- ☐ Low WBC
- ☐ Serious medical comorbidities, e.g. sepsis

High risk? Management:

- **<20 kcal per kg per day**
- **Monitor electrolytes twice daily**
- **build up calories swiftly**
- **avoid underfeeding**

Lower risk? Management:

- **Start at 1,400–2,000kcal per day (50 kcal/kg/day) and build by 200 kcal/day, to 2,400kcal/day or more**
- **Aim for weight increase of 0.5–1kg/week**
- **Avoid underfeeding**

Monitoring

- ☐ Electrolytes (especially P, K, glucose)
- ☐ ECG
- ☐ Vital signs
- ☐ BMI

Managing

Are medical and psychiatric staff collaborating in care?

Yes:

No: Psych. consultation awaited

Are nurses trained in managing medical and psychiatric problems?

Yes

No and appropriately skilled staff requested/training in place

Are there behaviours increasing risk?

- ☐ Falsifying weight
- ☐ Disposing of feed
- ☐ Exercising
- ☐ Self-harm, suicidality
- ☐ Family to stress/anxiety
- ☐ Safeguarding concerns

Mobilise psychiatric team to advise on management

Note:
%mBMI = mean percentage BMI

Please do not use BMI as a single indicator of risk

Source: The Royal College of Psychiatrists/The Royal College of Psychiatrists.

complications and can lead to seizures and heart failure. Close monitoring of bloods and physical observations are crucial (Royal College of Psychiatrists, 2023), and meal plans should be slowly increased. Even if the person wants to, they should not be allowed to eat more than their agreed meal plan, particularly in the first week of treatment, as it is essential that blood tests are reviewed for signs of refeeding syndrome prior to any increase in calories.

Refeeding syndrome

- Blood results show a drop in or low levels of phosphate (< 0.32 mmol/L), potassium (< 2.5 mmol/L) and magnesium (< 0.5 mmol/L)
- Oedema due to water and salt retention
- Extreme fatigue and weakness
- Confusion
- Seizures
- Heart failure

Other symptoms of eating disorders (Box 19.10).

Box 19.11 provides some information to consider when working with young people who are experiencing challenges with their mental health.

BOX 19.10 Helpful things to remember when working with young people experiencing mental health problems

A young person with an eating disorder may experience different physical health symptoms depending on their presentation. Most can be corrected with treatment.

- Weight loss – (significantly low against expected weight for height, recent weight loss of more than 1 kg a week for 2 weeks, or any rapid weight loss at any weight)
- Cognitive impairment – slow speech, poor memory recall, confusion

- Peripheral coldness due to inhibited circulation
- Postural hypotension
- Low blood pressure
- Low blood glucose
- Irregular periods/amenorrhea
- Bone density concerns
- Lanugo hair – fine hair on the body
- Losing hair, brittle nails and dull skin
- Constipation and stomach pain
- Muscle weakness
- Lack of expected growth
- Damage to tooth enamel, abrasions on knuckles (due to vomiting)
- Depletions in electrolytes such as potassium and sodium due to vomiting

Conclusion

Anyone can experience a mental health problem so you may meet children and young people in any area of your placement or future practice who are struggling with their mental health. It is important to be non-judgemental and empathetic in your approach, always considering your use of language. It is also important to look after your own mental health and ensure that you make use of supervision to ensure that you can be as effective as possible.

BOX 19.11 **Guidance related to young people who are experiencing challenges with their mental health**

Dos and Don'ts when working with young people experiencing mental health problems

Dos

- Take time to get to know the young person, not just their diagnosis.
- Talk about everyday things to put young people at ease.
- Be playful – play games, watch TV together, you do not have to be task-oriented.
- Share 'safe' information about yourself, e.g., pets, TV shows, hobbies, to help make a connection.
- Listen to the expertise of the family and young person – they know them best.
- Consider the young person's lived experience to avoid re-traumatising them.

Don'ts

- Don't avoid difficult questions or conversations.
- Don't feel the need to give answers or fill gaps in conversations, listening and letting the young person speak is important and silence is okay.
- Don't make promises that you can't keep, e.g., when they will be discharged.
- Don't forget to maintain professional boundaries and don't encourage an exclusive relationship.

References

American Psychiatric Association (2013). *Diagnostic and Statistical Manual of Mental Disorders*, 5th edn. American Psychiatric Association.

Autism Northern Ireland (2023). *Statistics.* https://autismni.org/what-is-autism/statistics (accessed 10 December 2024).

Autistic Girls Network (2022). *Autism, girls, & keeping it all inside.* https://autisticgirlsnetwork.org/keeping-it-all-inside.pdf (accessed 10 December 2024).

Barker, P. (1995). *The child and adolescent psychiatry evaluation: basic child psychiatry.* Blackwell Scientific, Inc, Oxford.

BEAT Eating Disorders (2025). *Tips for supporting somebody with an eating disorder.* https://www.beateatingdisorders.org.uk/get-information-and-support/support-someone-else/tips-for-supporting-somebody-with-an-eating-disorder/ (accessed 14 January 2025).

Berkshire Healthcare (2025) *Communication, sensory needs, emotions and behaviour.* https://www.berkshirehealthcare.nhs.uk/advice/adhd-and-autism/communication-sensory-needs-emotions-and-behaviour (accessed 22 January 2025).

Bommen, S., Nicholls, H., & Billings, J. (2023). Helper' or 'punisher'? A qualitative study exploring staff experiences of treating severe and complex eating disorder presentations in inpatient settings. *Journal of Eating Disorders* 11, 216 https://doi.org/10.1186/s40337-023-00938-1.

Centers for Disease Control and Prevention (2024). Prevalence and characteristics of autism spectrum disorder among children aged 8 years. *Surveillance Summaries* 72(2), 1–14 https://doi.org/10.15585/mmwr.ss7202a1.

Childline (2025). *Calm Zone.* https://www.childline.org.uk/toolbox/calm-zone/

Coady, C., Macqueen Black, G., Joseph, N. & Domakin, A. (2024). Using a needs-led eligibility framework to provide services to disabled children and their families. Council of Disabled Children and Research in Practice.

Connolly, S., Constable, H., & Mullally, S. (2023). School distress and the school attendance crisis: a story dominated by neurodivergence and unmet need. *Frontiers in Psychiatry* 14. https://doi.org/10.3389/fpsyt.2023.1237052.

Davies, J.A. (2022). Supporting children's nurses to deliver trauma-informed care. *Nursing Children and Young People* https://doi.org/10.7748/ncyp.2022.e1422.

Diggins, E., Heuvelman, H., Pujades-Rodriguez, M., *et al.* (2024). Exploring gender differences in risk factors for self-harm in adolescents using data from the Millennium Cohort Study. *Journal of Affective Disorders* 345, 131–140.

van Eeden, A.E., van Hoeken, D., & Hoek, H.W. (2021). Incidence, prevalence and mortality of anorexia nervosa and bulimia nervosa. *Current Opinion in Psychiatry* 34(6), 515–524 https://doi.org/10.1097/YCO.0000000000000739.

Elliot, J.G., & Place, M. (2019). Practitioner review: school refusal: developments in conceptualisation and treatment since 2000. *Journal of Child Psychology and Psychiatry* 60(1), 4–15 https://doi.org/10.1111/jcpp.12848.

Finning, K., Neochoriti Varvarrigou, I., Ford, T., *et al.* (2022). Mental health and school absenteeism in children with long-term physical conditions: a secondary analysis of the British Child and Adolescent Mental Health Surveys 2004 and 2007. *Child: Care, Health and Development* 48(1), 110–119.

Francesca, A.S.P., Stevens, K.S., Odar Stough, C.C., *et al.* (2025). Mealtime challenges from the perspectives of adolescents with anorexia nervosa and atypical anorexia nervosa and their caregivers enrolled in family-based treatment. *Eating Behaviors* 56 https://doi.org/10.1016/j.eatbeh.2025.101947.

Geulayov, G., Mansfield, K., Jindra, C., *et al.* (2024). Loneliness and self-harm in adolescents during the first national COVID-19 lockdown: results from a survey of 10,000 secondary school pupils in England. *Current Psychology* 43(15), 14063–11407.

Gnanavel, S., Sharma, P., Kaushal, P., & Hussain, S. (2019). Attention deficit hyperactivity disorder and comorbidity: a review of literature. *World Journal of Clinical Cases* 7(17), 2420–2426 https://doi.org/10.12998/wjcc.v7.i17.2420.

Gray, C. (2015). *The New Social Story Book*: 15th anniversary edition. Future Horizons Firm.

Hage, T.W., Rø, Ø., & Moen, A. (2015). "Time's up" – staff's management of mealtimes on inpatient eating disorder units. *Journal of Eating Disorders 3*, 13 https://doi.org/10.1186/s40337-015-0052-4.

Health and Care Act (2022). c. 31. https://www.legislation.gov.uk/ukpga/2022/31/contents (accessed 3 February 2025).

Hetrick, S.E., Subasinghe, A., Anglin, K., *et al.* (2020). Understanding the needs of young people who engage in self-harm: a qualitative investigation. *Frontiers in Psychology* 10, 2916.

Johnstone, L. (2018). Psychological formulation as an alternative to psychiatric diagnosis. *Journal of Humanistic Psychology* 58(1), 30–46 https://doi.org/10.1177/0022167817722230.

Kentrou, V., Livingston, L., Grove, R., *et al.* (2024). Perceived misdiagnosis of psychiatric conditions in autistic adults. *The Lancet* 71. https://doi.org/10.1016/j.eclinm.2024.102586.

Keski-Rahkonen, A., & Ruusunen, A. (2023). Avoidant-restrictive food intake disorder and autism: epidemiology, etiology, complications, treatment, and outcome. *Current Opinion in Psychiatry* 36(6), 438–442 https://doi.org/10.1097/YCO.0000000000000896.

Lange, K.W., Reichl, S., Lange, K.M., *et al.* (2010). The history of attention deficit hyperactivity disorder. *ADHD Attention Deficit and Hyperactivity Disorders* 2(4), 241–255 https://doi.org/10.1007/s12402-010-0045-8.

Le Grange, D. (2005). The Maudsley family-based treatment for adolescent anorexia nervosa. *World Psychiatry* 4(3), 142–146.

Lock, J., & le Grange, D. (2005). Family-based treatment of eating disorders. *The International Journal of Eating Disorders* 37(Suppl), S64–S89 https://doi.org/10.1002/eat.20122.

Marino, L.V., Merrin, J., Dodd, L., *et al.* (2024). Brief report early intervention in children with ARFID/ARFID-like symptoms. *Acta Paediatrica* 114(3), 665–667.5 https://doi.org/10.1111/apa.17527.

Martin, J. (2024). Why are females less likely to be diagnosed with ADHD in childhood than males? *The Lancet Psychiatry* 11(4), 303–310.

Mental Health Act 1983. (1983). https://www.legislation.gov.uk/ukpga/1983/20/contents.

Equality Act 2010 (c. 15). The Stationery Office.

National Autistic Society. (2025). *Demand avoidance*. https://www.autism.org.uk/advice-and-guidance/topics/behaviour/demand-avoidance (accessed 23 January 2025)

National Institute for Health and Care Excellence (2005). *Obsessive-compulsive disorder and body dysmorphic disorder: treatment (CG31)*. www.nice.org.uk/guidance/cg31 (accessed 2 January 2025).

National Institute for Health and Care Excellence (NICE) (2013). *Autism spectrum disorder in under 19s: support and management*. https://www.nice.org.uk/guidance/cg170 (accessed 23 January 2025).

National Institute for Health and Care Excellence (2018). *Attention deficit hyperactivity disorder: diagnosis and management (NG87)*. https://www.nice.org.uk/guidance/ng87 (accessed 23 January 2025).

National Institute for Health and Care Excellence (NICE) (2019). *Depression in children and young people: identification and management*. https://www.nice.org.uk/guidance/ng134/ (accessed 20 January 2025).

National Institute for Health and Care Excellence (2020). *NICE Guidance – Eating Disorders*. https://www.nice.org.uk/guidance/ng69/ifp/chapter/What-is-an-eating-disorder (accessed 15 March 2025).

National Institute for Health and Care Excellence (2022). *Self-Harm: Assessment, Management and Preventing Recurrence (NICE Guideline NG225).* https://www.nice.org.uk/guidance/ng225 (accessed 27 January 2025).

National Institute for Health and Care Excellence (2024a). *Attention deficit hyperactivity disorder: prevalence.* https://cks.nice.org.uk/topics/attention-deficit-hyperactivity-disorder/background-information/ (accessed 10 January 2025).

National Institute for Health and Care Excellence (2024b). *Eating Disorders.* National Institute for Health and Care Excellence. https://cks.nice.org.uk/topics/eating-disorders/background-information/prognosis/#:~:text=Mortality%20rates%20are%20over%20five%20times%20higher%20for,are%20cardiac%20complications%2C%20severe%20infection%2C%20and%20suicide%20%2820%25%29 (accessed 5 January 2025).

Newlove-Delgado T, Marcheselli F, Williams T, Mandalia D, Dennes M, McManus S, Savic M, Treloar W, Croft K, Ford T. (2023) Mental Health of Children and Young People in England, 2023. NHS England, Leeds.

NHS (2022). *What is autism?* https://www.nhs.uk/conditions/autism/what-is-autism/ (accessed 23 January 2025).

NHS (2023). Anxiety, fear and panic. https://www.nhs.uk/mental-health/feelings-symptoms-behaviours/feelings-and-symptoms/anxiety-fear-panic/ (accessed 17 January 2025).

OCD UK. (2025). *Types of OCD.* https://www.ocduk.org/ocd/types/ (accessed 23 January 2025).

PDA Society. (2022). *Identifying & assessing a PDA profile – practice guidance.* https://www.pdasociety.org.uk/resources/identifying-assessing-a-pda-profile-practice-guidance/.

PDA Society. (n.d.). Helpful approaches with PDA – children. https://www.pdasociety.org.uk/i-am-a-parent-carer/resources/helpful-approaches-for-children/ (accessed 23 January 2025).

Perry, Y., Krysinska, K., Byrne, S.J., *et al.* (2020). Best practice when working with suicidal behaviour and self-harm in primary care: a qualitative exploration of young people's perspectives. *BMJ Open* 10(10), e038855.

Pettersson, E., Lichtenstein, P., Larsson, H., *et al.* (2019). Genetic influences on eight psychiatric disorders based on family data of 4 408 646 full and half-siblings, and genetic data of 333 748 cases and controls. *Psychological Medicine* 49(7), 1166–1173 https://doi.org/10.1017/S0033291718002039.

Rosen, N.E., Lord, C., & Volkmar, F.R. (2021). The diagnosis of autism: from Kanner to DSM-III to DSM-5 and beyond. *Journal of Autism and Developmental Disorders* 51(12), 4253–4270 https://doi.org/10.1007/s10803-021-04904-1.

Royal College of Psychiatrists (2023). *College Report CR233: Medical Emergencies in Eating Disorders: Guidance on Recognition and Management.* Royal College of Psychiatrists.

Ruiz-Goikoetxea, *et al.* (2018). Risk of unintentional injuries in children and adolescents with ADHD and the impact of ADHD medications: a systematic review and meta-analysis. *Neuroscience and Biobehavioral Reviews* 84, 63–71 https://doi.org/10.1016/j.neubiorev.2017/11/007.

Schwartz, C., Barican, J.L., Yung, D., *et al.* (2019). Six decades of preventing and treating childhood anxiety disorders: a systematic review and meta-analysis to inform policy and practice. *BMJ Mental Health* 22(3), 103–110.

van Stralen, J. (2016). Emotional dysregulation in children with attention-deficit/hyperactivity disorder. *ADHD Attention Deficit and Hyperactivity Disorders* 8(4), 175–187 https://doi.org/10.1007/s12402-016-0199-0.

Thapar, A., Eyre, O., Patel, V., & Brent, D. (2022). Depression in young people. *Lancet* 400(10352), 617–631.

Thornicroft, G., Sunkel, C., Aliev, A.A., *et al.* (2022). The Lancet Commission on ending stigma and discrimination in mental health. *Lancet* 400(10361), 1438–1480.

UK Trauma Council (2022). *Complex trauma: evidence-based principles for the reform of children's social care. UK Trauma Council* https://uktraumacouncil.link/documents/UKTC-Complex Trauma-Principles.pdf (accessed 21 January 25).

Wade, T.D. (2019). Recent research on bulimia nervosa. *The Psychiatric Clinics of North America* 42(1), 21–32 https://doi.org/10.1016/j.psc.2018.10.002.

World Health Organization (2023). *Autism.* https://www.who.int/news-room/fact-sheets/detail/autism-spectrum-disorders (accessed 23 January 2025).

YoungMinds (2019). *How to make a self-soothe box.* https://www.youngminds.org.uk/young-person/blog/how-to-make-a-self-soothe-box/ (accessed 24 January 2025).

CHAPTER 20

Principles of end-of-life and palliative care

Louise McLaughlin and Sarah Brazel-Terris

AIM

The aim of this chapter is to develop an insight into the pathophysiological processes the baby, child or young person (BCYP) may experience during their palliative or end-of-life phases, and the impact this has on themselves as well as their families.

LEARNING OUTCOMES

On completion of this chapter, the reader will be able to:

- Discuss how healthcare professionals can support a baby, child or young person and their families with advanced care planning.
- Recognise common symptoms experienced at the end of life and how to manage these, noting the pathophysiological changes that may occur.
- Explain how to care for the person after death, with consideration of family and friends.
- Discuss the importance of communication with the child and young person as well as their family, including siblings.

KEYWORDS

- palliative
- life-threatening
- life-limiting
- symptom management
- pathophysiological changes
- advance care planning
- holistic
- death
- dying
- end of life

Test your knowledge

1. What are the benefits of advance care planning for babies, children and young people (BCYP) and their families?
2. What locations may be offered as the preferred place of death?
3. What non-pharmacological methods of pain relief could be offered to BCYP?
4. What symptoms might suggest a person is dying?
5. How should a person be cared for after their death?

Introduction

Together For Short Lives (TFSL) (2018) define children's palliative care for babies, children and young people (BCYP) with life-limiting or life-threatening conditions as from the point of diagnosis or recognition of a life-threatening event. It embraces physical, social, emotional and spiritual elements of care to enhance the quality of life of the baby, child or young person. Palliative care should include the management of symptoms through to bereavement care.

Throughout this chapter, the terms life-limiting and life-threatening will be used. It is important to understand the difference between these and the importance this bears on palliative care. The term life-limiting refers to a condition from which the BCYP is expected to die due to there being no reasonable hope of cure. On the other hand, life-threatening conditions are ones of which curative treatment is feasible but which may fail. These life-limiting and life-threatening conditions can be described in four groups, as described in Table 20.1.

Given the amount of uncertainty that comes when caring for a BCYP with life-limiting or life-threatening conditions, it is very important to parallel plan. Equally, the delivery of good-quality palliative care can often be hindered by late referrals to palliative and symptom management services. Therefore, early recognition is key. Figure 20.1 demonstrates how parallel planning can be delivered alongside palliative care.

It is important to recognise that BCYP with life-limiting conditions can be healthy and lead a good-quality life, with access to schooling and experiences that any other child should experience. Palliative care can be delivered alongside curative or active treatment.

The complexity of delivering palliative care alongside disease management with the aim of cure can be demonstrated in Fig. 20.2. This can be particularly helpful to conceptualise the different ways in which palliative care can be provided in different circumstances.

Epidemiology

The prevalence of children living with life-limiting conditions has increased over the years. In 2017, 86,625 children were living in the United Kingdom with a life-limiting condition, compared to 32,975 in 2001 (Fraser *et al.*, 2020). The prevalence in boys was significantly higher (72.5 per 10,000 in boys compared to 60 per 10,000 in girls). Whilst prevalence was higher in the under-ones, it was also noted that there is a growing number of young people surviving beyond their 19th birthday.

TABLE 20.1 Four groups of life-limiting and life-threatening conditions

Category 1	Life-threatening conditions for which curative treatment may be feasible but may fail – once the condition is cured or long-term remission has been achieved, palliative care is no longer required. Examples: Cancer, transplant and organ failure
Category 2	Conditions where premature death is inevitable – this may include periods of treatment/management of the disease with an aim to prolong life. The BCYP may have long periods of relatively good health, despite their disabilities. Examples: Spinal Muscular Atrophy type 1, Duchenne muscular dystrophy and cystic fibrosis
Category 3	Progressive treatments without curative treatments – treatment may be exclusively palliative, which can extend to several years. Examples: Mucopolysaccharides such as San Fillipo syndrome, metabolic conditions and Batten disease
Category 4	Irreversible but non-progressive conditions causing severe disability leading to susceptibility to health complications, causing premature death – palliative care may be required at any stage due to unpredictable episodes of care. Examples: Severe cerebral palsy, brain and spinal injuries

Source: Adapted from TFSL (2018).

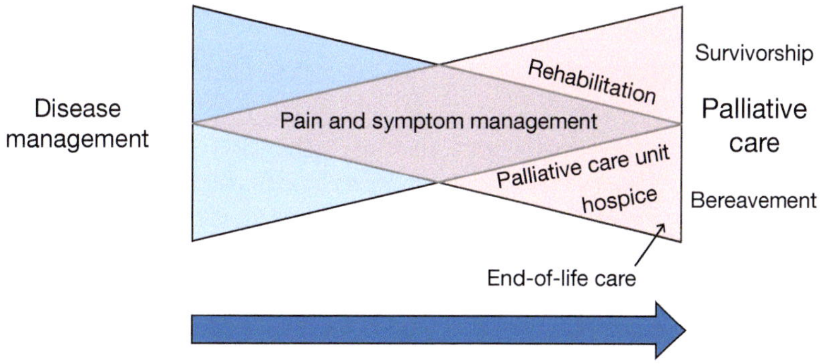

FIGURE 20.1 The bow tie model.
Source: Hawley, (2014)/with permission of Elsevier.

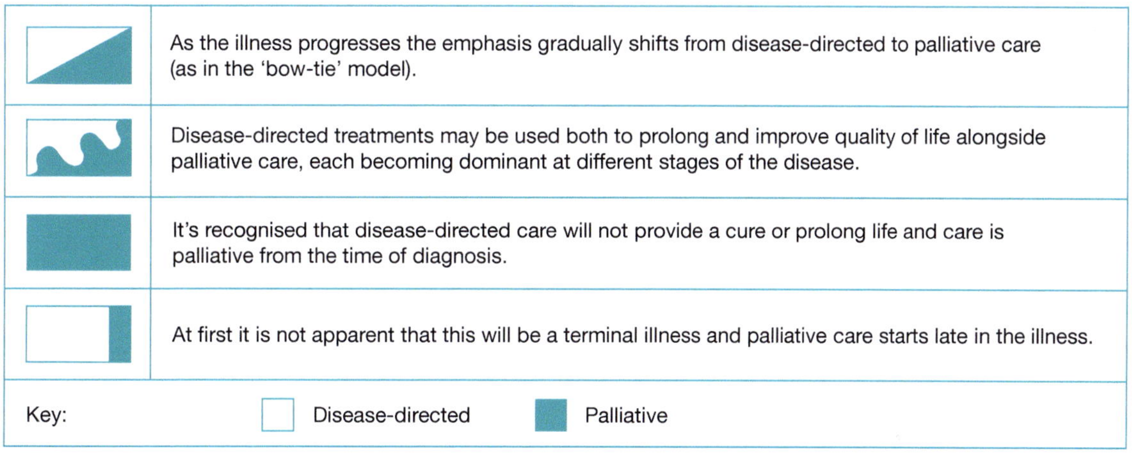

FIGURE 20.2 Examples of the relationship between palliative and disease-directed care (TFSL, 2018).

Advance care planning

National Institute for Health and Care Excellence (NICE) (2019) recommends that advance care plans (ACPs) should be developed for BCYP with a life-limiting condition. There is a misconception amongst some professionals and families that advance care planning means planning for the BCYP's death. Whilst planning for end of life and care after death is an important part of advance care planning, planning care to ensure the BCYP lives to their full potential with the support of professionals is also just as important. NICE (2019) explains that the following should be included within an ACP, which is explored in Table 20.2.

ACP discussions should take place when there is a change in the BCYP's condition or a change of circumstances/wishes. Where there is an antenatal diagnosis of a life-limiting condition, planning should start before the delivery of the baby. Midwives, obstetricians and neonatologists, as well as specialists within the life-limiting condition and paediatric palliative care, should be involved in these discussions (NICE, 2019).

ACP discussions empower CYP and their families to discuss their wishes and voice concerns, ensuring that the spiritual and social aspects of care are prioritised alongside the physical and emotional aspects.

Challenges in accessing palliative care

As part of the ACP discussions, children and their families should be offered choice in preferred place of care. As Liang (2024) discusses, clinicians themselves can be one

TABLE 20.2 Elements that should be included in an ACP

Housekeeping	• Demographic information about the child and family • Up-to-date contact information for the child and family, as well as all professionals involved in care (including school/college) • A statement outlining who has responsibility for giving consent • Agreed form of communication with the BCYP and family • A distribution list of the ACP
Details around the BCYP's diagnosis	A summary of the life-limiting condition
An outline of the BCYP's life ambitions and wishes	It is important to understand what is important to the BCYP and their family. This may include: • Social activities and participation • Education • Religious, spiritual, cultural beliefs and values • Family and friendship
Planning	• Agreed treatment plans and objectives. This will include discussing ceilings of care • Education plans if relevant.
Record of discussions	Discussions around the following should be included: • Preferred place of care • Preferred place of death (this may be different to the aforementioned) • Organ and tissue donation • Management of life-threatening events, including plans around resuscitation and advanced life support • Specific wishes around care of the body after death and funeral wishes

of the biggest hurdles BCYPs and their families face in accessing palliative care. Professionals are not always aware of the services available within the local area, particularly in relation to preferred place of death. Possible options are discussed herewith.

Home

The BCYP and their families may choose home as their preferred place of death for many reasons that are personal to them, such as the familiarity and the accessibility of a support network of friends and family without any limitations. A report by the National Child Mortality Database (NCMD) found that 15% of BCYP with a life-limiting condition died at home (NCMD, 2025). From a professional perspective, supporting the BCYP to die at home can be challenging in terms of managing symptoms and can be resource-heavy. In accordance with NICE (2019), BCYP should have access to a palliative care consultant and nursing care 24 hours a day, 7 days a week.

Hospice

Some BCYPs and their families may choose a hospice due to having a specialist palliative care nursing team around them who are able to offer symptom management and holistic care throughout their stay. However, due to a national funding crisis, challenges may arise with the availability of beds (TFSL, 2025). Geographically, some families live some distance from their local hospice, particularly in rural areas, which may offer challenges such as availability of a support network. Unsurprisingly, the NCMD (2025) reports 7% of BCYP with a life-limiting condition die in a hospice.

Ward and paediatric intensive care unit (PICU)

Care may need to de-escalate, and it may be appropriate for life-sustaining treatments/interventions to stop, and so the BCYP and family may feel the ward, or PICU may be the right place of care and death. For example, if a BCYP is intubated, it may be possible to withdraw care compassionately at home or the hospice; the family may choose the ward/PICU due to the familiarity of the environment and staff, or it may be that the BCYP is too unstable to move and may die during a transfer. The NCMD (2025) report found that 77% of BCYP with life-limiting conditions died in hospital.

Communication

Communication within palliative care is extremely important, particularly given the sensitivity some topics require. Consideration of the BCYP's communication needs will need to be considered as per NICE (2019) guidance, but the child should be involved in discussions as appropriate. Through involving the BCYP in discussions, they are more likely to want to become involved in their care and will improve adherence to care and treatment (Amery, 2016). BCYP and their families want direct and open communication, particularly in response to their questions (Zhang *et al.*, 2024). Figure 20.3 highlights the key skills which are essential in communicating in palliative care (adapted from TFSL, 2019).

Special considerations

Cultural, religious and spiritual beliefs form the foundation of family life. To communicate effectively, recognising and respecting the beliefs of the BCYP and family is crucial. To be culturally competent, nurses need to be open and curious about each patient's culture with some awareness of how it impacts their decision-making, coping responses and preferences for communication (Mack & Sisk, 2021).

Managing difficult conversations

Breaking bad news is one of the most challenging areas in communication for healthcare professionals. Often, nurses fear making the situation worse, or they may lack confidence in starting or exploring some of the issues raised. However, it is important to note how non-verbal communication may be interpreted, as well as avoidance of conversations. It is crucial that metaphors and euphemisms are avoided, particularly when communicating with children and young people. For example, if death is described as 'going to sleep', the child may be afraid to go to bed in case they do not wake up. Equally, if a sibling of a child who has died is told that their brother has gone to heaven in the clouds, the child may expect to see them when they board an aeroplane. The issue here is not that the child has gone to heaven, but heaven has been placed in the clouds, which is somewhere the sibling can visit.

A situation may arise when the CYP with a life-limiting or life-threatening condition approaches a conversation around death. This will usually occur when either they already know the answer to their question but want some confirmation, or that they have a confused and worrying idea of what may happen and would like it to be explained (Amery, 2016). A clear, honest and straightforward conversation is needed to avoid mistrust or further worry and confusion.

- Ensure you greet and introduce yourself – BCYPs will often have several different professionals involved in their care.
- Awareness of the importance of non-verbal language.
- The ability to be able to listen and understand the power of silence.
- Open but focused questions.
- Build trust with the BCYP and family. Remain respectful and polite.
- Understand the events that have unfolded and how the situation may change.
- Check they have understood.
- Safety net – ensure they know where to go for advice/questions following the conversation.

FIGURE 20.3 Essential skills in communication.

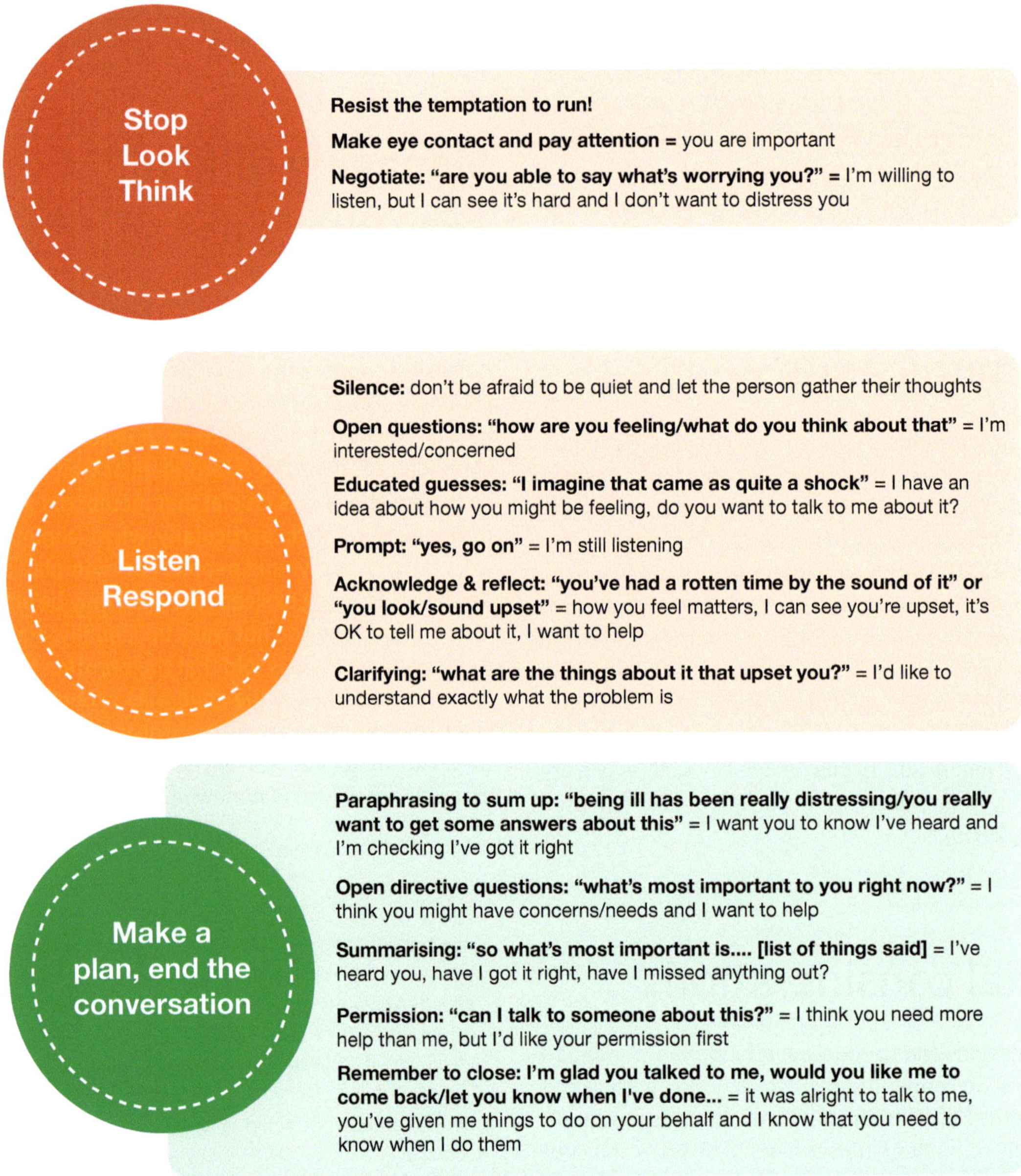
Stop Look Think
Resist the temptation to run!
Make eye contact and pay attention = you are important
Negotiate: "are you able to say what's worrying you?" = I'm willing to listen, but I can see it's hard and I don't want to distress you
Listen Respond
Silence: don't be afraid to be quiet and let the person gather their thoughts
Open questions: "how are you feeling/what do you think about that" = I'm interested/concerned
Educated guesses: "I imagine that came as quite a shock" = I have an idea about how you might be feeling, do you want to talk to me about it?
Prompt: "yes, go on" = I'm still listening
Acknowledge & reflect: "you've had a rotten time by the sound of it" or "you look/sound upset" = how you feel matters, I can see you're upset, it's OK to tell me about it, I want to help
Clarifying: "what are the things about it that upset you?" = I'd like to understand exactly what the problem is
Make a plan, end the conversation
Paraphrasing to sum up: "being ill has been really distressing/you really want to get some answers about this" = I want you to know I've heard and I'm checking I've got it right
Open directive questions: "what's most important to you right now?" = I think you might have concerns/needs and I want to help
Summarising: "so what's most important is.... [list of things said] = I've heard you, have I got it right, have I missed anything out?
Permission: "can I talk to someone about this?" = I think you need more help than me, but I'd like your permission first
Remember to close: I'm glad you talked to me, would you like me to come back/let you know when I've done... = it was alright to talk to me, you've given me things to do on your behalf and I know that you need to know when I do them

FIGURE 20.4 Framework for managing difficult conversations (TFSL, 2019).

Together for Short Lives (2019) suggests the following framework in managing difficult conversations (Fig. 20.4).

Assessment

Comprehensive assessment, leading to holistic individualised care, is pertinent in children's palliative care. A holistic assessment should include four components: physical, spiritual, psychological and social, which are now explored.

Physical

A physical assessment should be conducted in ways in which the patient is comfortable, with the aim of trying to control any symptoms that arise to enhance quality of life. Points to consider are mobility, sleep, fluid input and output, nutrition, skin integrity and any symptoms such as nausea, pain, breathlessness and so on. It is important to remember that comfort is the desired goal, and so some routine observations, such as blood pressure, may not be advisable if they do not influence management.

Spiritual

Brown *et al.* (2024) refer to spirituality as an intrinsic aspect of humanity, where the ultimate meaning and purpose of life are sought through relationships with their own self, family, community, society and nature and for some, a sacred or significant other. It is a way in which human beings make sense of the universe and their place within it. It is important to acknowledge that a child's cognitive ability, background and personality will influence their understanding of life and what happens beyond. For example, the western view of the life cycle consists of the foetus through to the elderly, with the belief that there is only one life cycle. However, Eastern views consider multiple lives with time for atonement. It is important to explore the BCYP narrative and the meanings that individuals develop for themselves, so professionals can collaborate with them and support them effectively. Assumptions should not be made that younger children, particularly babies and those with complex needs, do not have spiritual needs as they observe and interpret their parents' responses and have the need for nurture.

Psychological

The life-limiting condition of the BCYP will have an impact on their own lives and that of their family. It affects how other people may perceive and relate to them, and how unwell they perceive their ownself to be. A sense of burden may develop as their care needs heighten as well as mood disturbance and a low emotional state. It may be useful during the assessment to understand what the main priorities are for the BCYP and their families, such as symptom management. It is important that meaningful, honest and empathetic communication is offered whilst acknowledging that others within the multi-disciplinary team, such as psychologists, music therapists and art therapists, may be able to offer support in some of these areas.

Social

This part of the assessment can be varied and may include anything from family support to housing or financial issues. For example, the preferred place of care may be at home because the BCYP may want to be in a familiar environment. However, this may mean that a package of care will need to be in place to ensure the family receives support with care, for example. In turn, parents may need to take time off work to care for their BCYP, meaning that they may enter a period of financial or employment instability. When the wider impact is understood, relevant referrals and signposting, such as to social care, can be given to ensure the right support is offered.

Case study 20.1

Ash is 10 years old and has a diagnosis of Mucopolysaccharidosis type II (Hunter syndrome). Ash had enjoyed attending school and spending time with his friends up until 2 months ago, when he was admitted to PICU for a chest infection. Since this episode, Ash's care needs have increased, requiring nasogastric feeds as well as support with mobilisation and toileting. Previously, Ash used Makaton as a method of communication, but he is struggling to use this and communicate his needs effectively. Due to his increased care requirements, he has not been able to return to school full-time. His parents and carers are noticing that Ash is more withdrawn and having frequent outbursts.

Points to consider

- How would the four components of holistic assessment be assessed within this scenario?
- Is it appropriate to introduce or update a current ACP at this time?
- How would you ensure Ash's narrative is heard, despite his communication challenges?

The process of dying

Death, very much like birth, is a transition in which the body passes through, usually in phases. Not every person will experience the same symptoms leading up to their death; this may be very dependent on their diagnosis, as well as their general health and well-being. These changes can occur in the months, weeks, days and hours leading to their death. Recognition of the dying person is imperative to providing good end-of-life care as it allows the patient and family to recognise this themselves and prepare accordingly (Taylor *et al.*, 2017).

Eating less/loss of appetite

BCYP will experience reduced appetite because they require less calories due to reduced mobility and prioritisation of systems. Nausea and dry, painful mouths will make eating less appealing, so management of these symptoms is imperative. It is normal for the BCYP to lose weight during this phase, and their appearance may change due to muscle loss (cachexia) (Mahunt *et al.*, 2021). The BCYP should be encouraged to eat and drink where possible (NICE, 2019), but they should not feel pressured, as this can exacerbate other symptoms such as nausea and pain. Feeding interventions such as enteral feeding should only be introduced if agreed with the BCYP and their parents/guardians, that it is in their best interest.

Reduced bladder/bowel function

The digestive system is usually the first system affected in the natural dying process. It will usually start slowing down as the body prioritises systems that are required for the body to stay alive, such as the respiratory and cardiac systems. This, together with the reduced fluid and solid intake, will cause reduced urine output and constipation.

Feeling weaker and sleeping more

The BCYP may be spending more time resting, rather than participating in their normal everyday activities. They may require assistance with mobility and personal hygiene tasks, such as personal care. Communication may also be affected as they may not be able to hold a conversation or communicate in the way in which they usually would. This may be due to reduced intake of nutrients, but is most likely to be caused by the progression of disease and the body's prioritisation of systems. As time goes on, the BCYP will sleep for longer periods and will have less awake time. As death becomes closer, they may move into an unconscious state, which is part of the natural dying process.

Vital signs

Monitoring of routine observations is not supported at the end of life. With gentle touch and visual observations, any peripheral and central dysregulation can be observed with experience (Kinley and Sullivan, 2024).

Symptom management

The definition of symptom management is the use of medications or holistic therapies to alleviate the psychical and emotional symptoms of health conditions, including during end-of-life care. Together for Short Lives (2024) have developed a robust and nationally utilised manual, outlining medication and the doses that can be used to control the most notable symptoms during end of life for BCYP, which is outlined in Table 20.3. The Association for Paediatric Palliative Medicine (2024) should be consulted for specific prescribing recommendations.

Be aware of the use of non-steroidal anti-inflammatory (NSAIDs) medication in end-of-life care. These medications can reduce platelet count, thus resulting in a higher risk of bleeding. Furthermore, NSAIDs should not be administered orally without food, and if a BCYP has poor oral intake due to being end-of-life, this can result in stomach ulcers, pain and risk of bleeding.

Additionally, it is important to consider that all medications used in end-of-life care can still have side effects, which can cause further requirements for management. For example, the use of opiates may be effective in controlling pain but cause pruritus, which will need further management.

Symptom management plans and just-in-case medication

Symptoms should be anticipated ahead of time through a symptom management plan written by the palliative care team. This plan should address any symptoms that may occur due to the BCYP's condition (TFSL, 2018 and NICE, 2019). Any first-line medication named in the symptom management plan should be available in the preferred place of care/death. Any equipment that may be required should also be made available, such as syringe drivers, dark towels and syringes required to deliver medication via the required routes.

The symptom management plan and availability of drugs should be reviewed regularly, particularly when there has been a change in condition, to maximise comfort.

TABLE 20.3 Common palliative and end-of-life symptoms and their management

System	Symptoms	Pharmacological management	Non-pharmacological management and considerations	Pathophysiological changes
Respiratory	Excessive oral secretions and drooling (Sialorrhoea)	Hyoscine Butylbromide trans-dermal patch behind the ear to dry secretions and prevent nausea. Glycopyrronium Bromide can be given PO or IV dependant on where the patient is being cared for. This medication is often better tolerated and observed to be more effective than the patch.	Consider potential impact on skin integrity around the mouth – some BCYP may require additional skin care and barrier creams to prevent irritation.	Breathing will sound 'noisy', caused by a pooling of secretions at the back of their larynx. The BCYP may be too weak to cough or swallow to clear the secretions, and so the build-up of secretions can cause a loud rattling sound, which can be distressing for people nearby to hear, although not for the dying person.
	Dyspnoea	Benzodiazepines and opioids are commonly used for treatment of respiratory distress and are very effective. They can be administered in myriad ways, based on the clinical condition and location of the patient.	Administering oxygen as a comfort measure or creating movement of air with the use of an open window can relieve symptoms of dyspnoea in BCYP. Dyspnoea can often appear more distressing to those around them than it is for the BCYP. It is vital to ensure the patient is the focus of the treatment, and not the family.	Dyspnoea is a subjective experience and can be influenced by experiences such as anxiety. Chronic anaemia, which is often experienced in the palliative patient, may further exacerbate dyspnoea as it causes poor oxygen delivery, further weakening the muscles of the respiratory system, alongside heart failure and pulmonary oedema. There may be a change in pattern of breathing, such as irregular and shallow or agonal gasping respirations may occur (Kinley and Sullivan, 2024). An example of a typical breathing pattern that may be seen at the end of life is Cheyne-Stokes breathing, which likely indicates changes to the brainstem. Hockley (2015) describes this as delays between breaths, as though the BCYP is holding their own breath.

(Continued)

TABLE 20.3 *(Continued)*

System	Symptoms	Pharmacological management	Non-pharmacological management and considerations	Pathophysiological changes
Circulation	Bleeding	Compassionate blood products such as platelet transfusion or Fresh Frozen Plasma (FFP) to prevent haemorrhage in those who are at high risk. This would only be suitable in a hospital setting. Tranexamic Acid (TXA) is applied topically to sites of bleeding – particularly if localised to the mouth or nose. TXA can be administered intravenously (IV) or orally (PO) in cases of high risk of bleeding. If gastrointestinal bleeding is likely – ensure patient is on a Proton-Pump Inhibitor (PPI) such as Lansoprazole, administered PO or IV. In the event of a catastrophic and terminal haemorrhage, it is vital to administer buccal, intranasal, subcutaneous (SC) or IV Midazolam as soon as possible and repeat the dosing (or commence a continuous infusion) until the child is settled.	Consider colour of bedsheets and towels – using dark sheets can reduce visual impact of bleeding in the case of a catastrophic bleed. Whilst catastrophic bleeds in the death of BCYP are rare, they can occur, particularly in patients with leukaemia. Families and patients, where appropriate, must be advised of this risk, as this may impact where the BCYP will die.	As BCYP approach end of life, the body will no longer be able to effectively manage homeostasis. This applies to mechanisms such as the blood's ability to clot. When clotting factors become deranged and infective, BCYP can be at risk of excessive bleeding. Haemorrhage can also be secondary to underlying diseases, such as leukaemia or uncontrollable haemophilia. At the end of life, the body's ability to ensure effective circulation and perfusion will fail. A compensatory response and activation of sympathetic nervous system may lead to tachycardia in some patients, as well as an Electrolyte imbalance from reduced intake. Loss of brainstem function regulating respiratory function may lead to hypoxaemia. As blood pressure will reduce, resulting in poorly perfused extremities and progressing to poorly perfused organs. An abrupt drop in blood pressure may lead to difficulty in palpating a radial pulse (Hui & Mori, 2021).
Gastrointestinal	Dry mouth (Xerostomia)	Artificial saliva can be applied to the mouth using oral care sponges. Consider dosing of other medications that may be causing the dry mouth.	Regular mouth care and good oral hygiene. Additionally, consider using liquid the patient enjoys to moisten the mouth, such as flavoured juice. If the patient requires oxygen, consider if this can be humidified.	When a BCYP is at the end of life, appetite is often notably reduced. This is secondary to their need for food and drink reduces, as energy consumption within the body becomes less and less. Additionally, it may become too much effort to eat and drink. The swallowing mechanism may diminish, meaning the patient cannot swallow any solids, liquids or their own saliva.

	Constipation	Osmotic laxatives or stimulants may be used depending on the BCYP's tolerance. Some medications, such as opioids, may cause constipation.	Heat pads for abdominal pain associated with gastrointestinal issues – take care of positioning of this and risk of burns.	Poor oral intake, along with some medications such as opioids, contributes to drier faecal content and reduced motility, which can reduce the perception of rectal distention, causing the urge to defecate. The longer the stool remains in the colon, the drier it becomes. Some neurological and neuromuscular disorders that occur at the end of life, will also impact the BCYP's ability to defecate.
	Diarrhoea	Review of medication or feeds that may be causing diarrhoea. Treat pain that may be associated with muscle cramps.	Consider potential impact on skin integrity if the BCYP is in nappies, pads or immobile.	Impaired absorption of fluids and electrolytes may cause diarrhoea (Larkin, 2021). This may be secretory, where significant loss of fluid and electrolytes occurs in the jejunum, or osmotic, which usually occurs when the bowels are prevented from absorbing water and electrolytes (this can be seen in constipation management).
	Nausea and vomiting	Dependant on the cause of the nausea and vomiting will determine the treatment. As an example, if a BCYP continues on therapeutic chemotherapy, the prescribing centre will have specific anti-emetic pathways to follow. If the underlying cause of the nausea is unclear, Levomepromazine, administered either PO or IV, is often used as it acts on multiple receptors. Antiemetics work well in conjunction with each other, so many BCYP will require more than one to be effectively managed.	Avoid triggers such as strong-smelling foods or perfumes. Consider the role of anxiety in nausea, and whether this needs to be addressed separately.	The cause of nausea and vomiting can be multifaceted in palliative care. Changes in the autonomic nervous system, such as an increase in cortisol, as well as an increase in nervous system activity. In particular, gastric dysrhythmias may be triggered by motion or drugs such as morphine.
Neurological	Seizure	Anti-convulsant medication, such as Benzodiazepines, can be administered buccally, IV or rectally. Method of administration will depend on the location and clinical condition of the BCYP.	Airway positioning for comfort measures during or after seizure activity. Consider that those BCYP who are known to have seizures may have a medication plan in place.	Seizures may be caused by structural disease of the brain, such as cerebral lesions or infection, which may cause destruction and irritation of brain tissue as well as cerebral oedema and bleeding (Caraceni *et al.*, 2021). They may also be caused by metabolic derangement and drug toxicity.

(*Continued*)

TABLE 20.3 *(Continued)*

System	Symptoms	Pharmacological management	Non-pharmacological management and considerations	Pathophysiological changes
	Disordered sleep and insomnia	To note, medication to modulate sleep should only be used as a last resort. Melatonin is useful in assisting the BCYP to fall asleep; it is unlikely to improve quality or duration of sleep. Sedatives such as Chloral Hydrate or Benzodiazepines are more effective in prolonging unbroken sleep duration. Onset of sleep is a welcomed side effect of some antihistamines, which can influence medication choice if a BCYP is suffering from sleep disturbance and pruritus.	Sleep hygiene, such as low lighting, comfort measures, reduced screen time, aromatherapy and creating a relaxing environment, should be used in the first instance. Consider family education on sleep hygiene and how this can help the BCYP.	Some may experience a short surge of energy, referred to as 'terminal lucidity', although the physiology of this is not fully understood, but could be due to a surge in hormones or neurotransmitters (Kinley and Sullivan, 2024). This can be confusing for family members, as they may see this as the BCYP showing signs of recovery. If families are prepared well, they can use this time for final special moments such as reading a favourite book together or watching a favourite movie.
	Psychological	Anxiety – Benzodiazepines can be useful in treating anxiety, particularly in short-term outbursts. These medications are quick-acting and can be administered buccally, PO sublingually or per rectum (PR). For patients requiring longer-term management of anxiety, anti-psychotics can be considered. Depression – If non-pharmacological treatments are ineffective, Selective Serotonin Reuptake Inhibitors (SSRIs) are considered the safest class of medication to use. However, these medications can take 2–3 weeks to work, which means they can be ineffective in this patient cohort.	There must be an emphasis on correcting what is correctable –such as reviewing medications, optimising management of co-morbidities and managing other factors, such as distressing symptoms. Ensuring input from play teams, psychological team input and family-centred care. Ensuring that you offer the patient and their family space and time to talk. A holistic assessment is required to ensure any social or spiritual needs can be addressed.	Disease and treatment may cause some somatic symptoms attributed to depression. It may also be directly related to direct physiological results of the BCYP's conditions, such as medication effects, hypothyroidism and chronic uraemia (Kissane, 2021).

	Agitation	Benzodiazepines (particularly Midazolam) are very effective at relieving symptoms of agitation in BCYP. The route of administration will largely depend on the setting and can be administered in myriad ways. If a patient is at home and requires a continuous infusion of SC midazolam, this can be administered via syringe driver to ensure the safety of the patient, their family and the practitioner. Terminal agitation can also be treated with an anti-psychotic such as haloperidol, either in addition to a benzodiazepine or in replacement of.	Acute episodes of agitation are common towards the end of life. This can be secondary to hypoxia due to respiratory difficulties or generally neurological deficit. Non-pharmacological focus should be on ensuring there are no additional environmental factors that may be impacting the BCYP, and the patient is positioned as comfortably as possible.	The BCYP may appear agitated/restless at times. It is important to understand if there is an underlying physical factor, such as urine retention, constipation or hypoxia, that may be the underlying cause of this, which may require management if appropriate (Ijaopo et al., 2023).
Pain	Chronic and acute	Route of administration of pain relief will be patient specific – this can be SC, PO, PR, IV, Transdermal, buccal or intranasal. NICE (2019) recognise the first step for mild pain should be paracetamol/ibuprofen, escalating to opioids for moderate and severe pain. If a patient is at home and requires a continuous infusion of SC analgesia, this can be administered via syringe driver to ensure the safety of the patient, their family and the practitioner.	Ensuring the use of appropriate pain assessment tools and considering holistic pain assessment. Consider use of distraction, massage, imagery and Transcutaneous Electrical Nerve Stimulation (TENS) as examples.	Pain is more often caused by the pathophysiology of the cause of death. For example, patients with cancer may develop injury to somatic or visceral tissues or perhaps neural structures, causing neuropathic pain. Pain may also be associated with treatment, such as cytotoxic neuropathy, which is caused by chemotherapy-induced neuropathic pain (Dickenson and Gordon- Williams, 2021).

(*Continued*)

TABLE 20.3 *(Continued)*

System	Symptoms	Pharmacological management	Non-pharmacological management and considerations	Pathophysiological changes
Exposure/skin	Pressure sores	Consider need for pain management or specialised dressings.	Ensure regular repositioning of the patient to alleviate pressure points. Ensure close monitoring of skin and repositioning of medical devices such as oxygen tubing.	The BCYP's appearance will change as they move closer to death. This may start in the months leading up to their death, but there may be more significant changes the closer they become. Many of these changes occur due to the reduced cardiac function as the body prioritises blood flow to vital organs (Domeisen Benedetti, 2013). Mottling or change of colour of the skin may occur, particularly in the extremities, or if the patient has been lying in one position for a length of time. Extremities may also feel cool as the peripheral circulation diminishes, and the skin texture may become clammy and sweaty.
	Pruritus	Anti-histamines such as chlorphenamine can be effective for pruritus. Topical antipruritic creams and ointments can be effective in alleviating itching.	Consider a fan to alleviate pruritus. If the itching is secondary to dry skin, ensure that the BCYP is moisturised well after bathing. Consider reversible causes for itching, such as opiates or comorbidities.	When dying, the biochemistry will change, and symptoms such as increased confusion or decreased responsiveness to touch and other sensations may occur (Kinley and Sullivan, 2024).
	Fevers	Anti-pyretics (i.e., Paracetamol) administered PO, PR or IV.	Consider responding to how the patient is reporting to feel rather than what observations are telling you – for example, if the patient reports feeling cold even if febrile, allow them to have an extra blanket. The focus is on symptom management, not curative intent.	Episodes of fever are common when a BCYP is at the end of life. This can be secondary to infection, underlying disease or illness. Developing a fever may be the only part of the immune response that is functioning as it should be.

Source: Adapted from Together for Short Lives (2024) and The Association for Paediatric Palliative Medicine (2024).

Building an awareness of cultural and religious beliefs of the patient and their family will allow greater understanding of decision-making. As an example, rebirth is a central belief in Buddhism, and it is believed that the state of mind at the moment of death plays a key role in influencing the person's rebirth. Therefore, to preserve clarity and awareness, some Buddhist patients or their families may wish to avoid the use of analgesics nearing the time of death. Being aware of this will allow consideration and compassionate care from the nursing and allied health professional teams.

Siblings

A BCYP with a life-limiting or life-threatening condition may have siblings. It is important that their needs are not overlooked. They may be deprived of attention due to the ongoing needs of their sibling(s), which is preoccupying their parents. They may feel they want to be more involved with their sibling's care, but are not given the opportunity to. It may be difficult for siblings to feel their home is a 'safe haven' if their homes represent an environment in which their sibling is very ill or perhaps dying (Contro and Zimerman, 2021). They may also feel unable to share their own feelings, as this may exacerbate their parents' grief and sadness.

Ethical dilemmas

Ethical issues are especially relevant to the speciality of palliative care, given the type of patients and their stage of disease and illness. The practice of palliative care recognises that the physical sense is not the only aspect that is important when delivering care. Holistic care includes respecting the BCYP as a moral agent and allows them to express their moral choices, i.e., treating them ethically and allowing them to be ethical in their behaviour. Ethical principles remain the same for all ages; however, the way in which they are applied varies. According to Amery (2016), this may be because:

- They may not have a full understanding of their illness and treatment
- They may not have the means to communicate or be understood
- Their rights may not be well respected by adults
- The application of Gillick competency

Special considerations

Older children and young people of an adolescent age often can understand the world around them, yet parents are sometimes reluctant to share bad news about their illness and treatment with them. For example, a child who is diagnosed with cancer suddenly stops visiting the hospital for treatment, but is often visited at home by their Community Nurses and the Nurses from the hospice. They are often able to understand that the focus of their treatment has changed, along with perhaps the mood becoming solemn in the house, and lots of conversations happening in the house to which they are protected. This sometimes leaves the child or young person with questions that they feel they cannot have answered, which can lead to confusion and fear. In the situation where a parent does not want to tell a young person that they are going to die, it is important to explore the reason behind this and offer appropriate support. Often, it is the case that parents fear that their child will 'give up' if they knew they were going to die. It is important to navigate this fear with the parents and explore what the young person may be feeling or thinking.

Care after death

The BCYP should be cared for after death in accordance with their religious, cultural and spiritual wishes. If in accordance with their wishes, personal care of the body should happen 2–4 hours after death (Hospice UK, 2024). This is due to the pathophysiological changes that will occur.

Deterioration of the body – what to expect

Somatic death refers to the irreversible cessation of vital organs such as lungs and heart (Shedge *et al.*, 2023). A process known as molecular death follows this due to the lack of oxygen supplying the body. The following changes will occur over the following hours:

- **Algor mortis:** The body starts to cool down, both peripherally and centrally, within 2–8 hours (TFSL, 2019). This cooling process is important in slowing down the disintegration process, and so the BCYP should not be wrapped in heavy insulating blankets or clothes. The family should be allowed to hold and cuddle their child, but a balance will need to be struck between this and avoiding over-warming the body.

- **Pallor and loss of skin elasticity:** As the blood stops circulating, the skin will change colour. It is important to consider that the skin tone changes will appear different in all ethnicities. As an example, a white skin can become lighter, and their skin may become almost translucent. On the other hand, black skin can become darker and almost opaque. Moisture from the skin and lips may also be lost, and so they can become dry. Skin elasticity is lost within minutes of death, and so skin may be at risk of breakdown if constantly touched.
- **Ocular changes:** Most notably, there is a loss of pupillary and corneal reflex, and so the child may have their eyes open, which can be distressing for families. Eyelids should be gently closed immediately after death by gentle pressure on the eyelids.
- **Livor mortis:** Gravitational pooling of blood in the veins and capillary beds will start to occur around half an hour after cardiac circulation ceases. This will initially look like darker patches on the skin, eventually turning darker in colour, often reddish-purple and occupy larger areas. It is often seen on parts of the body in touch with an underlying surface, such as the back and buttocks, but is also often seen in the earlobes and fingernail beds.
- **Rigor mortis:** This is the stiffening of the body, which is a result of decreased adenosinetriphosphate (ATP) levels (Shedge *et al.*, 2023). It first appears 1–2 hours after death, but will disappear 36–48 hours after death. This is important to consider when parents request their child to be dressed in different clothes.
- **Leakage of bodily fluids:** This can occur at any time after death. Leakage of fluids, including blood, can occur from any orifice, such as the nose or ears. Urinal and faecal leaks are also possible. A pad should be placed under the body to contain this, and suction equipment should also be available.

A BCYP may be cared for in several places after death. Depending on any religious requirements, there is the option to use funeral directors if the family wishes to do so, or if the BCYP has died in hospital, the mortuary may also be an option. However, BCYP may also be cared for at home after death by using equipment that ensures the body is kept cool to prevent decomposition of the body, such as cooling mats. There may also be a designated bedroom available in Children's Hospices that can look after the BCYP after death (TFSL, 2019). However, before the body can be transferred, the death must be verified by a doctor or a nurse or a paramedic having been deemed competent. Some religions, such as the Muslim religion, require burial as soon as possible. It is important that as part of the advance care planning, this is known by the multi-disciplinary team so a death can be verified and certified as soon as possible.

There are times when a death may be unexpected. In these instances, the Coroner must be informed before the body is washed or any medical devices such as nasogastric tubes are removed. It may be a requirement that the body is sent for a post-mortem to investigate the cause of death, particularly when a death is unexpected or if there are concerns from the family surrounding medical negligence.

Pre-bereavement and post-bereavement

Loss is a universal human experience and is woven into everyday life (Archer and Machin, 2024). A family of a BCYP with a life-limiting or life-threatening condition will experience loss in the form of not having the life they once thought they would. When a CYP is diagnosed with a form of cancer requiring treatment, they will grieve for their normal life, which did not consist of feeling ill, being away from their friends and family and changes to their physical body such as weight gain/loss. Ways in which the BCYP and their families may react to loss are outlined in Table 20.4. This list is not exhaustive.

It is important to understand these reactions of loss, particularly in pre-bereavement, as these are not signs that the person is not coping; they are just experiencing the loss.

Children will experience grief differently from adults; occasionally, a child may appear in great distress and then ask a question such as 'what is for tea?', seemingly unbothered by what has or is happening. A child's grief will be influenced by those around them, particularly the adults. Siblings will have complicated feelings as their understanding of death will differ depending on their age (Portnoy and Ives-Baine, 2021). There may be a sense of guilt that they did something to cause their sibling's death, or there may be hope that now the family can return to some sort of normality.

TABLE 20.4 How people may react to loss

Dimension	Reactions
Emotional	Sadness, fear, anger, irritability, guilt, anxiety, apathy and envy
Physical	Restlessness, insomnia, menstrual irregularities, sensitivity to noise, hyperactivity or underactivity and pain such as chest, abdominal and headaches.
Cognitive	Thoughts are focused on the loss, and so they find it difficult to concentrate or think about other things.
Social and practical	Avoids contact and lacks interest in others
Spiritual	Existential questions raised – belief system and meaning of life challenged or reaffirmed.

Source: Adapted from Archer and Machin (2024) and Portnoy and Ives-Baine (2021).

Support for nurses and healthcare professionals

It is imperative that nurses and healthcare professionals feel supported in the delivery of palliative care, as well as during and after a BCYP death. Professionals may experience burnout in the sense of physical and emotional exhaustion caused by emotionally demanding workplace situations.

Case study 20.2

Aditi is an 8-year-old girl who lives with her mother, father and her 5-year-old twin siblings. Aditi was diagnosed with high-risk Acute Myeloid Leukaemia at 6 years of age after a short history of reduced appetite, weight loss and lethargy. After being successfully treated with chemotherapy, Aditi was well in herself and had returned to mainstream schooling.

Shortly before her eighth birthday, Aditi became unwell with shortness of breath, unexplained bruising and dizziness. She was diagnosed with relapsed Acute Myeloid Leukaemia and commenced intensive chemotherapy before undergoing a bone marrow transplant. The transplant was unsuccessful, and all other treatment options were unsuitable. The focus of Aditi's care turned to symptom management and palliation.

Aditi expressed a desire to die at home. Therefore, Aditi and her family were referred to the local hospice for input from their community team. Aditi was discharged from the hospital, predominantly symptom-free.

Over the coming weeks, Aditi's appetite began to reduce; she was eating less and less. Due to her reduced intake, Aditi began to lose weight rapidly and her appearance changed significantly. Aditi was on a high dose of oral steroids for disease management, which caused her to become aggressive at times. Aditi also developed gastric reflux, accompanied by intermittent vomiting. She had self-limiting nosebleeds daily.

Overnight, Aditi developed severe abdominal pain and became distressed. Her family called their community nursing team, who came to assess Aditi. On their arrival, Aditi was seen to be distressed and uncomfortable, with notable increased work of breathing. Aditi was given a dose of buccal Midazolam with minimal effect. The decision was made to commence Aditi on a subcutaneous continuous Midazolam infusion, which made Aditi more comfortable, although she became very sleepy and suppressed her breathing. Aditi's breathing became more laboured and slowed until she stopped breathing and died in the early hours of the morning with her parents and siblings with her.

Points to consider

- When could the palliative care team have been introduced to Aditi and her family?
- In the weeks leading to her death, how might Aditi's symptoms have been managed?
- Who may require support during and after Aditi's death? How can they be supported, and by whom?

Conclusion

This chapter has provided an insight into palliative and end-of-life care for BCYP with some of the pathophysiological changes that may occur. It has introduced Advanced Care planning, with emphasis on NICE guidance, and the importance of parallel planning with clear communication. This chapter has considered, although not a complete list, of the symptoms a BCYP may experience towards the end of their life, and pharmacological and non-pharmacological ways this can be managed. Emphasis has been placed on the four dimensions of care that require consideration and assessment.

References

Amery, J. (2016). *A Really Practical Handbook of Children's Palliative Care for Doctors and Nurses Anywhere in the World.* LuLu.

Archer, N. & Machin, L. (2024) Integrating new perspectives: working with loss and grief in palliative care. In Kitchen, R., Faull, C., Russell, S. & Wilson, J. (eds) *Handbook of palliative care.* 4th edn. pp 89–103. Wiley Blackwell.

Association for Paediatric Palliative Medicine (2024). *Association for Paediatric Palliative Medicine Formulary*, 6th edn. APPM Master Formulary.

Brown, E., Muckaden, M.A., & Mndende, N. (2024). Culture, spirituality and ritual. In: Goldman, A., Hain, R., Meiring, M., & Rapoport, A. (eds). *Oxford Textbook of Palliative Care for Children*, 3rd edn. Oxford University Press Academic UK, pp. 373–381.

Carceni, A., Simonetti, F., & Martini, C. (2021). *Neurological problems in advanced cancer.* In: Currow, D.C., Cherny, N.I., Fallon, M.T. *et al.* (eds). *Oxford Textbook of Palliative Medicine*, 6th edn. Oxford University Press Academic UK, pp. 872–889.

Contro, N., & Zimmerman, J. (2021). Assessment of the child. In: Goldman, A., Hain, R., Meiring, M., & Rapoport, A. (eds). *Oxford Textbook of Palliative Care for Children*, 3rd edn. Oxford University Press Academic UK, pp. 59–65.

Dickenson, A.H., & Gordon-Williams, R. (2021). *Pathophysiology of pain in cancer and other terminal illnesses.* In: Currow, D.C., Cherny, N.I., Fallon, M.T. *et al.* (eds). *Oxford Textbook of Palliative Medicine*, 6th edn. Oxford University Press Academic UK, pp. 321–332.

Domeisen Benedetti, F., Ostgathe, C., Clark, J., *et al.* (2013). International palliative care experts' view on phenomena indicating the last hours and days of life. *Support Care Cancer* 21, 1509–1517 https://doi.org/10.1007/s00520-012-1677-3.

Fraser, L. K., Gibson-Smith, D., Jarvis, S., Norman, P. & Parslow, R. (2020). 'Make Every Child Count' Estimating current and future prevalence of children and young people with life-limiting conditions in the United Kingdom. Together For Short Lives. Bristol.

Hawley, P.H. (2014). The bow tie model of 21st century palliative care. *Journal of Pain and Symptom Management* 47(1), 2–5 https://doi.org/10.1016/j.jpainsymman.2013.10.009.

Hockley, J. (2015). Intimations of dying: a visible and invisible process. *Journal of Palliative Care* 31(3), 166–171. https://journals.sagepub.com/doi/10.1177/082585971503100306.

Hospice UK (2025). *Cate after Death; Guidance for staff responsible for care after death*, 5th edn. Hospice UK.

Hui, D., & Mori, M. (2021). *Physiology of dying.* In: Currow, D.C., Cherny, N.I., Fallon, M.T. *et al.* (eds). *Oxford Textbook of Palliative Medicine*, 6th edn. Oxford University Press Academic UK, pp. 1094–1103.

Ijaopo, E.O., Zaw, K.M., Ijaopo, R.O., & Khawand-Azoulai, M. (2023). A review of clinical signs and symptoms of imminent end-of-life in individuals with advanced illness. *Gerontology and Geriatric Medicine* 9.

Kinley, J., & Sullivan, C. (2024). How to recognise the dying phase in palliative and end-of-life care. *Nursing Times* [online] 120, 9.

Kissane, D.W. (2021). Depression, demorilization and suicidality. In: Currow, D.C., Cherny, N.I., Fallon, M.T. *et al.* (eds). *Oxford Textbook of Palliative Medicine*, 6th edn. Oxford University Press Academic UK, pp. 747–754.

Larkin, P.J. (2021). *Constipation and diarrhoea.* In: Currow, D.C., Cherny, N.I., Fallon, M.T. *et al.* (eds). *Oxford Textbook of Palliative Medicine*, 6th edn. Oxford University Press Academic UK, pp. 545–555.

Liang, Y. (2024). Palliative care for infants, children and young people. In: Kitchen, R., Faull, C., Russell, S., & Wilson, J. (eds). *Handbook of Palliative Care*, 4th edn. Wiley Blackwell, pp. 218–229.

Mack, J., & Sisk, B. (2021). Communication. In: Hain, R., Rapoport, A., Meiring, M., & Goldman, A. (eds). *Oxford Textbook of Palliative Care for Children*, 3rd edn. Oxford University Press Academic UK, pp. 17–24.

Mahunt, S., Meiring, M., & Rapoport, A. (2021). Feeding, cachexia, and malnutrition in children's palliative care. In: Hain, R., Rapoport, A., Meiring, M., & Goldman, A. (eds). *Oxford Textbook of Palliative Care for Children*, 3rd edn. Oxford University Press Academic UK, pp. 231–243.

National Child Mortality Database (2025). Infants, children and young people with life-limiting conditions. *Learning from child death reviews on palliative and end of life care provision.* https://www.ncmd.info/publications/llc/

National Institute for health and Care Excellence (2019). *End of life care for infants, children and young people with life-limiting conditions: planning and management. NG61.*Overview | End of life care for infants, children and young people with life-limiting conditions: planning and management | Guidance | NICE (accessed 28 July 2025).

Portnoy, S., & Ives-Baine, L. (2021). Bereavement. In: Hain, R., Rapoport, A., Meiring, M., & Goldman, A. (eds). *Oxford Textbook of Palliative Care for Children*, 3rd edn. Oxford University Press Academic UK, pp. 126–134.

Shedge, R., Krishan, K., Warrier, V. & Kanchan, T. (2023). Postmortem Changes. StatPearls. https://www.ncbi.nlm.nih.gov/books/NBK539741/.

Taylor, P., Dowding, D., & Johnson, M. (2017). Clinical decision making in the recognition of dying: a qualitative interview study. *BMC Palliative Care* 16(11), 1–11 https://doi.org/10.1186/s12904-016-0179-3.

Together for Short Lives (2018). A guide to Children's Palliative Care: Supporting babies, children and young people with life-limiting and life-threatening conditions and their families. (4th edn.). Bristol.

Together for Short Lives (2024). *Basic symptom control in paediatric palliative care*, 10th edn. Bristol.

Together for Short Lives (2025). *Built to Last? The state of children's palliative Care in 2025.* The state of children's palliative care in 2025 - Together for Short Lives (accessed 28 July 2025).

Together for Short Lives (TFSL) (2019). Caring for a child at end of life: A guide for professionals on the care of children and young people, before death, at the time of death and after death). Bristol.

Zhang, M., Li, H., Li, F., & Zhang, Y. (2024). Facilitators and barriers to parent-child communication in pediatric palliative care: an integrative review. *International Journal of Nursing Sciences* 11(4), 495–503 https://doi.org/10.1016/j.ijnss.2024.08.001.

Index

Note: page numbers in *italics* refer to figures; those in **bold** to tables.